Methods in Cell Biology

VOLUME 49

Methods in Plant Cell Biology, Part A

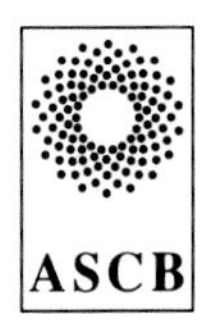

Series Editors

Leslie Wilson
Department of Biological Sciences
University of California, Santa Barbara
Santa Barbara, California

Paul Matsudaira
Whitehead Institute for Biomedical Research and
Department of Biology
Massachusetts Institute of Technology
Cambridge, Massachusetts

Methods in Cell Biology

Prepared under the Auspices of the American Society for Cell Biology

VOLUME 49

Methods in Plant Cell Biology, Part A

Edited by

David W. Galbraith

Department of Plant Sciences
University of Arizona
Tucson, Arizona

Hans J. Bohnert

Department of Biochemistry
University of Arizona
Tucson, Arizona

Don P. Bourque

Department of Biochemistry
University of Arizona
Tucson, Arizona

ACADEMIC PRESS

San Diego New York Boston London Sydney Tokyo Toronto

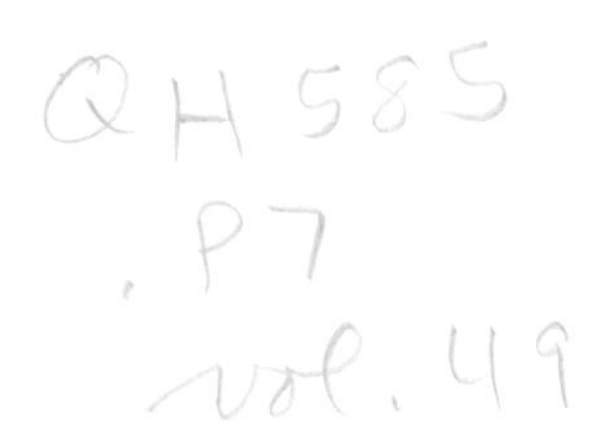

Cover photograph (paperback edition only): From Chapter 12 by McFadden.
For details see the legend to Fig. 2.

This book is printed on acid-free paper. ♾

Academic Press, Inc.
A Division of Harcourt Brace & Company
525 B Street, Suite 1900, San Diego, California 92101-4495

United Kingdom Edition published by
Academic Press Limited
24-28 Oval Road, London NW1 7DX

International Standard Serial Number: 0091-679X

International Standard Book Number: 0-12-564151-6 (hardcover)

International Standard Book Number: 0-12-273871-3 (comb)

PRINTED IN THE UNITED STATES OF AMERICA
95 96 97 98 99 00 EB 9 8 7 6 5 4 3 2 1

CONTENTS

PART III Signal Transduction and Information Transfer

CONTRIBUTORS

Numbers in parentheses indicate the pages on which the authors' contributions begin.

Frederick M. Ausubel (431), Department of Molecular Biology, Massachusetts General Hospital, Boston, Massachusetts 02114

Wendy F. Boss (543), Botany Department, North Carolina State University, Raleigh, North Carolina 27695

Lindy A. Brigham (377), Departments of Plant Pathology, and Molecular and Cellular Biology, University of Arizona, Tucson, Arizona 85721

Roy C. Brown (85), Department of Biology, University of Southwestern Louisiana, Lafayette, Louisiana 70504

Myeon H. Cho[1] (543), Department of Botany, University of Wisconsin, Madison, Wisconsin 53706

Joanne Chory (441), Plant Biology Laboratory, The Salk Institute for Biological Studies, San Diego, California 92186

Steven E. Clark (217), Division of Biology, California Institute of Technology, Pasadena, California 91125

Daniel J. Cosgrove (231), Department of Biology, Pennsylvania State University, University Park, Pennsylvania 16802

Veronica P. Counihan (515), Division of Biological Sciences, University of Missouri, Columbia, Missouri 65211

Christophe d'Enfert (417), Unité de Mycologie, Institut Pasteur, 75724 Paris, France

Marc De Block (153), Plant Genetic Systems N.V., G-9000 Gent, Belgium

Robert J. Ferl (391), Department of Horticultural Sciences, University of Florida, Gainesville, Florida 32611

L. C. Fowke (3), Department of Biology, University of Saskatchewan, Saskatoon, Saskatchewan, Canada S7N 0W0

K. Fritze (455), Max-Planck-Institut für Züchtungsforschung, D-50829 Köln, Germany

M. E. Galway (3), Department of Biology, The University of Michigan, Ann Arbor, Michigan 48109

Lawrence R. Griffing (109), Department of Biology, Texas A&M University, College Station, Texas 77843

Mark J. Guiltinan (143), Department of Horticulture and The Biotechnology Institute, The Center for Gene Expression, Pennsylvania State University, University Park, Pennsylvania 16802

H. Harling (455), Max-Planck-Institut für Züchtungsforschung, D-50829 Köln, Germany

[1] Present Address: Department of Botany, University of Wisconsin, Madison, Wisconsin 53706

Chris Hawes (33), RMC Centre for Electron Microscopy, School of Biological and Molecular Sciences, Oxford Brookes University, Oxford OX3 0BP, United Kingdom

Martha C. Hawes (377), Departments of Plant Pathology, and Molecular and Cellular Biology, University of Arizona, Tucson, Arizona 85721

J. W. Heckman, Jr. (3), Center for Electron Optics, Michigan State University, East Lansing, Michigan 48824

Martin J. Hodson (21), School of Biological and Molecular Sciences, Oxford Brookes University, Headington, Oxford OX3 0BP, United Kingdom

Mark A. Horn (531), Division of Biological Sciences, University of Missouri, Columbia, Missouri 65211

Inhwan Hwang (401), Plant Molecular Biology, and Biotechnology Research Center, Gyeongsang National University, Chinju, Kyeong Nam 660-701, South Korea

G. J. Hyde[2] (3), Department of Biology, York University, North York, Ontario, Canada M3J 1P3

Thomas Jacobs (355), Department of Plant Biology, University of Illinois, Urbana, Illinois 61801

Toshinori Kinoshita (501), Department of Biology, Faculty of Science, Kyushu University, Hakazaki, Fukuoka 812, Japan

Heather Knight (201), Department of Plant Sciences, University of Oxford, Oxford OX1 3RB, United Kingdom

Marc R. Knight (201), Department of Plant Sciences, University of Oxford, Oxford OX1 3RB, United Kingdom

Hiroaki Kodama (315), Department of Biology, Faculty of Science, Kyushu University 33, Fukuoka 812, Japan

Atsushi Komamine (315), Department of Chemical and Biological Sciences, Japan Women's University, Bunkyo-ku, Tokyo 112, Japan

François Lacroute (417), Centre de Génétique Moléculaire, CNRS, 91190 Gif sur Yvette, France

Betty E. Lemmon (85), Department of Biology, University of Southwestern Louisiana, Lafayette, Louisiana 70504

Xingxiang Li[3] (185), Institute of Biological Chemistry, Washington State University, Pullman, Washington 99164

Hsou-min Li (441), Plant Biology Laboratory, The Salk Institute for Biological Studies, San Diego, California 92186

Birong Liao (487), Department of Plant Biology, University of Illinois, Urbana, Illinois 61801

Hong Ma (471), Cold Spring Harbor Laboratory, Cold Spring, New York 11724

Frans J. M. Maathuis (293), Department of Biology, University of York, York YO1 5DD, United Kingdom

Barry Martin (33), RMC Centre for Electron Microscopy, School of Biological and Molecular Sciences, Oxford Brookes University, Oxford OX3 0BP, United Kingdom

[2] Present Address: School of Biological Sciences, University of New South Wales, Kensington NSW 2033, Australia

[3] Present Address: Department of Molecular and Cellular Biology, Harvard University, Cambridge, Massachusetts 02138

Geoffrey Ian McFadden (165), Plant Cell Biology Research Centre, School of Botany, University of Melbourne, Parkville, Victoria 3052, Australia

Lauren McHenry[4] (143), Department of Horticulture and The Biotechnology Institute, The Center for Gene Expression, Pennsylvania State University, University Park, Pennsylvania 16802

Elliot M. Meyerowitz (217), Division of Biology, California Institute of Technology, Pasadena, California 91125

A. J. Miller (275), Biochemistry & Physiology Department, Rothamsted Experimental Station, Harpenden, Hertfordshire AL5 2JQ, United Kingdom

Michèle Minet (417), Centre de Génétique Moléculaire, CNRS, 91190 Gif sur Yvette, France

Nobuyoshi Mochizuki (441), Plant Biology Laboratory, The Salk Institute for Biological Studies, San Diego, California 92186

Scott Moon (109), Department of Biology, Texas A&M University, College Station, Texas 77843

Patricia J. Moore (45), Division of Natural Sciences and Mathematics, Transylvania University, Lexington, Kentucky 40508

Thomas W. Okita (185), Institute of Biological Chemistry, Washington State University, Pullman, Washington 99164

M. V. Parthasarathy (57), Section of Plant Biology, Division of Biological Sciences, Cornell University, Ithaca, New York 14853

Anna-Lisa Paul (391), Department of Horticultural Sciences, University of Florida, Gainesville, Florida 32611

Roger I. Pennell[5] (123), Department of Biology, University College London, London WC1E 6BT, England

Thomas E. Phillips (515), Division of Biological Sciences, University of Missouri, Columbia, Missouri 65211

Betty Prewett (355), Department of Plant Biology, University of Illinois, Urbana, Illinois 61801

V. Raghavan (367), Department of Plant Biology, The Ohio State University, Columbus, Ohio 43210

T. Lynne Reuber (431), Department of Molecular Biology, Massachusetts General Hospital, Boston, Massachusetts 02114

Keith Roberts (123), Department of Cell Biology, John Innes Institute, Norwich NR4 7UH, England

Justin K. M. Roberts (245), Department of Biochemistry, University of California, Riverside, California 92521

Mark P. Running (217), Division of Biology, California Institute of Technology, Pasadena, California 91125

Francesco Salamini (331), MPI für Züchtungsforschung (Erwin-Baur-Institute), D-50829 Köln, Germany

[4] Present Address: Biology Department, Loyola College, Baltimore, Maryland 21210
[5] Present Address: Plant Biology Laboratory, Salk Institute, La Jolla, California 92037

Dale Sanders (293), Department of Biology, University of York, York YO1 5DD, United Kingdom

Melvin Schindler (71), Department of Biochemistry, Michigan State University, East Lansing, Michigan 48824

Jen Sheen (305), Department of Genetics, Harvard Medical School, and Department of Molecular Biology, Massachusetts General Hospital, Boston, Massachusetts 02114

Ken-Ichiro Shimazaki (501), Biological Laboratory, College of General Education, Kyushu University, Ropponmatsu, Fukuoka 810, Japan

Brenda W. Shirley (401), Department of Biology, Virginia Polytechnical Institute and State University, Blacksburg, Virginia 24061

Angelo Spena[6] (331), MPI für Züchtungsforschung (Erwin-Baur-Institute), D-50829 Köln, Germany

Josephine Taylor (109), Department of Biology, Stephen F. Austin University, Nacogdoches, Texas 75962

John F. Thain (259), School of Biological Sciences, University of East Anglia, Norwich NR4 7TJ, United Kingdom

Marco A. Villanueva[7] (109), Department of Biology, Texas A&M University, College Station, Texas 77843

R. Walden (455), Max-Planck-Institut für Züchtungsforschung, D-50829 Köln, Germany

John C. Walker (515, 531), Division of Biological Sciences, University of Missouri, Columbia, Missouri 65211

Catherine A. Weiss (471), Cold Spring Harbor Laboratory, Cold Spring, New York 11724

Ho-Hyung Woo (377), Departments of Plant Pathology, and Molecular and Cellular Biology, University of Arizona, Tucson, Arizona 85721

Jian-Hua Xia (245), Department of Biochemistry, University of California, Riverside, California 92521

Raymond E. Zielinski (487), Department of Plant Biology, University of Illinois, Urbana, Illinois 61801

[6] Present Address: Cattedra di Fisiologia Vegetale, University of Ancona, 60131 Ancona, Italy
[7] Present Address: Institute of Biotechnology, UNAM, Cuernavaca, Morelos 62271, Mexico

PREFACE

It is taken for granted that research scientists should employ the most powerful, most appropriate, and most up-to-date methods to investigate specific questions in biology. Yet biologists, as a group, have an ambivalent relationship with the methods they employ. This situation may reflect the observation that, in many cases, those methods providing the most powerful insights arise not from biology but from other scientific disciplines, notably physics, chemistry, and the mathematical sciences. Intelligent use of these techniques tends to require reeducation of the biologist in these disciplines, a process that often encounters a certain degree of inertia. It is also true that the emergence and widespread adoption of a particularly useful experimental method or instrument are not necessarily accompanied by a recognition of the difficulties inherent in the development and reduction to practice of this method. Consequently, the process of methods development within the biological sciences does not enjoy the general degree of support from the research community that is deserved in terms of the benefits that it provides. The elements of creativity, innovation, and sophistication in methods development are seldom appreciated and indeed are frequently the subject of active criticism.

Yet, if traced from the historical record, the biological sciences are replete with illustrations of the profound influence of novel methods and techniques on biological understanding. Few would question the impact of radioisotopes on studies of metabolism, or that of simple fixation solutions and embedding resins on revolutionizing techniques of visualizing cellular structure by transmission electron microscopy. Now readily accessible methods and equipment for computer-linked capture, storage, and manipulation of enormous amounts of data have further revolutionized microscopy, delivering a quantum leap in the provision of tools, again derived from other disciplines. Electrophysiological techniques have allowed increasingly greater insight into mechanisms of metabolite and ion transport in individual cells or cell membrane patches. Techniques for manipulation of DNA have fundamentally altered the ways in which biological questions are addressed. The amplification of specific gene fragments by iterative cycles of DNA annealing and synthesis has emerged as perhaps the single most powerful, yet elegantly simple, technique of modern biology, and such methods are well on their way to making an indelible mark on culture and society. It is not too difficult to predict that the continued development of computer and communications technologies will lead to increased use of computer-based modeling for analysis of biological questions. These tools should enhance the use and importance of theoretical, predictive approaches within the laboratory setting, in which experimental observation is used less to chart out and categorize unknown components and more to confirm or reject the predictions of these models.

The purpose of Volumes 49 and 50 in the series *Methods in Cell Biology* is threefold. First, we have brought together a comprehensive collection of different methods applicable to plant cell biology. This compilation should give researchers ready access to those methods that are most appropriate for their work. Second, we have attempted to demystify the individual methods by requesting from the authors a chapter format that clearly and succinctly explains the principles behind the individual methods, as well as providing a step-by-step "cookbook" approach to implementing these methods. Finally, we would like the reader to come away with an appreciation of the breadth and depth of sophisticated thought that went into the development of the individual methods. The diligence with which our colleagues have responded to our charge in dealing with the topics of their expertise is what makes these two volumes particularly important compilations of current technical knowledge. The authors have gone beyond the requisite provision of useful hints and tricks by lucidly explaining the conceptual framework of the techniques. Many chapters outline paths to future improvements. However, the essential theme reiterated within each chapter is that cutting-edge research in plant cell biology requires complex, multifaceted technical expertise and that interdisciplinary scientific efforts are integral to ensuring continued advancements in the field.

The Co-editors thank the Academic Press staff, past and present, for their expert help during the preparation of these volumes. We gratefully acknowledge the contributions of the authors, who promptly provided manuscripts requiring minimal editorial changes, and we look forward eagerly to the discoveries that will be made possible through the use of the methods within these volumes.

David W. Galbraith
Hans J. Bohnert
Don P. Bourque

PART I

Techniques for Examination of Cells within Tissues

CHAPTER 1

Advances in High-Pressure and Plunge-Freeze Fixation

M. E. Galway,[*] J. W. Heckman, Jr.,[†] G. J. Hyde,[‡] and L. C. Fowke[§]

[*]Department of Biology
The University of Michigan
Ann Arbor, Michigan 48109-1048

[†]Center for Electron Optics
Michigan State University
East Lansing, Michigan 48824-1311

[‡]Department of Biology
York University
North York, Ontario M3J 1P3, Canada

[§]Department of Biology
University of Saskatchewan
Saskatoon, Saskatchewan S7N 0W0, Canada

METHODS IN CELL BIOLOGY, VOL. 49

I. Introduction

A. Chemical Fixation versus Freeze Fixation

One of the conundrums facing cell biologists is that many of the methods that are employed for investigating the natural structure and function of living cells result in the injury and, in many cases, death of the cells that are being examined. In structural investigations, a compromise is sought, in which "fixation" is employed to kill the cells in a manner that stabilizes and preserves them in as lifelike a state as possible for subsequent investigation. Ideally, fixation should be achieved too rapidly for cells to react to the process. The effectiveness of fixation by reactive chemicals, for example, glutaraldehyde, which fixes cells via cross-linking proteins, depends on the speed of diffusion of the fixative into the specimen and on its reactivity with the molecules that it encounters. It has been found that chemical fixation is too slow to capture rapid cellular processes such as membrane fusion (Menco, 1986, and references therein). It has further been shown that cells can undergo dramatic structural changes between the time of first contact with chemical fixatives and completion of the fixation process, and that they are subject to loss or displacement of poorly fixed and water-soluble components (reviewed by Gilkey and Staehelin, 1986; Hyde *et al.,* 1991b; Kaminskyj *et al.,* 1992).

An alternative to chemical fixation is freeze fixation (cryofixation). The major advantage of cryofixation is that the physical structure of cells is stabilized much faster through reducing their thermal energy than through chemical cross-linking. Once frozen, further structural changes are almost completely inhibited in cells maintained below about −143°C (Bachman and Mayer, 1987). In order to prevent metabolic and structural changes from occurring in response to the falling temperature, the cooling rate during freezing should be very high. Water, the most abundant molecule in living cells, presents the major obstacle to achieving good cryofixation because the most thermodynamically stable state for frozen water is crystalline. Ice crystal growth during or after the freezing process severely disrupts cytoplasmic structure by displacing solutes and other cytoplasmic contents to the edges of the crystals. When the primary concern is the preservation of cellular ultrastructure in a lifelike state, the empirical goal of cryofixation is to freeze the samples so rapidly (about 10,000°C/s) that growth of ice crystals is restricted to less than about 10 nm in diameter (Gilkey and Staehelin, 1986; Moor, 1987; Dahl and Staehelin, 1989). These cause no detectable displacement or distortion of cellular contents at magnifications normally used for biological specimens in transmission electron microscopy. (TEM; magnifications are 20,000–40,000×).

Once successfully frozen, cells and tissues can be visualized and analyzed by a variety of techniques, including low-temperature scanning electron microscopy and low temperature TEM of ultrathin cryosections. Replicas can be made of freeze-fractured or freeze-etched specimens for study at normal temperature by electron microscopy, or the specimens can themselves be examined at room temperature after freeze drying or freeze substitution. These methods can be combined with various analytical methods, such as electron probe microanalysis, cytochemistry/immunocytochemistry, and autoradiography (reviewed by Plattner and Bachman, 1982; Menco, 1986; Steinbrecht and Zierold, 1987; Robards, 1991).

Recent advances in cryofixation have focused on improving the methods of heat removal from specimens, thereby increasing the size of specimens that can be successfully frozen. Here we describe the application of two rapid freezing methods for the successful preservation of plant cell ultrastructure. One of these, plunge freezing, is inexpensive and simple, but only in the outer 10-20-μm layer of a specimen will freezing be rapid enough to ensure good preservation. The other, high-pressure (hyperbaric) freezing, requires a specially designed apparatus, but is theoretically capable of preserving specimens that are 500–600 μm thick (Gilkey and Staehelin, 1986; Moor, 1987). Detailed discussions of the theory and techniques of freeze fixation can be found in Robards and Sleytr (1985), Gilkey and Staehelin (1986), Steinbrecht and Zierold (1987), Studer *et al.* (1989), Roos and Morgan (1990), and Robards (1991).

B. Plunge Freezing and High-Pressure Freezing

In plunge freezing, liquid nitrogen at its boiling point (−196°C) is used to cool a secondary cryogenic liquid, such as propane (which is liquid between −42 and −187°C). Specimens are frozen by plunging them rapidly and deeply into the secondary cryogen: the flow of cryogen over specimen surfaces ensures rapid dissipation of heat. The low boiling point of liquid nitrogen prevents it from being used directly on specimens in plunge freezing, since it boils on contact with the warm specimen. The resultant insulating layer of gas slows freezing sufficiently to allow large and disruptive ice crystals to form in cells (Sitte *et al.*, 1987). Even adiabatically frozen nitrogen slush (about −209°C) is unsuitable for any but the smallest specimens due to the limited heat capacity of the medium. Pressurization of liquid nitrogen inhibits boiling, allowing it to be used directly on specimens for high-pressure freezing (Moor, 1987). The concept and method of freezing biological specimens under high pressure were developed by Riehle, Moor, and their colleagues from the late 1960s to the 1980s and resulted in the design and manufacture of the Balzers HPM 010 high-pressure freezing machine (Moor, 1987). The technique and apparatus of high-pressure freezing continue to be refined, however, in response to new applications and results (Dahl and Staehelin, 1989; Studer *et al.*, 1989; Sartori *et al.*, 1993). Freezing specimens under high pressure protects them from ice crystal damage by lowering the freezing point of water and reducing the rate of ice crystal nucleation and growth (Moor, 1987; Dahl and Staehelin, 1989). The design and function of the HPM 010 is described by Moor (1987, and references therein). In brief, specimens are sandwiched between two small metal cups or plates, locked into a special holder which is inserted into the pressure chamber in the HPM 010 and then frozen in a 0.5-s burst of liquid nitrogen pressurized to 2100 atm. Rapid transfer of the frozen specimens to liquid nitrogen at normal pressure prevents rewarming after freezing. To prevent specimens from freezing before they are fully pressurized, warm isopropyl alcohol is injected into the chamber just ahead of the nitrogen burst. A temperature-controlled closed circuit water supply keeps the pressure chamber and alcohol supply from cooling during operation of the HPM 010.

C. Suitable Specimens for Freeze Fixation

In all rapid freezing methods, the quality of freeze fixation is affected by the water and solute content of the specimen. Formation of large damaging ice crystals is reduced in specimens with naturally low water content such as seeds or seed embryos. Naturally high solute levels in the cytoplasm of some cells like phloem sieve elements depresses the freezing point and reduces ice crystal formation. Similar cryoprotection can be obtained by deliberately adding such substances to specimens before freezing. Unfortunately many cryoprotectants (e.g., glycerol) can penetrate cells and perturb cellular structure and function, contrary to the goal of preserving cellular structure in its natural state (Plattner and Bachman, 1982; Gilkey and Staehelin, 1986). Some apparently inert and nonpenetrating cryoprotectants such as dextran, polyvinylpyrrolidone, and the paraffin oil 1-hexadecene, have been used in high pressure freezing to further reduce intracellular ice crystal formation by inhibiting the formation of extracellular ice crystals (Dahl and Staehelin, 1989; Studer *et al.,* 1989; Kiss *et al.,* 1990). However, these cryoprotectants have been rarely used for plunge freezing (Robards, 1991). One should check that cryoprotectants have no detectable effect on specimens of interest before routine use.

Since the content of free water is higher in vacuoles than in cytoplasm, highly cytoplasmic cells are, in general, better preserved by freezing than are vacuolated cells. Specimens should be as small and thin as possible, not exceeding 1 mm^3, so that they have a relatively large surface area (compared to volume) to contact the cryogen and dissipate heat. Examples of suitably shaped specimens are single cells (e.g., algae, pollen tubes), long thin organs like roots and fungal hyphae, excised pieces of thin tissues such as leaves, and cells projecting from the surface of organs such as hairs.

D. Hazards and Safety Precautions

It is important to understand the hazards of rapid freezing methods and to know what safety precautions are necessary before attempting freeze fixation (see Robards and Sleytr, 1985; Howard and O'Donnell, 1987; Sitte *et al.,* 1987; Roos and Morgan, 1990). Hazards include (*a*) freezing injuries due to splashed cryogens, (*b*) oxygen deprivation due to displacement of air by nitrogen gas from boiling liquid nitrogen, (*c*) explosion/fire hazard due to propane gas, or to condensation of oxygen from the air onto the surface of liquid propane, (*d*) breakage of brittle glass/plastic containers exposed to cryogenic liquids, and (*e*) pressure bursting of containers in which liquid cryogens have vaporized (e.g., liquid nitrogen may be inadvertently introduced into nitrogen-cooled specimen vials during plunge freezing experiments).

II. Plunge-Freeze Fixation

A. Materials and Method

1. Materials

Propane. Domestic propane gas contains sufficient adulterants to lower its freezing point to about −192°C. This feature along with the presence of olfactory indicators and low cost make it the medium of choice for routine use (Howard and O'Donnell, 1987; Ridge, 1988). Bulk propane from LP gas suppliers or propane in disposable 400-g cylinders works equally well.

Liquid nitrogen. Two to three liters of liquid nitrogen stored in a cryogenic Dewar flask should be sufficient for each freezing experiment.

Spark-free fume hood/cupboard in which to carry out plunge freezing, in order to prevent the accumulation of flammable heavy propane vapors.

Propane reservoir and Dewar flask. The reservoir consists of a 40-ml thimble, 50 mm deep, bored into the end of an aluminum rod, which can be placed in a Dewar flask for cooling in liquid nitrogen (Fig. 1). A tight-fitting aluminum cover is placed on the thimble when it is not in use to prevent condensation of atmospheric oxygen onto the propane.

Cryogenic vials and styrofoam container. Roots are freeze-substituted in small screw-capped centrifuge vials after plunge freezing. These can be weighted on the bottoms by fitting them with an ordinary 7/16-in. hex nut, and cooled in a suitably sized styrofoam container of liquid nitrogen before use.

Two or more pairs of fine forceps for plunging/manipulating roots during freezing.

Heavy metal rod for melting frozen propane.

Five- to six-day-old seedlings of *Arabidopsis thaliana* prepared according to Schiefelbein and Somerville (1990). In brief, surface-sterilized seeds are germinated and grown vertically for 5–6 days on the surface of agarose-solidified nutrient medium in sealed Petri plates under artificial illumination.

2. Method

The plunge freezing equipment is assembled inside a spark-free fume hood. The aluminum rod is immersed in a Dewar of liquid nitrogen and allowed to cool until bubbling of the nitrogen ceases. The surface of the nitrogen in the Dewar should be kept up to the level of the reservoir in the end of the rod. To

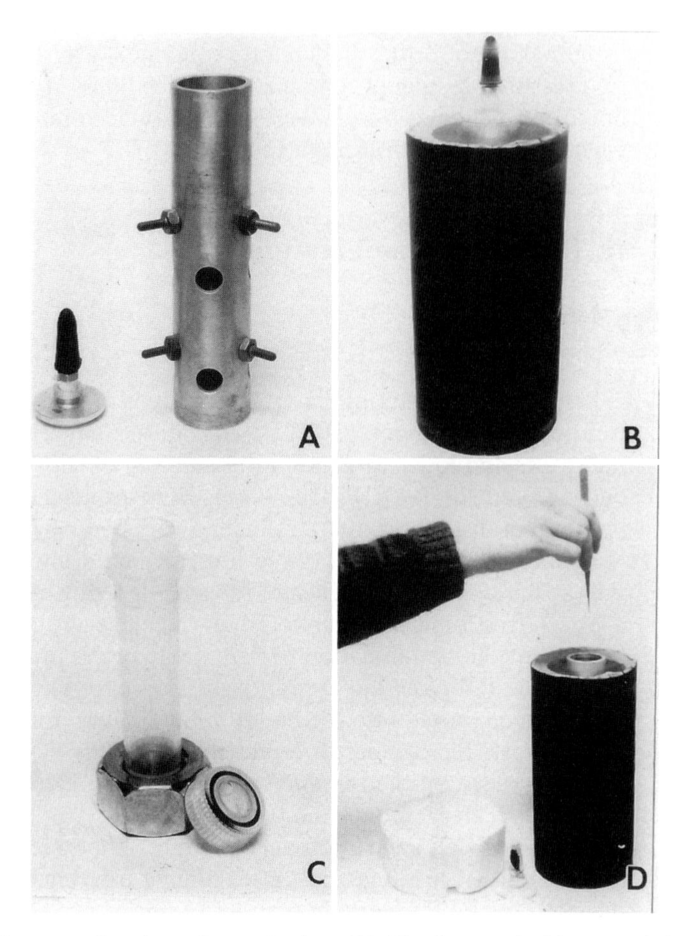

Fig. 1 Apparatus for plunge-freeze fixation. (A) Aluminum rod with reservoir bored in end at top for holding liquid propane; tight-fitting lid for excluding air from propane is shown at left beside rod. (B) Propane is liquified in the reservoir of the aluminum rod as it sits inside an ordinary wide-mouthed vacuum bottle liner filled with liquid nitrogen. (C) Cryogenic vial for specimen storage and freeze substitution is a modified microcentrifuge tube. Venting holes in cap prevent pressure build-up within from vaporized cryogens and allow forceps to be inserted and used as wrench for opening cold vial. The nut at base provides stability and holds vial upright in liquid nitrogen. (D) Plunge freezing of excised seedling roots. Specimens are quickly plunged straight down into the melting propane, held for 5–10 s, then rapidly transferred to precooled cryogenic vials for freeze substitution.

liquefy the propane, the tank valve is slightly opened and propane is gently introduced at a low flow rate so that it condenses on the cold walls of the reservoir. Once the thimble is full, the top is capped with a tight-fitting aluminum cover and the propane is cooled until frozen. Before use, the cover is removed and most of the frozen propane is melted with a heavy metal rod, and the liquid is stirred to achieve a uniform temperature (approximately −190°C) in the reservoir. While the propane is cooling, the weighted cryogenic vials are prepared for freeze substitution by adding to each 1 ml of 1% osmium tetroxide in acetone at −80°C. This solution is solidified by standing the vials upright (but not submerged) in a styrofoam box containing liquid nitrogen.

To initiate freezing, seedlings are rapidly removed from Petri plates using one pair of fine forceps and, after pinching off and discarding the cotyledons with a second pair of forceps, they are plunged root-first rapidly and deeply into the liquid propane. After holding each root in the propane for at least 5–10 s, to ensure it reaches liquid propane temperature, it is transferred as rapidly as possible onto the frozen surface of the osmium tetroxide/acetone mixture in an already opened cryogenic vial held at liquid nitrogen temperature in the styrofoam box. The vials are transferred in the styrofoam box into a −80°C freezer, and freeze-substitution is continued for 3 days. The samples are then rewarmed over an 8- to 12-h period in an insulated box. When the samples reach 0°C, they are washed three times in anhydrous acetone to remove unreacted osmium tetroxide, warmed to room temperature, infiltrated in a graded resin series, and embedded in Spurr's resin or a Quetol-based resin formulation (Kushida, 1974) for sectioning and TEM (see also Chapter 5, this volume).

B. Critical Aspects of the Procedure

The simple manual method of plunge freezing described here is subject to variability in a number of experimental conditions (e.g., speed and angle of plunge, exact temperature of propane) which are controlled in more sophisticated plunge-freeze devices (see Robards and Sleytr, 1985; Gilkey and Staehelin, 1986; Menco, 1986; Sitte *et al.*, 1987; Robards, 1991; and references therein). With practice, however, this method can yield good freezing of appropriate specimens (Fig. 2). Howard and O'Donnell (1987) and Ridge (1990) provide helpful illustrated descriptions of two other simple setups for manual plunge freezing of fungal and plant tissue in liquid nitrogen-cooled propane.

1. Specimen Preparation

Arabidopsis seedling roots are suitable specimens because they can be grasped easily in forceps and the cylindrical roots and root hairs provide large surface areas to contact the cold propane. Specimens should be surrounded by as little external liquid as possible when plunge frozen, since water is a poor thermal conductor and will slow freezing both by insulating the specimens from direct contact with the cryogen and by releasing heat during crystallization (Gilkey

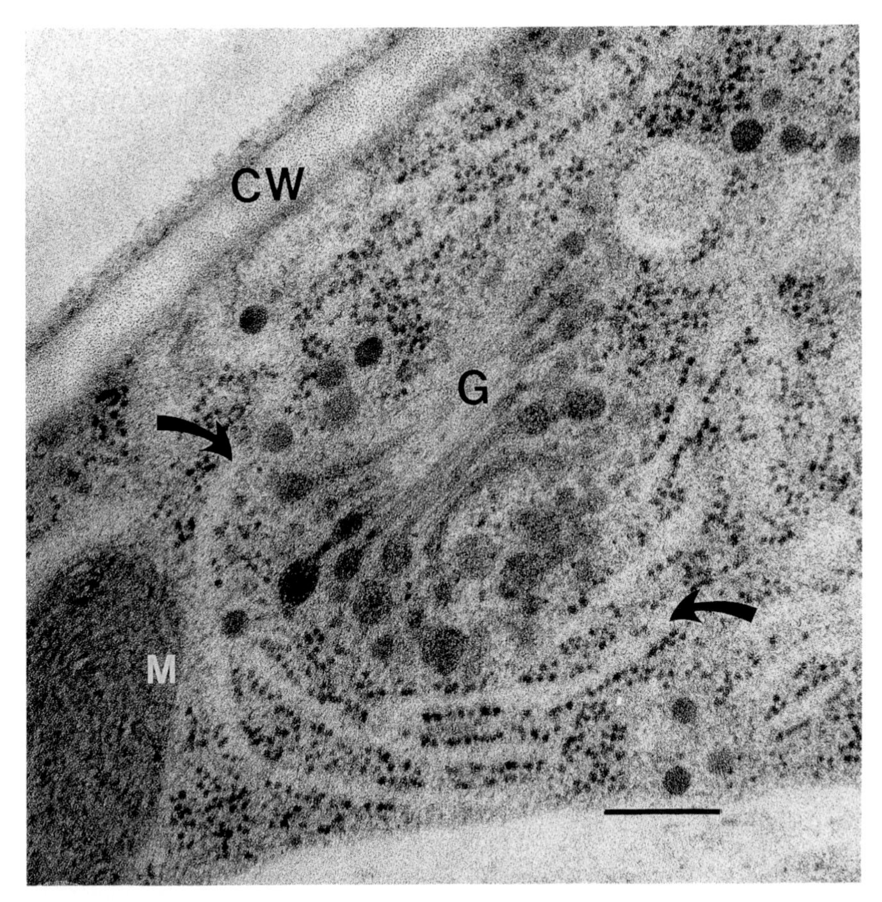

Fig. 2 Thin section from well-preserved root hair of short-haired mutant (rhd 3) of *Arabidopsis thaliana* depicts a Golgi body (G) with associated vesicles, mitochondrion (M), and rough endoplasmic reticulum (arrows). The cell wall (CW) is only lightly stained. The seedling root was plunge frozen in liquid propane and freeze substituted in 1% osmium tetroxide in acetone and embedded in Quetol-based resin mixture. Uranyl acetate and lead citrate staining. Bar, 200nm.

and Staehelin, 1986). It is preferable that some of the specimens be lost to desiccation, rather than that most be unusable due to being frozen under conditions that are too wet (Ridge, 1990). Growth of *Arabidopsis* seedlings on solidified agarose reduces the surface moisture of the roots. However, the root hairs will desiccate and collapse on removal from the high humidity of the Petri plates if not frozen with utmost speed.

2. Specimen Supports

The roots are held in very fine forceps of low thermal conductivity. This prevents heating the propane, which would retard specimen cooling (Robards and Sleytr 1985). Specimens that cannot be grasped directly in forceps require some form of support. Small Formvar-coated loops of fine wire seem to be the most successful design (Howard and O'Donnell, 1987; Ridge, 1990; Hyde *et al.*, 1991b, and references therein). To avoid inadvertantly wetting and/or precooling specimens, it is essential that forceps and loops be warm and dry before each use.

3. Plunge Freezing Technique

To be effective, manual plunge freezing requires constant monitoring of conditions. In order to prevent premature cooling of specimens in the cold vapor above the propane, insulated covers should be kept over the liquid nitrogen and propane, and the propane reservoir should be filled to the brim at all times. Best results are obtained when propane is maintained at a uniform temperature just above freezing point. This requires that (*a*) the surrounding bath of liquid nitrogen remain full, (*b*) the propane be allowed to recool after each addition of fresh propane and after freezing each specimen, (*c*) the propane be stirred frequently to abolish temperature gradients, and (*d*) if the propane begins to freeze, it be melted using a metal rod.

For best results, plunging specimens and transferring them to the cryogenic vials requires practice. Plunging should be a sudden, brisk movement that brings the sample into the cryogen as rapidly as possible. A deep propane reservoir helps, first, because it permits a longer flow of fresh cryogen over the specimen surface during the plunge, and, second, because the operator is not inhibited by fear of the specimen hitting the bottom of the reservoir.

III. High-Pressure Freeze Fixation

A. Materials and Method

1. Materials

Access to HPM 010 High Pressure Freezing Machine (Bal-Tec Products, Inc., Middlebury, CT; Balzers Union, Liechtenstein): eight of these are located in the United States.

Tank of liquid nitrogen, to supply HPM 010.

Isopropyl alcohol.

Wide-mouthed, shallow container of liquid nitrogen, in which to immerse the sample holder and remove frozen protoplasts after freezing (a styrofoam box is suitable).

Specimen cups forming a cavity 0.6 mm thick and 1 mm in diameter when sandwiched together (Craig *et al.,* 1987; Dahl and Staehelin, 1989).
Vegetable lecithin and chloroform, for coating specimen cups.
Silicone lubricant for O-ring on specimen holder.
Cryogenic vials for storage or freeze substitution of specimens after freezing.
Suspension of *Picea glauca* protoplasts in buffered osmoticum.
Ultra-low gelling temperature agarose (Sigma Type IX, Sigma Chemical Co., St. Louis, MO).

2. Method

Before starting to fill the 7-liter liquid nitrogen Dewar in the HPO 010, the supply of liquid nitrogen is checked to ensure it is sufficient for operating the machine, which has a consumption rate of 10–20 liters/h (Bal-Tec specifications for the HPM 010). The isopropyl alcohol reservoir in the HPM 010 is refilled, and the water level in the closed circulation water supply checked before switching it on. After startup on the automatic setting, the machine requires about 15 min to cool down with liquid nitrogen before use. Three preliminary test freezing runs are performed using a dummy sample holder with built-in temperature sensor (HPM 010 accessory). To ensure complete freezing of protoplasts during each burst of pressurized nitrogen, the monitoring system should show that pressure is maintained for 0.45–0.5 s, with a cooling time from 0 to −50°C of 10 ms. Temperature maintenance, which is an indicator of the time available to transfer the frozen protoplasts to liquid nitrogen before thawing, should be 5–9 s.

Protoplasts are isolated by enzymatic digestion of suspension-cultured white spruce embryos and resuspended in a buffered salt solution (Galway *et al.,* 1993) that includes 0.44 *M* sorbitol (as an osmoticum) and 0.5% ultra-low gelling temperature agarose (Sigma Type IX, Sigma Chemical Co.). The agarose holds protoplasts together during freeze substitution following freezing. Upper specimen support cups (designed by Craig *et al.,* 1987) are dipped in a freshly prepared solution of 100 mg/ml vegetable lecithin in chloroform and air-dried before use on a lint-free tissue. A drop of concentrated, suspended protoplasts is added to a lower specimen cup positioned in the fixed part of the unfolded hinged arm of the sample holder. The lecithin-coated upper cup is positioned on top of the lower cup, and the hinged arm is closed over the specimen cup "sandwich" and locked by rotation into the body of the handle. Protoplasts are then frozen immediately by inserting the sample holder into the pressure chamber of the HPM 010, locking it with the safety bolt and firing the nitrogen jet. The sample holder is then quickly removed and plunged into an adjacent liquid nitrogen container to prevent rewarming after freezing. The lecithin-coated upper specimen cup may separate from the specimen and the lower cup when the hinged arm is opened with forceps under liquid nitrogen; if not, the cups are separated using forceps or the sliding wedge device of Craig *et al.* (1987). The frozen tissue is then transferred to a vial for freeze substitution over 3 days at −79°C in 2%

osmium tetroxide in acetone, then rewarmed and embedded in Spurr's resin (see Galway *et al.,* 1993). The HPM 010 is allowed 5 min to reset before freezing another sample. Fresh silicone grease is applied to the O-ring of the specimen holder after every five freezing runs.

B. Critical Aspects of the Procedure

1. Specimen Preparation

Unlike manual plunge freezing, high-pressure freezing conditions are controlled automatically by the HPM 010. However, the preparation and handling of specimens can greatly influence the effectiveness of high-pressure freezing. Ideally, specimens should snugly fit the specimen cups to ensure the best thermal contact with the enclosing metal cups and to avoid damage (Kaeser *et al.,* 1989). A variety of specimen cups have been described for different types of specimens (Craig *et al.,* 1987; Moor, 1987; Welter *et al.,* 1988; Dahl and Staehelin, 1989; Studer *et al.,* 1989). The *P. glauca* protoplasts were frozen in interlocking specimen cups designed to prevent specimens from being blown out during pressurization (Craig *et al.,* 1987). Soft tissues and cell suspensions in particular may be blown out of noninterlocking cups (Craig *et al.,* 1987). If tissue must be excised or trimmed to fit the specimen cups, this is done just before freezing to minimize changes in cellular structure and function; the possibility of preparation-induced artifacts should be kept in mind.

In contrast to plunge freezing, specimens for high-pressure freezing are normally frozen in liquid, since the remaining space around the specimen in the cups is filled with a suitable air bubble-free fluid. This provides better thermal conductivity than air alone (Dahl and Staehelin, 1989; Kiss *et al.,* 1990), and if the viscosity of the fluid can be increased without affecting the specimens (for example, by adding agarose or a viscous cryoprotectant such as dextran: see below) it will help protect the specimens against physical damage from pressure-induced shearing or shock waves (Kiss *et al.,* 1990). Specimens containing air pockets such as leaves are vacuum-infiltrated to avoid deformation of tissue by the collapse of adjacent air pockets under pressurization (Welter *et al.,* 1988; Studer *et al.,* 1989).

2. Cryoprotectants

Despite the cryoprotective effects of high-pressure during freezing, many specimens frozen solely in distilled water or buffer will be severely damaged by ice crystal formation (Welter *et al.,* 1988; Studer *et al.,* 1989; Kiss *et al.,* 1990). Although information on the effectiveness of different nonpenetrating cryoprotectants is still limited, addition of 15% aqueous dextran (Kiss *et al.,* 1990) or replacement of water with 1-hexadecene (Studer *et al.,* 1989) can dramatically improve yields of well-preserved plant tissue.

IV. Results and Discussion

In root hairs, growth and cell expansion are restricted to the extreme tips of the cells. Unfortunately, these vacuolated cells are very sensitive to osmotic changes and, like many tip-growing cells, they are usually poorly preserved by chemical fixation (Ridge, 1988; Kaminskyj *et al.,* 1992). Seedling roots of *A. thaliana* (Columbia wild-type) average 110 μm in diameter. Root hairs are only about 20 μm in diameter at their widest, which is small enough for many to be well-preserved throughout by plunge freezing (Fig. 2), except at the highly vacuolated hair–root junction. Root hairs that are short (<0.5 mm long), either from young wild-type or mutant plants (Schiefelbein and Somerville, 1990), are better preserved than longer hairs that become bent against the roots during plunge freezing. The quality of cytoplasmic preservation in root epidermal cells varies between cells and between different roots but, in vacuolated mature cells, at best only a thin peripheral layer of cytoplasm is well preserved. Some phloem parenchyma and phloem companion cells were well preserved, probably due to the cryoprotective effect of concentrated solutes in phloem sap.

Attempts to plunge freeze protoplasts attached to various specimen supports including Formvar-coated wire loops resulted in severe ice damage. On the other hand, high-pressure freezing allowed us to recover a small proportion of well-preserved protoplasts (Fig. 3; see also Studer *et al.,* 1989; Galway *et al.,* 1993). It may be possible to increase the proportion of well-preserved protoplasts by adding dextran or other nonpenetrating cryoprotectants. Note that specimens frozen under high pressure may be more liable to ice damage caused by recrystallization during freeze substitution (Dahl and Staehelin, 1989). Although prolonged exposure to 2100 atm is lethal to living cells (Gilkey and Staehelin, 1986; Moor, 1987), cells frozen under high pressure have only 20–30 ms to react to high pressure before freezing occurs. Nevertheless, some known or suspected artifacts of high-pressure freezing have been identified in plant and fungal cells (Hyde *et al.,* 1991a; Galway *et al.,* 1993; and references therein).

Severe ice crystal damage causes unmistakable disruption of cell structure (e.g., Fig. 2G, Gilkey and Staehelin, 1986; Figs. 3, 4, Kaeser *et al.,* 1989). Milder ice crystal damage is also easily recognized in freeze-fixed specimens at intermediate magnifications in TEM (Fig. 4). The cytoplasm appears granular due to the localized aggregation of cytoplasmic contents such as ribosomes that are excluded from growing ice crystals. In addition, microtubules are collapsed, so that the distinct hollow cores are no longer visible in longitudinal sections (not shown).

The typical appearance of cytoplasm and organelles in thin sections of well-preserved plunge frozen root hairs and high-pressure frozen protoplasts is depicted in Figs. 2 and 3, respectively. The plasma membrane of root hairs is smooth and closely appressed to the cell wall (Fig. 2). In both cell types organelle profiles are smooth and rounded; Golgi body cisternae are straight and well

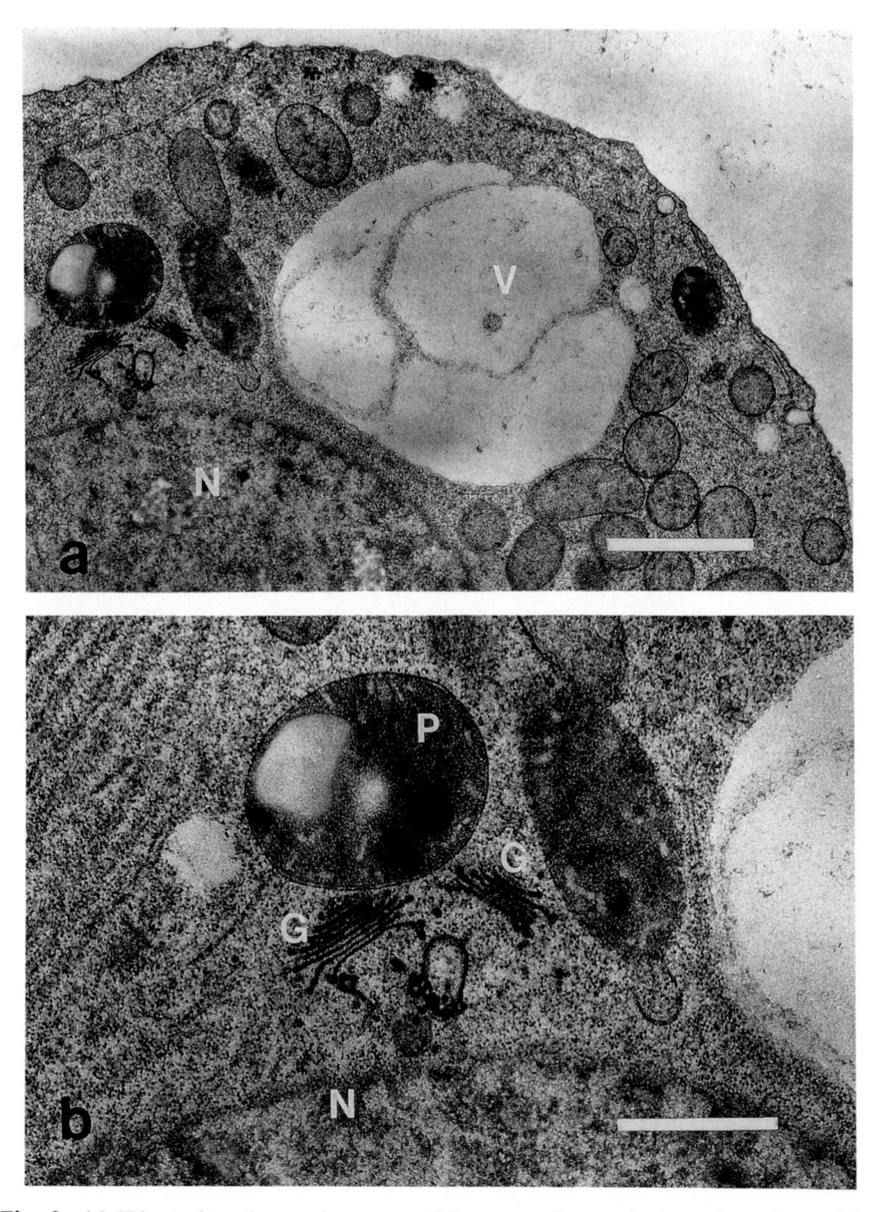

Fig. 3 (a) Thin section of protoplast prepared from an embryogenic suspension culture of *Picea glauca* frozen under high pressure in a Bal-Tec HPM 010, and then freeze-substituted in 2% osmium tetroxide in acetone and embedded in Spurr's resin. Note nucleus (N), Vacuole (V), and numerous plastids and mitochondria. Lead citrate staining. Bar, 1600 nm. (b) Enlargement shows details of nucleus (N), Golgi bodies (G), and plastid (P). Bar, 800 nm.

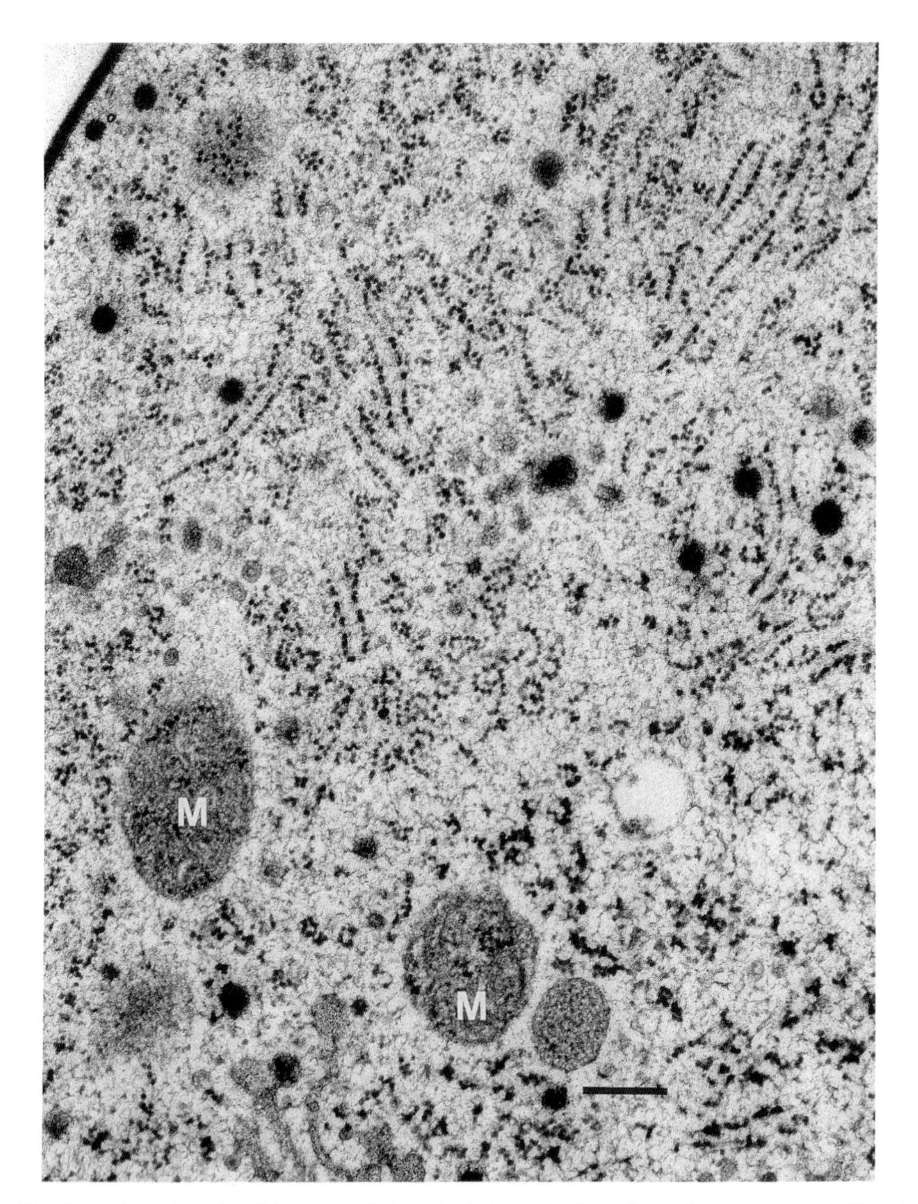

Fig. 4 Thin section of a wild-type root hair of *Arabidopsis thaliana* plunge frozen, freeze-substituted, and stained as in Fig. 1. A gradient of increasing ice damage extends through this hair from top to bottom of figure. Damaged cytoplasm at bottom appears granular and darkly stained due to the aggregation of cytoplasm into pockets between ice crystals. Note mitochondria (M). Bar, 200 nm.

defined (Figs. 2 and 3). Cytoplasmic ribosomes are uniformly distributed except when they are aligned along the surface of cross-sectioned endoplasmic reticulum. Contrast of endoplasmic reticulum and other cellular membranes was usually poor in stained sections of both root hairs and protoplasts. Membrane contrast, as well as the degree of extraction of cell contents, varies according to the freeze substitution and embedding protocol used (Howard and O'Donnell, 1987; Ridge, 1988, 1990; Kiss *et al.,* 1990).

V. Conclusions and Perspectives

Successful manual plunge freezing of suitable plant specimens, such as *Arabidopsis* root hairs, shows that rapid freezing does not require elaborate or expensive equipment. Other specimens that are not suitable for plunge freezing (such as protoplasts) can be conveniently freeze-fixed by high-pressure freezing in the Bal-Tec HPM 010. These methods undoubtedly preserved both root hairs and protoplasts in a more lifelike state than conventional chemical fixation and have been used to (*a*) confirm models of cellular processes derived from observation of chemically fixed cells (endocytosis in protoplasts: Galway *et al.,* 1993) and (*b*) obtain details of cytoplasmic organization that are destroyed by conventional chemical fixation (tip growth in *Arabidopsis* root hairs: Galway, Heckman and Schiefelbein, unpublished results). In many other cases, the application of freeze fixation methods has significantly changed our views of plant cell function and development (Dahl and Staehelin, 1989; Studer *et al.,* 1989; Kiss *et al.,* 1990; Robards, 1991; and references therein). The challenge now is to ensure that these methods come into routine use by more investigators, particularly for subcellular localization studies and for investigations of dynamic cellular processes where chemical fixation methods alone cannot be relied upon.

Acknowledgments

M.E.G. thanks Dr. John Schiefelbein at the University of Michigan, Ann Arbor, for the opportunity to study *Arabidopsis* root hair structure and development; Drs. Margaret McCully and Martin Canny for the introduction to plunge freezing methods; and Drs. Tom Giddings and Andrew Staehelin for the introduction to high-pressure freezing. G.J.H. thanks Peter Hepler, Sue Lancelle, and Dale Callahan for his introduction to plunge and high-pressure freezing, and Martin Müller for helpful advice on freezing methods. This work was supported by grants from the National Sciences and Engineering Research Council of Canada to L.C.F. and M.E.G. (NSERC Postdoctoral Award), and from the National Science Foundation to J. Schiefelbein.

References

Bachman, L., and Mayer, E. (1987). Physics of water and ice: Implications for cryofixation. *In* "Cryotechniques in Biological Electron Microscopy" (R. A. Steinbrecht and K. Zierold, eds.), pp. 3–34. Berlin: Springer-Verlag.

Craig, S., Gilkey, J. C., and Staehelin, L. A. (1987). Improved specimen support cups and auxiliary devices for the Balzers high pressure freezing apparatus. *J. Microsc.* **148,** 103–106.

Dahl, R., and Staehelin, L. A. (1989). High-pressure freezing for the preservation of biological structure: Theory and practice. *J. Electron Microsc. Tech.* **13,** 165–174.

Galway, M. E., Rennie, P. J., and Fowke, L. C. (1993). Ultrastructure of the endocytotic pathway in glutaraldehyde-fixed and high-pressure frozen/freeze-substituted protoplasts of white spruce (*Picea glauca*). *J. Cell Sci.* **106,** 847–858.

Gilkey, J. C., and Staehelin, L. A. (1986). Advances in ultrarapid freezing for the preservation of cellular ultrastructure. *J. Electron Microsc. Tech.* **3,** 177–210.

Howard, R. J., and O'Donnell, K. L. (1987). Freeze substitution of fungi for cytological analysis. *Exp. Mycol.* **11,** 250–269.

Hyde, G. J., Lancelle, S., Hepler, P. K., and Hardham, A. R. (1991a). Sporangial structure in *Phytophthora* is disrupted after high pressure freezing. *Protoplasma* **165,** 203–208.

Hyde, G. J., Lancelle, S., Hepler, P. K., and Hardham, A. R. (1991b). Freeze substitution reveals a new model for sporangial cleavage in *Phytophthora,* a result with implications for cytokinesis in other eukaryotes. *J. Cell Sci.* **100,** 735–746.

Kaeser, W., Koyro, H.-W., and Moor, H. (1989). Cryofixation of plant tissues without pretreatment. *J. Microsc.* **154,** 279–288.

Kaminskyj, S. G. W., Jackson, S. L., and Heath, I. B. (1992). Fixation induces differential polarized translocations of organelles in hyphae of *Saprolegnia ferax. J. Microsc.* **167,** 153–168.

Kiss, J. Z., Giddings, Th. H., Jr., Staehelin, L. A., and Sack, F. D. (1990). Comparison of the ultrastructure of conventionally fixed and high pressure frozen/freeze substituted root tips of *Nicotiana* and *Arabidopsis, Protoplasma* **157,** 64–74.

Kushida, H. (1974). A new method for embedding with a low viscosity epoxy resin "Quetol 651." *J. Electron Microsc.* (Jpn.) **23,** 197.

Menco, B. Ph. M. (1986). A survey of ultra-rapid cryofixation methods with particular emphasis on applications to freeze-fracturing, freeze-etching, and freeze-substitution. *J. Electron Microsc. Tech.* **4,** 177–240.

Moor, H. (1987). Theory and practice of high pressure freezing. *In* "Cryotechniques in Biological Electron Microscopy" (R. A. Steinbrecht and K. Zierold, eds.), pp. 175–191. Berlin: Springer-Verlag.

Plattner, H., and Bachmann, L. (1982). Cryofixation: A tool in biological ultrastructural research. *Int. Rev. Cytol.* **79,** 237–304.

Ridge, R. W. (1988). Freeze-substitution improves the ultrastructural preservation of legume root hairs. *Bot. Mag.* Tokyo **101,** 427–441.

Ridge, R. W. (1990). A simple apparatus and technique for the rapid-freeze and freeze-substitution of single-cell algae. *J. Electron Microsc.* **39,** 120–124.

Robards, A. W. (1991). Rapid-freezing methods and their applications. *In* "Electron Microscopy of Plant Cells" (J. L. Hall and C. Hawes, eds.), pp. 258–312. London: Academic Press.

Robards, A. W., and Sleytr, U. B. (1985). "Low Temperature Methods in Biological Electron Microscopy." Practical Methods in Electron Microscopy, Vol. 10 (A. M. Glauert, ed.). Amsterdam: Elsevier.

Roos, N., and Morgan, A. J. (1990). "Cryopreparation of Thin Biological Specimens for Electron Microscopy: Methods and Applications." RMS Microscopy Handbook No. 21, New York: Oxford Univ. Press.

Sartori, N., Richter, K., and Dubochet, J. (1993). Vitrification depth can be increased more than 10-fold by high-pressure freezing. *J. Microsc.* **172,** 55–61.

Schiefelbein, J. W., and Somerville, C. (1990). Genetic control of root hair development in *Arabidopsis thaliana. The Plant Cell* **2,** 235–243.

Sitte, H., Edelmann, L., and Neumann, K. (1987). Cryofixation without pretreatment at ambient pressure. *In* "Cryotechniques in Biological Electron Microscopy" (R. A. Steinbrecht and K. Zierold, eds.), pp. 87–113. Berlin: Springer-Verlag.

Steinbrecht, R. A., and Zierold, K. (1987). "Cryotechniques in Biological Electron Microscopy." Berlin: Springer-Verlag.

Studer, D., Michel, M., and Müller, M. (1989). High pressure freezing comes of age. *Scanning Microsc.,* Suppl. **3,** 253–269.

Welter, K., Müller, M., and Mendgen, K. (1988). The hyphae of *Uromyces appendiculatus* within the leaf tissue after high pressure freezing and freeze substitution. *Protoplasma* **147,** 91–99.

CHAPTER 2

Ion Localization and X-Ray Microanalysis

Martin J. Hodson
School of Biological and Molecular Sciences
Oxford Brookes University
Gipsy Lane, Headington
Oxford OX3 0BP, United Kingdom

I. Introduction

Plant scientists interested in mineral relations often wish to extend their observations at a whole plant level to investigate ion localization at a cellular or even subcellular level. Techniques for the localization of ions within plant tissues have advanced considerably in the last 20 years. Many, but not all, of these have been based on the technique of electron probe X-ray microanalysis. X-ray microanalysis has been well described by Russ (1978), and only a brief account is given here. Most biological X-ray microanalysis is now carried out in SEM, TEM, or STEM to which energy dispersive X-ray microanalysis (EDX) equipment has been fitted. When electrons are fired at or through the specimens in these machines they interact with the atoms of material, resulting in the emission of X-rays that are characteristic for the elements present. Nearly all equipment will detect only those elements with the atomic number of sodium or above. Microanalysis can be quantified, but cannot indicate what form or combination the element is in. In principle X-ray microanalysis is highly sensitive and capable of detecting 10^{-18} g of an element (Russ, 1978). The problems confronting a plant scientist interested in using microanalysis are not with the machinery, but with the methods of preparing plant material prior to analysis. This chapter will concentrate on the problems of producing plant material for microanalytical investigations.

II. Plant Materials

Before considering the methods that are available for the localization of ions in plant tissue, some consideration should be given to the types of study in which microanalysis is commonly used. Spurr (1980) reviewed the applications of X-ray microanalysis in botany, and provided a comprehensive account of the literature prior to that date. Harvey (1986) identified four major topics in plant science that have been investigated using X-ray microanalysis: the effects of salinity; effects of pollutants; distribution of silica; and analysis of seeds and protein bodies. The majority of publications published since 1986 have also fallen into these categories. A recent example concerning the effects of salinity on higher plants is the work of Leigh and Storey (1993) on intercellular compartmentation of ions in the leaves of salt stressed barley plants. The localization of aluminium in plant tissues has recently become an important topic (Hodson and Sangster, 1993). Hodson and Sangster (1990) reviewed the literature concerning microanalysis of silicon in higher plants. Studies of the protein globoids of seeds have continued, a recent example being the work of West and Lott (1993) on the seeds of 11 *Pinus* species.

III. The Choice of Methods

Figure 1 shows a summary of the main approaches to the preparation of plant tissues for X-ray microanalysis that have evolved over the last 15 years. When considering a microanalytical study, there are now two major procedures. SEM coupled with EDX is usually employed when distinguishing ion contents between different cell types or layers within the plant tissue is required. Higher resolution is normally needed if localization at the subcellular level is the aim, and TEM

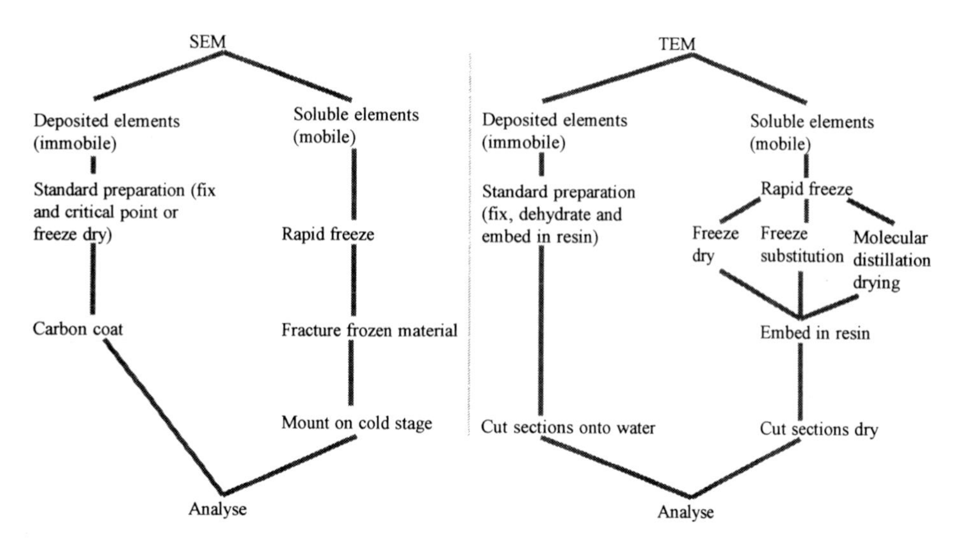

Fig. 1 Summary of techniques used to prepare plant tissues for X-ray microanalysis.

(or STEM) fitted with EDX will be preferred. The other main dichotomy concerns whether the elements of interest are deposited and immobile, or soluble and mobile. When minerals are in a deposited form it is often possible to use conventional preparative techniques for SEM (freeze or critical point dry, coat with carbon, mount on a stub, and analyze on a stage at room temperature) or TEM (fix in glutaraldehyde/osmium tetroxide, dehydrate, embed, and cut onto water). Much useful information on silica deposition in plants (Hodson and Sangster, 1990) and the protein globoids of seeds (West and Lott, 1993) has been obtained in this way. However, when the investigation concerns soluble elements (e.g., sodium, potassium, and chloride) far more care is required with the preparative techniques. It has been shown that conventional aqueous preparation leads to considerable ion loss from the tissue (Morgan *et al.,* 1978), and it can be assumed that any ions remaining in the tissue after such a procedure will not be in their original *in vivo* locations. After much experimentation two major methods have emerged for the localization of soluble elements in higher plants: analysis of the fracture faces of frozen material on a cryostage of an SEM and freeze substitution as a method for preparing material for analysis in TEM. It is with these two techniques that the majority of this chapter is concerned.

IV. Cryo-SEM and X-Ray Microanalysis

Where analysis that distinguishes between the ion contents of different cells in a tissue is required, the method of choice is cryo-SEM, and microanalysis of frozen tissue. A typical procedure (Hodson and Sangster, 1990) is shown in Fig. 2, but there are many variations and these are discussed below.

A. Freezing and Fracturing

The topic of freezing plant tissue as a preparative procedure is complex, and is covered in more detail in Chapter 1 of this volume. Freezing rates are somewhat less critical when preparing tissues for cryo-SEM and microanalysis than for other procedures. Provided that ion movement from cell to cell is prevented, the technique should give good results. The majority of workers have used the following protocol: Segments of plant material (usually root or leaf) 4–5 mm long are quickly mounted on aluminium or copper stubs, using a conductive carbon cement. The mounted specimens are then frozen by plunging into supercooled nitrogen slush (approximately −210°C), and are then transferred while frozen to a precooled cryopreparation chamber. Here specimens are fractured transversely using a cold knife. Routinely specimens that do not show a reasonably flat fracture plane are rejected. Most recently, Huang *et al.* (1994) have developed a procedure for planing frozen hydrated plant specimens to form a flat face.

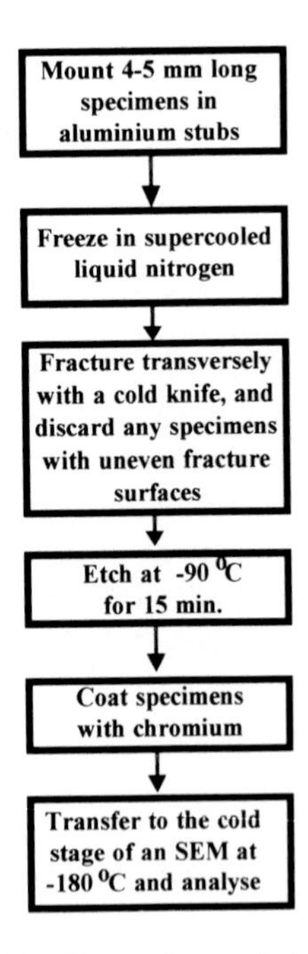

Fig. 2 Preparation of plant material for X-ray microanalysis on the cold stage of an SEM. Method based on that of Hodson and Sangster (1990).

B. Etching and Coating

Some controversy surrounds both etching and coating. Frozen hydrated specimens are difficult to visualize under SEM unless a certain amount of water is removed from their fractured surfaces. Etching involves the sublimation of a small amount of water from the specimen surface, and almost all workers have carried out this procedure to some extent. Times and temperatures for etching vary markedly: Hodson and Sangster (1989, 1990) etched for 15 min at −90°C; Drew *et al.* (1990) etched for 2 min at −82°C; Leigh and Storey (1993) raised their samples to −86°C through a temperature profile; Frensch *et al.* (1992) performed their analyses on "slightly etched specimens"; and McCully *et al.* (1987) did not etch their samples. The problem with etching is that it involves the removal of water from the specimen surface, and thus the concentration of ions in the cells exposed at the fracture face increases. This creates considerable difficulties in quantification of the results.

Specimen charging is usually a problem unless the specimen is coated with a conductive material. Drew *et al.* (1990) used carbon coating, whereas Hodson and Sangster (1989, 1990) and Leigh and Storey (1993) preferred chromium. Coating with chromium has the advantage that the metal is a good conductor, but it may also decrease the X-rays emitted from the specimen.

C. Analysis and Quantification

The majority of cryo-SEM and X-ray microanalysis investigations have not attempted full quantification of the results, and have given presence/absence data, or semiquantitative peak/background ratios. There are a number of reasons for this. First, it is difficult to obtain totally flat specimens. For quantification it is essential that a constant geometry among the specimen, the incident electron beam, and the X-ray detector be maintained. When the cryoplaning technique of Huang *et al.* (1994) becomes more widely available it should eliminate this problem. Second, etching, as noted above, increases ion concentrations. It is hard to ensure that this increase is constant in all cell types, and between different specimens. Third, the electron beam, even in flat specimens, will penetrate to different depths into the tissue depending on the matrix. It is also difficult to be certain what is being analyzed beneath the surface of a fractured specimen. By far the greatest problem, however, is the production of suitable standards. The matrix of the standards should be as close in properties to the tissue as possible. McCully *et al.* (1987), working on potassium in the metaxylem of maize roots, drew out the cell contents under vacuum, and replaced it with standard KCl solutions. They then treated these roots in the same way as the sample roots. Absolute concentrations were obtained by comparison with carbon slurry standards containing appropriate amounts of potassium. The peak/background ratios of the standards were then compared with the sample roots and those that had been perfused with potassium. Most recently, Muralitharan *et al.* (1993) used colloidal graphite standards with 9.5% carbon. It does appear that the use of this type of standard is becoming accepted practice, particularly for the analysis of vacuoles or other large homogeneous areas. However, it should be remembered that the matrix of the material analyzed can vary markedly between and within samples. Work on mineralized tissues presents particular difficulties (Hodson and Sangster, 1989), as mineralization itself changes the matrix of the sample. The topic of quantification is covered in detail by Van Steveninck and Van Steveninck (1991).

V. Freeze Substitution and TEM

With this technique the aim is often to locate ions at the subcellular level. Figure 3 shows a typical procedure (Hodson and Sangster, 1990), but again there are quite a number of variations on the basic technique.

A. Freezing

Again tissue freezing rates are not regarded as critical here as in work where ultrastructural detail is required. Most commonly 1- to 2-mm segments of tissue are rapidly frozen by dunking in 8% (v/v) methylcyclohexane in 2-methylbutane cooled to −170°C by liquid nitrogen (Harvey *et al.,* 1976), or in super cooled liquid propane at −186°C (Hodson and Sangster, 1989). The latter technique is hazardous, as oxygen/propane mixtures are potentially explosive. After freezing, specimens can be placed in steel mesh bags, which are then sealed to prevent the escape of material during further processing.

B. Substitution

Harvey (1982) reviewed the technique of freeze substitution. After freezing, the specimens are transferred to a precooled, anhydrous solvent in a sealed container in a deep freeze at −70 to −80°C. The solvent is kept anhydrous by the inclusion of activated molecular sieve. Choice of the solvent is dictated by the solubility of the ions that are the major subject of interest. Ideally the ions should be totally insoluble in the solvent used. The most common substitution solvents used are acetone and diethyl ether, but others are available (Harvey, 1982). The length of time needed to complete substitution varies according to the solvent and the tissue investigated. Typical substitution times are 3 days in acetone and 14–21 days in diethyl ether. For ion localization work, fixatives such as glutaraldehyde or osmium tetroxide are rarely added into the substitution medium. Loss of soluble ions from the tissue during substitution has been shown to be negligible, provided that care is taken to use the correct solvent, and that anhydrous conditions are maintained. There is, however, no definitive proof that some redistribution within the tissue does not take place.

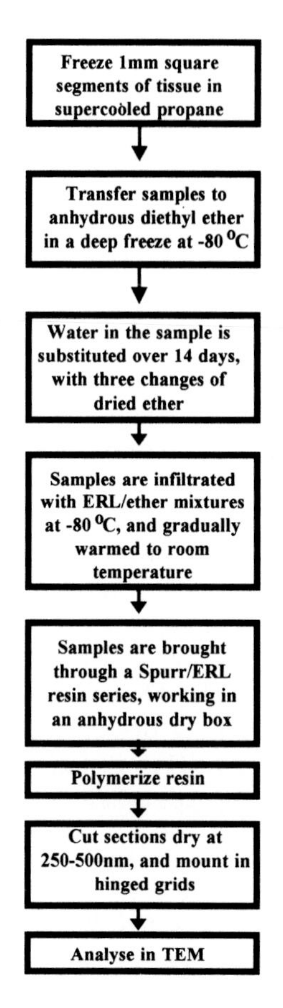

Fig. 3 Preparation of plant material for X-ray microanalysis in TEM using freeze substitution. Method based on that of Hodson and Sangster (1990).

C. Embedding in Resin

Despite its known toxicity, the majority of workers have preferred to use Spurr (1969) resin for microanalytical work involving freeze substitution as the preparative procedure. This has the advantage that it is possible to start resin infiltration at low temperature (−40 to −80°C depending on the workers), by introducing the specimens to mixtures of the ERL4206 component and solvent (Hodson and Sangster, 1990). In the present author's opinion it is also the best resin available when dry cut sections are required. All resin/solvent mixtures must be predried with activated molecular sieve. The temperature of the specimens is gradually raised to room temperature, and the concentration of the resin is also gradually increased. From then on all operations must take place in a dry atmosphere, preferably in a specially constructed dry box. Once the specimens have been infiltrated with complete medium, the resin is polymerized and the blocks are stored in a dry environment prior to cutting.

Recently, Hajibagheri and Flowers (1993) compared Nanoplast MUV116 resin (a UV-polymerized aminoplastic medium) with Spurr resin as media for embedding plant material after freeze substitution. Ion contents were marginally higher after embedding in Nanoplast than in Spurr resin, and the authors preferred Nanoplast, as it can be polymerized at low temperatures.

D. Cutting Sections

Cutting freeze-substituted sections onto water has been shown to lead to substantial ion loss from the section (Harvey *et al.*, 1976). Despite some interest in the idea of cutting sections onto solvents other than water, almost all of the published work has been carried out using dry sections. Cutting thin dry sections is technically difficult, but Harvey *et al.* (1981) found that it was possible to cut them at 100 nm. With mineralized material thicker (250–500 nm) sections can be used, particularly if a TEM with a high accelerating voltage is available (Hodson and Sangster, 1989). Usually the dry sections are loaded into folding grids prior to analysis, but Fritz (1990) has suggested that adhesive coated grids may be preferable. Hodson and Sangster (1989, 1993) have obtained useful results by mounting dry cut specimens onto stubs and then carrying out the analysis in SEM. This technique is particularly valuable when working with mineralized materials where X-ray maps at low magnification are required.

E. Analysis and Quantification

In this case, most investigations in the last 10 years have been quantitative. The vast majority of these have concerned salt tolerance and toxicity, with Harvey *et al.* (1981) being the first of a whole series of papers to present quantitative data on this topic. Quantification essentially depends on the production of suitable standards in the same resin that the tissue analyzed is embedded in. It is very important that the matrix of the sample match that of the standard. Standards in Spurr (1969) resin are available for sodium, potassium, and chlorine (Harvey *et al.*, 1980), and for a variety of other elements. Unfortunately there are several elements for which suitable standards are not available (e.g., silicon and aluminium), and this has limited investigations of these elements to semiquantitative results. Again mineralization of the material presents considerable difficulties for quantification (Hodson and Sangster, 1989). Even if a suitable standard for an element is available (e.g., for potassium), results obtained from biomineralized areas of the sample (e.g., silicified areas) will be considerably influenced by the change in matrix properties caused by mineralization.

VI. Other Preparative Techniques

In addition to the two major techniques for the localization of soluble elements outlined above, a number of less common methods have also been used. Several workers have used analysis of microdrops to investigate sap collected either from the xylem (e.g. Gartner *et al.*, 1984) or from cell vacuoles using a modified pressure probe (Malone *et al.*, 1991). These are useful techniques, but the majority of papers have concerned analysis of intact tissues.

If this review had been written 10 years ago, a considerable part of it would have been taken up in discussing various methods of precipitating ions during fixation using precipitants such as silver salts for the localization of chloride ions or pyroantimonate for a variety of cations (see Spurr, 1980, for a review). Intensive investigations pointed out a number of problems with these techniques, principally that they do not prevent ion movement and loss, and that they are impossible to quantify. It is a measure of the progress that has been made in this field that hardly any recently published investigations have used these methods.

Plant tissues have also been prepared for microanalysis in TEM using freeze drying and molecular distillation drying (Fig. 1). The former technique involves rapid freezing, the removal of water from the specimen by freeze drying, and embedding in a suitable resin. This may be a useful method in nonvacuolated tissues, but its use for highly vacuolated plant tissues has been criticized by Harvey (1986): "It is difficult to envisage how the deposition of ions from evacuated spaces onto the nearest membrane or support can be avoided during freeze-drying."

Molecular distillation drying (MDD) is the latest method to be used for the preparation of plant material for X-ray microanalysis, and so far only one paper on ion localization in the alga *Dunaliella parva* is available (Hajibagheri and Flowers, 1993). The authors defined MDD as "drying samples within an apparatus which has the condenser surfaces in direct line of sight of the samples." In this technique the samples are rapidly frozen and transferred while under liquid nitrogen to the specimen chamber in the dryer. Once the chamber reaches 10^{-7} mbar, a slow heating and drying cycle is commenced. After nearly 4 days drying, the samples are infiltrated with Spurr resin (without the accelerator) under vacuum. After transfer to fresh resin with accelerator, polymerization is carried out at 60°C for 16 h. Hajibagheri and Flowers compared the results of preparing material using MDD with those obtained from freeze substitution in acetone. Quantitative X-ray microanalysis revealed that sodium and chloride concentrations in material prepared by MDD were 82% of the values for freeze-substituted material. The authors could not explain the lower values obtained, but considered that it may be related to differences in tissue volume produced as a result of the different preparative techniques. It is difficult to assess this new procedure when only one investigation has been carried out, and more work is required before its use can be recommended for the routine preparation of samples for microanalysis.

VII. Other Machinery Used for Ion Localization

Besides electron probe X-ray microanalysis several other types of machine have been used to study ion localization in plant tissues. Proton-induced X-ray emission (PIXE) operates on principles similar to those for EDX, except that protons are used to excite atoms in the specimen. PIXE is more sensitive than EDX, but has a lower spatial resolution. Maenhaut (1988) reviewed the literature concerning the applications of this technique in biology. Electron energy loss spectroscopy (EELS) has a better spatial resolution than EDX and is more sensitive than EDX, particularly for elements of low atomic number. However, its use is restricted to ultrathin (30 nm) sections, which cannot realistically be cut dry. Rogerson *et al.* (1987) used EELS to investigate the localization of soluble silicon in the diatom *Thalassiosira pseudonana.* They claimed that soluble silicon was associated with lipid inclusions and ribosomes, but the results must be considered suspect, as they used conventional aqueous fixation procedures and cut their sections onto water. Laser microprobe mass analysis (LAMMA) has thus far been little used by plant scientists (see Van Steveninck and Van Steveninck, 1991, for references). One feature of many of the published investigations using these machines is that preparation of the plant material for analysis is often fairly primitive. Ion loss and movement during preparation are frequently neglected. If suitable preparative techniques are used, then PIXE, EELS, and LAMMA all show some promise for the future, but they are expensive and not available in most laboratories.

VIII. Conclusions

Considerable progress has been made in the preparation of plant material for microanalytical investigations involving soluble elements. In particular almost all of the serious work in this field now uses rapid freezing as the first stage in tissue preparation. Far more studies are attempting quantification of their results. In the future new preparative techniques such as MDD will undoubtedly improve matters even further. Other types of machinery, such as PIXE, EELS, and LAMMA, have the potential to increase analytical sensitivity, analytical resolution, or both. The fact that most of these machines will not be available to nearly all plant scientists should not be too disheartening, as very good quantitative results are now possible using either of the two main techniques outlined in this chapter.

References

Drew, M. C., Webb, J., and Saker, L. R. (1990). Regulation of K^+ uptake and transport to the xylem in barley roots; K^+ distribution determined by electron probe x-ray microanalysis of frozen-hydrated cells. *J. Exp. Bot.* **41,** 815–825.

Frensch, J., Stelzer, R., and Steudle, E. (1992). NaCl uptake in roots of *Zea mays* seedlings: Comparison of root pressure probe and EDX data. *Ann. Bot.* **70,** 543–550.

Fritz, E. (1990). The use of adhesive-coated grids for the x-ray microanalysis of dry-cut sections in the TEM. *J. Microsc.* **161,** 501–504.

Gartner, S., LeFaucheur, L., Roinel, N., and Paris-Pireyre, N. (1984). Preliminary studies on the elemental composition of xylem exudate from two varieties of wheat by electron probe analysis. *Scanning Electron Microsc.* **1984/IV,** 1739–1744.

Hajibagheri, M. A., and Flowers, T. J. (1993). Use of freeze-substitution and molecular distillation drying in the preparation of *Dunaliella parva* for ion localization studies by x-ray microanalysis. *Microsc. Res. Tech.* **24,** 395–399.

Harvey, D. M. R. (1982). Freeze-substitution. *J. Microsc.* **127,** 209–221.

Harvey, D. M. R. (1986). Applications of x-ray microanalysis in botanical research. *Scanning Electron Microsc.* **1986/III,** 953–973.

Harvey, D. M. R., Flowers, T. J., Hall, J. L., and Spurr, A. R. (1980). The preparation of calibration standards for sodium, potassium and chlorine analyses by analytical electron microscopy. *J. Microsc.* **118,** 143–152.

Harvey, D. M. R., Hall, J. L., and Flowers, T. J. (1976). The use of freeze-substitution in the preparation of plant tissue for ion localisation studies. *J. Microsc.* **107,** 189–198.

Harvey, D. M. R., Hall, J. L., Flowers, T. J., and Kent, B. (1981). Quantitative ion localisation within *Suaeda maritima* leaf mesophyll cells. *Planta* **151,** 555–560.

Hodson, M. J., and Sangster, A. G. (1989). Subcellular localization of mineral deposits in the roots of wheat (*Triticum aestivum* L.). *Protoplasma* **151,** 19–32.

Hodson, M. J., and Sangster, A. G. (1990). Techniques for the microanalysis of higher plants with particular reference to silicon in cryofixed wheat tissues. *Scanning Microsc.* **4,** 407–408.

Hodson, M. J., and Sangster, A. G. (1993). The interaction between silicon and aluminium in *Sorghum bicolor* (L.) Moench: Growth analysis and x-ray microanalysis. *Ann. Bot.* **72,** 389–400.

Huang, C. X., Canny, M. J., Oates, K., and McCully, M. E. (1994). Planing frozen hydrated specimens for SEM observation and EDX analysis. *Microsc. Res. Tech.* **28,** 67–74.

Leigh, R. A., and Storey, R. (1993). Intercellular compartmentation of ions in barley leaves in relation to potassium nutrition and salinity. *J. Exp. Bot.* **44,** 755–762.

Maenhaut, W. (1988). Applications of ion beam analysis in biology and medicine, a review. *Nuc. Instrum. Methods Phys. Res.* **B35,** 388–403.

Malone, M., Leigh, R. A., and Tomos, A. D. (1991). Concentrations of vacuolar inorganic ions in individual cells of intact wheat leaf epidermis. *J. Exp. Bot.* **42,** 305–309.

McCully, M. E., Canny, M. J., and Van Steveninck, R. F. M. (1987). Accumulation of potassium by differentiating metaxylem elements of maize roots. *Physiol. Plant.* **69,** 73–80.

Morgan, A. J., Davies, T. W., and Erasmus, D. A. (1978). Specimen preparation. *In* "Electron Probe Microanalysis in Biology" (D. A. Erasmus, ed.), pp. 94–147. London: Chapman & Hall.

Muralitharan, M. S., Chandler, S. F., and Van Steveninck, R. F. M. (1993). Physiological adaptation to high ion concentrations or water deficits by callus cultures of highbush blueberry, *Vaccinium corymbosum*. *Aust. J. Plant Physiol.* **20,** 159–172.

Rogerson, A., DeFreitas, A. S. W., and McInnes, A. G. (1987). Cytoplasmic silicon in the centric diatom *Thalassiosira pseudonana* localized by electron spectroscopic imaging. *Can. J. Microbiol.* **33,** 128–131.

Russ, J. C. (1978). Electron probe x-ray microanalysis—Principles. *In* "Electron Probe Microanalysis in Biology" (D. A. Erasmus, ed.), pp. 5–36. London: Chapman & Hall.

Spurr, A. R. (1969). A low viscosity epoxy resin embedding medium for electron microscopy. *J. Ultrastruct. Res.* **26,** 31–43.

Spurr, A. R. (1980). Applications of x-ray microanalysis in botany. *Scanning Electron Microsc.* **1980/II,** 535–564.

Van Steveninck, R. F. M., and Van Steveninck, M. E. (1991). Microanalysis. *In* "Electron Microscopy of Plant Cells" (J. L. Hall and C. Hawes, eds.), pp. 415–455. New York/London: Academic Press.

West, M. M., and Lott, J. N. A. (1993). Studies of mature seeds of eleven *Pinus* species differing in seed weight. II. Subcellular structure and localization of elements. *Can. J. Bot.* **71,** 577–585.

CHAPTER 3

Freeze-Fracture Deep-Etch Methods

Chris Hawes and Barry Martin
RMC Centre for Electron Microscopy
School of Biological and Molecular Sciences
Oxford Brookes University
Oxford OX3 0BP, United Kingdom

I. Introduction

The quick-freeze, deep-etch technique for the preparation of rotary shadowed replicas of unfixed biological material was pioneered by John Heuser at the beginning of the last decade (Heuser *et al.,* 1979; Heuser, 1981, 1983; Hirokawa and Heuser, 1981). The method avoids the use of both chemical fixatives and cryoprotectants and results in the production of a three-dimensional replica of the etched surface of the specimen. Samples are ultra-rapidly frozen and fractured, the ice is sublimed under vacuum from the fracture surface (deep-etched), and the specimen is replicated. Using this technique, great advances have been made in our understanding of the structure and molecular make up of animal cell

METHODS IN CELL BIOLOGY, VOL. 49

cytoplasm. Over the years the technique has been adapted to permit replication of extracted or isolated cytoskeletons (Heuser and Kirschner, 1980; Hirokawa and Heuser, 1981), fracture surfaces (Heuser, 1981; Hirokawa, 1982), isolated organelles (Heuser, 1981), and macromolecules (Heuser, 1989). Deep-etching can even be combined with immunogold labeling techniques giving excellent localization of cytoskeletal proteins (Lawson, 1984). Thus, the technique has enormous potential for the study of plant cells and it is something of a disappointment that this methodology has never been fully exploited by plant cell biologists, with only a handful of papers having appeared in the recent literature. This situation is probably more attributable to the lack of access to the necessary equipment rather than problems with the successful freezing and fracturing of plant material. To date, deep-etching has been used to study the ultrastructure of algal and higher plant cell walls (Goodenough and Heuser, 1985; McCann *et al.,* 1990; Satiat-Jeunemaitre *et al.,* 1992; Tamura and Senda, 1992), the cytoskeleton (Hawes and Martin, 1986; Kachar and Reese, 1988; McLean and Juniper, 1988), and plant clathrin-coated pits and vesicles (Hawes and Martin, 1986; Coleman *et al.,* 1987).

II. Materials

The one main advantage of the rapid-freeze deep-etch technique is that very little prior preparation of material is needed other than that required by the experiments that are being carried out. Therefore, most of the material requirements are in the instrumentation, and accessability to the necessary freezing and fracturing equipment is often the major limitation in the application of this technique. The procedure can be split into two separate events: freezing, followed by the fracturing, etching, and replication of the frozen material. Specimens can be frozen and stored under liquid nitrogen for any length of time prior to the fracturing procedure.

There are many different rapid freezing devices on the market ranging from the extremely expensive high-pressure freezing apparatus to metal mirror slammers that can be cooled by liquid nitrogen or liquid helium, propane jet freezers, and propane or ethane plungers (see Robards, 1991, and Chapter 1, this volume). In many cases satisfactory freezing can be obtained by manual plunging of the sample into liquid propane or ethane. However, it should be remembered that liquid propane and ethane are extremely dangerous cryogens and considerable care must be taken with their handling and disposal. Liquid propane has a flash point of −104°C and ethane can be ignited at −130°C. Thus, the cryogens should always be kept near their freezing point with liquid nitrogen and if possible handled under a nitrogen gas atmosphere and at all times in a spark-free fume cupboard. If a tailor-made burner is not available for disposal of the coolant then it is safest to allow slow evaporation in the fume cupboard. Remember that spilt propane/ethane can linger, as it is heavier than air, and poses a potential hazard. The reader is referred to Ryan and Liddicoat (1987) for further details on the handling of flammable coolants.

For fracturing and replication a high vacuum freeze-fracture unit with a rotary specimen stage is required and if possible it should be fitted with electron beam evaporation guns. A window in the specimen chamber is necessary so that the fracturing process can be monitored and an air lock into the specimen chamber is an advantage, as a high vacuum can be retained during specimen change over, which prevents frosting of both the specimen and the chamber. Replica thickness is best controlled by a quartz crystal monitor.

III. Methods

A. Specimen Freezing

As mentioned above there are various rapid freezing techniques that can be applied to material that is to be freeze-fractured. The one important criterion is that the material be mounted on a planchette or stub that is compatible with the stage of the freeze-fracture unit to be used. However, as advocated by Heuser (1981), in our experience freeze-slamming onto nitrogen or helium cooled copper blocks is the most appropriate freezing technique prior to fracturing and deep-etching (Hawes and Martin, 1986). The depth of good freezing into the specimen will depend on both the freezing technique used and the nature of the specimen being studied but may only extend to a couple of cells from the freezing front. It may well be advisable to parallel the deep-etch preparation with freeze-substitution of the specimen in order to ascertain the depth of acceptable freezing from sectioned material. For further details on rapid-freezing techniques the reader is referred to Chapter 1 in this volume.

B. Fracture and Deep-Etch

The fracturing and replication procedure is relatively straightforward once the intricacies of the freeze-fracture unit are learned. The specimen must be transferred from storage in liquid nitrogen on the specimen fracturing planchette without any significant heating. It is also important to keep the specimen covered with a small shroud or hat to minimize any ice crystallization on or warming of the specimen surface. The basic procedures for fracturing and replication are given in the following protocol.

1. Protocol 1: Rapid-Freeze, Deep-Etch of Plant Cells

1. Ultra-rapidly freeze tissue or thick cell suspension on a suitable stub or pins designed for the freeze-fracture (FF) apparatus to be used. Remove as much water from around the specimen as possible just prior to freezing.

2. Transfer the specimen at liquid nitrogen temperatures through the air lock into the freeze-fracture unit.

3. Gently remove the shroud covering the specimen with the knife and fracture the specimen at −110°C in the freeze-fracture unit with the cold knife at −196°C. It is important not to fracture deep into the specimen, as only well-frozen cells are useable. This in most cases means a simple scrape over the surface of the specimen.

4. Maneuver the cold knife over specimen to act as a condensing surface for sublimed ice and etch at −100°C for 10–30 min.

5. Low-angle rotary shadow at 26° with platinum/carbon at −100°C.[1]

6. Rotary replicate at 70° with carbon at −100°C.[2]

7. Remove specimens from the freeze-fracture apparatus and float replica onto DW. Alternatively, a more gentle procedure is to place the planchette with the replica still frozen onto a block of frozen water (frozen in liquid nitrogen) and allow it to thaw slowly.

8. Clean replica in 70% H_2SO_4, followed by 70% bleach over 2 to 3 days.[3] Replicas can be transferred between solutions by picking up with a platinum loop or picking up on the end of a glass pipette that has been heat fused to form a solid "blob" of glass.

9. Wash on filtered distilled water 3× 5 min.

10. Collect on Formvar- or carbon-coated grids.[4]

2. Deep-Etch Replication of Isolated Cell Walls

Besides whole cells and tissues, isolated fragments of cell walls can be fractured and cell wall structure analyzed. This has been successfully achieved by McCann *et al.* (1990), who sequentially chemically extracted the pectic and hemicellulose polymers of onion cell wall fragments prior to replicating the remaining structure. Thus, by comparing rapid-freeze deep-etch replicas of wall material at different stages of chemical extraction, a three-dimensional picture of wall construction was obtained. The protocol used by McCann *et al.* (1990) follows.

3. Protocol 2: Preparation of Isolated Plant Cell Walls for Deep-Etching

This protocol was developed for onion parenchyma, but can be modified for other tissues.

[1] Determine film thickness with a quartz crystal monitor; 1.5–2 nm should be adequate.

[2] Carbon film should be 10–35 nm thick.

[3] Replicas of deep-etched material can take much longer to clean than conventional freeze-fracture replicas.

[4] Deep-etch replicas are more fragile than conventional freeze-fracture replicas, so great care must be taken in handling.

1. Peel away the concave epidermis of onion bulb scales and remove the convex epidermis and visible veins with a razor blade.

2. Chop the remainder of each scale and liquidize in a homogenization buffer[5] in a Waring or similar blender at 0°C.

3. Filter through Miracloth (Calbiochem, California) and wash with buffer over the Miracloth.

4. Grind in liquid nitrogen to produce a fine white powder.

5. Sonicate in homogenization buffer for 15 min to break open the remaining cells.

6. Wash in buffer and collect wall fragments by centrifugation.[6]

7. Sequentially extract the cell wall material as follows:

a. 0.05 *M* *trans*-1,2-diaminocyclohexane-*N,N,N′,N′*-tetraacetic acid (Na^+ salt, pH 6.5) at 20°C for 6 h and in fresh solution for 2 h.
b. 0.05 *M* Na_2CO_3 at 1°C overnight followed by 3 h at 20°C in fresh solution.
c. 1 *M* KOH at 20°C for 2 h and a further 2 h in fresh 1 *M* KOH.
d. 4 *M* KOH at 20°C for 2 h and a further 2 h in fresh KOH.
e. Finally, extract the α-cellulosic residue with acidified chlorite at 70°C for 2 h.

8. At any stage during the extraction procedure remove a pellet of cell wall material, wash in distilled water, and rapidly freeze on a freeze-fracture planchette.

9. Carefully scrape away the surface ice from the frozen pellet with the cold knife in the freeze-fracture unit and etch and rotary replicate as described in Protocol 1.

C. Taking Stereo-Pair Micrographs

Perhaps the best method of recording micrographs from deep-etch replicas is to take stereo-pairs (Hawes, 1991). Replicas can be extremely complex, especially when cast on overlapping fibrillar structures such as cell walls (Satiat-Jeunemaitre *et al.,* 1992). Taking the stereo-pair is a simple operation, as due to the rotary shadowing there are no unidirectional shadows on the replica, which is the case with conventional freeze-fracture replicas. Therefore, prealignment of the specimen with the tilt axis to adjust for the direction of shadow is not required. There is no hard and fast rule for the best tilt angle to be used. Between 7 and 10 degrees should suffice in most instances (Heuser, 1989). It is important, however, not to use too great a tilt angle, otherwise the excessive parallax created will not permit optical fusion of the stereo-pair.

[5] Homogenization buffer: 0.1 *M* Hepes, 0.3 *M* sucrose, 3 m*M* potassium metabisulfite, 10 m*M* calcium chloride.

[6] Cell wall fragments can be checked by differential interference contrast light microscopy or electron microscopy.

D. Printing the Micrographs

Negatives of deep-etch replicas give a positive image of the original fractured specimen and they cannot be printed directly, as this will give rise to a negative print. There are several ways in which this problem can be overcome. An internegative back onto EM film can be made (Heuser, 1989). This inevitably increases the contrast of the image, so either an adjustment to the contrast of the microscope image (higher kV, larger objective aperture) and/or change in exposure of the film must be made or the development of the internegative must be controlled to reduce contrast. A simple, although slightly less controllable, technique is to print directly onto reverse contrast paper such as Kodak Kodagraph Transtar.

IV. Critical Aspects of the Procedure

A. Specimen Freezing

The most important aspect of specimen freezing is to ensure rapid and efficient thermal transfer between the specimen and the cryogen. Generally this means having as little water or buffer around the specimen as possible without exposing the specimen surface to air-drying. It is advisable to mount the specimen on the freezing stub wet and just prior to freezing to dab the edge of the material with filter paper to draw off an excess liquid. If the specimen is in the form of a suspension (i.e., cells, protoplasts), make the suspension as concentrated as possible and, if freeze-slamming, mount onto a small disc of filter paper on the freezing stub. A deep-etch replica of a well-frozen carrot suspension culture cell is shown in Fig. 1. The etched cytoplasm is regularly granular and shows no evidence of resolvable ice crystal damage. The major organelles are clearly defined, including those that are membrane-bounded such as the Golgi apparatus and endoplasmic reticulum.

B. Fracturing the Specimen

As mentioned above, it is important that the specimen is well frozen and that all precautions be taken to minimize ice crystal damage, such as partially drying the specimen surface immediately prior to freezing. In reality with most specimens this means that only the cells at the freezing front will be suitable for fracturing and replication. In deep-etch replicas, as opposed to conventional freeze-fracture replicas, even minor ice crystal damage is very apparent. Figure 2 shows an example of a poorly frozen cell with extensive ice crystal damage to the cytoplasm even though the membrane bounding an organelle remains relatively intact. Therefore, unless the specimens have been high-pressure frozen the fracture procedure is a simple scraping of the cooled knife across the surface of the specimen breaking no more than a few micrometers into the tissue. In this respect fracture units with knives whose cutting stroke circumscribes a shallow arc are

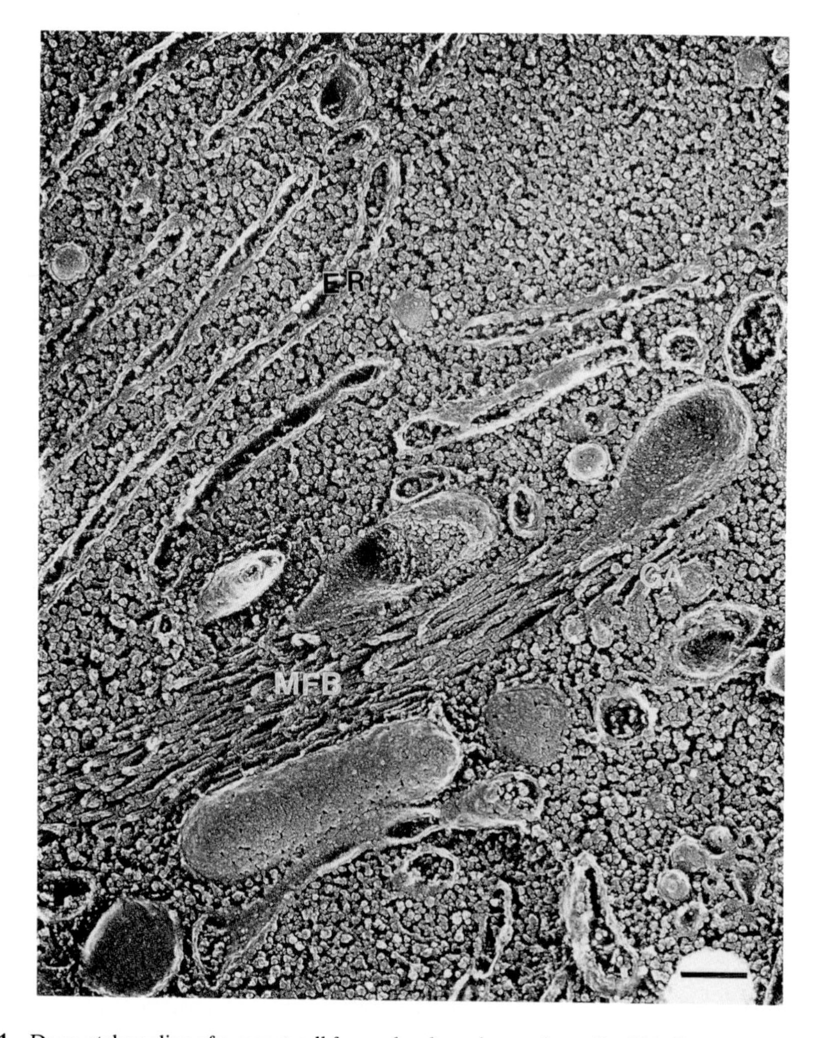

Fig. 1 Deep-etch replica of a carrot cell frozen by slamming against a liquid helium cooled copper mirror at −263°C. Note the total lack of ice crystal damage to the cytoplasm and that all major organelles are well preserved. ER, endoplasmic reticulum; GA, Golgi apparatus; MFB, microfibrillar bundle. Bar, 22 nm.

useful in that the fracture surface will vary in depth, thus increasing the likelihood of at least several well-preserved areas of cytoplasm in the replica.

C. Handling Deep-Etch Replicas

Deep-etch replicas tend to take longer to clean and are more fragile than conventional freeze-fracture replicas. Material can often prove to be resistant

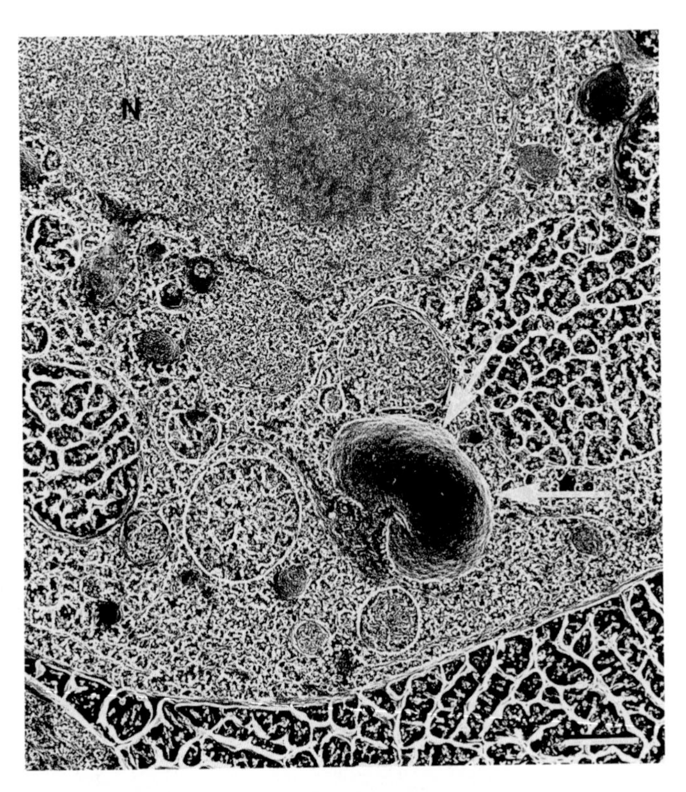

Fig. 2 Deep-etched carrot suspension cell protoplast showing poor freezing. Note the extensive ice crystal damage in the nucleus (N) and the cytoplasm. In contrast, the membrane of a protruding organelle is relatively undamaged (arrows). Bar, 1.5 μm.

to hypochlorite or weak acids, but perseverance and strong solutions of sulfuric acid and even chromic acid will eventually dissolve most plant material. Final washing after transfer through weak acid to water can be in 70% hypochlorite followed by several washes on filtered distilled water. Replicas tend to fragment during prolonged cleaning due to expansion of the tissue during digestion and this effect is enhanced in deep-etch replicas. However, even the smallest visible fragments can hold valuable data, and should be kept and mounted on grids.

The use of fixed material can often make the production of intact replicas easier. However, this is not a recommended strategy, as one of the major aims of the technique is to observe the ultrastructure of chemically untouched material. Replicas can be strengthened by depositing a thicker layer of carbon, but this can reduce resolution. Another method is to coat them with a plastic film such as parloidion (Bordi, 1979) or "Lexan" polycarbonate plastic (Steere and Erbe, 1983) to support the replica while the biological material is dissolved away.

D. Interpretation of Artifacts

As in any microscopical procedure, it is important that the potential of creating artifacts be fully appreciated. These may be easy to recognize, such as compression of the specimen during freeze-slamming, and this can be compensated for by adjusting the thickness of the sponge or biological support on the freezing stubs. Membrane damage is common in deep-etch material, as during the freeze-drying procedure sheets of membrane such as the plasma membrane can become pitted and ruptured as water molecules are effectively sucked through them (see

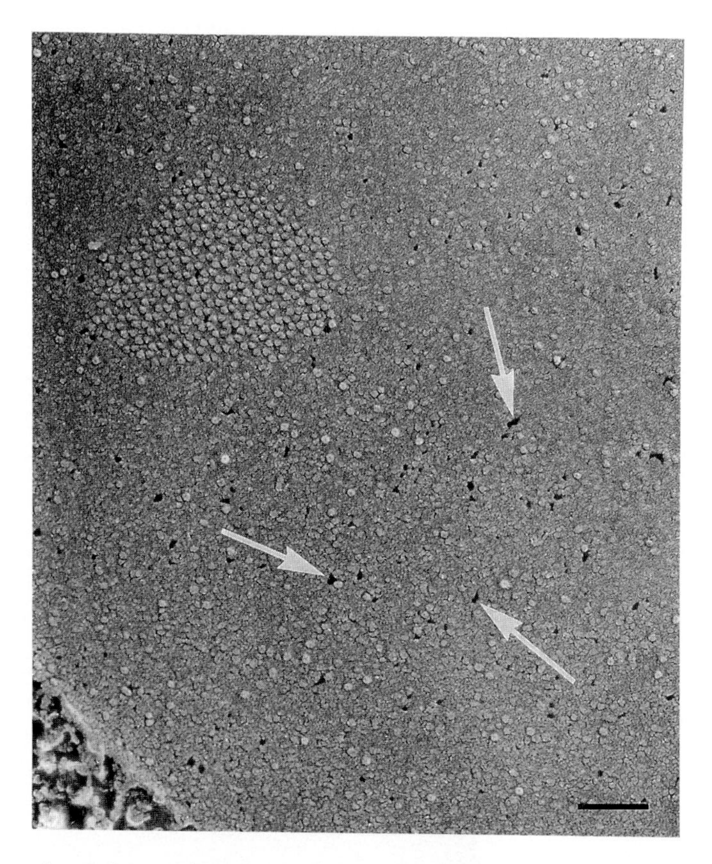

Fig. 3 Protoplasmic fracture face of a carrot protoplast plasma membrane showing damage due to ice sublimation through the membrane (arrows). Bar, 100 nm.

Fig. 3). Sheets of membrane often have a "shredded" appearance and can easily be mistaken for cytoskeletal elements (see Fig. 4).

V. Conclusions

The freeze-fracture deep-etch methodology is ideal for producing high-resolution information on the structure of chemically unfixed plant cell cytoplasm and cell walls. The great advantage over other techniques for interpreting the three-dimensional nature of the specimen is that it permits surface views of cytoplasmic contents complete with overlap and obstruction, thus avoiding a lot of the confusion arising in the interpretation of a thick resin section of comparable depth. We are, however, still awaiting its successful application to the study of isolated plant organelles and macromolecules. It is to be expected that the technique will also soon be combined with specific labeling of cellular antigens by immunocytochemical methods and used for direct epitope mapping on purified organelles and structural proteins.

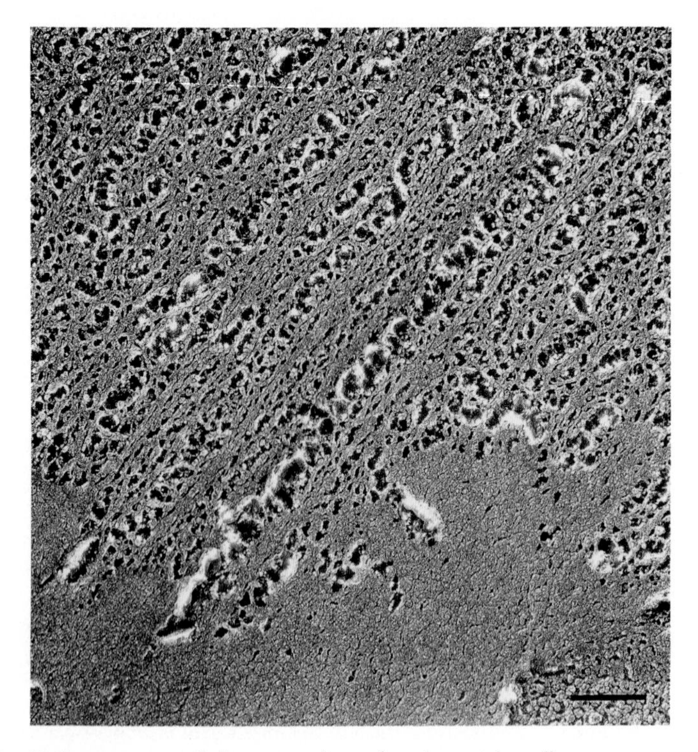

Fig. 4 Shredded appearance of plasma membrane in a deep-etch replica, a common artifact. Bar, 150 nm.

Acknowledgment

We thank Dr. Maureen McCann for advice on the cell wall preparative procedures and Dr. Béatrice Satiat-Jeunemaitre for critical reading of the manuscript.

References

Bordi, C. (1979). Parlodion coating of highly fragile freeze-fracture replicas. *Micron* **10,** 139–140.

Coleman, J., Evans, D., Hawes, C., Horsley, D., and Cole, L. (1987). Structure and molecular organisation of higher plant coated vesicles. *J. Cell Sci.* **88,** 35–45.

Goodenough, U. W., and Heuser, J. E. (1985). The *Chlamydomonas* cell wall and its constituent glycoproteins analysed by the quick-freeze, deep-etch technique. *J. Cell Biol.* **101,** 1550–1568.

Hawes, C., and Martin, B. (1986). Deep-etching of plant cells: Cytoskeleton and coated pits. *Cell Biol. Int. Rep.* **10,** 985–992.

Hawes, C. (1991). Stereo-electron microscopy. *In* "Electron Microscopy of Plant Cells" (J. L. Hall and C. Hawes, eds.), pp. 67–84. London: Academic Press.

Heuser, J. (1981). Quick-freeze, deep-etch preparation of samples for 3-D electron microscopy. *Trends Biochem. Sci.* **6,** 64–68.

Heuser, J. E. (1983). Procedure for freeze-drying molecules adsorbed to mica flakes. *J. Mol. Biol.* **169,** 155–195.

Heuser, J. (1989). Protocol for 3-D visualization of molecules on mica via the quick-freeze, deep-etch technique. *J. Electron Microsc. Tech.* **13,** 244–263.

Heuser, J. E., Reese, T. S., Dennis, M. J., Jan, Y., Jan, L., and Evans, L. (1979). Synaptic vesicle exocytosis captured by quick freezing and correlated with quantel transmitter release. *J. Cell Biol.* **81,** 275–300.

Heuser, J. E., and Kirschner, M. W. (1980). Filament organization revealed in platinum replicas of freeze-dried cytoskeleton. *J. Cell Biol.* **86,** 212–234.

Hirokawa, N. (1982). Cross-linker system between neurofilaments, microtubules, and membranous organelles in frog axons revealed by the quick-freeze, deep-etching method. *J. Cell Biol.* **94,** 129–142.

Hirokawa, N., and Heuser, J. E. (1981). Quick-freeze, deep-etch visualization of the cytoskeleton beneath surface differentiation of intestinal epithelial cells. *J. Cell Biol.* **91,** 399–409.

Kachar, B., and Reese, T. S. (1988). The mechanism of cytoplasmic streaming in Characean algal cells: Sliding of endoplasmic reticulum along actin filaments. *J. Cell Biol.* **106,** 1545–1552.

Lawson, D. (1984). Distribution of epinemin in colloidal gold-labelled, quick frozen, deep-etched cytoskeletons. *J. Cell Biol.* **99,** 1451–1460.

McCann, M. C., Wells, B., and Roberts, K. (1990). Direct visualisation of cross-links in the primary cell wall. *J. Cell Sci.* **96,** 323–334.

McLean, B., and Juniper, B. E. (1988). Fine structure of *Chara* actin bundles, using rapid-freezing and deep-etching. *Cell Biol. Int. Rep.* **12,** 509–517.

Robards, A. W. (1991). Rapid-freezing methods and their applications. *In* "Electron Microscopy of Plant Cells" (J. L. Hall and C. Hawes, eds.), pp. 257–312. London: Academic Press.

Ryan, K. P., and Liddicoat, M. I. (1987). Safety considerations regarding the use of propane and other liquified gases as coolants for rapid freezing purposes. *J. Microsc.* **147,** 337–340.

Satiat-Jeunemaitre, B., Martin, B., and Hawes, C. (1992). Plant cell wall architecture is revealed by rapid-freezing and deep-etching. *Protoplasma* **167,** 33–42.

Steere, R. L., and Erbe, E. F. (1983). Supporting freeze-etch specimens with "Lexan" while dissolving biological remains in acids. *In* "Proceedings of the 41st Annual Meeting of the Electron Microscopy Society of America" (G. W. Bailey, ed.), pp. 618–619. San Francisco: San Francisco Press Inc.

Tamura, S., and Senda, T. (1992). Fine structure of the cell wall of carrot parenchyma revealed by quick-freeze, deep-etch electron microscopy. *J. Electron Microsc.* **41,** 91–98.

CHAPTER 4

Advances in Immunoelectron Microscopy

Patricia J. Moore
Division of Natural Sciences and Mathematics
Transylvania University
Lexington, Kentucky 40508

I. Introduction

Immunoelectron microscopy allows researchers to precisely locate specific macromolecules within cells. The successful application of immunoelectron microscopy depends on acheiving a balance between structural preservation and retention of the antigenicity of the molecules to which the antibodies bind. There are three basic approaches to this problem. The most widely utilized technique is antibody labeling of thin-sectioned, resin-embedded samples. Although the fixation and plastic embedding necessary to obtain good structural preservation can be deleterious to antibody binding, it is often possible to find the right conditions for tissue preparation that will lead to positive results. A second technique that has been used for immunoelectron microscopy is to apply antibodies prior to embedding. This approach involves a mild fixation of the material to be labeled, followed by permeabilization to allow the antibodies access to the cell interior. Although antigenicity is preserved, this technique is hindered by poor structural preservation due to permeabilization and the obstruction to diffusion of large molecules, such as antibodies, presented by the cell wall. It can, however, be an effective technique for examining the location of cell surface molecules. A third approach, one that also overcomes the problem of retention of antigenicity, is to immunostain ultrathin frozen sections (Tokuyasu, 1986). However, the preparation of ultrathin frozen sections requires specialized equipment, and in the case of plant cells, it is difficult to obtain high quality sections. This chapter will present protocols only for the preparation and immunolabeling of thin-sectioned, resin-embedded tissues. VanderBosch (1991) presents an excellent review of the alternatives to the post-embedding labeling technique. For other reviews of immunogold techniques see Hayat (1989b), Kiss and McDonald (1993), VanderBosch (1991) and Verkleij and Leunissen (1989).

II. Tissue Preparation

A. Fixation

The goal of immunoelectron microscopy, to localize molecules in their native site, can be realized only if two conditions are met. First, the *in vivo* condition of the tissue must be maintained; not only should morphology be retained but ideally ions and other small molecules would also be preserved (Bullock, 1983; Dahl and Staehelin, 1989). Second, the fixation cannot eliminate the ability of the antibody to recognize the antigen. The best protocol for fixation, one that balances the preservation of cellular structure and antigenicity of the molecule of interest, will depend to a large extent on the system under study. The method used will need to be determined empirically. Knowledge of the nature of the molecule to be localized and of the reactivity of the antibody will greatly aid in the initial choices of protocols to test.

The most widely used fixatives are the aldehydes. Glutaraldehyde, a dialdehyde, results in better cross-linking of proteins than the monoaldehyde paraformaldehyde, and thus results in better perservation of ultrastructure. However, both glutaraldehyde and paraformaldehyde can produce severe antigen modification that reduces protein antigenicity (Bullock, 1984; Craig and Goodchild, 1982). Glutaraldehyde fixation is not always an obstacle, since some antibodies will react with glutaraldehyde-fixed antigen. This in fact represents the ideal situation, as it permits the use of antibodies under conditions in which the best structural preservation can be attained. The reactivity of antibodies against antigen immobilized on nitrocellulose and treated with fixative is a fairly good predictor of antigenicity in fixed tissue (VanderBosch, 1991).

Postfixation of tissues with osmium tetroxide yields optimal ultrastructural preservation. Again, osmium fixation can block antibody binding sites. These binding sites can sometimes be unmasked with the use of the oxidizing agent sodium metaperiodate (Bendayan and Zollinger, 1983). One drawback to this method is that, under acidic conditions, sodium metaperiodate will destroy some carbohydrate moities by cleaving vicinal hydroxyl groups (Woodward *et al.*, 1985). Since many plant antigens are either highly glycosylated or are pure carbohydrates, treatment of sections with sodium metaperiodate will eliminate antibody binding to these antigens. However, carbohydrates do not react to any great extent with osmium, and cell wall carbohydrates have been successfully immunolocalized in osmium-postfixed tissues without the use of the sodium metaperiodate treatment (Moore, 1989). A further problem with osmium fixation is that it interferes with the use of the UV light for the polymerization of resins developed for use in immunocytochemistry.

An exciting alternative of chemical fixation for immunoelectron microscopy is the use of cryofixation followed by freeze substitution (Dahl and Staehelin, 1989; Kiss and McDonald, 1993). The advent of the high-pressure freezing technique has expanded the types of tissues to which cryofixation can be applied. Cryofixation has the advantage over chemical fixation because fixation is extremely rapid and cellular components are stabilized simultaneously. Cryofixation also appears to improve immunocytochemical localization. The use of cryofixation and freeze substitution for immunoelectron microscopy is reviewed in Kiss and McDonald (1993).

B. Embedding

Several resins are currently available for use in immunocytochemical studies. Although epoxy resins such as Epon/Araldite or Spurr's provide excellent structural preservation, they often are not amenable to immunoelectron microscopy due to the loss of antigenic sites (Craig and Goodchild, 1982). Currently, the most frequently used resins are LR White and Lowicryl K4M. These resins are hydrophilic in nature, allowing molecules to retain their shell of hydration and thus a more native state. Alcohol dehydration can stop at 70% with LR White, although plant materials typically require a greater degree of dehydration (VanderBosch, 1991). Besides the hydrophilic nature of these resins, they also have the advantage of having a low viscosity and can be used to infiltate and embed samples at low temperature. Low-temperature embedding may increase antigen retention.

LR White is typically used at room temperature, but can be used for low-temperature embedding (see VanderBosch, 1991). LR White can be polymerized with heat, and thus can be used in conjunction with osmium postfixation if the antigen is heat stable. At room temperature LR White infiltrates well into plant tissues. LR White blocks are relatively easy to section. LR Gold, a related resin available from the London Resin Co., is less viscous at low temperatures than

LR White. Both LR White and LR Gold can be polymerized with UV light if the catalyst benzoin methyl ester is added.

Lowicryl K4M is the resin most often used where low-temperature dehydration and embedding is required. The density of immunolabeling is often dramatically increased with the use of Lowicryl K4M at low temperatures over embedding in LR White at room temperature. The denisty of gold label over the Golgi apparatus in clover root tip cells immunolabeled with an anti-hemicellulose antibody increased 4.5 times when Lowicryl K4M was used (Moore, 1989). In addition, antibody label against a viral movement protein in transgenic tobacco was virtually undetectable in LR White-embedded samples. Other after tissues were embedded in Lowicryl K4M at low temperatures could the protein be localized to the plasmodesmata (Fig. 1). Problems exist with Lowicryl K4M, however. Infiltration of plant materials is often very slow at low temperatures. Infiltration times of up to a week may be required for good penetration. Lowicryl K4M-embedded tissues can also be difficult to section. Additionally, structural preservation may not be optimal, especially for membranous structures, due to the inability to use an osmium postfixation.

A modification of the technique of low-temperature embedding that provides good membrane contrast without sacrificing antigenicity has been published (Berryman and Rodewald, 1990). Aldehyde-fixed, non-osmicated rat intestine was postfixed in 2% uranyl acetate. This tissue was then dehydrated in acetone and embedded at −20°C in LR Gold. Following on-grid immunolabeling the sections were stained in 2% aqueous osmium tetroxide and counterstained in lead citrate. This technique provide good ultrastructural preservation, especially of membranous structures, as well as enhancing localization of antigens. Although this technique was not developed for botanical materials, it may be a worthwhile modification for researcher especially interested in membrane structure and function.

III. On-Grid Section Labeling

A. Antibodies

The success of any immunocytochemical study will depend to a large extent on the specificity and reactivity of the antibody being used. It is essential that the antibody bind to the antigen with a moderately high titer. It is advantageous if the antibody will react with glutaraldehyde-fixed antigen, allowing for the best preservation of ultrastructure. In addition to these factors, a knowledge of the exact nature of the epitopes to which the antibody binds will allow a more precise interpretation of the results of section labeling. It is also important to characterize how antibody reactivity may be affected by the conditions used in section labeling.

An example of the importance of understanding how the chemicals used during the immunolabeling procedure can effect antibody reactivity comes from a study by Swords and Staehelin (1993) on the immunolocalization of the cell wall

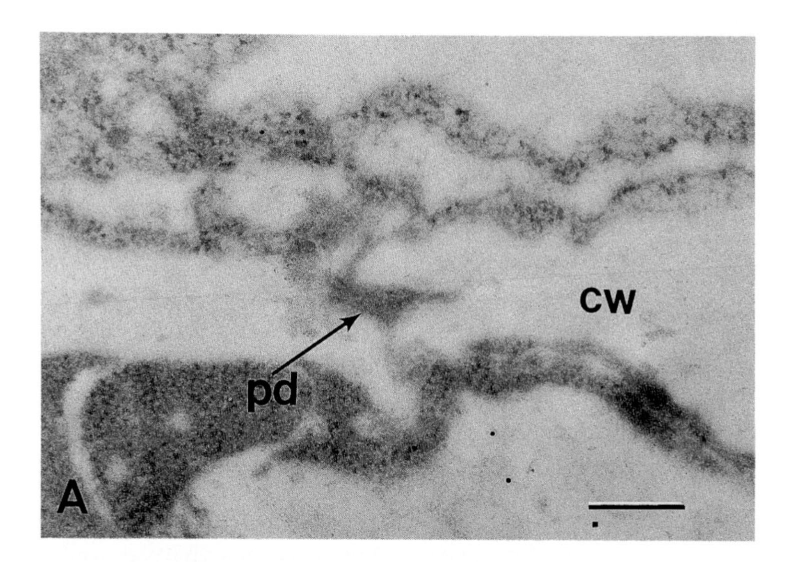

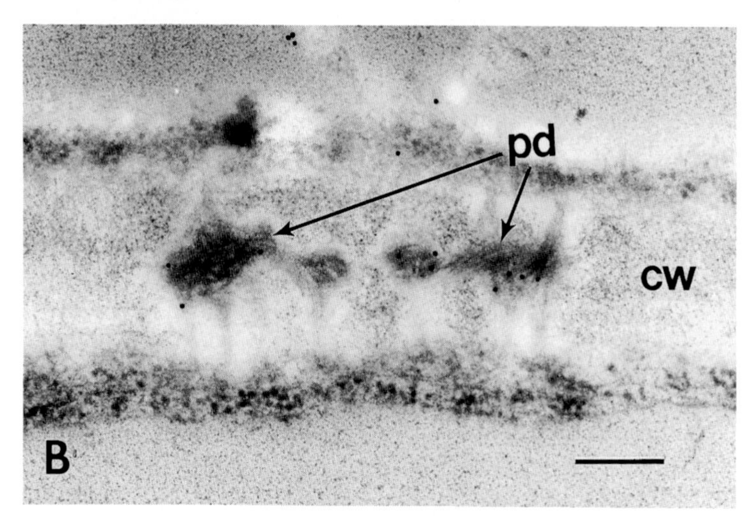

Fig. 1 Comparison of embedding procedures on anti-tobacco mosaic virus movement protein (TMV-MP) antibody binding in sections of transgenic tobacco plants expressing the TMV-MP (Deom *et al.,* 1987). The antigenicity of the TMV-MP was affected by the conditions used to prepare the tissue for immunoelectron microscopy in the resin LR White (A). Little or no specific antibody binding was detected in leaf tissue embedded in LR White. Leaf tissue embedded at low temperature in the resin Lowicryl K4M (B), however, showed significantly more antibody binding and demonstrated the localization of the TMV-MP in the plasmodesmata (pd) of the transgenic tobacco leaf tissue (Moore *et al.,* 1992). cw, cell wall. Bar, 0.25 μm.

glycoproteins extensin-1 and extensin-2 in carrot tap root. Because both extensin-1 and extensin-2 are highly glycosylated, Swords and Staehelin tested the effect of sodium metaperiodate treatment on antibody reactivity against these antigens. The reactivity of the anti-extensin-1 antibody, which recognizes terminal sugar residues, was abolished by periodate treatment. The binding of the anti-extensin-2 antibody, however, which recognizes internal sugars of the oligosaccharide side chains of both extensin-1 and extensin-2, was insensitive to periodate treatment prior to Western blot analysis. However, periodate treatment during on-grid immunolabeling led to a change in labeling patterns with the anti-extensin-2 antibody. On sections labeled without periodate treatment, anti-extensin-2 label was found strictly at the cell corners of the cell walls. Periodate treatment of sections prior to antibody labeling unmasked anti-extensin-2 binding sites on extension-1 molecules and led to antibody label over the cellulose region of the cell wall. Thus, if periodate-treated sections only had been examined, misleading results for the location of extensin-2 would have been obtained. The accurate localization of extensin-2 in the cell walls required information gained from Western blot analysis of antibody reactivity as well as section labeling under various conditions.

A second example demonstrating how the exact nature of the epitopes to which antibodies bind can influence immunolabeling results comes from Zhang and Staehelin (1992). They investigated the labeling patterns over the Golgi apparatus of an antibody that recognizes the cell wall pectic polysaccharides polygalacturonic acid and rhamnogalacturonan I (anti-PGA/RGI, Moore *et al.*, 1991). Moore and co-workers had previously used this antibody to localize PGA/RGI to the *cis* and medial cisternae of the Golgi. It had subsequently been determined that anti-PGA/RGI only recognizes deesterified PGA/RGI (Lynch and Staehelin, 1992). Zhang and Staehelin found that treatment of sections with Na_2CO_3 to deesterify methylesterified PGA resulted in much heavier labeling over the Golgi apparatus with the anti-PGA/RGI antibody, and that the overall labeling shifted toward the medial and *trans* cisternae and the *trans* Golgi network. Further quantitative analysis of the labeling pattern showed that deesterification uncovered cryptic anti-PGA/RGI epitopes in the later compartments of the Golgi apparatus, and demonstrated that these pectic polysaccharides do indeed traverse the entire Golgi stack on their way to the cell surface. Thus, the greater knowledge of epitope recognition and subsequent experiments arising from that knowledge allowed a more precise determination of the biosynthetic pathway of these pectic polysaccharides.

B. Gold Markers

A variety of electron opaque markers can be employed in immunocytochemistry, including colloidal gold, ferritin, and diaminobenzidine staining of peroxidase activity. Colloidal gold has become the marker of choice for antibody labeling of thin sections. It is extremely electron-dense and can be distinguished even at low magnifications by its uniform appearance. In addition, colloidal gold can be conjugated to many types of macromolecules, including enzymes and antibodies, that retain their biological activity. The most commonly used probe for immunoelectron microscopy is colloidal gold conjugated to protein A. A potential problem with the use of protein A–gold as a probe is the low affinity binding of protein A to IgGs from some species, notably rats, mice, and goats. Therefore, for immunolocalization of monoclonal antibodies and polyclonal antibodies raised in rats, mice, or goats, secondary antibodies raised against IgGs from the appropriate species and conjugated to colloidal gold should be used.

Gold probes, conjugated either to protein A or to a secondary antibody, can be purchased from a commercial supplier or prepared in the laboratory. The preparation of uniform suspensions of colloidal gold is relatively straightforward (Slot and Geuze, 1985). The advantage of preparing the gold probe in the laboratory is that, using a minimal number of reagents, a large number of different-sized probes can be produced, allowing for greater flexability in choice of probe size and at a very reasonable cost. Commercial probes, although more expensive, are available in a wide range of colloidal gold sizes and as a variety of protein conjugates. Further information on gold probes is available in Hayat (1989a) and Verkleij and Leunissen (1989).

C. Immunocytochemical Controls

A number of controls must be done in order to confirm the cellular site of a molecule localized through immunocytochemistry. The first type of control is to immunostain the sections with preimmune serum from the animal in which the antibody was raised. This will confirm that there are no preexisting antibodies in the serum that label the cells under study. Alternatively, if no preimmune serum is available, the primary immune serum can be preabsorbed with purified antigen prior to section labeling. The immunolabeling protocol should also be performed with the omission of the primary antiserum. This is due to the reactivity some secondary probes (both secondary antibodies and the protein A as well as the colloidal gold itself) can have with tissue sections. If extraneous label occurs with the secondary probe alone, it may be necessary to switch to an alternate type of probe.

An excess of background labeling often can be reduced with more stringent wash conditions. In the first labeling attempts with any antibody it is best to use low stringency conditions, i.e., a low concentration of the detergent Tween-20. For the initial labeling experiments the wash solution should be the same as the solution the antibody is diluted in. One example is the phosphate-buffered saline solutions used in the following protocols. The antibody and secondary probes are diluted in a 10 m*M* sodium phosphate buffer, pH 7.2, with 500 m*M* NaCl and 0.1% Tween-20. After a positive antibody reaction has been verified in the microscope, background staining can be reduced or eliminated in subsequent section labeling by increasing the concentration of Tween-20 in the wash buffer, up to 0.5% or even 1%.

Some background labeling can be tolerated if the density of specific labeling is high enough. If it becomes impossible to eliminate completely background labeling even in the negative controls, it may be necessary to use quantitative analysis to subtract nonspecific antibody binding. Additionally, the quantitation of labeling patterns over different cellular structures can often lead to important insights into subtle differences in localization that might not be obvious from individual micrographs.

IV. Protocols

The following protocols are representative of those used successfully for immunolocalization of a variety of molecules in plant tissues. Modifications may be necessary for any particular tissue.

A. Embedding Plant Tissues in LR White (from Moore, 1989)

1. Fix tissue in 2.5% glutaraldehyde in 50 m*M* $NaPO_4$, pH 7, for 2 h at room temperature. Fixation conditions may need to be modified for any particular sample. Vacuum infiltration of the fixative may be necessary for highly vacuolated tissues. Also, glutaraldehyde and paraformaldehyde are osmotically active, thus the osmolarity of the buffer may need to be adjusted for optimum structural preservation.
2. Wash the tissue three times for 5 min each in 50 m*M* $NaPO_4$, pH 7.
3. Postfix the tissue in 1% aqueous osmium tetroxide for 1 h at room temperature, then rinse the tissue three times for 5 min each with distilled water.
4. Dehydrate the tissue in an ethanol series (30, 50, 70, 95, and 100% twice) for 20 min each step at room temperature. If it is necessary to leave the tissue in ethanol for a long time period, leave it in the 70% ethanol step at 4°C.
5. Infiltrate in LR White as follows:

2 parts ethanol : 1 part LR White	1 h RT
1 part ethanol : 2 parts LR White	2 h RT
100% LR White	16 h 4°C

6. Embed samples in 100% LR White in gelatin or BEEM capsules and polymerize for 16 h at 50°C.

B. Embedding Plant Tissues in Lowicryl K4M at Low Temperature (from Moore *et al.*, 1992)

1. Fix tissue in 2.5% glutaraldehyde in 50 m*M* $NaPO_4$, pH 7, for 16 h at 4°C.
2. Wash the tissue three times for 5 min each in 50 m*M* $NaPO_4$, pH 7, at 4°C.

3. Dehydrate the tissue through the following steps:

30% ethanol, 50% ethanol	30 min each step	0°C
70, 95, 100% ethanol	45 min each step	−20°C

4. Infiltrate the tissue with Lowicryl K4M as follows:

2 parts ethanol : 1 part Lowicryl K4M	2 h	−20°C
1 part ethanol : 2 parts Lowicryl K4M	2 h	−20°C
100% Lowicryl K4M	7 days, change resin every 48 h	−20°C

5. Embed samples in Lowicryl K4M in BEEM capsules and polymerize for 48 h in a styrofoam cooler lined with aluminum foil and filled with dry ice with a long-wave UV lamp (4W, 366 nm) positioned 10 cm above samples. Alternatively, samples may be placed in a freezer with the UV lamp for polymerization.

NOTE

It is important when using Lowicryl K4M to exclude oxygen from the resin, as it will inhibit polymerization. After mixing the resin components, bubble nitrogen through the resin for 10 to 15 min. Resin mixure should have nitrogen bubbled through it again immediately prior to using it to embed the tissue. Lowicryl K4M should be stored in an amber bottle in the freezer.

C. On-Grid Immunolocalization

The following is a general on-grid labeling protocol that has been used for immunolocalization of cell wall carbohydrates (Moore, 1989) and cell wall glycoproteins (Moore *et al.,* 1991) using polyclonal antibodies. Some modifications may be required for other types of antigens and antibodies and I have tried to point out steps at which alterations to the protocol may be needed. All steps are carried out at room temperature.

1. Cut 70- to 100-nm-thick sections and pick up sections on Formvar–carbon-coated nickel grids. The Formvar coating is necessary to support the LR White and Lowicryl sections, which tend to be unstable in the electron beam. Nickel grids are required so that the metal grids do not react with solutions used in later steps.

2. For specimens fixed with OsO_4, treat grids in a saturated solution of aqueous sodium metaperiodate ($NaIO_4$) for 10 min to unmask proteinaceous antigenic sites. $NaIO_4$ will destroy carbohydrate antigenic sites; therefore if the antibody being used recognizes a carbohydrate moity, omit this step.

3. Treat grids with 0.1 *N* HCL for 10 min to remove glutaraldehyde from the sections.

4. Block nonspecific binding sites on the sections by incubating the grids in a freshly prepared blocking solution of 5% low fat dried milk powder (Carnation Co., Los Angeles, CA) in PBST (10 m*M* sodium phosphate buffer, pH 7.2, 500 m*M* NaCl, 0.1% Tween-20). Since protein A–gold will bind to Formvar, grids should be sunk in the blocking solution to block all possible binding sites. Other blocking solutions may be desirable with different antibodies. Alternatives to low-fat milk powder include bovine serum albumin (10 mg/ml), ovalbumin (10 mg/ml), and fetal calf serum (10%).

5. Remove blocking solution by blotting grid with Whatman Grade 1 filter paper.

6. Incubate grids in primary antiserum diluted in PBST for 1 h.

7. Wash grids for 30 s in a continuous stream of PBST containing 0.5% Tween-20. The increased concentration of Tween-20 reduces background staining.

8. Incubate grids for 30 min in a protein A–gold solution that is diluted to a very pale pink color with PBST. When choosing a colloidal gold marker, keep in mind that smaller gold particles will bind at a higher density, but are more difficult to distinguish. Gold particles between 5 and 12 nm usually work well.

9. Rinse grids in PBST plus 0.5% Tween-20, followed by a distilled water rinse. It is very important never to allow the grids to dry during the immunolabeling procedure prior to this water rinse.

10. Counterstain grids with 2% aqueous uranyl acetate and lead citrate.

D. Double Immunogold Localization

Often it is useful to localize two antigens on a single section so that the locations of these two molecules can be directly compared. This is possible to do, even using polyclonal antibodies raised in the same species employing protein A–gold as the probe. The following is a protocol modified from that of Titus and Becker (1985) that has proven successful with several different combinations of antibodies (see for example Moore *et al.,* 1991).

1. Prepare grids as described in the protocol for on-grid immunolabeling, steps 1–4.

2. Incubate grids in the first primary antiserum diluted in PBST for 1 h. The first antiserum should be against the least abundant antigen.

3. Wash grids for 30 s in a continuous stream of PBST containing 0.5% Tween-20.

4. Incubate grids for 30 min in the smaller protein A–gold solution (5 to 8 nm in diameter).

5. Wash grids for 30 s in a continuous stream of PBST containing 0.5% Tween-20.

6. Incubate grids in an excess of protein A (0.2 mg/ml in PBST) and blot to remove excess solution. It may also be helpful to include a second blocking step at this point.

7. Incubate grids in the second primary antiserum diluted in PBST for 1 h.

8. Wash grids for 30 sec in a continuous stream of PBST containing 0.5% Tween-20.

9. Incubate grids for 30 min in the larger protein A–gold solution (14 to 17 nm in diameter).

10. Wash grids for 30 s in a continuous stream of PBST containing 0.5% Tween-20.

11. Rinse grids in PBST plus 0.5% Tween-20, followed by a distilled water rinse.

12. Counterstain grids with 2% aqueous uranyl acetate and lead citrate.

V. Conclusions and Perspectives

Immunoelectron microscopy provides a powerful tool for the researcher interested in studying cellular structure and function. The precise localization of a specific macromolecule, along with biochemical data, can provide detailed information about the functions of the cell. The development of new reagents for immunocytochemistry makes this technique more widely applicable than ever before.

Acknowledgments

I thank Drs. L. Andrew Staehelin and Allen J. Moore for critical reading of the manuscript and Dr. John Kiss for helpful discussions. The author was supported by a grant from the National Science Foundation (DIR-9114968) to P.J.M.

References

Bendayan, M., and Zollinger, M. (1983). Ultrastructural localization of antigenic sites on osmium-fixed tissues applying the protein A-gold technique. *J. Histochem. Cytochem.* **31,** 101–109.

Berryman, M. A., and Rodewald, R. D. (1990). An enhanced method for post-embedding immunocytochemical staining which preserves cell membranes. *J. Histochem. Cytochem.* **38,** 159–170.

Bullock, G. R. (1984). The current status of fixation for electron microscopy: A review. *J. Microsc.* **133,** 1–15.

Craig, S., and Goodchild, D. J. (1982). Post-embedding immunolabeling. Some effects of tissue preparation on the antigenicity of plant proteins. *Eur. J. Cell Biol.* **28,** 251–256.

Dahl, R., and Staehelin, L. A. (1989). High pressure freezing for the preservation of biological structure: Theory and practice. *J. Electron Microsc. Tech.* **13,** 165–174.

Deom, C. M., Oliver, M. J., and Beachy, R. N. (1987). The 30-kilodalton gene product of tobacco mosaic virus potentiates virus movement. *Science* **337,** 389–394.

Hayat, M. A., ed. (1989a). "Colloidal Gold: Principles, Methods, and Applications," 2 vols. San Diego: Academic Press.

Hayat, M. A., ed. (1989b). "Principles and Techniques of Electron Microscopy: Biological Applications," 3rd Ed. Boca Raton, FL: CRC Press.

Kiss, J. Z., and McDonald, K. (1993). Electron microscopy immunocytochemistry following cryofixation and freeze substitution. *In* "Methods in Cell Biology," vol. 37. San Diego: Academic Press.

Lynch, M. A., and Staehelin, L. A. (1992). Domain-specific and cell-type-specific localization of two types of cell wall matrix polysaccharides in the clover root tip. *J. Cell Biol.* **118,** 467–479.

Moore, P. J. (1989). Immunolocalization of specific components of plant cell walls. *In* "Modern Methods of Plant Analysis New Series," vol. 10, Plant Fibers (H. F. Linskens and J. Jackson, eds.). Berlin/Heidelberg: Springer-Verlag.

Moore, P. J., Fenczik, C., Deom, C. M., and Beachy, R. N. (1992). The expression of the TMV p30 protein alters plasmodesmatal structure in a developmentally dependent fashion. *Protoplasma* **170,** 115–127.

Moore, P. J., Swords, K. M. M., Lynch, M. A., and Staehelin, L. A. (1991). Spatial organization of the assembly pathways of glycoproteins and complex polysaccharides in the Golgi apparatus of plants. *J. Cell Biol.* **112,** 589–602.

Slot, J. W., and Geuze, H. J. (1985). A new method of preparing gold probes for multiple labelling cytochemistry. *Eur. J. Cell Biol.* **38,** 87–93.

Swords, K. M. M., and Staehelin, L. A. (1993). Complementary immunolocalization patterns of cell wall hydroxyproline-rich glycoproteins studied with the use of antibodies directed against different carbohydrate epitopes. *Plant Physiol.* **102,** 891–901.

Titus, D. E., and Becker, W. M. (1985). Investigation of the glyoxysome-peroxisome transition in germinating cucumber cotyledons using double-label immunoelectron microscopy. *J. Cell Biol.* **101,** 1288–1299.

Tokuyasu, K. T. (1986). Immunocytochemistry on ultra-thin frozen sections. *Histochemistry* **12,** 381–403.

VanderBosch, K. A. (1991). Immunogold labelling. *In* "Electron Microscopy of Plant Cells" (J. L. Hall and C. Hawes, eds.). San Diego: Academic Press.

Verkleij, A. J., and Leunissen, J. L. M., eds (1989). "Immuno-Gold Labeling in Cell Biology." Florida: CRC Press, Boca Raton,

Woodward, M. P., Young, W. W., and Bloodgood, R. A (1985). Detection of monoclonal antibodies specific for carbohydrate epitopes using periodate oxidation. *J. Immunol. Methods* **78,** 143–153.

Zhang, G. F., and Staehelin, L. A. (1992). Functional compartmentation of the Golgi apparatus of plant cells. *Plant Physiol.* **99,** 1070–1083.

CHAPTER 5

Freeze-Substitution

M. V. Parthasarathy

Section of Plant Biology
Division of Biological Sciences
Cornell University
Ithaca, New York 14853

I. Introduction

Although chemical fixation is the routine method of preserving biological materials for electron microscopy, chemical fixatives penetrate cells slowly, take several seconds to minutes to immobilize cellular structures, and can also destroy or cause morphological changes in organelles. Rapid freezing, or cryofixation, is considered to be the best method for immobilizing biological specimens in their natural state since it can physically stabilize cellular components in a few milliseconds (see Chapter 1, this volume, for freezing methods). For example, labile actin filaments in plant cells that are difficult to preserve with chemical fixation can be readily visualized after cryofixation with jet-freezing and freeze-substitution (Ding *et al.,* 1991a,b,c).

II. Freeze-Substitution

Good cryofixation of a specimen is an obvious prerequisite for successful results with freeze-substitution. Freeze-substitution is a technique that combines

METHODS IN CELL BIOLOGY, VOL. 49

the advantages of cryofixation with those of sectioning at room temperature. In this procedure, the ice in the frozen specimen is substituted with an organic solvent at low temperatures (−80 to −90°C) to prevent secondary ice-crystal growth. Depending on the kind of information needed from the cryofixed specimen, the organic solvent to be used may or may not contain chemical fixatives. For example, addition of chemical fixatives is avoided if the specimen is to be used for elemental analysis or for preserving the antigenicity of certain highly sensitive antigens for immunogold labeling. If the purpose is mainly to investigate the ultrastructure of cells, addition of chemical fixatives may be necessary to prevent excessive lipid extraction and to improve image contrast. After the substitution with the organic solvent is complete, the specimen can either be brought to room temperature, infiltrated with embedding resin, embedded in the resin mixture and then polymerized in an oven, or the specimen can be infiltrated with resin at cold temperatures, embedded, and polymerized under UV light at cold temperatures (Fig. 1).

A. Substitution

1. Materials

An ultracold freezer or a cold chest capable of maintaining temperature at about −85°C, a standard refrigerator, a shaker, suitable specimen baskets for processing the frozen specimens, insulated forceps, screw-cap vials of 20- to 30-ml capacity that are wide enough to accommodate the specimen baskets, insulated gloves for handling material at cold temperatures, safety eye-goggles, respirator, LN_2, Dewars insulted containers, acetone, molecular sieves, a high-temperature oven for drying molecular sieves, osmium tetroxide crystals, uranyl acetate (optional), tannic acid (optional), anhydrous glutaraldehyde (optional).

2. Specimen Basket for Processing Frozen Material

Frozen specimens stored in LN_2 and large enough to be handled with forceps can be collected in a 1- or 1.5-ml Eppendorf-type tube that is modified by cutting away the tapered bottom and the hinge and heat-fusing stainless-steel or nylon mesh of appropriate size (e.g., Cell Microsieves-BioDesign, Inc., or Nicro) to the cut end (Fig. 2). Similarly, a hole punched in the middle of the cap can be covered by heat-fusing either an EM grid or the mesh. A platinum wire looped through a pair of small holes pierced in the cap, with its ends twisted, provides a "handle" for easy and quick retrieval of the basket from LN_2 storage or for transfer from one solvent container to another during freeze-substitution. If the mesh size of the specimen basket is very small, the basket will tend to float in the liquid or will sink in very slowly in solutions. To avoid this, one or two clean stainless-steel ball bearings, which have been precooled to LN_2 temperature, can

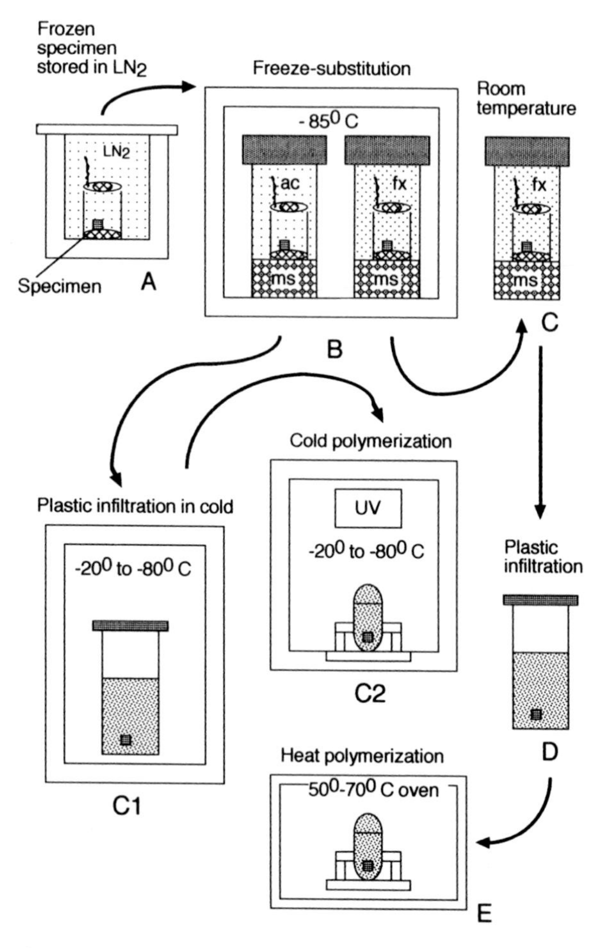

Fig. 1 An overview of the freeze-substitution, embedding, and polymerization procedures. ac, acetone only; fx, acetone with fixative; ms, molecular sieves.

be placed in the basket with the specimen. Specimens can also be processed by just keeping them in an Eppendorf-type tube with its cap removed and ensuring that the tube does not tip over during substitution. But this has limitations if more than one fixative/substitution fluid is to be used in the protocol (e.g., tannic acid/acetone → osmium tetroxide/acetone).

3. Solvents for Substitution

The advantages and disadvantages of various solvents for substitution have been well discussed by Steinbrecht and Müller (1987). Acetone and methanol are the most commonly used solvents. Methanol can substitute specimens even

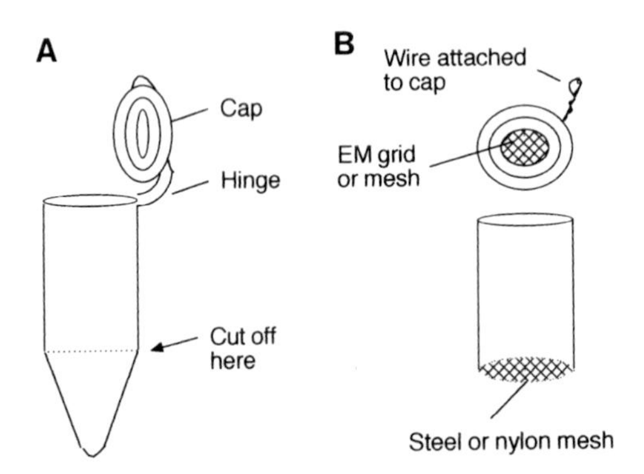

Fig. 2 Baskets for processing specimens. An Eppendorf-type tube (A) can be modified by cutting away the bottom end and heat-fusing to it an appropriate size metal or nylon mesh (B). The cap with the hinge removed can be modified by heat-fusing an EM grid. A wire attached to the cap facilitates quick transfer of capped baskets during freeze-substitution.

in the presence of relatively large amounts of water and substitutes more rapidly at lower temperatures than acetone. This allows one to choose a wide range of chemical fixatives including aqueous acrolein and glutaraldehyde during substitution. However, plant cells substituted with methanol in general yield poorer results compared to those substituted in acetone. The use of molecular sieves is recommended (e.g., Division Chemical, Grade 514) when using acetone as solvent (ACS grade). The molecular sieves will have to be baked for 2–3 h in an oven at the "self-cleaning" setting, before use. If a screw-cap glass vial (about 30-ml capacity) is about one-third filled with molecular sieves, this is normally enough to ensure that the substitution fluid will remain anhydrous. There should be sufficient space for the substitution fluid over the top of molecular sieves to immerse completely the specimen basket. If wire loops with a Formvar or agar film are used to freeze single cells with plunge-freezing, they can also be processed by placing them in the specimen basket. Alternatively, the loops can be placed directly into the substitution vial that has a piece of well-dried filter paper placed on top of the molecular sieves (Lancelle *et al.*, 1986). This will prevent direct contact between the molecular sieves and the loops and avoid possible loss of film/sample.

4. Adding Fixatives for Ultrastructural Studies

The most commonly used fixative/substitution fluid for ultrastructural studies is 2% osmium tetroxide in acetone. **Osmium should be handled with care in a fume hood.** The solution is unstable at room temperature and has to be transferred to a freezer immediately after osmium crystals are dissolved. A mixture of 2% osmium tetroxide/1–2% uranyl acetate/acetone yields even better results. Most of the uranyl acetate salt will dissolve in acetone if left in a tightly covered beaker over a stir-plate for 1–2 h. Uranyl acetate/acetone is first prepared and then the osmium crystals are added to the solution. Acrolein/acetone (e.g., Bridgman and Reese, 1984) can be used for elemental localizations but is in general not very good for ultrastructure. Glutaraldehyde/acetone followed by osmium/acetone can also be used (Howard and Aist, 1979). Anhydrous glutaraldehyde can be commercially obtained (e.g., Electron Microscopy Sciences, Fort Washington, PA). Some of the best results have been obtained by using 0.1% tannic acid/acetone followed by 2% uranyl acetate/2% osmium tetroxide/acetone (Ding *et al.,* 1991a). Figures 3 and 4 are examples of plant specimens that were propane jet-frozen (Müller *et al.,* 1993) and freeze-substituted using this protocol.

5. Adding Fixatives for Immunogold Localization

Successful use of fixatives during freeze-substitution for immunolocalization depends on the sensitivity of antigens to fixatives at low temperature. Excellent ultrastructure as well as good immunogold localization can be obtained if the antigen is present in large quantities and retains some of its antigenicity after osmium tetroxide/acetone substitution (e.g., Kandasamy *et al.,* 1991). Although substitution with pure acetone alone may yield images of low contrast, it would be desirable for immunogold localizations in specimens where the antigenicity is lost due to osmium treatment (e.g., Lancelle and Hepler, 1989; Lichtscheidl *et al.,* 1990). Depending on the antigen to be labeled, substitution with glutaraldehyde/acetone can also yield good results (Ding *et al.,* 1992). If low-temperature-embedding resins are to be used for UV polymerization, osmium tetroxide should not be included in the freeze-substitution solution.

6. Equipment and Method

The fixative/substitution fluids in the 30-ml vials can be placed in rack or in an aluminum block. The aluminum block has holes drilled in it to accommodate the vials. A small amount of ethanol in the holes will fill the gaps between the vials and the aluminum block and ensure good thermal conductivity. Such a setup can help keep temperature fluctuations to a minimum during specimen transfers. The metal block with the vials can then be left overnight in an ultracold freezer (e.g., Forma, Revco) at −80 to −85°C before use. A relatively simple temperature-controlled device can also be constructed with a LN_2 Dewar, temperature sensor, thermocouple, and some lab equipment (e.g., Hess *et al.,* 1983). A simpler but more crude method for attaining about a −80°C temperature without an ultracold freezer is to place a well-sealed specimen vial in a mixture of dry ice and acetone held in a suitable container. The container can then be placed in a flame-proof freezer at −20°C. To prevent condensation of water, the basket with the frozen specimen that is in LN_2 should be transferred as quickly as possible into the precooled vial containing the fixative/substitution fluid. **Protective eye-**

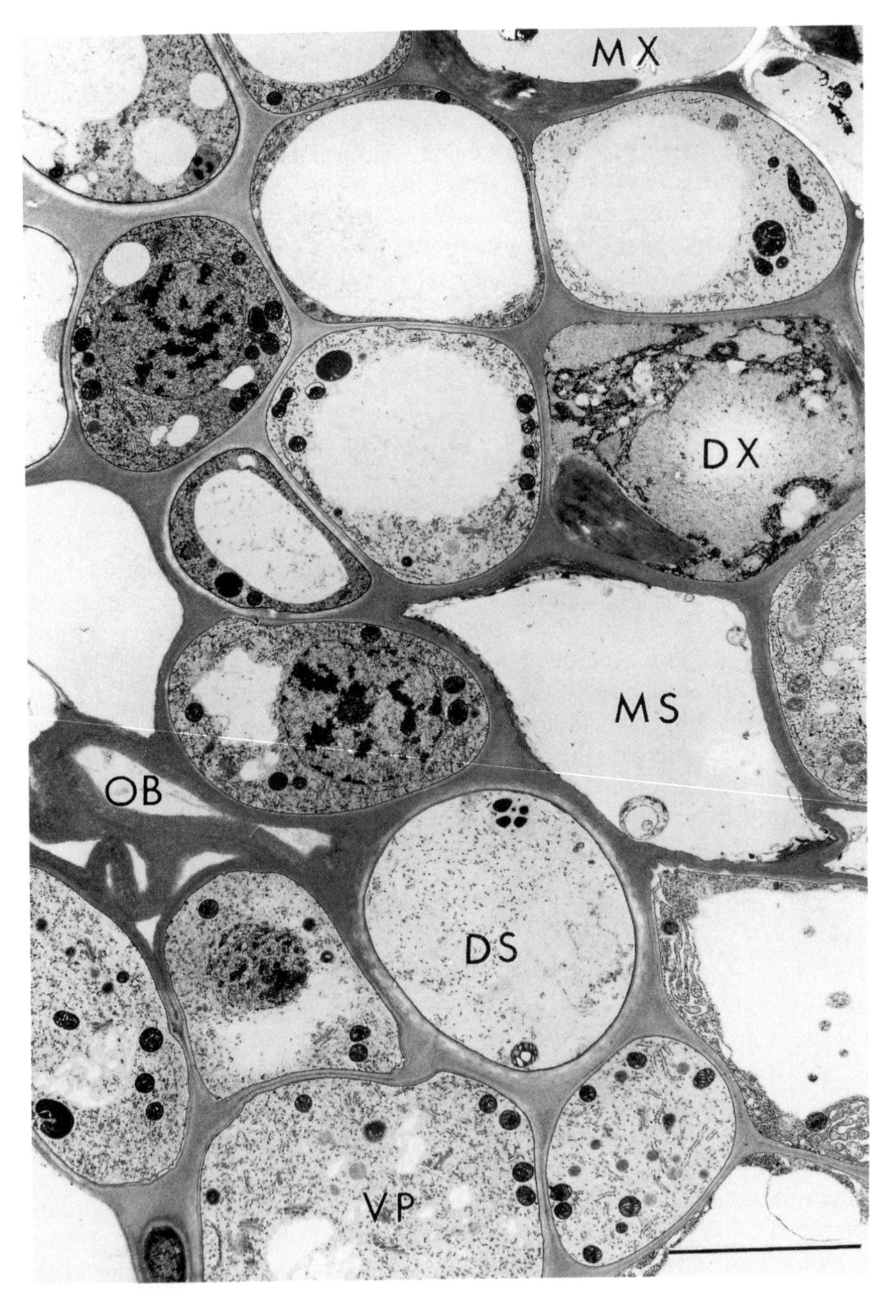

Fig. 3 Transverse section of freeze-substituted vascular tissue in an oat coleoptile that was propane jet-frozen after treatment with 0.2 *M* buffered sucrose and sandwiched between two 0.5-mm copper specimen carriers. The specimen was freeze-substituted in 0.1% tannic acid/acetone followed by 2% uranyl acetate//2% osmium tetroxide/acetone and embedded in Spurr medium. DS, differentiating sieve element; DX, a nearly mature xylem element containing disintegrating protoplast; MS, mature sieve element; MX, mature xylem element; OB, obliterated protophloem; VP, vascular parenchyma. Scale bar, 5 μm

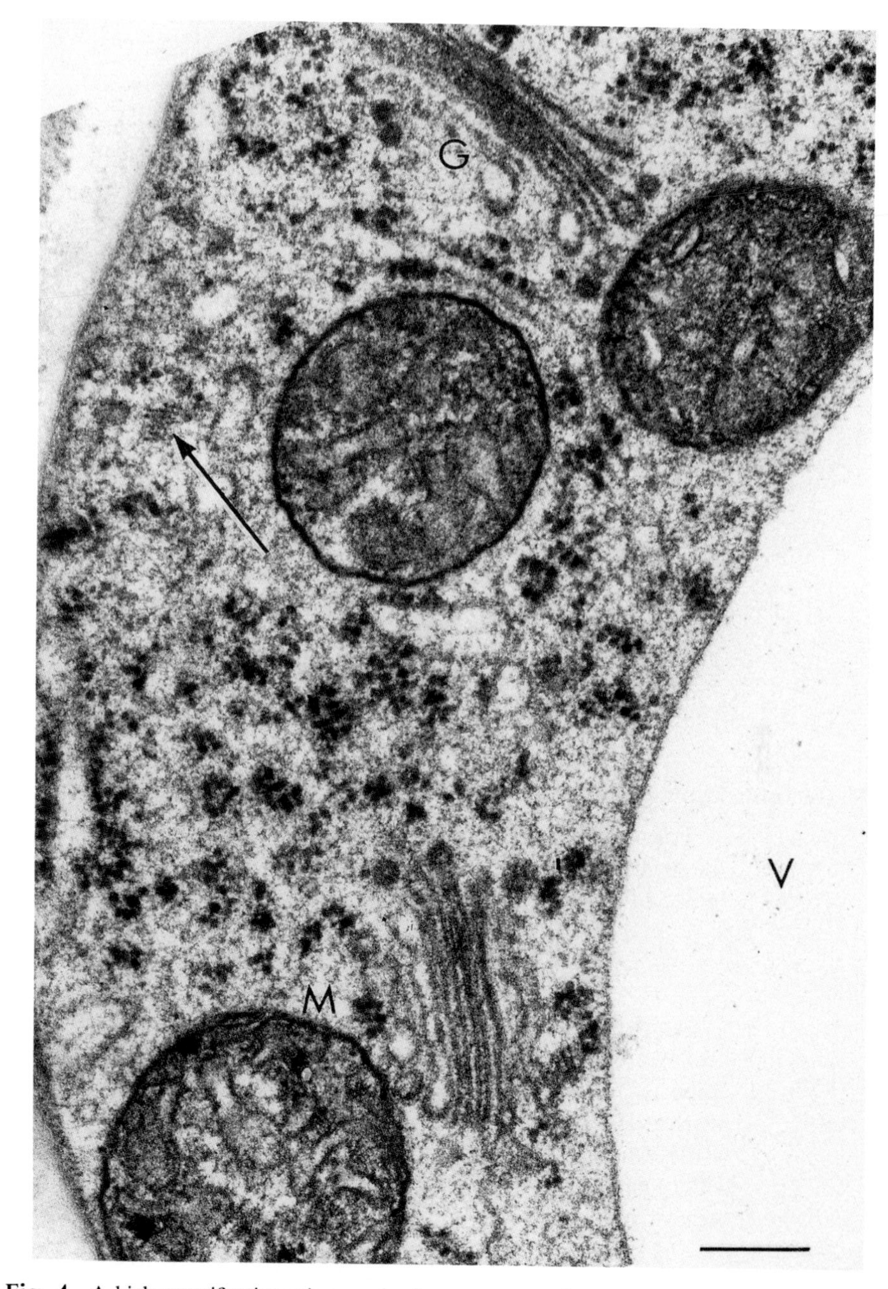

Fig. 4 A high-magnification micrograph of an oat coleoptile vascular parenchyma cell that was freeze-substituted using the same protocol as in Fig. 3. However, the specimen was sandwiched between 0.025-mm-thick titanium specimen holders and propane jet-frozen without any prior treatment with sucrose. G, Golgi body; M, mitochondrion; V, vacuole; arrow, microfilament bundle. Scale bar, 0.2 μm

goggles and respirator should be used if the fixative/substitution fluid contains osmium. The recommended substitution temperature is between −80 and −85°C.

7. Substitution Time

Depending on the specimen and the solvent used, the substitution time can vary from 24 to 72 h. If acetone is used, at least 2 days of substitution time would normally be required for mature plant tissues and 1 day for single cells before gradually warming the specimen (over an 8- to 12-h period) to 4°C. If tannic acid is used during the substitution, the specimen is first left in tannic acid/ acetone for 1 or 2 days at −85°C, then transferred to osmium/acetone 1 day at the same temperature, and gradually warmed to 4°C. There is commercial equipment available for controlled warming but in the majority of cases the controlled gradual warming may be unnecessary. Transferring the substituted specimen held at −85°C to a standard refrigerator freezer held at −20°C for 4–8 hr, followed by transfer to 4°C for 2–4 h in a refrigerator is usually sufficient. For normal ultrastructural studies, the specimens can then be transferred to precooled (4°C) pure acetone and then brought to room temperature. After two more rinses in pure acetone, the specimens can be processed for resin infiltration and embedment. If only osmium/acetone is used during substitution, the image contrast can be improved by staining the specimen en bloc for 2h in 5% uranyl acetate in pure methanol followed by a rinse in pure methanol. The specimen can then be transferred again to acetone before resin infiltration.

B. Resin Infiltration and Embedding

For normal ultrastructural studies, resin infiltration of freeze-substituted specimens at room temperature followed by heat polymerization of the epoxy resin-embedded specimen in an oven yields excellent results.

1. Materials

An oven (50–70°C), a rotary mixer, a centrifuge if particulate materials (single cells) are to be processed, a top loading balance, graduated cylinders, vials, pipettes, acetone, one of the commercially available epoxy resin embedding kits such as Epon 812 (or its substitutes LX-112, Poly/Bed 812, Pelco Medcast, Embed 812), Quetol 651, or Spurr (also known as Vinylcyclohexene dioxide, and ERL 4206) embedding medium, and rubber-silicone flat embedding molds, polyethylene or polypropylene capsules (both commercially available) for embedding.

2. Resin Infiltration

All resin embedding kits are supplied with the necessary flexibilizer, hardener, and accelerator and instructions for mixing the embedding medium. Since infiltration of resin in freeze-substituted plant cells can be difficult, a low-viscosity embedding medium such as the Spurr medium (the final mixture has a viscosity of 140 cP) is recommended. Although LR White, another low-viscosity embedding medium, can also be used instead of Spurr, it is generally used for immunogold localization studies. Freeze-substituted plant cells generally require more gradual and prolonged infiltration times than those that are chemically fixed. The infiltration is usually done on a slowly rotating shaker. **All expoxy resin formulations are toxic and skin contact with them could lead to allergic reactions. Disposable gloves should be worn when handling the resin.** Polymerized blocks, however, can be handled normally. A typical protocol for Spurr embedding resin at room temperature for the infiltration of plant tissue freeze-substituted with tannic acid/acetone followed by osmium tetroxide/uranyl acetate/acetone is given in Table I.

Resin infiltration of woody tissues can be difficult. Ristic and Ashworth (1993) report that a gradual hydration of freeze-substituted woody material followed by a treatment with sodium phosphate buffer before dehydrating it again in acetone improves resin infiltration. In addition, the authors recommend using acidified DMP during the final stages dehydration.

3. Embedding and Polymerization

Specimens that have been infiltrated with resin mixture/accelerator can be embedded in either the capsules or rubber–silicone molds. The capsules need a stand to hold them upright; one can readily be made in lab with either thin metal strips or heat-resistant plastic strips. The advantage of the flat embedding mold is that specimens can be easily positioned to obtain the desired orientation for

Table I
Typical Infiltration and Embedding Schedule for Freeze-Substituted Plant Specimens

Infiltration steps	Time
4 parts acetone/1 part Spurr[a,b]	1 h
3 parts acetone/1 part Spurr[b]	1 h
2 parts acetone/1 part Spurr[b]	1 h
1 part acetone/1 part Spurr[b]	2 h
1 part acetone/2 parts Spurr[b]	Overnight
1 part acetone/3 parts Spurr[b]	4 h
1 part acetone/4 parts Spurr[b]	4 h
Pure Spurr[b]	Overnight
Pure Spurr with the accelerator	3 h
A second change of pure Spurr with accelerator	3 h

[a] This part of the infiltration is done very gradually by adding drops of the resin into acetone containing the specimen.

[b] Accelerator is not added in the Spurr mixture during these steps.

sectioning prior to polymerization. A toothpick or a straightened paperclip is a good disposable "tool" for manipulating the specimens in embedding medium. After ensuring that there are no air bubbles, the embedded material can be left in an oven overnight for polymerization. Recommended polymerization temperature for most epoxy resin mixtures is 60°C, although a temperature of 70°C is recommended for Spurr embedding medium. The polymerized blocks should be brought to room temperature before trimming and sectioning.

C. Immunogold Localization and Low-Temperature Embedding

Freeze-substitution can significantly improve the antigenic preservation in plants (e.g., Kandasamy *et al.*, 1991). Epoxy resins such as Epon or Spurr are generally not suitable for immunogold localizations since they react with side chains of biomolecules, which then become an integral part of the polymer. Thus specimens, embedded in epoxy resins, tend to yield sections in which the epitopes are masked by a thin layer of resin. On the other hand, acrylic resins (e.g., LR White) and acrylic–methacrylate resins (Lowicryls) tend to cleave along the interface between the resin and the antigens, leaving the epitopes exposed for efficient labeling (Kellenberger and Hayat, 1991). The protocols for embedding, polymerizing, and immunogold labeling of chemically fixed specimens is covered else where in this book (Chapter 4, this volume). The same protocols can also be used for freeze-substituted specimens that are warmed to −20°C or to room temperature before embedding. Only very low temperature embedding (−35 to −80°C) of freeze-substituted material is considered in this section.

1. Materials

A top-loading balance, vials, and glassware for mixing resin formulations, Lowicryl resins, a rotator, a cold chest capable of maintaining temperatures from −35 to −80°C, is low-temperature digital thermometer for measuring temperatures to −90°C (e.g., Omega 450 digital thermometer), a 2× 15-W 360-nm UV lamp, capsules made of gelatin, polyethylene, or polypropylene for embedding, disposable plastic gloves.

2. Low-Temperature Embedding in Lowicryls

Lowicryl K4M, HM20, K11M, and HM23 are highly cross-linked acrylate—methacrylate-based embedding media formulated to provide low viscosity at low temperatures. The Lowicryls come with a monomer, a cross-linker and an initiator. Formulations for embedding are supplied with the kits. **Since the Lowicryls emit a foul odor, infiltration and embedding should be done in a fume hood. Like epoxy resins, these resins can also cause allergic reactions if they come in contact with skin.** Polymerized blocks can be handled normally. Since K4M and K11M are polar (hydrophilic) resins, they are usually the preferred embedding media for immunogold labeling. HM20 and HM23 are nonpolar resins that are frequently used to produce high-contrast images of unstained sections. Lowicryls are miscible with acetone and depending on the embedding medium used, the specimen can be gradually warmed after the freeze-substitution step to the desired temperatue for resin infiltration. Resin infiltration and UV polymerization of Lowicryl K4M can be done at −35°C, HM20 at −50°C, K11M at −60°C, and HM23 at −80°C (Villiger, 1991). Below −35°C, the embedding media become more viscous and the infiltration times need to be prolonged. For such low temperatures, the infiltration schedule suggested for embedding in K11M and HM23 at −60 and −80°C, respectively, by Villiger (1991) can be followed. Proper orientation of specimens during embedding can pose some difficulty since the specimens exhibit no contrast in the embedding medium. The cold temperatures can promote condensation and further compound the problem. Good lighting in the fume hood and rapid execution of all the steps are essential. Equipment for the UV polymerization of Lowicryl-embedded sepcimens at low temperatures is commercially available. However, it is relatively easy to achieve good polymerization by using an ultracold freezer or chest (−35 to −80°C depending on the type of Lowicryl) as a polymerizing chamber and placing a 2 × 15-W 360-nm UV lamp about 30–40 cm from the embedded specimens (see also Chapter 4, this volume). Although LR White is still the resin of choice for immunolocalization studies among plant biologists, the use of Lowicryls is gaining acceptance both for that purpose (e.g., Vallon *et al.,* 1987; Herman, 1989; Sato, 1990; Grote, 1991; Testillano *et al.,* 1993; Trembley and Lafontaine, 1991) and for *in situ* hybridization studies (e.g., Motte *et al.,* 1991; Lin *et al.,* 1993). Thin sectioning and immunolabeling procedures for LR White- and Lowicryl-embedded plant material is described in Chapter 4 (this volume).

III. Conclusion and Perspectives

Although cryofixation/freeze-substitution procedures are costlier and technically more demanding than conventional techniques, the superior preservation of labile structures and antigenicity should make it an attractive technique for many cell biologists. The possibility of carrying out embedding and polymerization at near freeze-substitution temperature (−80°C) with Lowicryl HM23 adds a new dimension to the freeze-substitution technique. Lipid extractions can be kept to a minimum during substitution/resin embedding and the preservation of labile structures and image contrast further improved. In addition, the anhydrous processing of cryofixed material at very low temperatures should make this a technique of choice for elemental microanalysis (e.g., Warblewski *et al.,* 1991).

References

Bridgman, P. C., and Reese, T. S. (1984). The structure of cytoplasm in directly frozen cultured cells. I. Filamentous meshworks and cytoplasmic ground substance. *J. Cell Biol.* **99,** 1655–1668.

Ding, B., Turgeon, R., and Parthasarathy, M. V. (1991a). Routine cryofixation of plant tissues by propane jet freezing for freeze substitution. *J. Electron Microsc. Technique* **19,** 107–117.
Ding, B., Turgeon, R., and Parthasarathy, M. V. (1991b). Microfilament organization and distribution in freeze substituted tobacco plant tissues. *Protoplasma* **165,** 96–105.
Ding, B., Turgeon, R., and Parthasarathy, M. V. (1991c). Microfilaments in the preprophase band of freeze-substituted tobacco root cells. *Protoplasma* **165,** 209–211.
Ding, B., Haudenshield, J. S., Hull, R. J., Wolf, S., Beach, R. N., and Lucas, W. J. (1992). Secondary plasmodesmata are specific sites of localization of the tobacco mosaic virus movement protein in transgenic tobacco plants. *Plant Cell* **4,** 915–928.
Grote, M. (1991). Immunogold electron microscopy of soluble proteins localization of BET v I major allergen in ultrathin sections of birch pollen after anhydrous fixation techniques. *J. Histochem. Cytochem.* 1395–1402.
Herman, M. A. (1989). Colloidal gold labeling of acrylic resin-embedded plant tissues. *In* "Colloidal Gold. Principles, Methods, and Applications" (M. A. Hayat, ed.), Vol. 2, pp. 303–323. New York: Academic Press.
Hess, M. W., and Glaser, A. (1993). A simple and inexpensive device for freeze substitution at 183 K/−90°C. *Biotech. Histochem.* **68,** 211–214.
Howard, R. J., and Aist, J. R. (1979). Hyphal tip ultrastructure of the fungus Fusarium: Improved preservation by freeze substitution. *J. Ultrastruct. Res.* **66,** 224–234.
Kandasamy, M. K., Parthasarathy, M. V., and Nasarallah, M. E. (1991). High pressure freezing and freeze substitution improve immunolabeling of S-locus specific glycoproteins in the stigma papillae of Brassica. *Protoplasma* **162,** 187–191.
Kellenberger, E., and Hayat, M. A. (1991). Some basic concepts for the choice of methods. *In* "Colloidal Gold: Principles, Methods, and Applications" (M. A. Hayat, ed.), Vol. 3, pp 1–30. New York: Academic Press.
Lancelle, S. A., Callaham, D. A., and Hepler, P. K. (1986). A method for rapid freeze fixation of plant cells. *Protoplasma* **131,** 153–165.
Lancelle, S. A., and Hepler, P. K. (1989). Immunogold labelling of actin on sections of freeze substituted cells. *Protoplasma* **150,** 72–74.
Lichtscheidl, I. K., Lancelle, S. A., and Hepler, P. K. (1990). Actin-endoplasmic reticulum complex in *Drosera. Protoplasma* **155,** 116–126.
Lin, N. S., Chem, C. C., and Hsu, Y. H. (1993). Post embedding in-situ hybridization of viral nucleic acid ultra-thin sections. *J. Histochem. Cytochem.* **41,** 1513–1519.
Motte, P. M., Loppes, R., Menager, M., and Deltour, R. (1991). Three-dimensional electron microscopy of ribosomal chromatin in two higher plants. A immunocytochemical and insitu hybridization approach. *J. Histochem. Cytochem.* **39,** 1495–1506.
Müller, T., Moser, S., Vogt, M., Daugherty, C., and Parthasarathy, M. V. (1993). Optimization and application of jet-freezing. *Scanning Microsc.* **7,** 1295–1310.
Ristic, Z., and Ashworth, E. N. (1993). New infiltration method permits use of freeze substitution for preparation of wood tissues for transmission electron microscopy. *J. Microsc.* **171,** 137–142.
Sato, S. (1990). Estimation of RNA content of the nucleolus and nuceolus-derived structures in *Vicia faba* mitotic cells embedded in Lowicryl resin using RNAse gold labeling. *J. Electron Microsc.* **39,** 382–387.
Steinbrecht, R. A., and Müller, M. (1987). Freeze substitution and freeze drying. *In* "Cryotechniques in Biological Electron Microscopy" (R. A. Steinbrecht and K. Zierold, eds.), pp. 150–172. New York/Berlin: Springer-Verlag.
Testillano, P. S., Sanchez-Pina, M. A., Omedilla, A., Fuchs, J. P., and Risueno, M. C. (1993). Characterization of the interchromatin region as the nuclear domain containing SNRNPs in plant cells. A cytochemical and immunoelectron microscopy study. *Eur. Curr. J. Cell Biol.* **61,** 349–361.
Trembley, S. D., and Lafontaine, J. G. (1991). Immunochemical localization of nuclear antigens in the unicellular alga *Chlamydomonas reinhardii* processes by cryofixation and freeze-substitution. *Protoplasma* **165,** 189–202.

Vallon, O., Hoyerm H. G., and Simpson, D. J. (1987). Photosystem II and cytochrome B-559 in the stroma lamellae of barley. *Carlsburg Res. Commun.* **52,** 405–421.
Villiger, W. (1991). Lowicryl resins. *In* "Colloidal Gold. Principles, Methods, and Applications" (M. A. Hayat, ed.), Vol. 3, pp. 59–69. New York: Academic Press.
Warblewski, J., Worblewski, R., Mory, C., and Colliex, C. (1991). Elemental analysis and fine structure of mitochondrial granules in growth plate condrocytes studied by electron energy loss spectroscopy and energy dispersive X-ray microanalysis. *Scanning Microsc.* **5,** 885–894.

CHAPTER 6

Cell Optical Displacement Assay (CODA)—Measurements of Cytoskeletal Tension in Living Plant Cells with a Laser Optical Trap

Melvin Schindler

Department of Biochemistry
Michigan State University
East Lansing, Michigan 48824

I. Introduction

The cytoskeleton of plant and animal cells has been demonstrated to be a transducer and effector of cell signaling mechanisms (Herman and Pledger, 1985; Landreth *et al.,* 1985; Luna and Hitt, 1992; Tan and Boss, 1992; Williamson, 1993). Pathways for proliferation, transformation, differentiation, chemotaxis, stimulated secretion, migration, and adhesion all involve stimulus-coupled rearrangements of actin- and tubulin-based structures within the cytoplasm (Pfeuty

METHODS IN CELL BIOLOGY, VOL. 49

and Singer, 1980; Herman and Pledger, 1985; Luna and Hitt, 1992; Ridley and Hall, 1992; Schliwa *et al.*, 1984; Shariff and Luna, 1992; Williamson, 1993). Rearrangements of the cell cytoskeleton and altered expression of cytoskeletal proteins appear diagnostic for specific types of neoplasms (David-Pfeuty and Singer, 1980; Osborn, 1983; Schliwa *et al.*, 1984). These changes in filament organization have been demonstrated to occur as a result of signal-mediated alterations in subunit interactions, e.g., actin monomer–polymer equilibria, modifications in the pattern and extent of association with the family of actin, and/or tubulin binding proteins, e.g., profilin, myosin, microtubule-associated proteins (MAPs), and differences in the degree of interaction with plasma membrane components, e.g., polyphosphoinositides, transmembrane proteins (Edelman, 1976; Goldschmidt-Clermont *et al.*, 1990; Luna and Hitt, 1992; Schliwa *et al.*, 1984; Shariff and Luna, 1992; Williamson, 1993). A diverse group of biochemical assays has provided considerable information concerning the regulation, post-translational modifications, specificity, and kinetics associated with the monomer–polymer transitions within the actin/tubulin networks, and the modulatory influence of associated proteins and phospholipids (Adams and Pollard, 1989; Giuliano *et al.*, 1992; Goldschmidt-Clermont *et al.*, 1990; Koledney and Elson, 1993; Luna and Hitt, 1992; Ridley and Hall, 1992; Shariff and Luna, 1992). Electron and fluorescence microscopy have provided powerful optical tools to examine the spatial distribution of cytoskeletal components (Giuliano and Taylor, 1994; Landreth *et al.*, 1985; Schliwa *et al.*, 1984; Wang, 1984). Fluorescence-based imaging and microinjection methods have proven essential for real-time visualization of the spatial reorganization of these networks and redistribution of associated proteins in living cells. Changes in organization are examined as a consequence of (*a*) exposure to biosignaling molecules, (*b*) progression through the cell cycle or differentiation programs, and (*c*) cell transformation.

Given all these analytical approaches, it is significant that only a limited body of data exists to describe the physical parameters most directly associated with these polymorphic cellular networks, their viscoelastic and mechanochemical properties. For the most part, examinations of tension, compression, and viscoelasticity have been pursued in model systems comprising solutions of actin and tubulin (Elson, 1988; Kasai *et al.*, 1960; Kerst *et al.*, 1990; Zaner and Stossel, 1982). Such studies have provided the basis for present knowledge on the relationship between the polymer organization of actin and tubulin networks and their thixotropic properties (Kerst *et al.*, 1990). Considerably less information, however, is available concerning the mechanical properties of these networks under conditions that maintain their *in vivo* connections, interactions, and three-dimensional spatial organization.

Some of the first efforts to pursue *in vivo* investigations of the viscoelastic properties of the cytoskeleton were initiated to study the physical properties of cytoplasm. This involved the phagocytosis of small magnetic particles by living cells (Crick and Hughes, 1950). These incorporated particles could then be moved in the cytoplasm by means of an externally applied magnetic field. These measurements were successful in demonstrating that the relaxation time of the magnetic particle, when displaced a defined distance, is a function of the shear, in essence, that the cell cytoplasm could be modeled after a thixotropic gel. Support for this view was provided by centrifugation experiments in which the displacement of intracellular organelles could be used to probe the viscoelastic properties of the cell cytoplasm (DeGaetano and Schindler, 1987; Elson, 1988; Galatis *et al.,* 1984; Kamitsubo *et al.,* 1989; Marc *et al.,* 1989). Evidence that the viscoelastic properties of cytoplasm were a function of the organization of cytoskeletal networks emerged from work using red blood cells (Elson, 1988; Evans and LaCelle, 1975), then fibroblasts and lymphocytes (Pasternak and Elson, 1985; Petersen *et al.,* 1982). In one experimental approach, a small segment of the plasma membrane of an erythrocyte was sucked into a micropipette (Evans and LaCelle, 1975; Hochmuth *et al.,* 1979). These pinched membrane segments could be physically manipulated to demonstrate their extensibility. The availability of a variety of chemical methods to alter the cytoskeleton organization of erythrocytes was central in demonstrating that the elastic properties observed for the plasma membrane were a consequence of the organization and membrane association of a spectrin–actin cortical cytoskeletal network (Elson, 1988; Smith and Hochmuth, 1982; Weed *et al.,* 1969). Similar efforts with fibroblasts and lymphocytes, using surface "pokers" rather than "suckers," demonstrated that the elastic and contractile properties of cells are a function of the physicochemical state of at least two topologically distinct actin- and tubulin-based cytoskeleton networks: one multicomponent assemblage (cytoplasmic cytoskeleton) within the cytoplasm and the other in proximity to the plasma membrane (cortical cytoskeleton) (Elson, 1988; Pasternak and Elson, 1985; Petersen *et al.,* 1982). As useful as these methods have been for measurements of cytoskeletal properties in living cells, they are low resolution in their ability to (*a*) distinguish between contributions of actin and tubulin networks in defining the elastic properties of the cytoskeleton and (*b*) discriminate between the tension and elasticity produced by domains within the cytoskeletal network, e.g., nuclear actin cage, Golgi actin network. Understanding the response of subcellular cytoskeletal domains to stimulation by global and localized chemical effectors and the mechanisms by which these localized responses are integrated into the transcellular cytoskeletal network is essential for elucidating the signal transduction pathway.

Recently, a new experimental technique has entered the analytical armory that has provided the opportunity to push the resolution for rheological investigations to the sub-micrometer scale. The technique has been termed optical trapping (Ashkin and Dziedzic, 1989; Block, 1992; Chu, 1991), and it is the purpose of this chapter to demonstrate its unique and powerful role as a quantitative tool for measuring the elasticity of individual actin cables in living plant cells.

II. Optical Trapping—A Tool for Cellular Measurements and Manipulations

A. Optical Trap

Working with a focused beam of laser light and small particles [with refractive indices greater than the surrounding medium (water)], Ashkin and Dziedzic (1989) demonstrated that the particles aggregate and become immobilized or trapped at the focal point of a three-dimensional light gradient formed by a focused laser beam. Movement of these particles to the focal point occurs as a result of induced dipole moments in the particles produced by exposure to the laser beam. The interaction of these dipoles with the electric field of the light gradient results in a force on the particle that directs it toward the brighter region (focal point) of the incident light. This principle can also be utilized in reverse to repel particles from the focal point and requires the use of particles with a refractive index lower than that of the surrounding medium; such particle repelling has been demonstrated on air bubbles in water. The size of trapped objects has ranged from the nanometer to the micrometer scale (Block, 1992; Chu, 1991). The strength of the trap is related to the intensity of light that can be focused to the focal point. The power employed for trapping has been from several milliwatts to several watts, which results in a force on samples of micrometer size, from ten to hundreds of piconewtons. Because of the high power fluxes that may be required for trapping, Ashkin and Dziedzic (1989) introduced the use of an infrared laser since light at these wavelengths is not readily absorbed by biological material. Another recent adaptation for optical trapping has been the creation of multiple optical trap sites within a sample through the use of a single fast-scanning trap (Visscher *et al.*, 1993).

B. Optical Trap Measurements in Plant Cells

Ashkin and Dziedzic (1989) were the first to utilize the optical trap to immobilize or trap long thin filaments within the cytoplasm of scallion cells. These filaments, because of their higher index of refraction, were readily visible under phase contrast illumination. Displacement of the sample plane in *x*, *y*, or *z*, relative to the fixed laser beam, resulted in the intracellular displacement of the filament from its normal position. The displacement length, the laser power required to maintain the filament within the trap, and the speed and extent of rebound were found to be dependent on the velocity of displacement. This dependency was closely analogous to the viscoelastic properties observed for the non-Newtonian mechanical properties of polymers and actin/actin–tubulin networks (Elson, 1988). This work clearly highlighted the ability of this technique to pursue high resolution analysis of the viscoelastic properties of transvacuolar strands, predominantly composed of actin and associated binding proteins, within topologically defined regions of the plant cell. It is noteworthy that the plant cell wall, until the introduction of this technique, precluded the possibility of direct and topologically defined manipulation of cytoskeletal components to measure quantitatively tension, as was performed in fibroblasts, lymphocytes, and erythrocytes (Elson, 1988; Evans, 1975; Pasternak and Elson, 1985; Peterson *et al.*, 1982). The introduction of the optical trap technique to plant cells makes the cell wall barrier operationally transparent for experiments to measure directly tension within transvacuolar strands and the cortical cytoskeletal network of the cell.

III. Cell Optical Displacement Assay (CODA)—A Quantitative Tool for Tension Analysis in the Cytoskeleton of Living Plant Cells

A. Cell Optical Displacement Assay—Method and Instrumentation

A typical measurement is performed in the following manner. Soybean (*Glycine max* L. Merr. cv. Mandarin) root cells (48–72 h of growth) are washed with 1B5C medium (Metcalf *et al.*, 1983) and then placed on a slide in a 10-μl drop with media. A coverslip is applied and then sealed with paraffin wax. The slide, coverslip face down, is placed on the computer-controlled stage of an ACAS 570 Fluorescence interactive laser cytometer (Meridian Instruments, Okemos, MI; Wade *et al.*, 1993). The cells are viewed under phase illumination with an oil immersion 100× (1.4 N.A.) objective. A video camera captures the images, which are then observed on a monitor and recorded on videotape. To initiate trapping, the sample is moved, by manipulating the two-dimensional scanning stage, to a transcytoplasmic strand that can be identified either by its higher index of refraction or by associated vesicles. Light from either an infrared Nb:YAG (1064 nm) or argon ion (488 nm) laser beam is focused onto the fiber or an associated vesicle. This is facilitated by the parfocality of the beam and the imaging plane. The intensity of the trapping laser beam is then monotonically increased to a level that can maintain the optical trapping of the strand at its initial position as the stage is moved through a defined displacement at a constant velocity. For transvacuolar strands, measurements are performed in 20 different cells. The maximum trapping intensity to achieve a successful displacement in all 20 attempts does not vary from day-to-day use by more than 5 mW, as recorded at the laser head (12% variation). The trapping beam is positioned at a point on the filament between the nucleus and the membrane/wall for each attempt in the assay. To ensure that the trapping intensity does not damage the fibers, each displacement at a particular power setting is performed five times and, in all instances, the fiber is required to rebound to the original position following termination of the trap. All trapping experiments can be recorded on videotape and individual pictures can be prepared frame-by-frame from the tapes. Although the technique is described for plant cells grown in suspension culture, this technique can also be extended to whole plant measurements in root cells and root hairs (unpublished results). This capability facilitates the use of this technology for measurements in plants that have been subjected to a variety of genetic manipulations and environmental conditions. It can also be exploited to measure changes in the cytoskeleton during infection thread formation that occurs following the attachment of *Bradyrhizobium japonicum* to soybean root hairs (Wang *et al.,* 1993).

B. Tension and Elasticity Measured in the Transvacuolar Strands of Soybean Cells

An examination of the actin-based network in soybean cells demonstrates an extensive transvacuolar network of cables, filaments, and fibers. A distinct cortical network is also observed at the cell periphery (Lloyd, 1989). Dynamic interactions between the nuclear and the cortical networks are apparently transduced through the transvacuolar strands. These rearrangements appear to be essential for the organization of the division plane and site of new cell wall formation during mitosis (Lloyd, 1989). A high-resolution, three-dimensional view of this network is presented in Fig. 1. Soybean root cells were fixed, permeabilized, and stained [bodipy–phallacidin (Molecular Probes, Eugene, OR), an F-actin fluorescent stain, was used instead of rhodaminyl lysine phallotoxin] as previously described (Traas *et al.,* 1987). Individual optical sections of the fluorescence distribution of the probe were acquired with an InSight bilateral laser scanning confocal microscope (Meridian Instruments). Fifteen optical sections obtained at intervals of 0.5 μm were then recombined using the simulated fluorescence process (SFP) algorithm, as previously described for bacterial imaging (Loh *et al.,* 1993). The result is a three-dimensional reconstruction of the actin network in the soybean root cell (Fig. 1A). These images can be examined with an electronic zoom function to provide a higher degree of magnification (Figs. 1B–1E). A view (1×) of one cell is shown in Fig. 1B. A magnified view of the actin cables that constitute the transvacuolar strands is observed in Figs. 1C (2×) and 1D [slightly rotated (3×)], while the actin cage surrounding the nucleus (2×) is shown in Fig. 1E. The connections (contact points) on the nuclear actin cage and the cortical network that are formed by the transvacuolar actin strands are indicated by the arrowheads in the figures.

The CODA is performed by focusing the diffraction-limited laser beam onto a transvacuolar strand as described in the text. An argon-ion laser was used for all these studies. The displacement of a vesicle associated with the nuclear cage and a transvacuolar strand is shown in Figs. 2 and 3, respectively. In Fig. 2A, the trap is initiated by focusing to the surface of the vesicle (arrow). The stage is moved and the vesicle associated with the strand remains trapped by the beam, resulting in the displacement of the vesicle and the associated strand from its original position near the nucleus (Figs. 2B, 2C). The strand (observed by its higher index of refraction; double arrowhead) that is associated with the vesicle is stretched (Figs. 2B, 2C). Terminating the trap results in the rebound of the

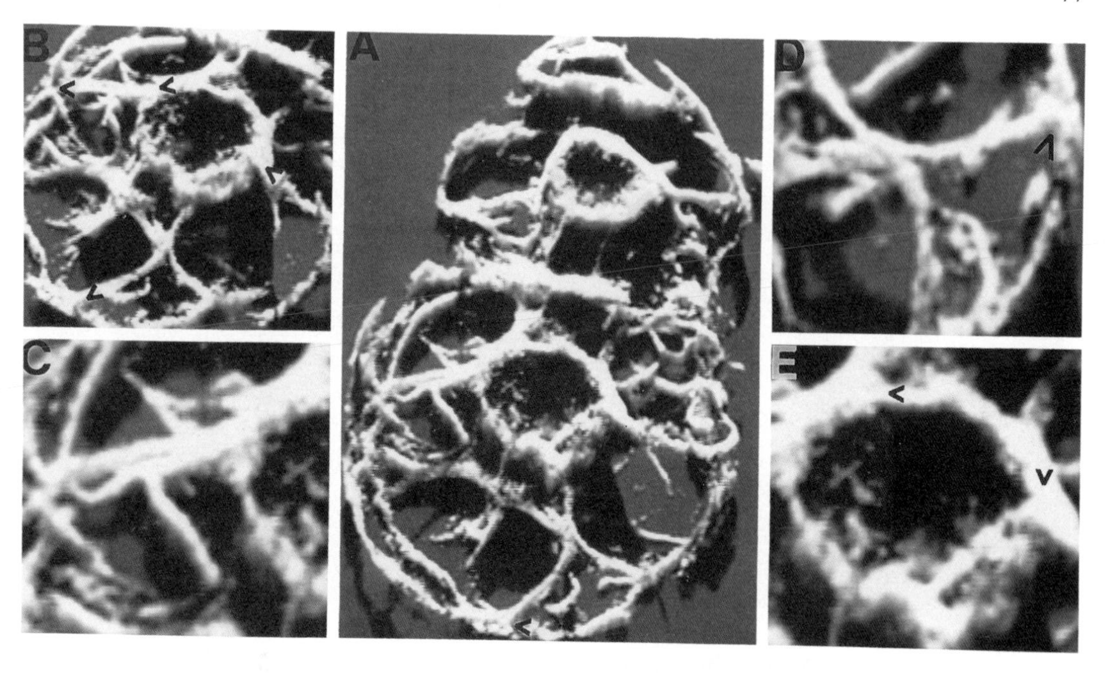

Fig. 1 Confocal fluorescence imaging and three-dimensional reconstruction of F-actin distribution in soybean root cells. Cells were permeabilized and stained with bodipy–phallacidin (F-actin-specific fluorescent probe) (Molecular Probes, Eugene, OR) (Traas *et al.*, 1987). A total of 15 sections (at 0.5-μm intervals) were scanned to generate the 3D reconstructions (Loh *et al.*, 1993). (A) Two soybean root cells permeabilized, fixed, and stained for F-actin. Actin cables are observed to extend from a nuclear actin cage to the periphery. Finer actin filaments are also observed. (B) Single cell view of image in (A). Arrowheads point to connections between transvacuolar actin strands and the nuclear and cortical actin networks. (C) A 2× magnification of (A) showing multiple actin cables of a transvacuolar strand in close proximity. (D) A 3× and rotated view of a section of (A) showing close association between the transvacuolar actin cable and the cortical actin network. (E) A 2× magnification of (A) showing close association between transvacuolar actin cables and the nuclear actin cage.

vesicle and the associated strand to the original position (Fig. 2D). This displacement and rebound can be observed following multiple experiments and provides strong evidence that the viscoelastic properties of the strand are not altered by the intensity of the trapping beam during the course of these experiments. Figure 3 shows the type of strand with associated vesicles that is utilized in the performance of CODA. The trapping beam is focused on a vesicle located toward the center of the strand (Fig. 3A, arrow). The stage is moved and the strand is displaced in a manner reminiscent of an intracellular "sling-shot" (Fig. 3B, arrow). This position can be maintained as long as the trap is focused on the vesicle, in this instance 20 s (Fig. 3C, arrow). When the trap is terminated, the sling-shot is released and the strand with its associated vesicle returns to the original position (Fig. 3D, arrow). Although the power levels required for trap-

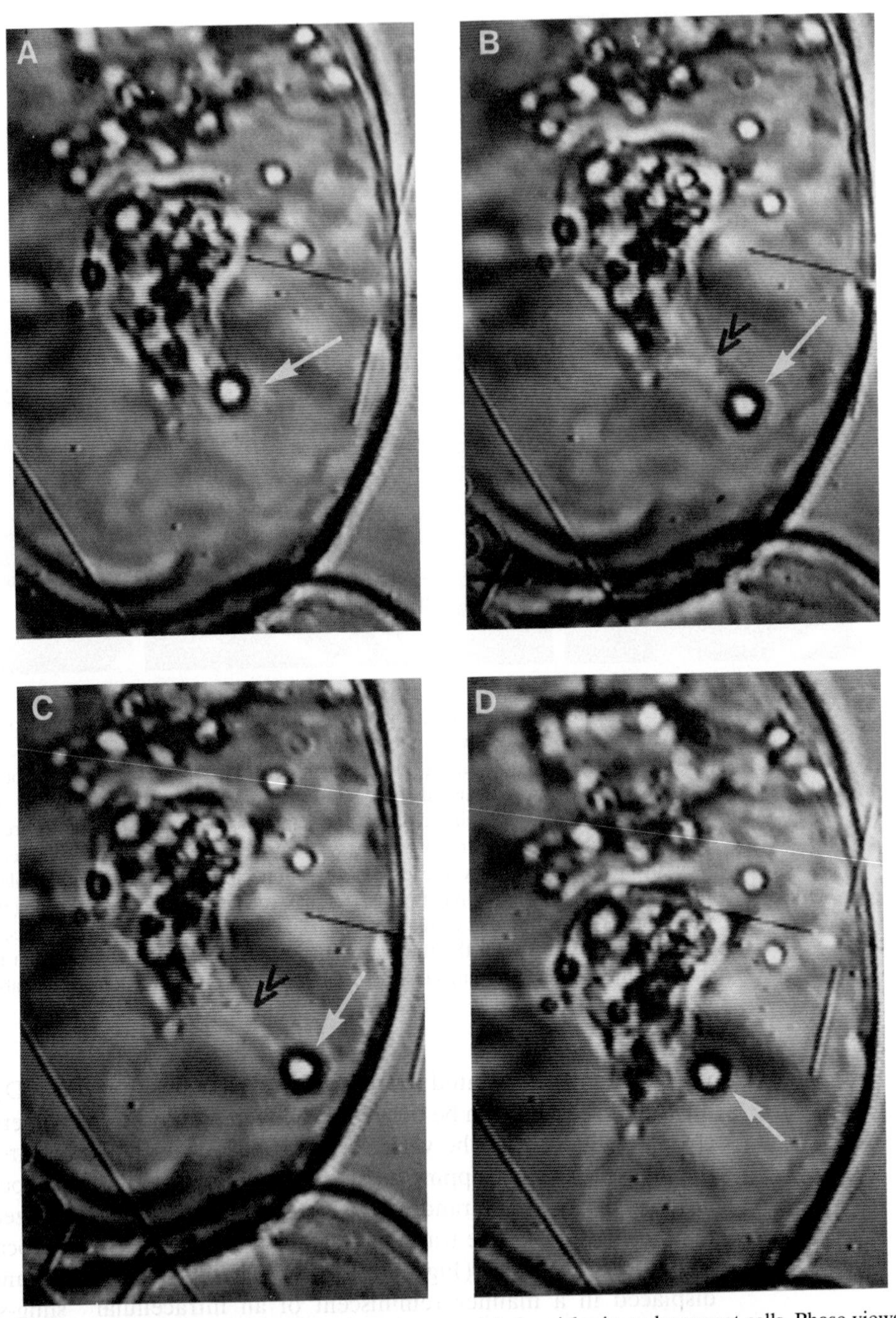

Fig. 2 Optical displacement of nuclear cage-associated vesicles in soybean root cells. Phase views of a single soybean root cell grown in suspension culture. (A) The optical trap is focused on a vesicle attached to the nuclear actin cage (arrow). (B) The vesicle (arrow) is displaced and the associated strand(s) is stretched (double arrowhead) from its original position within the cytoplasm by moving the sample as described in the text. (C) A greater displacement results in increased stretching. (D) Removal of the optical trap results in the rebound of both the vesicle and the associated strand to the original position. These displacements can be performed multiple times without apparent damage.

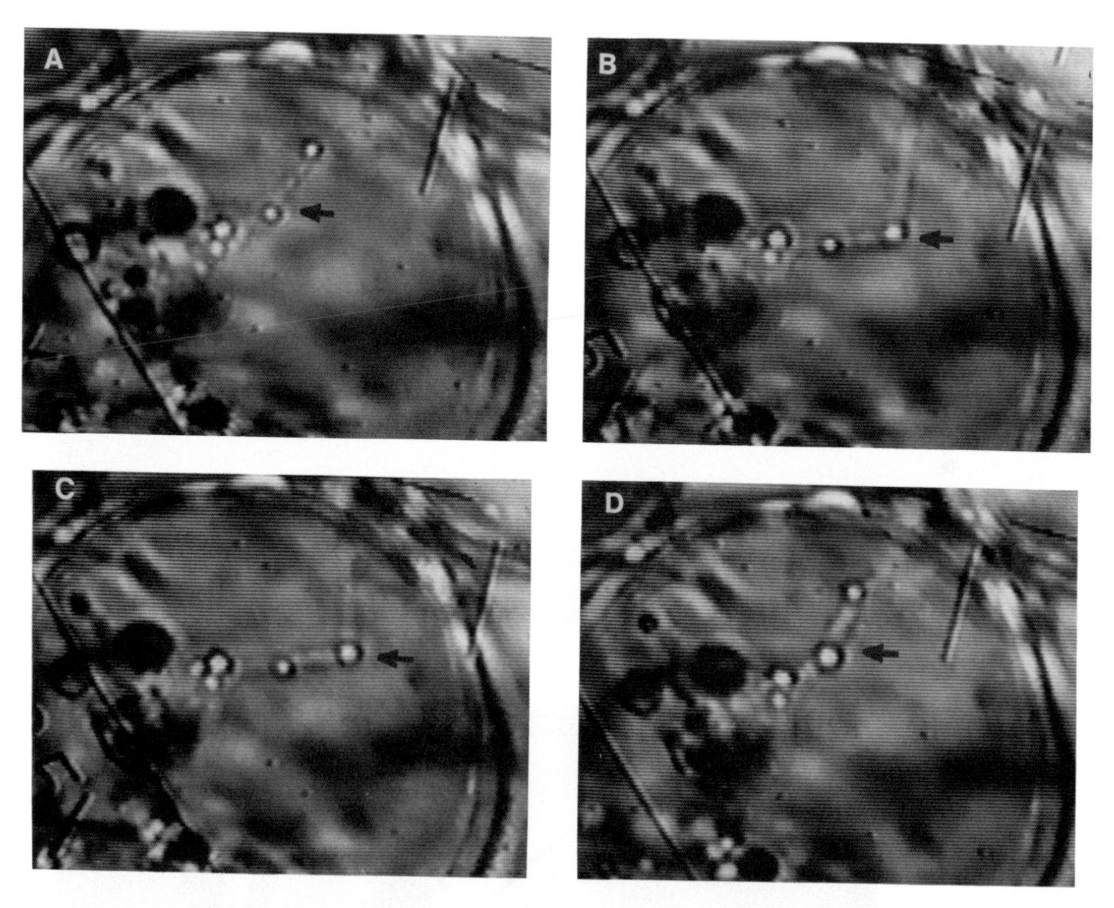

Fig. 3 Optical displacement of transvacuolar strands in soybean plant root cells. Phase views of a single soybean root cell grown in suspension culture. The optical trap is initiated on a vesicle associated with the central portion of a transvacuolar strand. Images (A–D) demonstrate the displacement of the strand with its associated vesicle (arrow).

ping (10–30 mW) do not appear to result in irreversible damage of the strands, measurements of elasticity under conditions that can enhance tension may require significantly higher trapping intensities (100–250 mW). Under these conditions, in isolated instances, the optical trap can cause noticeable damage (Fig. 4). This light-induced damage has been termed opticution by Ashkin and Dziedzic (1989), and it is readily observed as an explosion of light that occurs with a concomitant bubbling of the media and burning of the strand (Figs. 4A, 4B). Strands that have been subjected to opticution are no longer elastic. This provides confidence that the potential damaging effects of the method can be appropriately diagnosed, both by visual inspection during trapping and by multiple displacements of a strand.

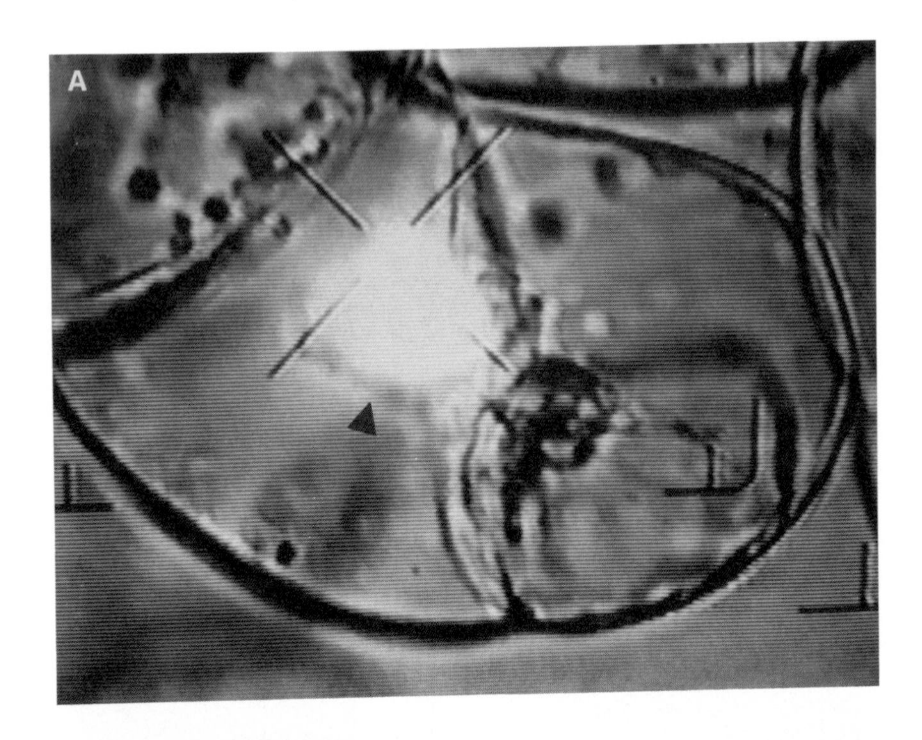

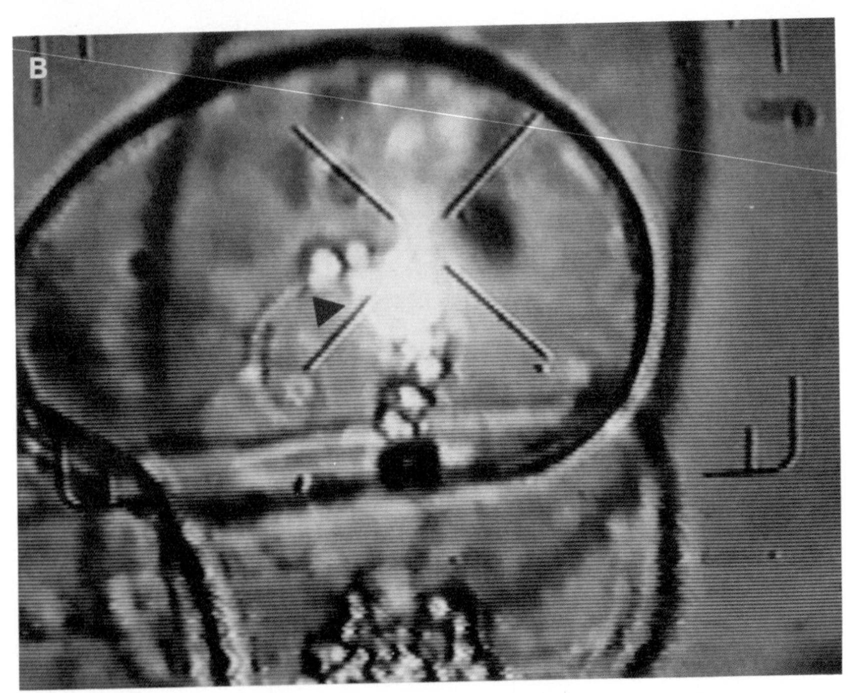

Fig. 4 Opticution of a soybean root cell (A,B). The intensity of the trapping beam has been increased to a level (250 mW at the laser head) to induce heating and concomitant cellular damage.

Quantitation of the displacements observed in Figs. 2 and 3 is performed as described above and is shown in Fig. 5. CODA response curves are presented for normal strands and for strands in cells treated with pectinase (EC 3.27.25; Sigma, St. Louis, MO) or cellulysin (Calbiochem, La Jolla, CA) (Baron-Epel *et al.*, 1988). The linear relationship observed for strand displacement vs power is characteristic for viscoelastic materials. Treatment of the cells with pectinase (Baron-Epel *et al.*, 1988) resulted in a decrease in strand tension that is represented by a shift to lower trapping intensities to produce a constant displacement. This decrease in tension was observed to be a function of the time of exposure of the cells to the enzyme. In contrast, treatment of cells with cellulysin does not appear to cause any significant changes in strand tension. These results may have relevance to a number of observations, suggesting that modifications of the cell wall can influence trans-wall porosity (Baron-Epel *et al.*, 1988) and initiate the activation of phospholipases that may then release bioactive signaling molecules (Tan and Boss, 1992). The CODA results provide the first direct evidence that changes in the organization and state of the wall can have a significant influence on the physical properties of the cytoskeletal network. Recently, similar experiments have provided evidence that lipids, Ca^{2+}, and pH can trigger significant changes in the viscoelastic properties of the actin network in plant cells (Grabski *et al.*, 1994).

IV. CODA and the Plant Cell—Conclusions

The development of the CODA for use in plant cells was motivated by the unique challenges inherent in attempting to measure viscoelastic properties through the barrier of the rigid cell wall. In the course of these studies, it became apparent that the plant cell had a number of particular advantages for pursuing general cellular questions of cytoskeletal organization, function, and integration. The central vacuole creates an intracellular space that excludes intracellular organelles. Individual transvacuolar strands, composed predominantly of actin, myosin, and associated regulatory proteins, provide for distinct contractile structures that are isolated within the transvacuolar space. These topologically distinct strands can be easily imaged by conventional microscopic approaches. In many ways, these isolated strands are reminiscent of isolated muscle preparations that have been extensively employed to explore the effects of substances that moderate the processes of tension and relaxation in muscle contraction. In addition to the advantages of this technique for plant studies, it is believed that plant cells may provide a useful *in vivo* model system for general studies of the physical properties of a dynamic and integrated cytoskeletal network.

The CODA offers a powerful new tool to pursue these noninvasive examinations of the viscoelastic properties of topologically distinct cytoskeletal domains. The ability to both focus a beam of light to specific coordinates in space and simultaneously monitor rates of extension for cytoskeletal elements places this

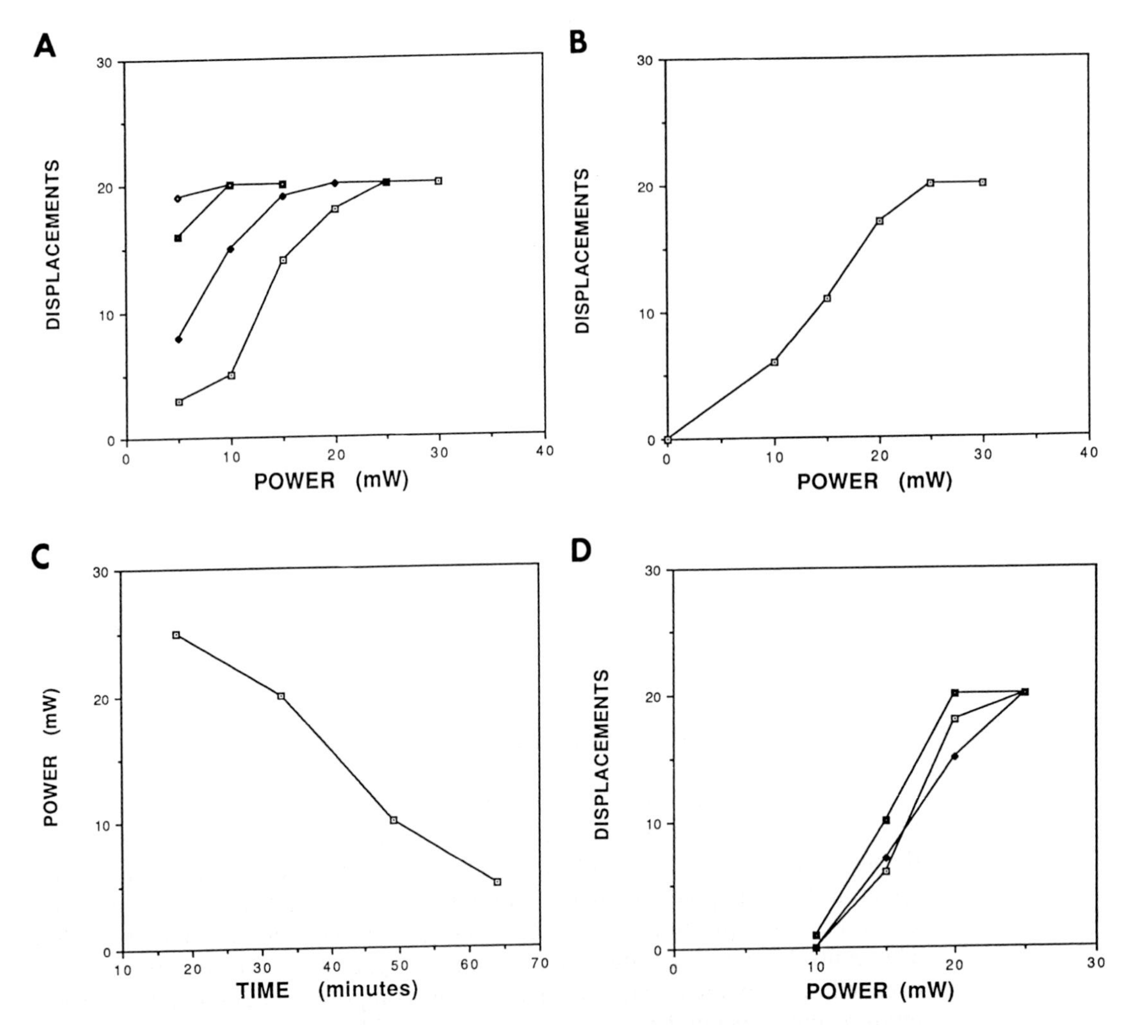

Fig. 5 Quantitation of strand elasticity using the cell optical displacement assay (CODA). CODA was performed as described in the text. (A) The curves represent the following incubation conditions for cells treated with 0.5 mg/ml pectinase in 1B5C medium (Baron-Epel *et al.*, 1988) and measured 10–27 min (⊡), 27–40 min (◆), 41–56 min (■), and 57–71 (◇) after the addition of pectinase. Curves represent the average time of each measurement interval. (B) The curve (⊡) represents the displacement of strands in cells treated with cellulysin (5 mg/ml in 1B5C for 65 min). Results were the same for 1, 5, 10, and 20 mg/ml cellulysin. (C) The curve shows the decrease in tension observed as a function of time that results from treatment with pectinase (0.5 mg/ml). Each point on the curve represents the average time for each measurement interval as described in (A). (D) Effect of culture age on the tension of transvacuolar strands. Curves are: 1-day-old (■), 2-day-old (⊡), and 4-day-old (■) cells in suspension culture.

technique in the expanding arsenal of optically based analytical methods capable of pursuing four-dimensional biochemistry in living cells.

Acknowledgments

Thanks go to L. Lang for superior secretarial assistance, S. Grabski for technical help, and to Dr. J. F. Holland for technical discussions (Department of Biochemistry, Michigan State University).

References

Adams, R. J., and Pollard, T. D. (1989). Inhibition of synaptosomal serotonin uptake by ketalar. *Nature* (*London*) **340,** 565–568.

Ashkin, A., and Dziedzic, J. M. (1989). Internal cell manipulation using IR laser trays. *Proc. Natl. Acad. Sci. USA* **86,** 7914–7918.

Baron-Epel, O., Gharyal, P. K., and Schindler, M. (1988). Pectins as mediators of wall porosity in soybean cells. *Planta* **175,** 389–395.

Block, S. M. (1992). Making light work with optical tweezers. *Nature* **360,** 493–495.

Chu, S. (1991). Laser manipulation of atoms and particles. *Science* **253,** 861–866.

Crick, F. H. C., and Hughes, A. F. W. (1950). The physical properties of cytoplasm. *Exp. Cell Res.* **1,** 37–80.

DeGaetano, D., and Schindler, M. (1987). Enucleation of normal and transformed cells. *J. Cell. Physiol.* **130,** 301–309.

Edelman, G. (1976). Antibody structure and molecular immunology. *Science* **192,** 218–226.

Elson, E. (1988). Cellular mechanics as an indicator of cytoskeletal structure and function. *Annu. Rev. Biophys. Chem.* **17,** 397–430.

Evans, E. A., and LaCelle, P. L. (1975). Mechanics of bilayer membranes. *Blood* **45,** 29–43.

Galatis, B., Apostolakos, P., and Katsaros, C. (1984). Experimental studies on the function of the cortical cytoplasmic zones of the preprophase microtubule band. *Protoplasma* **122,** 11–26.

Giuliano, K. A., and Taylor, D. L. (1994). Fluorescent actin analogs with a high affinity for profilin in vitro exhibit an enhanced gradient of assembly in living cells. *J. Cell Biol.* **124,** 971–983.

Giuliano, K. A., Kolega, J., DeBiasio, R., and Taylor, D. L. (1992). Patterns of elevated free calcium and calmodulin activation in living cells. *Mol. Biol. Cell* **3,** 1037–1048.

Goldschmidt-Clermont, P. J., Machesky, L. M., Baldassare, J. J., and Pollard, T. D. (1990). The actin binding protein profilin binds to PIP_2 and inhibits its hydrolysis by phospholipase C. *Science* **247,** 1575–1577.

Grabski, S., Xie, X., Holland, J. H., and Schindler, M. (1994). Lipids trigger changes in the elasticity of the cytoskeleton in plant cells: A cell optical displacement assay for live cell measurements. *J. Cell Biol.* **126,** 713–726.

Herman, B., and Pledger, W. J. (1985). Platelet-derived growth factor-induced alterations in vinculin and actin distribution in BALB/c-3T3 cells. *J. Cell Biol.* **100,** 1031–1040.

Hochmuth, R. M., Worthy, P. R., and Evans, E. A. (1979). Red cell extensional recovery and the determination of membrane viscosity. *Biophys. J.* **26,** 101–114.

Kamitsubo, E., Ohashi, Y., and Kikuyama, M. (1989). Cytoplasmic streaming in intermodal cells of *Nitella* under centrifugal acceleration: A study done with a newly constructed centrifugal microscope. *Protoplasma* **152,** 148–155.

Kasai, M., Kawashima, H., and Oosawa, F. (1960). Structure of F-actin solutions. *J. Polym. Sci.* **XLIV,** 51–69.

Kerst, A., Chmielewski, G., Livesay, C., Buxbaum, R. R., and Heidemann, S. (1990). Liquid crystal domains and thixotrophy of filamentous actin suspensions. *Proc. Natl. Acad. Sci. USA* **87,** 4241–4245.

Koledney, M. S., and Elson, E. L. (1993). Correlation of myosin light chain phosphorylation with isometric contraction of fibroblasts. *J. Biol. Chem.* **268,** 23850–23855.

Landreth, G. E., Williams, L. K., and Rieser, G. D. (1985). Association of the epidermal growth factor receptor kinase with the detergent-insoluble cytoskeleton of A431 cells. *J. Cell Biol.* **101,** 1341–1350.

Lloyd, C. W. (1989). The plant cytoskeleton. *Curr. Op. Cell Biol.* **1,** 30–35.

Loh, J. T., Ho, S.-C., deFeijter, A. W., Wang, J. L., and Schindler, M. (1993). Carbohydrate binding activities of *Bradyrhizobium japonicum* III. Unipolar localization of the lectin BJ38 in the bacterial cell surface. *Proc. Natl. Acad. Sci. USA* **90,** 3033–3037.

Luna, E. J., and Hitt, A. L. (1992). Cytoskeleton-plasma membrane interactions. *Science* **258,** 955–963.

Marc, J., Mineyuki, Y., and Palevitz, B. (1989). Development of the preprophase band from random cytoplastic microtubules in guard mother cells of *Allium cepa L. Planta* **179,** 539–540.

Metcalf, T. N., III, Wang, J. L., Schubertz, K. R., and Schindler, M. (1983). Lectin receptors on the plasma membrane of soybean cells. Binding and lateral diffusion of lectins. *Biochemistry* **22,** 3969–3975.

Osborn, M. (1983). Intermediate filaments as histologic markers: an overview. *J. Invest. Dermatol.* **81,** 104s–109s.

Pasternak, C., and Elson, E. L. (1985). The effect of salivary amylase on the viscosity behavior of gelatinised starch suspensions and the mechanical properties of gelatinised starch granules. *J. Cell Biol.* **100,** 860–872.

Petersen, N. O., McConnaughey, W. B., and Elson, E. L. (1982). Dependence of locally measured cellular deformability on position on the cell, temperature, and cytochalasin B. *Proc. Natl. Acad. Sci. USA* **79,** 5327–5331.

Pfeuty-David, T. D., and Singer, S. J. (1980). Altered distributions of the cytoskeletal proteins vinculin and α-actinin in cultured fibroblasts transformed by Rous sarcoma virus. *Proc. Natl. Acad. Sci. USA* **77,** 6687–6691.

Ridley, A. J., and Hall, A. (1992). The small GTP-binding protein rho regulates assembly of focal adhesions and actin stress fibers in response to growth factors. *Cell* **70,** 389–399.

Schliwa, M., Nakamura, T., Porter, K. R., and Euteneur, U. (1984). The cytoskeleton: An introductory survey. *J. Cell Biol.* **99,** 1045–1059.

Shariff, A., and Luna, E. J. (1992). Diacylglycerol-stimulated formation of actin nucleation sites at plasma membranes. *Science* **256,** 245–247.

Smith, L., and Hochmuth, R. M. (1982). Effect of wheat germ agglutinin on the viscoelastic properties of erythrocyte membrane. *J. Cell Biol.* **94,** 7–11.

Tan, Z., and Boss, W. F. (1992). Association of phosphatidylinositol kinase, phosphatidylinositol monophosphate kinase, and diacylglycerol kinase with the cytoskeleton and F actin fractions of carrot (*Daucus curota L.*) cells grown in suspension culture. *Plant Physiol.* **100,** 2116–2120.

Traas, J. A., Doonan, J. H., Rawlins, D. J., Shaw, P. J., Watts, J., and Lloyd, C. W. (1987). An actin network is present in the cytoplasm throughout the cell cycle of carrot cells and associates with the dividing nucleus. *J. Cell Biol.* **105,** 387–395.

Visscher, K., Brakenhoff, G. J., and Krol, J. J. (1993). Micromanipulation by "multiple" optical traps created by a single fast scanning trap integrated with the bilateral confocal scanning laser microscope. *Cytometry* **14,** 105–114.

Wade, M. H., deFeijter, A. W., Frame, M. K., and Schindler, M. (1993). Quantitative fluorescence imaging techniques for the study of organization and signaling mechanisms in the cell. *Bioanal. Instrumen.* **37,** 117–141.

Wang, J. L., Schindler, M., and Ho, S.-C. (1993). Carbohydrate binding activities of *Bradyrhizobium japonicum.* III. Lectin expression, bilateral binding and nodulation efficiency. *Trends Glycosci. Glycotech.* **5,** 331–342.

Wang, Y. L. (1984). Reorganization of actin filament bundles in living fibroblasts. *J. Cell Biol.* **99,** 1478–1485.

Weed, R. I., LaCelle, P. L., and Merrill, E. W. (1969). Metabolic dependence of red cell deformability. *J. Clin. Invest.* **48,** 795–809.

Williamson, R. E. (1993). Ethylene, microtubules and root morphology in wild-type and mutant *Arabidopsis* seedlings. *Annu. Rev. Plant Physiol. Plant Mol. Biol.* **44,** 181–202.

Zaner, K. S., and Stossel, T. P. (1982). Some perspectives on the viscosity of actin filaments. *J. Cell Biol.* **93,** 987–991.

CHAPTER 7

Methods in Plant Immunolight Microscopy

Roy C. Brown and Betty E. Lemmon

Department of Biology
University of Southwestern Louisiana
Lafayette, Louisiana 70504-2451

METHODS IN CELL BIOLOGY, VOL. 49

I. Introduction

The purpose of this chapter is to describe methods for preparing plant cells and tissues for immunolight microscopy. Immunocytochemistry takes advantage of the immune reaction between antibody and antigen to identify and localize molecules in cells and tissues. Since antibodies can be made to virtually every biological molecule, this method is at the core of modern cell biology and is rapidly advancing with innovations in microscopy and biochemistry. For aspects of immunocytochemistry that are beyond the scope of this paper, the reader is referred to specific treatments on the isolation of proteins (Hames and Rickwood, 1981; 1990), production and characterization of antibodies (Harlow and Lane, 1988; Liddell and Cryer, 1991; Borrebaeck, 1992; Peters and Baumgarten, 1992; Asai, 1993), theory and practice of fluorescence and confocal microscopy (Pawley, 1989; Matsumoto, 1993), and computer enhancement of images (Inoué, 1986).

In order to detect a target molecule with immunolight microscopy, it is necessary to use an antibody conjugated to an easily recognized tag. The most widely used method is to label an antibody either directly or indirectly with a fluorochrome, a chemical that upon excitation at a specific wavelength will fluoresce in another (lower) wavelength. This signal is seen with the fluorescence microscope and the method is known as the fluorescent antibody or immunofluorescence technique. The design of a simple microscope that illustrates the principles of fluorescence microscopy as well as a sound introduction to fluorescence microscopy is found in O'Brien and McCully (1981). In practice, most laboratories will have integrated systems supplied by various microscope manufacturers. The selection of filters appropriate to separate wavelengths of fluorescence excitation and emission is crucial to the success of fluorescence microscopy. Fortunately, the spectral characteristics of fluorophores are well known and the manufacturers of molecular probes and filters are a rich source of information. Epifluorescence microscopy is the most effective system; this involves focusing the light used for excitation onto the specimen using the objective lens, which is also used to collect the fluorescent light that is emitted. This arrangement simplifies alignment, and reduces the background.

In most applications, indirect immunofluorescence is used. This technique involves at least two antibodies, the primary antibody made against the antigen to be localized, and the secondary antibody made against the immunoglobulins (usually IgGs, or in a few cases IgMs) of the animal in which the primary antibody was produced. The primary antibody attaches to specific sites of the immunogen. The secondary antibody, which is conjugated to a fluorochrome, most commonly fluorescein, attaches to the primary antibody. This method both intensifies signal and allows a single secondary antibody to label any of the primary antibodies produced in the same kind of host. Since monoclonal antibodies are produced in both rat and mouse, it is useful to have on hand secondary antibodies against both rat and mouse IgGs.

Although most work has been done using antibodies conjugated to fluorochromes, there is rapid development of immunogold microscopy where antibodies are conjugated to colloidal gold particles of known diameter (e.g., deMey *et al.,* 1982; Molè-Bajer *et al.,* 1988; Moore, this volume). The immunogold localization can be viewed in the electron microscope and in the light microscope using darkfield illumination or, after silver enhancement, in brightfield or differential interference contrast. This latter technique is particularly effective when combined with computer enhancement of the image. The advantage of this technology is that preparations can be viewed with visible light, are relatively permanent, and can be counterstained with biological stains, allowing the new immunolight methods to be combined with more classical techniques of histochemistry.

It must be emphasized that immunolight microscopy is a very dynamic field at the interface of biology and technology. Conventional epifluorescence microscopy (Fig. 1) is increasingly being supplemented, and in some cases replaced, by confocal laser scanning microscopy (Fig. 2). For treatment of this topic, see Pawley (1989), Gunning (1992), Matsumoto (1993), and the chapter by Running *et al.* (Chapter 15, this volume). The optical sectioning capability of confocal microscopy allows enhanced resolution through elimination of out-of-focus information and permits reconstruction of three-dimensional information for presentation in stereo. Confocal images are displayed on monitors, making this method especially valuable in teaching and presentation. The sensitivity of confocal microscopy has enabled development of techniques for microinjection into living cells of fluorochrome-conjugated cytoskeletal proteins (Hepler *et al.,* 1993) and other vital stains (Haugland, 1992). This provides direct visualization of dynamic aspects of organization and function. Technically this is not immunolight microscopy since antibodies are not necessarily employed, but the methods have much in common with immunofluorescence techniques. The combination of static images from fixed cells with dynamic images of living cells is yielding a more complete understanding of development and organization in plant cells.

This chapter is concerned with the indirect immunofluorescence localization of cytoskeletal proteins in isolated plant cells and in intact tissues. However, the fundamental technique can be used to localize other target molecules for which antibodies are available; examples include phytochromes, seed storage proteins, extracellular matrix or cell wall constituents, integrin, calmodulin, and centrin. Techniques for studying plant cells with immunolight microscopy were derived from methods originally worked out for animal cells. Plant cells, however, present unique difficulties. For example, the cell wall presents a barrier to entrance of antibodies, numerous autofluorescent compounds can be present in both the wall and cytoplasm, and many heavily walled or highly vacuolate plant cells are difficult to fix properly. The protocols for the indirect immunofluorescence microtechnique that we present have been thoroughly worked out and tested on numerous and diverse plants ranging from bryophytes to orchids, and from root tips to pollen and spores. At each step of the procedure, suggestions for overcoming the inherent difficulties of plant materials are included and the user

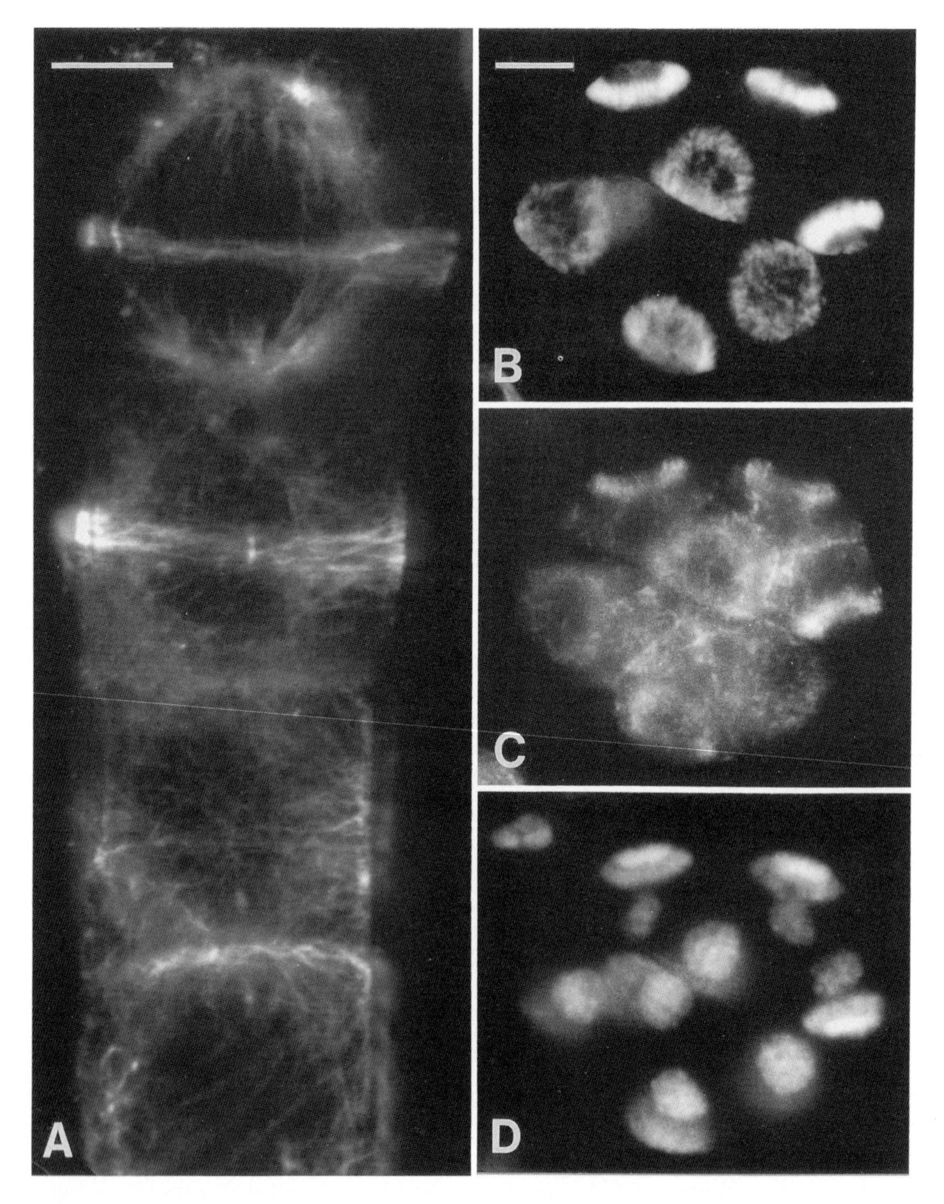

Fig. 1 Conventional epifluorescence micrographs. (A) This column of cells showing stages in development of the preprophase band of microtubules in the root tip of broad bean was isolated from neighboring cells by enzymatic treatment as described herein. Cells were stained by the indirect immunofluorescence method (monoclonal antibody to tubulin produced in rat, followed by anti-rat IgG conjugated to fluorescein). Scale bar, 10 μm. (B–D) Pollen mitosis in persistent tetrads of the moth orchid showing a combination of staining methods with each fluorochrome viewed in a different channel. Scale bar, 5 μm. (B) Microtubules were stained by indirect immunofluorescence. (C) Actin was stained by direct fluorescence with rhodamine phalloidin. (D) Nuclei stained with the DNA stain Hoechst 33258.

is encouraged to select the technique that seems best for the tissue/cells at hand. The major steps discussed are dissection, buffers, fixation, adhering cells to coverslip, wall removal, permeabilization, primary and secondary antibodies, nuclear staining, mounting media, and controls. A technique for embedding, sectioning, and dewaxing sections of intact plant tissues for immunolight microscopy is provided as a separate section. All reagents, except when noted, are available from large supply houses such as Sigma Chemical.

The general schedule for immunofluorescence staining is given here with details of each step provided in the following sections.

1. Dissection
2. Fixation

   -----For thick and complex tissues such as root tips, reverse steps 3 and 4
3. Attachment of individual cells to coverslips

   Buffer washes, 3 × 5 min
4. Enzymatic removal of walls, 15–20 min

   Buffer washes, 3 × 5 min
5. Extraction with detergent, 30 min–1 h

   Buffer washes, 3 × 5 min
6. Incubation in primary antibody, 1–6 h

   Buffer washes, 3 × 5 min
7. Secondary antibody, 1–6 h

   Buffer washes, 3 × 5 min

   -----If double labeling, repeat steps 6–7 with different set of antibodies followed by buffer washes, 3 × 5 min

   -----If necessary, wash with ethanol to reduce autofluorescence
8. Nuclear stain, 15–30 s

   d-H_2O wash, 5 min
9. Mount coverslip to slide and store in dark at room temperature for 3 h–overnight before viewing.

II. Preparing Isolated Cells for Immunostaining

A. Buffers, Fixatives, and Protease Inhibitors

Buffers: Standard buffers such as phosphate-buffered saline (PBS), usually adjusted to pH 6.8–7, can be used successfully for immunostaining of most antigens. However, various modifications are recommended for the stabilization of microtubules. Most of these microtubule stabilizing buffers contain ethylene glycol-bis-(β-aminoethyl ether)*N,N,N′N′*-tetraacetic acid (EGTA) and/or magnesium salts.

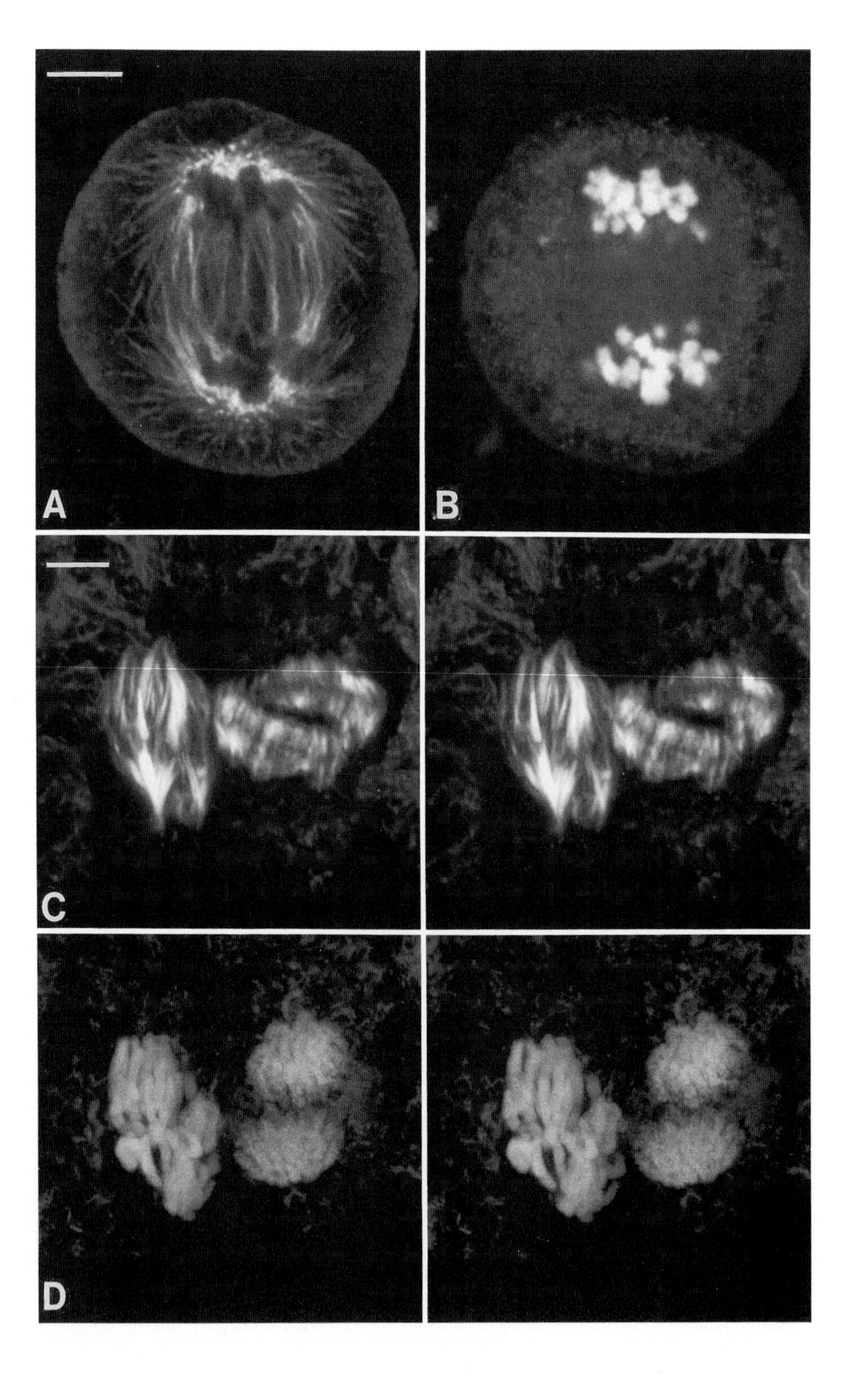
A
B
C
D

PHEM buffer (Schliwa and van Blerkom, 1981) is an excellent microtubule-stabilizing buffer that can also be used successfully in processing cells for localization of other antigens as well as tubulin. PHEM buffer contains 60 m*M* Pipes (piperazine -*N,N'*-bis [2-ethane-sulfonic acid]), 25 m*M* Hepes (*N*-2-hydroxyethyl-piperazine-*N'*-2-ethane-sulfonic acid), 2 m*M* $MgCl_2$, 10 m*M* EGTA. A simple way to prepare PHEM is to weigh separately and place in a 1000-ml beaker the following:

Pipes	18.14 g
Hepes	5.95 g
EGTA	3.80 g (may be omitted when staining calcium-sensitive antigens)
$MgCl_2$	0.41 g

Add 800–900 ml of d-H_2O and a stir bar to the beaker and place on a stirrer. The solution may appear cloudy, but will clear when the pH is adjusted to 6.8 or higher. Add 10 *N* NaOH drop-wise, testing until the desired pH (usually 6.9) is reached. Adjust the volume of the buffer to 1000 ml using d-H_2O. The buffer can be stored in a plastic container in the refrigerator for long periods. For immunolocalizations, we add 5 ml DMSO (dimethyl sulfoxide) to 95 ml of PHEM and store the PHEM/DMSO buffer for shorter periods (no longer than a week or so) in the refrigerator.

We use PBS at pH 7.2 for diluting antibodies, and at pH 8.5 for making the mounting medium. To make PBS pH 7.2, weigh the following and bring to 1 liter with d-H_2O. Adjust pH.

NaCl	7.9 g
KCl	1.8 g
Na_2HPO_4	1.4 g
KH_2PO_4	0.2 g

To make PBS pH 8.5, omit the KH_2PO_4, and adjust the pH with 10 *N* NaOH.

Fixatives: The ideal fixative for immunolight microscopy preserves all cell components as they were in the living cell, preserves antigenicity, and does not introduce artifacts and/or background fluorescence. For discussion of fixatives used in immunolight microscopy, see Wick and Duniec (1986). Although glutaral-

Fig. 2 Confocal laser scanning micrographs. Hard copy of computer images were generated using Bio-Rad software and a Lasertechnics continuous tone laser printer. (A,B) Double stained microtubules (A) and chromosomes (B) in telophase of the first meiotic division in daylily. The microsporocytes were expressed directly into a drop of fixative, covered by an A-G film and processed according to the method described herein. Scale bar, 10 μm. (C,D) Stereo pairs of microtubules (C) and chromosomes (D) in dividing cells of aleurone in the developing grain of barley. The tissue was sectioned in Steedman's wax as described herein, dewaxed, and double-stained for microtubules (indirect immunofluorescence) and nuclei (propidium iodide). The specimen was optically sectioned at 1-μm intervals with a Bio-Rad MRC-600 coupled to a Nikon Optiphot with a planapochromatic 60× oil immersion objective. Stereo pairs were produced with Bio-Rad software by projecting images with −1 pixel shift left and +1 pixel shift right. Scale bar, 5 μm.

dehyde is an excellent fixative in many respects, it penetrates slowly and has the additional disadvantage of resulting in a high level of background fluorescence. For this reason, formalin or freshly prepared formaldehyde (from paraformaldehyde) is widely used. The two aldehydes can be used together to take advantage of the best qualities of each, but best results are obtained when the mixture contains a final concentration of no more than 1% glutaraldehyde. Higher percentages of glutaraldehyde require subsequent treatment with sodium borohydride ($NaBH_4$) to reduce background fluorescence. The recommended treatment of 3 × 5 min washes with a 0.5% solution of $NaBH_4$ in buffer is rather harsh, and can dislodge and damage cells. In most cases, formalin will fix the tissues adequately so that, in addition to preserving antigenicity, distribution of the antigen in the cell can be interpreted accurately. To prepare a 4% (w/v) solution of formaldehyde, add 1 g paraformaldehyde to 12.5 ml d-H_20 and heat to 60–70°C for 20 min in a fume cabinet. Gloves should always be worn when handling fixatives and other toxic substances. Add three drops of 1 *N* NaOH to clear. Dilute 1 : 1 with PBS or PHEM buffer. Formaldehyde can be used as soon as it cools and should not be kept more than a day.

The fixative routinely used in our laboratory for all types of plant cells is 3.7% reagent grade formaldehyde stabilized with methanol (formalin) in PHEM/DMSO buffer pH 6.9. This mixture is freshly prepared each day. Formaldehyde should not be refrigerated nor agitated. To make 10 ml of 3.7% fixative, carefully draw off 1 ml of 37% formaldehyde from well above the sediment that accumulates at the bottom and combine with 9 ml of PHEM/DMSO. Cells should remain in the fixative for 30–60 min at room temperature. Many plant materials can be allowed to fix overnight in the refrigerator for convenience of the technician. A change of fixative should be made if material is to be fixed overnight.

Protease Inhibitors: Certain antigens may be sensitive to degradation by proteases, which either may be abundant in specific plant tissues or can be introduced as contaminants in wall-digesting enzymes. EGTA serves as an inhibitor of calcium-dependent proteases, and gelatin acts as an alternative substrate, consequently reducing effects of protease activity. Specific protease inhibitors can also be added following fixation. Phenylmethylsulfonyl fluoride (PMSF) and leupeptin are commonly used. All protease inhibitors are toxic and should be mixed under a fume hood and aliquoted to avoid prolonged handling. Both stock solutions can be frozen in small aliquots to avoid repeated thawing and freezing.

PMSF: make a 30 m*M* stock solution by dissolving 0.015 g in 3 ml DMSO. To use, dilute to 0.3 m*M*.

Leupeptin: make a 1 mg/ml aqueous (d-H_2O) stock solution. To use, dilute to 10 μg/ml.

B. Dissection of Plant Materials

Almost all plant materials require dissection before they can be adequately fixed. Dissecting in fixative is a possibility but can defeat the purpose if cells in the interior of the plant tissue die prior to arrival of the fixative. We recommend fixation after dissection, with the goal being to make a quick clean cut that does not injure adjacent cells, and to subsequently submerge the living cells in fixative as quickly as possible. One needs to assemble the following: a dissecting microscope with good (preferably cool) light, fine-tip forceps, new single-edge razor blades that have been degreased by wiping with acetone before use, wooden toothpicks, fixative, and a place to keep the plant healthy (cool, moist, etc.) during dissection.

Root tips or similar structures should be sliced longitudinally. This is best done by holding the root tip (approximately 1 cm long) lengthwise with a fine forceps and slicing lengthwise between the prongs of the forceps. Very small roots can be sliced into halves and larger roots into three or more slices. Since it is important that the slices be transferred immediately into fixative without drying, it is convenient to dissect on a depression slide with fixative in the well so that no time is lost in the transfer. Once the material is fixed (30–60 min), it can be trimmed and all but the meristematic region discarded. The now very small pieces of tissue are washed in PHEM/DMSO. This can be done by replacing the fixative in the well with buffer or by transferring the tissue to a small container of buffer with a splinter of wood (a flat toothpick cut at an angle with a single edge razor blade). After three changes of buffer, the root tips are incubated in an enzyme mixture (see section on Enzymatic Removal of Walls) for about 10–15 min to break down the cell walls. When the root tips are soft, but still intact, they are transferred to the coverslip (see Section C below), which will serve as a carrier for all subsequent steps of processing. This method assures that no cells will be lost as they slough off. As the walls are further broken down, the cells can be separated mechanically with forceps or a wood splinter, or another coverslip can be placed over the root tips and gentle pressure applied. In the latter case, both coverslips can be processed if cells remain attached to both. By either method, the goal is to have only isolated cells on the coverslip and all debris removed before processing. If it becomes difficult to pick out large clumps of debris, a small drop of buffer can be added. This type of preparation results in isolated cells, although packets of several cells may remain together as in Fig. 1A.

Free cells, such as pollen (Fig. 1B), microsporocytes (Figs. 2A and 2B) or cells in suspension culture, can be fixed in a drop of fixative directly on the coverslip so that they are never transferred, or they may be expressed into small tubes and concentrated by gentle centrifugation. In some cases, slices of an anther can be fixed in a small container without a serious loss of cells. The availability of cells determines the method of handling. When cells are few in number and/or difficult to obtain, either because of the developmental stage or experimental pretreatment, the more care must be taken not to lose them during subsequent processing.

C. Attaching Cells to Coverslips

The coverslip serves as a carrier for the multiple steps in the immunostaining procedure described here. This distinguishes the protocol from those in which materials are processed on a slide. The advantages of using coverslips are that the cells are adjacent to the glass surface through which the image is collected, the material can be easily located, and the amounts of antibodies used can be controlled by the size of the coverslip. The quality of the coverslip is even more critical than the slide in epifluorescence light microscopy since the light is transmitted through the coverslip, absorbed by the fluorochromes in the specimen, and fluorescence emitted again through the coverslip.

Preparation of Coverslips and Slides: A good choice for coverslips is grade $1\frac{1}{2}$ and size 18 × 18 mm. These can be scored with a diamond scribe and broken to half or quarter size when necessary to conserve antibodies or when material to be processed is limited. The smaller (9 × 18 mm) size is convenient for fitting into microfuge tubes.

Since the quality of slides and coverslips is critical in all types of light microscopy, it is convenient to have a supply of cleaned slides and coverslips on hand. They should be washed in dishwashing detergent such as Alconox, thoroughly rinsed and wiped with 70% ethanol, and stored in a dust-free container, usually the original box. If agar–gelatin films are to be used with coverslips, better adherence can be obtained by etching the border of the coverslips with glass-etching solution. Glass-etching cream (e.g., Armour Etch, Part No. 15-0200, Armour Products, Midland Park, NJ) is available from craft and hobby stores. Follow the instructions on the bottle. Paint a narrow border 2–3 mm on the coverslip. After etching, wash the coverslips as described above the store in a dust-free container.

Adhesives: Many types of cells will adhere to coverslips coated with an adhesive such as poly-L-lysine, polyethylenimine, or Mayer's albumen; others may require covering with a thin film of agarose–gelatin (A-G). The latter method is preferable whenever cells are particularly precious, as it ensures that none will be lost during subsequent processing.

Poly-L-lysine: (300,000 NW). Make a 1 mg/ml solution in d-H_2O. Coverslips or microslides are spread with a thin film, or are submerged by dipping. Incubate for 1 h in a moist chamber before using.

Polyethylenimine: Dilute to 0.01–0.001% in distilled d-H_2O. Use as above.

Mayer's Albumen Adhesive: This is a simple, fast, and inexpensive adhesive for many plant materials. Although it has the disadvantage of being stained by many histological stains, it exhibits minimal background fluorescence. It can be used for both free cells and sections. The solution can be kept for several months in the refrigerator and should be replaced when it becomes cloudy or loses its effectiveness as an adhesive. To prepare, mix with a stir bar the following:

White of fresh egg (active ingredient)	50 ml
Glycerine (to prevent drying)	50 ml
Sodium salicylate (antiseptic)	0.1 g

Put a very small drop on a clean coverslip, spread evenly with a clean finger until a thin film remains. Free or isolated cells can be placed directly on the surface and allowed to dry. Plastic sections are placed in a small drop of water and dried immediately on a hotplate. Wax sections are placed on a slide warming table with temperature adjusted to just below the melting point of the wax until the sections flatten and dry.

A small drop of fixative (or buffer if cells are prefixed) is placed on each coverslip to receive the cells. This step is best accomplished by working under a dissecting microscope. It is convenient to attach the coverslips (with coated or etched sides upward) to a microscope slide with a small drop of water so that they can be moved about without danger of slipping off the slide, particularly when very small coverslips are used. The slide with coverslips can be examined (cells in liquid uppermost) with the low-power objective of a standard light microscope, or with higher power objectives of an inverted microscope, to monitor the number of cells, and to make certain that they are spread properly. The spread droplet containing the cells is now allowed to evaporate until dry. If the cells are not to be covered with an agarose/gelatin film, they should be allowed to dry at room temperature (avoid heating the cells) for at least an hour or more to assure adhesion. If the cells are to be covered with agarose–gelatin, they need not be dried completely.

Agarose–Gelatin Films: Cells or dissected tissues can be covered with a thin film of A-G for processing. Although this technique takes practice to master, it is worth the effort, as it ensures that no cells will be lost during processing. In addition, this technique allows processing of cells without drying, thereby minimizing artifacts induced by collapse and distortion. A-G presents no background fluorescence and does not appreciably increase incubation and staining times. Thin A-G films were particularly effective in studies of stomatogenesis, where it was necessary to prevent distortion of delicate systems of microtubules and F-actin on the inner and outer periclinal walls of guard cells (Cleary *et al.*, 1992). For this study, thin strips of tissue containing epidermal cells with underlying mesophyll were placed on the coverslip, secured with an A-G film while still moist, processed, and mounted on a slide with spacers to prevent squashing the cells. Since the tissue was adjacent to the coverslip, there was no difficulty in examining the thick preparation under high-power oil-immersion objectives.

Prepare a solution of 0.75% agar and 0.75% gelatin in d-H_2O. Osmality can be adjusted by the addition of glucose. Vegetative cells do well in about 1% glucose, whereas sporocytes and pollen may require up to 10% or more. Heat the mixture in a water bath until liquid. In working with fixed materials, we use the A-G stock solution repeatedly, adding water as it is lost through evaporation. When working with very delicate living endosperm, it is recommended that the mixture be stored in small aliquots and reheated only once (Molè-Bajer and Bajer, 1968). Experience will determine what is best for each application.

Glass beakers or deep petri dishes that can be placed in a water bath for heating are good containers for A-G. The container should be wide enough to accommodate easily the loop, which will be used to collect a thin film. The loop itself must be larger than the coverslip. A loop can be made from a standard microbiological inoculation wire by bending platinum wire into the desired shape and tightening it into the holder. We use the open handle of the sturdy and smooth chromium loops, used in the early days of transmission electron microscopy (TEM) for manipulating ultrathin sections. The instrument is bent at right angles to fit into a beaker and is reversed so that it is held by the small end and the original handle forms a rectangular loop.

Cells are placed on the coverslip, preferably one with etched borders, and allowed to dry until little moisture remains. The coverslip is elevated in some way, such as on a small-diameter cork, so that the loop with a film can be passed over it. Casting a good quality film requires some skill. The quality of the film will depend upon a number of factors including temperature of the A-G, speed at which the film is cast, and thickness of the wire. It is best to keep the A-G at a medium temperature to avoid thick streaks if the mixture is too cool, or bubbles in the film if it is too hot. The loop should be clean and raised slowly so that a film will form. It is possible to cover a faulty film with a second film, but the preparation is seldom as clean. When working with living cells or very delicate cells, it may also be necessary to first coat the coverslip with a thin film of A-G before cells are placed on it. Alternatively, the film may be combined with other methods and coverslips subbed with an adhesive.

Once the cells are covered with a film the coverslip is removed to a slightly elevated surface for processing (film upward). The film covering the cells is allowed to cool 30–60 s and then covered with buffer so that it does not shrink away from the edges. From this point on it is important that the film be kept moist. The various liquids are dropped onto the film and drained off by tipping the coverslip. The advantage of keeping the coverslip slightly elevated is that surface tension will keep the fluids from spreading beyond the edges of the coverslips. If conservation of antibodies is not a concern the coverslips can be processed flat on a glass slide or in a petri dish. Standing coverslips vertically in a staining jar is risky because of the increased chance that the film will slip off.

D. Enzymatic Removal of Walls

Plant cells, except of the brief coenocytic stage of endosperm and some tapeta, are surrounded by walls that must be removed, at least partially, before incubation in antibodies.

Root Tips and Related Vegetative Tissues: The primary walls of vegetative tissues consist principally of complex polysaccharides and protein cross-linkers and are broken down by cellulase, pectinase, and glucuronidase. Enzymes are stored in a desiccator in the freezer; even so, it is best to purchase enzymes in small quantities to assure freshness. Since working with enzymes is imprecise and different lots may vary in activity, one must experiment with the tissue at hand to determine the proper concentration and time for digestion. The usual enzyme mixture, which should be freshly prepared, consists of 0.1% cellulase, 0.1% glucuronidase, and 0.1% glucose (or any osmoticum) in buffer or d-H_2O.

EGTA in the buffer may enhance the wall disruption by chelating calcium. These proportions are starting points that should be varied as necessary to remove walls in 15–20 min and to match osmality of the cell type. As discussed in the section on dissection, it is desirable to slice the tissue so that, as much as possible, all cells are affected at the same time. The purpose of the enzyme treatment is to separate the cells and partially digest the walls. Too much enzymatic activity can destroy the integrity of the cells. Therefore, it is a good plan to monitor the progress of enzymatic treatment by teasing apart the cells to check degree of separation.

Sporocytes/Microsporocytes: Prior to meiosis, plants lay down a sporocyte wall within the cellulosic wall, which subsequently breaks down to release the sporocytes. Thus, the enzyme cellulase is omitted. The sporocyte walls of lower plants such as bryophytes are digested by the glucuronidase, but microsporocyte walls of angiosperms are principally callose and require the addition of 0.1% lyticase for removal.

The enzyme mixture is dropped onto the film of A-G on the coverslips, or directly onto cells if no film is used. Removal of the sporocyte walls can be monitored by placing the coverslip with cell/A-G film side up on a slide for viewing with an inverted microscope or with a long working distance objective on an upright microscope.

E. Detergent Extraction

Entry of antibodies into the cell is facilitated by permeabilizing the plasma membrane using a detergent. Plant cells usually tolerate and, for optimal staining, often require as much as 1.0% Triton X-100 (v/v) in PHEM/DMSO. Permeabilization typically requires 15 min, and the detergent should be removed with at least 3×5 min washes of PHEM/DMSO. Longer treatments with detergent (up to 60 min) can be used to reduce offending autofluorescence from compounds such as oils.

III. Immunostaining

A. Primary Antibody

The quality of the primary antibody is of paramount importance to the success of immunolight microscopy. If the specificity of the antibody is not known, it should be determined by immunoblotting (Otto, 1993). A good antibody has both high binding strength and high titer. This allows for greater dilution of the antibody, which helps to reduce contaminating proteins, dilutes out nonspecific antibodies, and is economical. These are not necessarily important considerations if monoclonal antibodies are used, since unwanted reactions are negligible and the supply is unlimited. Antibodies sold commercially are sent with recommendations for dilution, or instructions can be requested from the supplier. Since recommendations are usually based on experimentation with animal cells, it is advisable to make the antibody stock at the lowest recommended dilution, and then experiment with further dilutions to determine what is most effective for the plant tissue at hand. Once the initial dilution has been made, the antibodies should be stored in a freezer in small aliquots to avoid repeated thawing and freezing. A convenient container is a standard BEEM capsule (size 00) sold for TEM embedding. Each BEEM capsule will hold 0.5 ml, an amount adequate for processing two to four standard 18-mm-square coverslips, or more if the antibody is diluted further at the time of use.

The time allowed for incubation of antibodies depends upon the plant material and can vary from 1 h to overnight at room temperature. For long incubations, it is important to keep the coverslips in a moist chamber to prevent drying.

Plant cells are notorious for containing various compounds that autofluoresce. Autofluorescence can seriously detract from meaningful signal. With unknown material it is advisable to check the coverslip (cell side up and uncovered with low-power objective or with an inverted microscope) at this stage for unwanted fluorescence. It is possible to bleach chlorophyll and some oils by washing the preparation in absolute ethanol after the secondary antibody. This treatment usually does not damage the immunostaining, even when a graded series of steps is skipped. However, it is advisable to experiment with one coverslip before treating all. As stated earlier, selection of the fluorophore and filters is important in minimizing autofluorescence. In some cases, addition of histological stains such as toluidine blue O reduces autofluorescence (Baluska *et al.,* 1992).

B. Secondary Antibody

Imaging the immune reaction by fluorescence microscopy depends upon following the primary antibody, which attaches to target molecules in the cell, with a secondary antibody conjugated to a fluorescent dye, which specifically recognizes the primary antibody. Absorption and emission wavelengths and fluorescence intensities are important properties to consider in fluorophore selection. Autofluorescence is reduced by using fluorophores that are excited at wavelengths longer than 500 nm. For a thorough discussion of the optical properties of fluorophores, see Haugland (1992) and Brelje *et al.* (1993). [The secondary antibody is typically directed against immunoglobulins (usually IgGs) of the animal in which the primary antibody was produced. Thus, a secondary antibody against mouse IgG can be used with any primary IgG made in mouse, and a secondary against rat can be used with any primary IgG made in rat. By having on hand two of each, one conjugated to a green dye such as fluorescein and the other to a red dye such as Texas Red, the technician can readily set up double labeling of target molecules.]

An alternative method involves the use of the avidin/biotin-labeling system. This three-step method, which is based on the high affinity of egg white avidin for biotin, is highly specific and can result in increased label when the antigen is present in low concentrations. The secondary antibody is conjugated to biotin (biotinylation) and the reporter fluorophore is conjugated to the avidin.

Commercially available secondary antibodies are usually supplied lyophilized. They should be reconstituted with d-H_2O according to the manufacturer's recommendation, aliquoted as 0.005-ml drops into BEEM capsules or Eppendorf tubes, and frozen. Just before use, the concentrated antibody is further diluted. Filling a BEEM capsule, which holds 0.5 ml, results in a 1:100 dilution.

As with the primary antibody, the time of incubation in the secondary antibody will vary with the plant material. In our experience, it is not necessary to extend the time to more than 3–4 h.

C. Controls

Controls are important since they increase confidence in the specificity of immunostaining. Commonly used controls for the specificity of the primary antibody include the following:

1. Preabsorb the primary antibody with the antigen. No staining should occur.
2. Preabsorb with an inappropriate antigen (e.g., actin with anti-tubulin). Staining should not be affected.

Controls that test specificity of the secondary antibody include:

1. Omit the primary antibody.
2. Use nonimmune serum in place of the primary antibody.
3. Use an inappropriate primary antibody.

In all cases, no staining should be observed.

D. Double-Labeling

Any two antigens can be stained in the same preparation so long as the primary antibodies to them were produced in different animal species, and the secondary antibody to each is conjugated to a dye that fluoresces at a different wavelength. Secondary antibodies that exhibit minimal cross-reactivity with non-host IgGs are commercially available. Follow the staining of the first antigen with a thorough buffer wash, incubate in the next primary and secondary antibodies, and wash again.

For targeting plant microtubules, we use a monoclonal antibody produced in rat against yeast tubulin, YOL $\frac{1}{34}$, (Accurate Chemical and Scientific Corporation, Westbury, NJ). For localizing plant actin, we use a monoclonal antibody raised in mouse (Amersham, Arlington Heights, IL). Actin also can be stained directly with phalloidin (a fungal toxin) linked to a fluorochrome such as rhodamine or fluorescein.

E. Nuclear Staining

Plant cells stained with one or more antibodies can be counterstained with various dyes to contrast chromosomes and nuclei. A detailed discussion of DNA fluorochromes can be found in Haugland (1992). The three dyes listed below will also stain organellar DNA; plastid and mitochondrial DNA is seen as fluorescent dots surrounding the spindle in Fig. 2B. In all cases, 1% aqueous stock solutions are kept in lightproof containers in the refrigerator and are diluted to suitable concentrations by experimentation with the cells/tissue at hand. Most cells require no more than a 0.001% solution to stain chromosomes/nuclei in 10–30 s, even through an A-G film. The DNA stain can be added after the last buffer wash and followed by a d-H_2O wash before mounting the preparation.

Propidium iodide fluoresces red with the same filters and wavelengths used to view green fluorescence of fluorescein. This is convenient for viewing with the standard fluorescence microscope and the red/green image can be recorded with color film. For photography with black and white film, which does not distinguish red from green, the images can be separated by using a barrier filter to exclude red from the green image, and the red image can be viewed exclusively with green light excitation. The CLSM will collect the red and green emission signals separately. The Hoechst dyes (33258 and 33342) and DAPI fluoresce blue-white under ultraviolet illumination; this contrasts well with green and red fluorochromes. At present, these dyes are most widely used with conventional mercury arc lamp fluorescence since many confocal microscopes lack a UV laser.

IV. Mounting

A. Mounting Medium

After the final washing, coverslips with processed cells are inverted in a drop of mounting medium on a clean slide. Glycerol is a simple mounting medium but has the disadvantage of remaining liquid. Before viewing under oil-immersion, the edges of the coverslip must be sealed. The medium of choice is Mowiol 4-88 (Calbiochem Corp., La Jolla, CA), a water-miscible plastic that hardens within a few hours and requires no further sealing. A stock of Mowiol is prepared by combining 20 g Mowiol with 100 ml PBS, pH 8.5, and stirring with a stir bar for several hours; it is stored at 4°C. Ignore the few flecks of undissolved Mowiol that may remain on the bottom; these should be avoided by pipetting from the upper part of the solution.

B. Antifade Agents

Fading of fluorescent dyes can be retarded by the addition to the mounting medium of various agents such as *p*-phenylenediamine (Johnson *et al.*, 1982), *n*-propyl gallate (Giloh and Sedat, 1982), or DABCO (Johnson *et al.*, 1982). Several commercial mounting media containing antifade agents are also available. We obtain consistently good results with *p*-phenylenediamine in Mowiol, and this justifies the effort of preparation. Cells can be repeatedly photographed (even through several confocal Z-series) without appreciable reduction of signal. The following method was developed to avoid some of the difficulties involved in getting the extremely light-sensitive chemical into solution in cold Mowiol.

Weigh 0.005 g *p*-phenylenediamine and put into a small snap cap vial with a drop of d-H_20. Add a tiny stir bar and stir until the flake(s) of *p*-phenylenediamine breaks up and goes into solution, or nearly so. Then add 5 ml of stock Mowiol and stir briefly. Allow a few minutes for air bubbles to clear from the mixture. The solution, which is very pale straw color, will darken quickly if exposed to light, but can be kept for a few days (or even weeks) in a lightproof container in the freezer. Larger amounts can be aliquoted into small containers (BEEM capsules or Eppendorf tubes) to avoid repeated thawing and freezing. The mixture will go through a series of color changes and will eventually darken to a deep burgundy-black. The antifading agent is still effective when the color is light (peach to brick color); however, the mixture should be replaced when it darkens further. Another method is to put the *p*-phenylenediamine flakes into solution in PBS, aliquot into small containers, freeze, and add to Mowiol just before use.

Mounting: To mount the coverslip, place a generous bubble-free drop of Mowiol on a clean slide. Gently wipe dry the cell free surface of the coverslip. If the coverslip is covered with an A-G film, avoid wiping the edges to prevent pulling the film off with the Kimwipe. Invert the coverslip onto the drop of Mowiol. Do not blot away extra mounting medium unless it is really excessive (and reduce size of the drop in future), to allow for shrinkage of Mowiol with drying. Keep the finished slides flat in a dark box for several hours, preferably overnight, at room temperature to allow time for the Mowiol to harden and the antifading agent to become most effective. Preparations may remain brightly stained for several weeks if stored in the dark, or longer if frozen. If necessary, hardened Mowiol can be cleaned from the surface of the coverslip by wiping with a damp tissue, or the coverslip can be completely removed by soaking in water.

V. Image Recording

Methods of recording images for study and publication are dependent upon the type of microscopy used. In any case, the signal will be of low intensity. The microscope should be operated in a semidarkened room, and eyes allowed to become dark-adapted. For conventional photography, it is desirable to have a microscope configurated to deliver 100% of the light to the camera. Since film is not sensitive in the same wavelengths as human vision and the film is recording points of light on a black background, a test strip should be made with exposures that bracket the times indicated by the exposure meter. For black and white negatives, we use Kodak technical plan film, exposed at ASA 100, and developed according to specifications given for the film. Photobleaching can be a significant problem and can be minimized through the use of antifade additives and reducing exposure times by using high ASA (fast) films. Many of these problems are eliminated in video microscopy where the low light detection cameras reduce the adverse effects of fading. Extensive treatments of photomicroscopy are found in O'Brien and McCully (1981), Inoué (1986), and in the Eastman Kodak publication "Photography Through the Microscope."

VI. Sectioning Intact Tissues for Immunostaining

A. Steedman's Wax

Steedman's wax is a useful embedding material for plant materials that require sectioning before immunostaining (Brown *et al.,* 1989). Sectioning may be required either when dealing with intact tissues, or when encountering cell walls resistant to enzymatic digestion. Steedman's wax melts at a relatively low temperature (37°C) and can be serially sectioned with a glass or metal knife. The sections can be manipulated in H_2O and subsequently dewaxed by washing in absolute ethanol prior to immunostaining. Additionally, Steedman's wax can be cut ultrathin to permit observation with the TEM.

The components of Steedman's wax are polyethylene glycol (PEG) 400 distearate and 1-hexadecanol. To prepare the wax, put the bottle of PEG distearate in an oven or water bath at 40°C. When melted, pour about 200–250 ml into a preweighed plastic container; we use a 400-ml plastic widemouth container with a snap-cap cover. The PEG distearate will harden quickly. Weigh the container of PEG distearate, subtract the weight of the container, and add one-ninth the amount of 1-hexadecanol powder. Place the mixture in the oven just long enough for it to melt. Stir to mix, and store covered at room temperature.

To use the wax: Shave off a small amount and place in a small beaker or shell vial in the oven just prior to using. Do not melt more wax than you need at the time and do not remelt it repeatedly nor keep it molten for long periods (days). These practices adversely affect the sectioning characteristics of the wax. As with any wax technique, prepare ahead everything you will need, including a container for waste wax so that the oven door is left open no longer than necessary.

To prepare the material: Fix according to the protocol given above. The addition of 1 m*M* dithiothreitol (DTT) to all solutions used in washing and dehydrating may enhance stainability, perhaps by preventing degradation of proteins by free radicals and/or inhibiting protease activity. After fixation, you may want to stain lightly the material so that it is possible to orient the material in the opaque wax and locate it again for sectioning. After the buffer wash, stain the tissue with an aqueous solution of 1% acid fuchsin. Material may be dehydrated directly or preembedded in agar. If the material is small or difficult to see, it may be preembedded in agar and the entire agar block dehydrated and infiltrated with wax.

To preembed in agar: Make stock agar by adding 0.37 g purified agar (not agarose) to 25 ml d-H_2O in a small flask. Cover with aluminum foil and put into solution in a water bath brought to boiling. The stock agar can be stored in a refrigerator, but one should avoid concentrating it by evaporating water away in repeated reheatings. To use, liquify in a water bath brought to boiling, then reduce the heat to keep it just above the melting point. Leave a pipette in the agar to stay warm, as agar will solidify in a cold pipette. Distribute material in buffer into small embedding molds. You may place several pieces in each mold, but be certain to leave enough space between them to cut them apart later. We find that the caps of size 00 BEEM embedding capsules for electron microscopy are a convenient size. Remove buffer and replace immediately with warm agar to fill the container. After a few minutes the agar hardens and the entire cap is dropped into a vial of buffer. From this point on, the entire cap containing the material embedded in agar will be processed. The vial should be large enough to hold as many caps as you plan to process in a generous amount of fluid.

B. Dehydration, Infiltration, and Embedding

Dehydrate in a graded ethanol series, 20 min in each change of 15, 30, 50, 70, and 90% and three changes of 100%. We routinely dehydrate tissues at room temperature (ca. 20°C), although lowering the temperature to 0°C can reduce autofluorescence due to oxidization, and may help to stabilize mechanically delicate specimens (O'Brien and McCully, 1981). For some plant tissues, the addition of 1 m*M* DTT to the dehydrating series can improve staining.

Infiltration: Specimens are gradually infiltrated in a 40°C oven. Scrape off small flakes of wax from the stock and add to the vial containing material in 100% ethanol. Continue to add wax every hour until the mixture is about 1:1, then draw off some of the volume and discard. Keep the pipette in the oven, since the wax will solidify quickly in a cold pipette. Add melted wax for a 3:1 mixture. After 1 h replace with pure wax. Make three changes of pure wax, providing 1 h between each change. Vacuum evacuation at the pure wax stage may be helpful in removing the final traces of ethanol.

Embedding: If the material was preembedded in agar, skip this step. Pieces of material are transferred to molds of suitable size containing pure wax. The molds with wax should be kept on a heating table. Be sure to anticipate the eventual plane of sectioning since it is more difficult to reorient material after embedding. Position the material against the bottom of the mold with the surface to be sectioned lowermost. Remove from heat and allow to cool at room temperature.

If material was preembedded in agar, remove molds from the oven, place on paper toweling to remove excess wax from bottom of the molds, and allow to cool at room temperature.

C. Sectioning

Material embedded in Steedman's wax will section in same manner as paraffin-embedded material. Detailed instructions for paraffin sectioning are found in standard treatments of microtechnique such as O'Brien and McCully (1981). Material is removed from embedding molds and a pyramidal block cut with a razor blade. The block is attached to a block holder that fits a microtome chuck. We use a cylinder of plexiglass to hold the block. You can also recycle plastic cylinders previously used for TEM embedding, or use metal rods or wood dowels of similar diameter. The wax is attached to the block holder with cyanoacrylate cement ("superglue"). After sectioning, the used up blocks are cut from the holder with a razor blade and the holders recycled by renewing the surface with a fine toothed file.

The block is now ready for final trimming before microtomy. A histological microtome is adequate for sectioning. Steedman's wax exhibits minimal solubility in water so sections can be sectioned on a dry knife or wet into a boat. A histological steel microtome knife is adequate, although for convenience we use disposable Ralph-type glass knives. It is desirable to optimize conditions so that a ribbon of sections can be obtained. This facilitates handling and allows analysis of serial sections if desirable. Sections are cut from 2 to 15 μm in thickness, depending on the size of cells and other characteristics such as autofluorescence of the sample. Sections should be thin enough so that most cells are cut open to facilitate even access of antibodies. Optical sectioning capabilities of confocal microscopy allows observation of several cell layers, and very informative three-dimensional images can be produced (Figs. 2C and 2D).

D. Mounting Ribbons of Sections

Mounting the sections to substrate to prevent loss during lengthy staining procedures is critical to the success of any histological procedure. The ribbon of sections is removed from the knife using a fine camel hair brush, single bristle, or microtomist's hair. The ribbon is placed in a lint-free container until it is mounted and stained. How long the ribbon can be kept has not been determined, but sections held for several days can still be immunostained successfully. The ribbons can be mounted on either coverslips or glass slides. The advantage of coverslips is that volumes of solutions are easily controlled and more importantly, the section is immediately against the coverslip so epifluorescence is maximized while absorption and diffusion of light is at a minimum.

Coat clean coverslips with a thin film of Mayer's albumen (see section on Adhesives) and attach them (adhesive side up) with a small drop of water onto a glass slide for ease in handling. Place a drop of d-H_2O on the adhesive and float the ribbons of sections on the water. The ribbons will expand considerably, so allow enough space. Arrange the sections and allow to dry on a slide warmer maintained at a temperature just below the melting point of the wax (37°C). The ribbons can be further manipulated after expansion on the slide warmer by moving the wax around, but the tissue itself is extremely fragile and must not be touched directly. Once the sections have expanded and are aligned, excess water can be removed by carefully blotting with absorbent paper. The sections will adhere to the adhesive when dry and need not be covered with an A-G film. If sections do not adhere properly, prepare a fresh batch of Mayer's albumen adhesive.

E. Dewaxing and Immunostaining

Steedman's wax is removed from the sections with absolute ethanol. The sections are less likely to float off of the coverslip if completely dried onto the coverslip. Although coverslips can be placed vertically in a staining jar, it is safer to add the enthanol to the surface of a horizontal coverslip. The alcohol is poured off and more added several times until no wax is visible, then rinsed a few more times. It is important that the solvent be completely anhydrous, as even the slightest amount of moisture may result in sections with residual wax. After dewaxing, the sections are allowed to dry. Sections should not require treatment with enzymes to remove walls or detergent treatment for permeabilization if all cells have a cut surface. In practice, however, it is wise to do both before immunostaining as described above, especially if walls exhibit autofluorescence. We have not experimented with critical-point-drying after staining, a step which may be necessary if the sections are used for electron microscopy.

A general schedule for staining dewaxed sections for immunolight microscopy is as follows:

1. Enzymatic wall removal, 5 min. This step is optional.
   Buffer wash, 3 × 5 min
2. Extraction with detergent, 5 min. Again, this is optional.
   Buffer wash, 3 × 5 min
3. Incubation in primary antibody, 1–2 h
   Buffer wash, 3 × 5 min
4. Incubation in secondary antibody, 1–2 h
   ----to double label, repeat steps 3 and 4 with another set of antibodies.
   Buffer wash, 3 × 5 min
5. Nuclear stain
   d-H_2O wash, 5 min
6. Mount coverslip to slide

VII. Perspectives

Immunohistochemistry is a basic tool in cell and molecular biology. The methods described in this chapter have been tested on a diversity of plant cell types ranging from algae to orchids. The methods allow detection of antigen in isolated cells and intact tissues. These basic methods will be continually refined with developments in cellular and molecular biology, immunology, and imaging technology. Interesting new applications, such as the detection of *in situ* hybridization, in addition to demands for stronger and more permanent signals, should lead the way to further rapid improvements and exciting new dimensions in the field of immunolight microscopy.

Acknowledgments

We thank Drs. Ann L. Cleary and Tom Pesacreta for help is developing techniques, Dr. O.-A. Olsen for providing fixed and embedded young barley seeds, and Linda LeBlanc for image processing and photography. The author's research has been supported by grants from the NSF, most recently by DCB-9104528.

References

Anonymous. (1988). "Photography through the Microscope," 9th Ed. Rochester, NY: Eastman Kodak Corp.

Asai, D. J., ed. (1993). "Methods in Cell Biology," Vol. 37. San Diego: Academic Press.

Baluska, F., Parker, J. S., and Barlow, P. W. (1992). Specific patterns of cortical and endoplasmic microtubules associated with cell growth and tissue differentiation in roots of maize (*Zea mays* L.). *J. Cell Sci.* **103,** 191–200.

Borrebaeck, C. A. K., ed. (1992). "Antibody Engineering: A Practical Guide." New York: W. H. Freeman.

Brelje, T. C., Wessendorf, M. W., and Sorenson, R. L. (1993). Multicolor laser scanning confocal immunofluorescence microscopy: Practical application and limitations. *Methods Cell Biol.* **38,** 97–181.

Brown, R. C., Lemmon, B. E., and Mullinax, J. B. (1989). Immunofluorescent staining of microtubules in plant tissues: Improved embedding and sectioning techniques using polyethylene glycol (PEG) and Steedman's wax. *Bot. Acta* **102,** 54–61.

Clearly, A. L., Brown, R. C., and Lemmon, B. E. (1992). Establishment of division plane and mitosis in monoplastidic guard mother cells of *Selaginella. Cell Motil. Cytoskel.* **23,** 89–101.

De Mey, J., Lambert, A.-M., Bajer, A. S., Moremans, M., and de Brabander, M. (1982). Visualization of microtubules in interphase and mitotic plant cells of *Haemanthus* with the immunogold staining method. *Proc. Natl. Acad. Sci. U.S.A.* **79,** 1898–1902.

Giloh, H., and Sedat, J. W. (1982). Fluorescence microscopy: Reduced photobleaching of rhodamine and fluorescein protein conjugates by *n*-propyl gallate. *Science* **217,** 1252–1255.

Gunning, B. E. S. (1992). Use of confocal microscopy to examine transitions between successive microtubule arrays in the plant cell division cycle. *In* "Proceedings of the VII International Symposium (Cellular basis of growth and development in plants)" (H. Shibaoka, ed.), pp. 145–155. Osaka, Japan: Osaka University Press.

Hames, B. D., and Rickwood, D. eds. (1981). "Gel Electrophoresis of Proteins: A Practical Approach." Oxford: IRL Press.

Hames, B. D., and Rickwood, D., eds. (1990). "Gel Electrophoresis of Proteins: A Practical Approach," 2nd Ed. Oxford: IRL Press.

Harlow, E., and Lane, D. (1988). "Antibodies: A Laboratory Manual." Cold Spring, NY: Cold Spring Harbor Laboratory.

Haugland, R. P. (1992). "Handbook of Fluorescent Probes and Research Chemicals," 5th Ed. Eugene, Oregon: Molecular Probes.

Hepler, P. K., Cleary, A. L., Gunning, B. E. S., Wadsworth, P., Wasteneys, G. O., and Zhang, D. H. (1993). Cytoskeletal dynamics in living plant cells. *Cell Biol. Int.* **17,** 127–142.

Inoué, S. (1986). "Video Microscopy." New York: Plenum.

Johnson, G. D., Davidson, R. S., McNamee, K. C., Russell, G., Goodwin, D., and Holborow, E. J. (1982). Fading of immunofluorescence during microscopy: A study of the phenomenon and its remedy. *J. Immunol. Methods* **26,** 231–242.

Liddell, J. E., and Cryer, A. (1991). "A Practical Guide to Monoclonal Antibodies." New York: Wiley.

Matsumoto, B., ed. (1993). Cell biological applications of confocal microscopy. "Methods in Cell Biology," Vol. 38. San Diego: Academic Press.

Molè-Bajer, J., and Bajer, A. S. (1968). Studies of selected endosperm cells with the light and electron microscope. The technique. *Cellule* **67,** 257–265 + 5 plates.

Molè-Bajer, J., Bajer, A. S., and Inoué, S. (1988). 3-dimensional localization and redistribution of F-actin in higher plant mitosis and cell plate formation. *Cell Motil. Cytoskel.* **10,** 217–228.

O'Brien, T. P., and McCully, M. E. (1981). The study of plant structure. "Principles and Selected Methods." Melbourne, Australia: Termarcarphi Pty, Ltd.

Otto, J. J. (1993). Immunoblotting. *Methods Cell Biol.* **37,** 105–117.

Pawley, J., ed. (1989). "The Handbook of Biological Confocal Microscopy." Madison, Wisc.: IMR Press.

Peters, J. H., and Baumgarten, H., eds. (1992). "Monoclonal antibodies." New York: Springer-Verlag.

Schliwa, M., and van Blerkom, J. (1981). Structural interaction of cytoskeletal components. *J. Cell Biol.* **90,** 222–235.

Wick, S. M., and Duniec, J. (1986). Effects of various fixatives on the reactivity of plant cell tubulin and calmodulin in immunofluorescence microscopy. *Protoplasma* **133,** 1–18.

CHAPTER 8

Confocal Epipolarization Microscopy of Gold Probes in Plant Cells and Protoplasts

Lawrence R. Griffing,[*] Marco A. Villanueva,[*] Josephine Taylor,[†] and Scott Moon[*]

[*] Department of Biology
Texas A&M University
College Station, Texas 77843-3258

[†] Department of Biology
Stephen F. Austin University
Nacogdoches, Texas 75962-3003

I. Introduction

Since its initial application to immunocytochemistry in 1983 (de Mey, 1983), nonconfocal epipolarization microscopy of colloidal gold or silver-enhanced colloidal gold has been widely used (Scopsi, 1989; Hacker, 1989). Many of the objects in biological samples weakly reflect epi-illumination, but only highly ordered structures change its polarization. If reflective gold or silver crystals, which repolarize the light, are introduced into the sample, then they appear bright on a dark backgound, when viewed under crossed epipolarizing filters. Epipolarization microscopy of gold–antibody or gold–ligand conjugates requires relatively large, 20- to 40-nm, gold particles (Ellis *et al.,* 1988; de Brabander *et al.,* 1986). However, gold clusters as small as 1.4 nm (Nanogold; Hainfield and Furuya, 1992) can be detected with epipolarization microscopy if they are made larger by *in situ* silver enhancement, the process whereby gold provides a nucleation site for silver crystallite growth under reducing conditions.

A major strength of colloidal gold as a cellular probe is the ability to visualize it with both light and electron microscopy. Gold particle sizes that are optimal for use with immunoelectron microscopy, 5 to 15 nm, can be silver-enhanced for direct correlative studies of tissue distribution with light microscopy (Stout and Griffing, 1993; VandenBosch, 1990). The purpose of this chapter is to describe, by example, how the cellular distribution of colloidal gold can be imaged in three dimensions at the light level using confocal laser scanning microscopy (CLSM) in the epipolarization mode (confocal laser scanning epipolarization microscopy, CLSEM).

The conventional use of CLSM in biological samples has been for fluorescence analysis (White *et al.,* 1987; Brackenhoff *et al.,* 1989). Confocal laser scanning fluorescence microscopy (CLSFM) gives much sharper images because out-of-focus fluoresced light, scatter, and flare are reduced (Wilson, 1990). By providing sharp optical sections in the *z* dimension, a better understanding of the 3D organization of the structure is possible. Although suggestions have been published concerning the possibility of using epipolarization optics in confocal laser scanning microscopes (Sarafis, 1990), it has only recently been reported (Villanueva *et al.,* 1993a,b; Taylor *et al.,* 1995).

Applications of CLSEM described here include (*a*) fluid phase uptake of gold colloids by plant protoplasts, (*b*) analysis of ligand–gold binding to plant cells and protoplasts, and (*c*) determination of cytoplasmic and wall delivery of biolistic gold beads. All of these applications have been developed to overcome challenges posed by the structure and physiology of the plant cell, i.e., the cell wall-imposed limitation of delivery of macromolecules to the cell surface and cytoplasm and the presence of anion-carriers on the plasma membrane and tonoplast that efficiently scavenge and compartmentalize fluorescent anions such as fluorescein isothiocyanate (FITC), carboxyfluorescein, and lucifer yellow CH (LY), which are frequently used, either free or in conjugated form, for the study endocytic processes.

II. Configuring a Confocal Laser Scanning Microscope for Epipolarization

Just as CLSFM uses an optical configuration similar to conventional epifluoresence microscopy, so CLSEM (Fig. 1A) uses a configuration similar to conventional epipolarization microscopy (Fig. 1B). Unlike conventional epipolarization, however, no initial polarizer is needed, since the laser source is usually polarized.

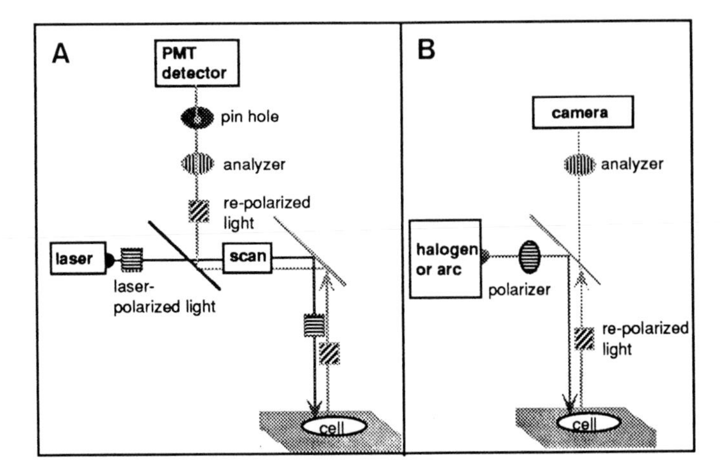

Fig. 1 Comparison of confocal laser-scanning epipolarization microscopy (CLSEM) configuration (A) with that of conventional, nonlaser epipolarization microscopy (B). For simplicity intermediate optical elements including projection lenses and objectives are not shown.

In some machines, however, the laser light is circularly polarized by a quarter wave plate in order to avoid orientation effects (Brakenhoff *et al.,* 1990).

Configuration of a fluorescence confocal microscope for epipolarization is done by simply installing the analyzer (dichroic sheet polarizer) in the emission-side filter holder and aligning the azimuth of polarization orthogonal to that of the laser. The analyzer alignment would be identical to that empirically found when the polarizing filter is placed on the sample stage and turned to the point of maximum extinction (i.e., the position at which transmitted laser light is lowest).

The analyzer is placed in the light path before the pinhole (Fig. 1A) and reflective objects that repolarize the light are seen with high contrast (Fig. 2A). The azimuth of polarization of the analyzer is critical, as seen by comparing images of an agarose-embedded gold bead preparation in reflection and epipolarization modes (Fig. 2). Figure 2B shows total reflection (analyzer azimuth $\|$ laser polarization), whereas Fig. 2A shows epipolarization (analyzer azimuth $\perp$ laser polarization). The intensity of total reflection from the sample is proportional to the difference in refractive indices of the sample and its surround (Cheng and Summers, 1990). Although the difference between the refractive index of biological objects and that of the aqueous surround is small, it is significant; e.g., it provides the basis for contrast formation in phase contrast microscopy. In Fig. 2B, the gold bead reflects strongly, but the image is very noisy because particles of the agar matrix also reflect and scatter light. The gold bead, however, repolarizes the incident light, and can thereby be distinguished from all the other reflective components with high contrast when viewed with epipolarization (Fig. 2A).

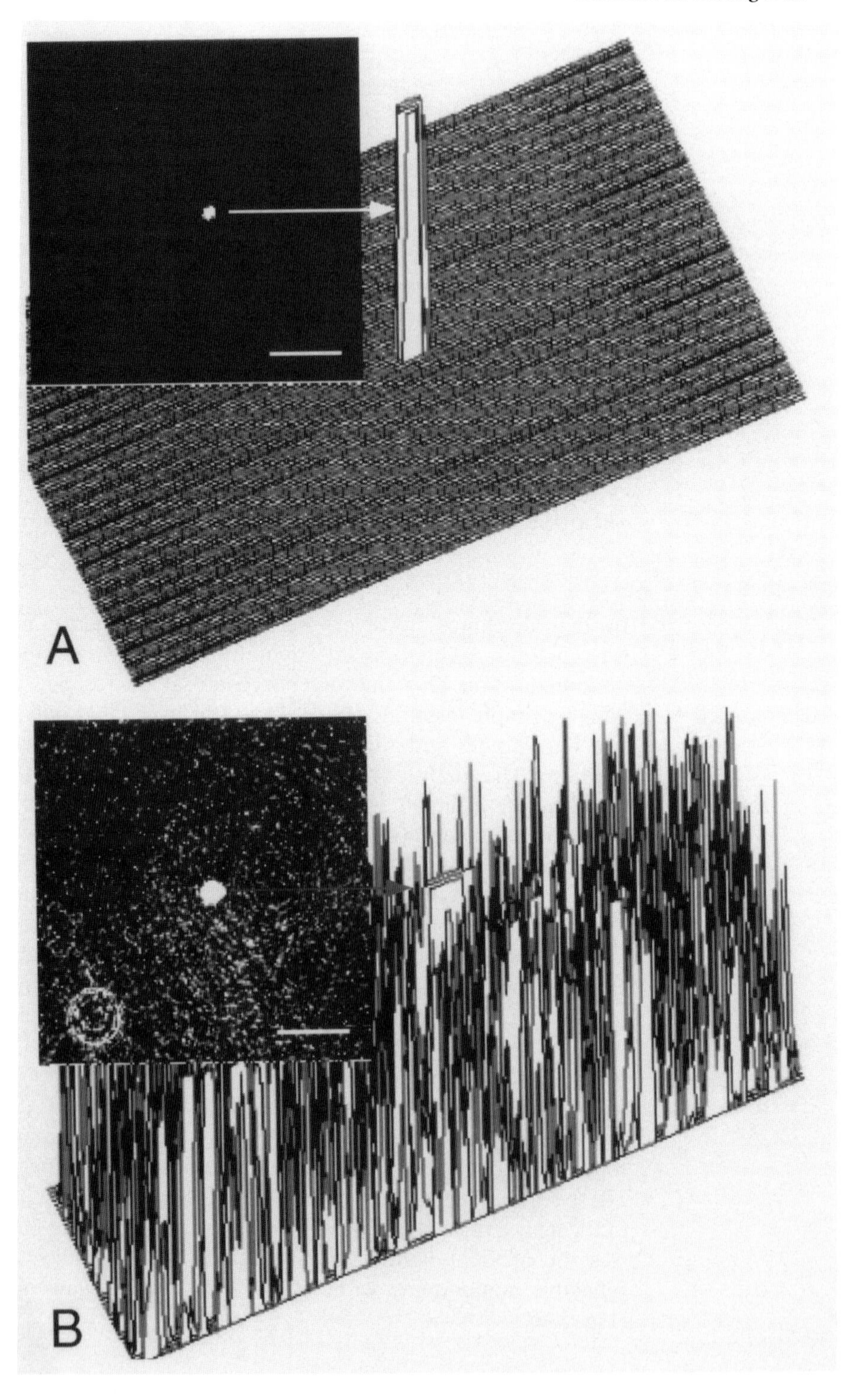
A
B

Although there are several reports of the application of confocal laser scanning reflection microscopy (CLSRM) to living (Cheng and Summers, 1990) and nonliving, fixed tissues (Van den Pol, 1989; Boyde, 1993), few have used epipolarization. Cheng and Summers (1990) show an optical arrangement that includes a quarter wavelength retardation plate positioned near the objective in combination with a standard polarizer and analyzer configuration. This is used for the reduction of reflection from internal components of the optical system. It is not epipolarization in the sense used here because the quarter wave plate circularly polarizes the beam before and after it hits the object. A similar optical configuration is described by Masters and Kino (1993) for Nipkow disk-based scanning systems, which use incandescent or arc light sources.

The major advantage of CLSEM is the use of reflection instead of fluorescence. Reflectance analysis of planar objects provides intrinsically higher signal and axial resolution over fluorescence analysis (Sheppard *et al.*, 1992). Consequently, in fixed, silver-enhanced tissues, CLSEM could give better results than CLSFM. It provides another channel for analysis with little cross-talk into other channels used for fluorescence (for an example of dual reflectance/fluorescence analysis, see below). Furthermore, it does so without changing lasers.

III. Imaging Colloidal Gold in Protoplasts

A. Fluid Phase Uptake of BSA–Colloidal Gold

Two current goals in the study of plant endocytosis are to determine the basal level of uptake and to show how the plant deals with occupied cell surface receptors of cell signaling molecules. Initial studies on the rate of fluid phase endocytosis in plants employed FITC-dextran and LY (Griffing, 1988; Wright and Oparka, 1989). Although a component of fluorescent probe uptake may arise from vesicle-mediated internalization, a large component comes from uptake via anion channels of free FITC or LY. This was initially discovered in yeast, where endocytosis was measured with preparations of FITC-dextran that were probably contaminated with free FITC. This FITC was shown to enter via nonvesicular means (Preston *et al.*, 1987). Although endocytosis has been shown with well-prepared FITC conjugates in plants in both protoplasts (Griffing, 1988) and intact cells (Cole *et al.*, 1990), the other probe routinely used for endocytosis

Fig. 2 Comparison of CLSM epipolarization signal with CLSM total reflectance signal from a gold bead in agarose. (A) CLSEM: Density plot of image inset taken with azimuth of analyzer polarization at 90° to azimuth of polarization of laser. White arrow points from bead image to density plot of bead image. (B) CLSRM: Density plot of image inset taken with azimuth of analyzer polarization at 0° to azimuth of polarization of laser. Gray arrow points from bead image to density plot of bead image. Scale bars on image insets, 10 μm. Plotted values show 8-bit signal, with peak at 256 gray levels plotted in z dimension.

measurements in yeast and animal cells (Griffiths *et al.*, 1989), LY, is frequently sequestered into the vacuole in plants via plasma membrane and vacuolar anion channels (Oparka, 1991).

Bovine serum albumin (BSA) coupled to colloidal gold, Table I, has been widely used and accepted as a probe for fluid phase endocytosis in animal cell systems (Hermo *et al.*, 1985; Griffiths *et al.*, 1989). We have demonstrated that it can also be used as a fluid phase marker with soybean protoplasts (Villanueva *et al.*, 1993a). Protoplasts were incubated in BSA–gold at various concentrations for various times, fixed with 1% (v/v) glutaraldehyde, and silver-enhanced *en bloc,* Table III. Uptake was visualized using CSLEM (Fig. 3, see Color Plates). Quantitation could be done by adsorbing protoplasts onto nitrocellulose, silver-enhancing the blot, and determining the relative amount of silver-enhanced gold using video densitometry. The uptake was shown to be nonsaturable with time and concentration (Villanueva *et al.*, 1993a; Taylor *et al.*, 1995) and temperature-dependent.

B. Plant Receptor Ligands Conjugated to Colloidal Gold

Surface receptors and their fate have been very difficult to visualize in plants. To approach this problem, gold probes have been developed for ligands to specific receptors on the plant plasma membrane, Tables I and II (Villanueva *et al.*, 1993b; Taylor *et al.*, 1995). The two ligands that have been chosen are

Table I
Stabilization of 10 nm Colloidal Gold with BSA and Fusicoccin-Conjugated BSA (FC-BSA)[a]

1. Place 1 ml of 1 mg/ml BSA (globulin-free, Catalog No. A-7638, Sigma Chemical Co. St. Louis, MO) on the bottom of a flask or a new sterile plastic tube.[b]
2. Add 10 ml of the colloidal gold solution (Slot and Geuze, 1985) at once and swirl for 2 min.
3. Add 250 μl 1% (w/v) polyethylene glycol (1,500–12,000 MW) solution and swirl for 1 min.
4. Add 100 μl of 50 mg/ml BSA solution and swirl for 1 min.
5. Add 500 μl 0.1 *M* sodium phosphate buffer, pH 6.9, and swirl for 1 min.
6. Test the stability by mixing 100 μl of the solution with 100 μl 10% (w/v) NaCl in a small tube; a stable solution will remain bright pink whereas nonstabilized gold will flocculate and form a purple to steel blue solution.
7. Store the solution at 4°C; do not add any preservatives and use promptly.
8. Just before incubation with the cells wash three times by centrifugation at 44,000 $\times$ *g* and resuspension of the mobile pool in the appropriate buffer. In our particular case we use Sorb/Mes-1B5, pH 5.8 (Villanueva *et al.*, 1993a,b).
9. Miniprep for FC–BSA: The above steps can be converted to a miniprep procedure in which the reagents are reduced to one-tenth of the volume.

[a] FC–BSA was made according to the procedure of Pini *et al.* (1979)

[b] The procedure is carried out at 25°C; if the solutions are cold, allow them to reach the adequate temperature.

Table II
Stabilization of 10 nm Colloidal Gold with a β-Glucan Oligosaccharide Elicitor

1. Place 520 μl of a 1 mg/ml Pre-A glucan[a] solution in a flask.
2. Add 20 ml of the colloidal gold solution and swirl for 2 min.
3. Add 500 μl of 1% PEG and mix for 1 min.
4. Add 200 μl of a 50 mg/ml BSA solution and mix for 1 min.
5. Add 1 ml of 0.1 *M* sodium phosphate buffer, pH 7.
6. Steps 6, 7, and 8 as with the BSA–gold conjugate in Table I.

Miniprep:
As with BSA–gold, we have successfully made the probe using a miniprep procedure in which the reagents are reduced to one-tenth of the volume.

Additional Suggestions:
1. Use newly made gold colloid; even when the colloidal gold can be stored sterile and at 4°C, the amount of conjugate recovered decreases with time of storage of the colloid.
2. Use freshly prepared conjugates. Conjugates should not be stored frozen and (of course) metabolic poison preservatives cannot be used for *in vivo* work.
3. Check the concentration of ligand required for gold stabilization by making serial dilutions of the ligand at the appropriate pH (for proteins, a pH value 0.5 units above the pI; Slot and Geuze, 1985). Add 250 μl of gold sol to 250 μl of each dilution, then test for stability by adding 500 μl of 10% sodium chloride.

[a] Pre-A glucan is a 10–20 mer mixture of a β1-6, β1-3 glucose oligosaccharide (Cheong *et al.*, 1991) and was a kind gift of Dr. Michael G. Hahn (Complex Carbohydrate Research Center, University of Georgia, Athens, GA).

fusicoccin, a diterpene glucoside, and a β-glucan oligomer that elicits a defense response in soybean. Both of these present certain difficulties for gold labeling. Fusicoccin is a very small molecule and adsorption to a large colloid particle might sterically hinder the binding site. The glucan elicitor is an oligosaccharide, very few of which have been adsorbed to colloidal gold (an exception is the mannan discussed in Horisberger and Rosset, 1977). The use of gold probes for studying endocytosis of ligand–receptor complexes overcomes the potential problem of loss or dislocation of fluorophores from the ligand. This is particularly important when studying ligands that may come to reside in the vacuole (Horn *et al.*, 1989), since the fluorophores may ultimately be sequestered there via anion channels (Oparka, 1991).

Gold probes labeled with fusicoccin have been made by first conjugating fusicoccin to BSA, then coupling BSA to gold, Table I. The fusicoccin–BSA conjugate is physiologically active in the same concentration range as free fusicoccin (Feyerabend and Weiler, 1989). CLSEM of FC–BSA gold in protoplasts shows extensive binding to the cell surface (Fig. 4, see Color Plates) and, ultimately, perinuclear localization (Villanueva and Griffing, unpublished observations).

Glucan elicitor derived from *Phytophthora megasperma* f.sp. *glycinea* is conjugated to colloidal gold through a modification of the technique used for proteins, Table II. When added to plant protoplasts, CLSEM reveals that it binds to the plasma membrane (Fig. 5, see Color Plates) and is ultimately delivered to the vacuole (Taylor *et al.,* 1995).

C. Experimental Conditions for CLSEM of Colloidal Gold

Colloidal gold particles of very uniform size can be prepared for use as probes by the tannic acid method of Slot and Geuze (1985). The size of the colloid varies between 10 and 15 nm, depending on the amount of tannic acid used. The colloids are unstable in high ionic strength solutions until coated with macromolecules. Acid-cleaned, silanized glassware is essential in colloid production and conjugation.

When incubating protoplasts in gold conjugate, several conditions must be controlled in order to minimize gold flocculation. We have found the following to be most important: (*a*) the freshness and sterility of the colloid conjugate, (*b*) the pH of the incubation media, and (*c*) the physical integrity of the protoplasts.

The colloidal gold solutions should be stored aseptically at 4°C. BSA conjugated with older colloidal gold solutions not maintained sterile will bind to the plasma membrane and give higher values for "uptake" than BSA conjugated with freshly prepared colloid. To avoid this artifact a fresh solution of colloidal gold is essential for conjugation with the protein. If storage is necessary, the freshly made colloidal gold solution can be filter-sterilized through a 0.22-μm filter and kept in a sterile plastic tube for about 4 months. After 4 months, new colloidal gold solution should be prepared to assure freshness.

The pH of the incubation medium influences the nonspecific association of stabilized colloidal gold sols. This is a particularly important point for plant cells, where the external pH is 5.5–6. At pH values lower than 5, gold conjugates clump or flocculate in solution and associate strongly with the plasma membrane of protoplasts in a nondissociable manner. Behnke *et al.* (1986) and Geoghegan (1988) have shown this to be disadsorption of the conjugate from gold at low pH. The gold then flocculates and associates with the membrane through hydrophobic interactions.

Any cellular debris can trap gold particles and form a surface for additonal nonspecific adsorption. Its elimination is achieved through gentle handling of protoplast suspensions (wide-mouth pipettes, no air bubbles) and through floatation on 8% (w/v) dextran (Galbraith and Northcote, 1977; Villanueva *et al.,* 1993a). Only intact protoplasts float to the dextran-wash medium interface, while debris sediments. At the end of the gold–conjugate treatment and just prior to fixation, the cells can be floated again in Eppendorf tubes, collected from the interface of dextran-wash medium and fixed.

D. *En bloc* or Whole Mount Silver Enhancement of Colloidal Gold or Nanogold

The silver enhancement step is a very critical one. There are several options for the preparation of a silver-enhancer (Stierhof *et al.,* 1992). These include an acidic silver lactate reagent, a neutral silver lactate reagent, a silver lacetate reagent and the commercial kits Intense M, pH 7.3, from Amersham, Inc. (Arlington Heights, IL), and the R-Gent, pH 5.5, from Aurion (Wageningen, The Netherlands). The commercial kits have the advantage that the initiator and the enhancer are supplied and they only require mixing prior to the silver-enhancing step. In addition, they can be handled safely in daylight, whereas others are light sensitive and should be handled under a red safelight (Stierhof *et al.,* 1992).

Protoplasts are fixed in 1% w/v glutaraldehyde overnight at 4°C prior to *en bloc* silver enhancement of the internalized gold conjugate. After several water washes, the IntenseM silver-enhancement kit from Amersham is used, as described in Table III. Time and temperature of enhancement have to be controlled, as outlined in the protocol below, in order to obtain silver crystallite sizes that provide adequate reflectance signal for CLSEM but do not mask cellular components. Furthermore, protoplasts are fragile and rough handling during silver enhancement alone can disrupt them, leading to the presence of clumped nonspecific (nongold) nucleation sites on cell fragments. This is aggravated by lower pH values (i.e., pH 4). Low temperature is used to stop the reaction as immediately as possible, because removal of the reagents through washing would take more than 5 min.

E. Image Acquisition and Processing

Silver-enhanced gold-labeled protoplasts can be examined with CLSEM in a small droplet of water under a coverslip "bridge." When intact cells are viewed, suspension in 1% low-melting-temperature agarose is recommended. This avoids the problem of cell movement during optical sectioning.

The initial settings on the machine for optimal epipolarization signal can be adjusted using an unlabeled control cell or tissue. The "control" or "blank" tissue should be carried through steps identical to those of gold-treated tissue, but without the gold-labeling step. Silver-enhanced "controls" have little more

Table III
***En bloc* or Whole-Mount Silver Enhancement of Colloidal Gold and Nanogold in Fixed Plant Protoplasts or Cells with IntenseM (Amersham, Inc.)**

1. Allow the "initiator" and the "enhancer" solutions to reach room temperature.
2. Add 400 μl of the "enhancer" mixture to the tubes containing the fixed protoplast pellets; resuspend the cells immediately.
3. Incubate at 24°C for 10–15 min in waterbath or agitator, carefully monitoring the pellets. As soon as they become visibly light gray, start the centrifugation step (below) immediately.
4. Cool to 4°C and wash four times in cold water[a] ($100 \times g_{av}$).

[a] If instead of cold temperature, 2.5% w/v sodium thiosulfate or 1% v/v acetic acid is used to stop the silver deposition, some label is removed.

epipolarization background signal than cells, but it is important to carry out this step, if there is some structure that acts as a nucleating site for silver which is not the gold probe. Suitable brightness (voltage) and contrast (gain) settings are empirically determined for sample examination by adjusting them to a point just below detectability in the controls. Images from control samples should be acquired and analyzed for pixel intensities with a gray level higher than 1. If there are any, this level should be subtracted from the images of the gold-treated tissue that are acquired. We routinely acquire images in the epipolarization mode that are then thresholded to the gray level of the "noise" found in the control tissues. The thresholded images are then converted into binary files, which are then superimposed in a single bit onto 8-bit DIC (differential interference contrast) or fluorescence images of the cell. That bit can then be pseudo-colored to red for optimal visual contrast for presentation.

The laser used for reflectance can be chosen based on the gold particle sizes used. Large (>1 μm) gold particles reflect red more strongly, whereas the smaller particles reflect blue or green (Sarafis, 1990). The same laser for fluorescence and reflectance can be used with appropriate filter and photomultiplier tube settings.

When analyzing the fate of ligands that have been internalized by cells, it is necessary to set a criterion for discriminating between internal and external label. The criterion that we have used is that in order to be classed as "internal," the label must be 6 μm from the DIC-determined cell periphery in optical sections. This is based on the empirical uncertainty of the precise cell boundary in DIC optical sections (up to 2 μm in a median section), the axial resolution of the microscope (twice the lateral resolution of about 400 nm), and the size of the silver grain or gold particle (up to 1.5 μm, depending on enhancement time).

A method that provides inherently more contrast of the outer boundary of the cell is through fluorophore label of cellular proteins, Table IV. We have applied this method to both suspension cultures of soybean and roots from soybean seedlings. The presence of free aldehyde groups after aldehyde fixation of the cells is exploited and an amine- containing fluorophore (Texas Red cadaverine, Table IV) is introduced. This fluorophore is linked covalently to the free

Table IV
Labeling the Cytoplasm of Fixed Plant Cells and Protoplasts with Texas Red

1. Aldehyde-fixed and silver-enhanced cells or tissues are washed once by centrifugation and resuspension in 0.1 *M*, pH 8, phosphate buffer.
2. Resuspend cells in 1 ml 0.1 *M* phosphate buffer, add 4.5×10^{-4} nmol TRSC[a] (Texas Red sulfonyl cadaverine, Molecular Probes, Inc., Eugene, OR), and mix well in this suspension.
3. Incubate 1 h in the dark on ice.
4. Wash the cells as above three times with 1% (w/v) ammonium chloride and two times with water.
5. Resuspend the cells in 500 μl water and analyze immediately.

[a] TRSC can be conveniently dissolved in ethanol as a stock from which the equivalent amounts can be added.

aldehydes of fixative that has only partially reacted with cellular proteins. Optical sections of the fluorescence are acquired before epipolarization analysis in order to avoid bleaching of the fluorophore. The signal from the fluorescent molecule is not detected by the photomultiplier in epipolarization mode adjusted to the epipolarization signal detection parameters and with epi-illumination from the 488-nm argon laser.

IV. Imaging Biolistically Delivered Gold Beads

A common method for getting foreign DNA into walled plant cells is to use DNA-coated metal beads explosively delivered into the cytoplasm or nucleus, i.e., biolistics (Klein *et al.,* 1992). The explosive force is sufficient to carry the particles through the cell wall and outer membrane and into the nucleus and cytoplasm of the outer layers of cells of the tissue. The disposition of the beads, once delivered has not been well studied beyond the initital description that they do, indeed, get into the cytoplasm (Klein *et al.,* 1987). CLSEM has been employed recently to reveal the disposition of the beads introduced into onion epidermal cells (Fig. 6, see Color Plates).

Gold particles (1.5 μm) were introduced into the epidermal cells as described in the instruction manual of the Biolistic PDS-1000/He particle delivery system (Bio-Rad Laboratories, Richmond, CA). The cells were then incubated in fluorescein diacetate (FDA) and viewed with the HeNe laser for epipolarized reflectance and with the Argon laser for FDA fluorescence. The fluorescein was sequestered into the peripheral ER system as described by Quader and Schnepf (1986). In Fig. 6A, the total distribution of the gold particles on the tissue can be seen. Most of the gold remains in the outer wall. The presence of the gold particles just outside the wall is shown in Fig. 6B, where the gold is shown as white-gold and the ER system is seen as red.

V. Conclusions

CLSEM provides a convenient alternative to labeling strategies that would otherwise require the addition of another laser for multichannel laser-scanning confocal analysis of biological specimens. The three-dimensional information on the location of gold probes that derives from CLSEM complements the information that can be derived from silver-enhanced gold-treated sections at the light level and the ultrastructural studies done with electron microscopy. CLSEM could be used to advantage in many of the present widespread applications of gold probes to immunolocalization and ligand binding at the cellular level. In the future, this technique will be easily applied to newly introduced direct-view confocal systems.

Acknowledgements

We thank Rhône-Poulenc Agrochemie and the Texas Applied Research Program for financial support. The Texas A&M Biological Imaging Laboratory and EMC provided access to instrumentation. Comments from Georges Freyssinet, Jean Varagnat, and Kate VandenBosch were much appreciated. Richard Stout and Michael Hahn graciously provided critical reagents.

References

Behnke, O., Ammitzboll, T., Jessen, H., Klokker, M., Nilausen, K., Tranum-Jensen, J., and Olsson, L. (1986). Non-specific binding of protein-stabilied gold sols as a source of errror in immunocytochemistry. *Eur. J. Cell Biol.* **41,** 326–338.

Boyde, A. (1993). Real-time direct-view laser scanning microscopy. *In* "Electronic Light Microscopy" (D. Shotton, ed.), pp. 289–314. New York: Wiley-Liss.

Brakenhoff, G. J., van Spronsen, E. A., van der Voort, H. T. M., and Nonninga, N. (1989). Three dimensional confocal fluorescence microscopy. *Methods Cell Biol.* **30,** 379–398.

Brakenhoff, G. J., van der Voort, H. T. M., and Oud, J. L. (1990). Three-dimensional representation in confocal microscopy. *In* "Confocal Microscopy" (T. Wilson, ed.), pp. 185–197. London: Academic Press.

Cheng, P. C., and Summers, R. G. (1990). Image contrast in confocal light microscopy. *In* "Handbook of Biological Microscopy" (J. B. Pawley, ed.), pp. 179–195. New York/London: Plenum.

Cheong, J. J., Birberg, W., Fugedi, P., Pilotti, A., Garegg, P. J.. Hong, N., Ogawa, T., and Hahn, M. G. (1991). Structure-activity relationships of oligo-β-glucoside elicitors of phytoalexin accumulation in soybean. *Plant Cell* **3,** 127–136.

Cole, L. Coleman, J. Evans, D., and Hawes, C. (1990). Internalization of fluorescein isothiocyanate and fluorescein isothiocyanate-dextran by suspension-cultured plant cell. *J. Cell Sci.* **96,** 721–730.

de Brabander, M., Nuydens, R., Geuens, G. Moeremans, M., and De Mey, J. (1986). The use of submicroscopic gold particles combined with video contrast enhancement as a simple molecular probe for the living cell. *Cell Mot. Cytoskel.* **6,** 105.

de Mey, J. (1983). Colloidal gold probes in immunocytochemistry. *In* "Immunocytochemistry. Practical Applications in Pathology and Biology" (J. Polak and S. Van Noorden, eds.), pp. 82–112. Bristol/London: Wright PSG.

Ellis, I. O., Bell, J., and Bancroft, J. D. (1988). An investigation of optimal gold particle size for immunohistological immunogold and immunogold-silver staining to be viewed by polarized incident light (epipolarization) microscopy. *J. Histochem. Cytochem.* **36,** 121–124.

Feyerabend, M., and Weiler, E. (1989). Photoaffinity labeling and partical purification of the putative plant receptor for the fungal elicitor toxin, fusicoccin. *Planta* **178,** 282–290.

Galbraith, D. W., and Northcote, D. H. (1977). The isolation of plasma membrane from protoplasts of soybean suspension cultures. *J. Cell Sci.* **24,** 295–310.

Geoghegan, W. D. (1988). Immunoassays at the microscopic level: Solid phase colloidal gold methods. *J. Clin. Immunoassay* **11,** 11–23.

Griffing, L. R. (1988). Fluid-phase and membrane-bound transport to the endocytic compartment in plants. *Curr. Top. Plant Bioch. Physiol.* **7,** 101–111.

Griffiths, G., Back, R., and Marsh, M. (1989). A quantitative analysis of the endocytic pathway in baby hamster kidney cells. *J. Cell Biol.* **109,** 2703–2720.

Hacker, G. W. (1989). Silver-enhanced colloidal gold for light microscopy. *In* "Colloidal Gold: Principles, Methods, and Applications" (M. A. Hayatt, ed.), Vol. 1, pp. 297–321. San Diego/London: Academic Press.

Hainfield, J. F. and Furuya, F. R. (1992). A 1.4 nm gold cluster covalently attached to antibodies improves immunolabeling. *J. Histochem. Cytochem.* **40,** 177–184.

Hermo, L., Clermont, Y., and Morales, C. (1985). Fluid-phase and adsorptive endocytosis in ciliated epithelial cells of rat ductili efferentes. *Anat. Rec.* **211,** 285–294.

Horisberger, M., and Rosset, J. (1977). Colloidal gold, a useful marker for transmission and scanning electron microscopy. *J. Histochem. Cytochem.* **25,** 295–305.

Horn, M., Heinstein, P., and Low, P. (1989). Receptor-mediated endocytosis in plant cells. *Plant Cell* **1,** 1003–1009.

Klein, T. M., Arentzen, R., Lewis, P. A., and Fitzpatrick-McElligott, S. (1992). Transformation of microbes, plants and animals by particle bombardment. *Bio/Technology* **10,** 286–291.

Klein, T. M., Wolf, E. D., Wu, R., and Sanford, J. C. (1987). High velocity microprojectiles for delivery of nucleic acids into living cells. *Nature* **327,** 70–73.

Masters, B. R., and Kino, G. S. (1993). Charge-coupled devices for quantitative nipkow disk real-time scanning confocal microscopy. *In* "Electronic Light Microscopy" (D. Shotton, ed.), pp. 315–327. New York: Wiley-Liss.

Oparka, K. J. (1991). Uptake and compartmentation of fluorescent probes by plant cells. *J. Exp. Bot.* **42,** 565–579.

Pini, C., Vicari, G., Ballio, A., Federico, R., Evidente, A., and Randazzo, G. (1979). Antibodies specific for fusicoccins. *Plant Sci. Lett.* **16,** 343–353.

Preston, R. A., Murphy, R. F., and Jones, E. W. (1987). Apparent endocytosis of fluorescein isothiocyanate-conjugated dextran by *Saccharomyces cerevisiae* reflects uptake of low molecular weight impurities, not dextrans. *J. Cell Biol.* **105,** 1981–1988.

Quader, H., and Schnepf, E. (1986). Endoplasmic reticulum and cytoplasmic streaming: Fluorescence microscopical observations in adaxial epidermis cells of onion bulb scales. *Protoplasma* **131,** 250–252.

Sarafis, V. (1990). Biological perspectives of confocal microscopy. *In* "Confocal Microscopy" (T. Wilson, ed.), pp. 325–337. New York/London: Academic Press.

Scopsi, L. (1989). Silver-enhanced colloidal gold method. *In* "Colloidal Gold: Principles, Methods, and Applications;; (M. A. Hayat, ed.), Vol. 1, pp. 251–295. San Diego/London: Academic Press.

Sheppard, C. J. R., Gu, M., and Roy, M. (1992). Signal-to-noise ratio in confocal microscope systems. *J. Microsc.* **168,** 209–218.

Slot, J. W., and Geuze, H. J. (1985). A new method for preparing gold probes for multiple-labeling cytochemistry. *Eur. J. Cell Biol.* **38,** 87–93.

Stout, R., and Griffing, L. R. (1993). Transmural secretion of a highly-expressed cell surface antigen of oat root cap cells. *Protoplasma* **172,** 27–37.

Taylor, J., Villanueva, M. A., Aliaga, G. R., Hahn, M. G., and Griffing, L. R. (1995). Binding and receptor-mediated endocytosis of *Phytophthora megasperma* glucan elicitor-colloidal gold conjugates of soybean protoplasts. Submitted for publication.

VandenBosch, K. A. (1990). Immunogold labelling. *In* "Electron Microscopy of Plant Cells" (J. Hall and C. Hawes, eds.), pp. 181–218. London: Academic Press.

van den Pol, A. N. (1989). Neuronal imaging with colloidal gold. *J. Microsc.* **155,** 27–59.

Villanueva, M. A., Taylor, J., Sui, X., and Griffing, L. R. (1993a). Endocytosis of plant protoplasts: Visualization and quantitation of fluid-phase endocytosis using silver-enhanced bovine serum albumin-gold. *J. Exp. Bot.* **44s,** 275–281.

Villanueva, M. A., Stout, R., and Griffing, L. R. (1993b). Fusicoccin binding and internalization by soybean protoplasts. *In* "Molecular Mechanisms of Membrane Traffic" (D. J. Morré, K. E. Howell, and J. J. Bergeron, eds.), pp. 111–112. Berlin: Springer-Verlag.

White, J. G., Amos, W. B., and Fordham, M. (1987). An evaluation of confocal versus conventional imaging of biological structures by fluorescence light microscopy. *J. Cell Biol.* **105,** 41–48.

Wilson, T. (1990). Confocal microscopy. *In* "Confocal Microscopy" (T. Wilson, ed.), pp. 1–64. London: Academic Press.

Wright, K., and Oparka, K. (1989). Uptake of lucifer yellow CH into plant cell protopasts: A quantitative assessment of fluid-phase endocytosis. *Planta* **179,** 257–264.

CHAPTER 9

Monoclonal Antibodies to Cell-Specific Cell Surface Carbohydrates in Plant Cell Biology and Development

Roger I. Pennell* and Keith Roberts†

* Department of Biology
University College London
Gower Street
London WC1E 6BT, England

† Department of Cell Biology
John Innes Institute
Colney Lane
Norwich NR4 7UH, England

METHODS IN CELL BIOLOGY, VOL. 49

I. Applications

A. Introduction

Monoclonal antibodies (MAbs) to cell-specific cell surface carbohydrate epitopes are versatile molecular probes with multiple applications for plant cell biology and development, for plant molecular biology, and for plant cell and tissue culture. MAbs have been essential probes for identifying and characterizing developmentally regulated cell surface epitopes in plants, and now can be used for the manipulation of the cells in which they are expressed. Although reports have appeared of the production and characterization of cell-specific polyclonal antisera (Moore *et al.,* 1986; Cassab and Varner, 1987; Stafstrom and Staehelin, 1988; Ryser and Keller, 1992; Condit, 1993; Swords and Staehelin, 1993), MAbs retain the unique advantage of monospecificity, and this is particularly useful when they are produced via immunizations with complex mixtures of nonpurified antigens, such as plant extracts (Anderson *et al.,* 1984) or plant cell protoplasts (Knox *et al.,* 1989; Pennell *et al.,* 1991). Monospecificity turns out to be critical in the analysis of carbohydrate eptiopes within glycoproteins and polysaccharides, since these types of epitopes are frequently mingled with other epitopes within the same molecules. This makes it difficult, if not impossible, to purify them as would be required for production of monospecific polyclonal antisera.

Our interest has centered on the use of MAbs for the purification and characterization of cell- and tissue-specific carbohydrate antigens, and for the manipulation of defined cellular targets. In this work, we typically have employed indirect immunolabeling techniques, in which the MAb is first bound to the antigen then, after washing to remove surplus MAb, is tagged with an enzyme, radioisotope, fluorochrome, electron-opaque particle, or paramagnetic bead. In this chapter, we illustrate the variety of ways in which MAb technology can be used for the analysis of cell- and tissue-specific carbohydrate antigens present at the surfaces of plant cells. Principles and full technical details of MAb production techniques can be found elsewhere (Goding, 1986; Harlow and Lane, 1988).

The surfaces of plant cells are dynamic cellular domains involving plasma membranes and cell walls, and these possess many cellular and developmental functions (Roberts, 1989, 1990). We, and others, have used MAb technology to identify and study the different kinds of antigen present at the plasma membrane/cell wall interface. This has been achieved through immunization using heterogeneous mixtures of antigens. The resultant MAbs have then been studied individually, by assaying their binding properties, by analyzing the purified antigens chemically and biochemically, and by using the MAbs to demonstrate complex patterns of developmental regulation at the plant cell surface. From this has emerged the important observation that the regulated epitopes in the vast majority are composed of carbohydrate, and the expression patterns signify collectives of different kinds of cells, which vary with plant species.

Broadly, the MAbs represent two classes of cell surface antigens, the hydroxyproline-rich glycoproteins (HRGPs) termed arabinogalactan-proteins

COLOR PLATES

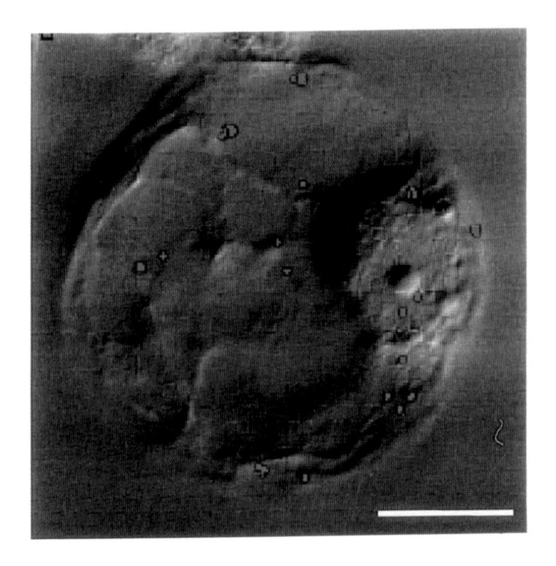

Chapter 8, Fig. 3 CLSEM/DIC combined image of BSA–gold in protoplast after silver enhancement. Protoplast was treated with BSA–gold for 2 h at 24°C. Epipolarization signal is superimposed on DIC image of the protoplast in red. Bar, 10 μm.

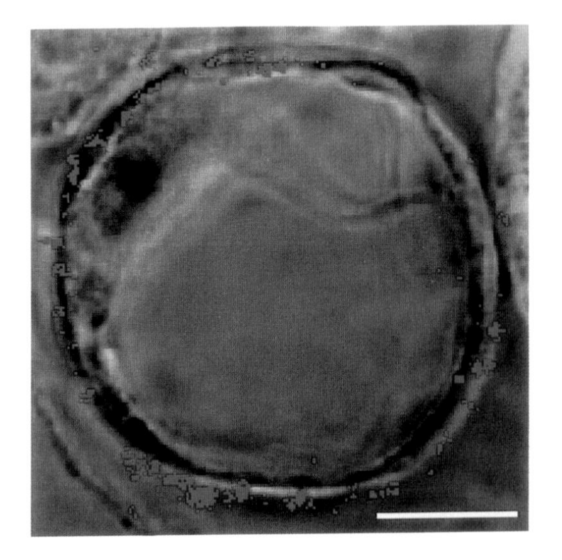

Chapter 8, Fig. 4 CLSEM/DIC combined image of FC–BSA–gold bound to the surface of a protoplast. The gold has been silver-enhanced. Protoplast was treated with FC–BSA–gold for 30 min at 24°C. Epipolarization signal is superimposed on DIC image of the protoplast in red. Bar, 8 μm.

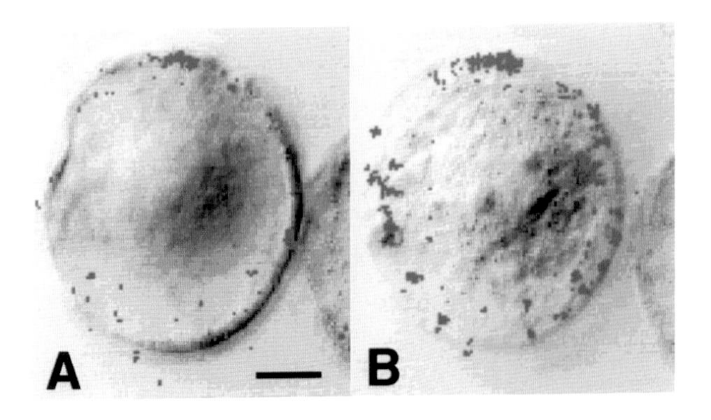

Chapter 8, Fig. 5 CLSEM/DIC combined image of elicitor-gold bound to the surface of a protoplast which had been treated with elicitor-gold for 30 min at 24°C. The gold has been silver-enhanced. Epipolarization signal is superimposed in red on the DIC image. Scale bar, 10 μm.

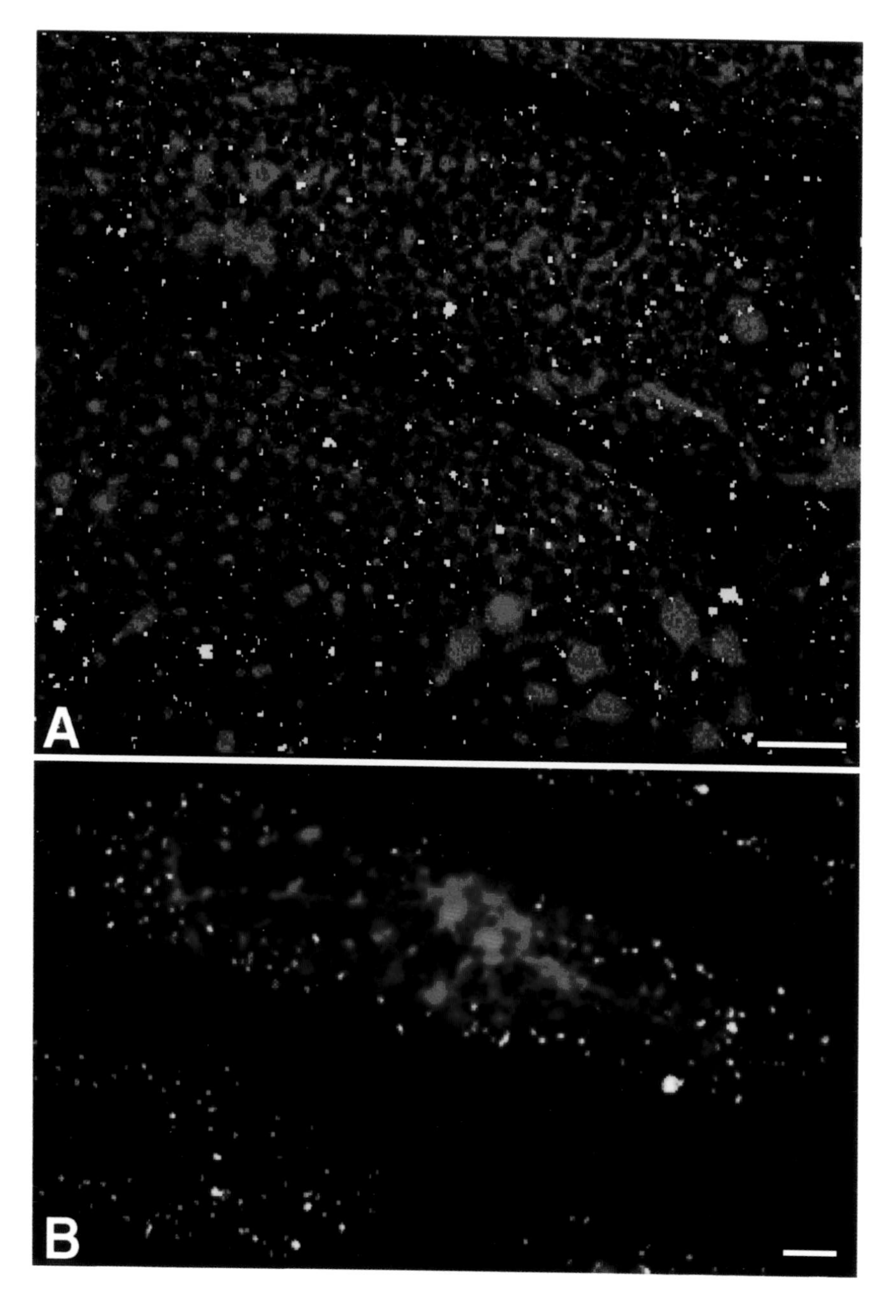

Chapter 8, Fig. 6 CLSEM/CLSFM combined images of nonenhanced gold particles biolistically delivered to the surface of onion epidermal cells that have been vitally stained with fluorescein diacetate. (A) Composite reprojected front view (ray-tracing algorithm, NIH Image) of 10 optical sections 2 μm thick. Epipolarization signal is shown in white-gold, fluorescence in red/red-orange. Scale bar, 20 μm. (B) Single optical section of outer cortical region and wall of onion epidermal cell. Epipolarization signal is shown is white-gold. Cortical ER fluorescence is shown in red/red-orange. Scale bar, 5 μm.

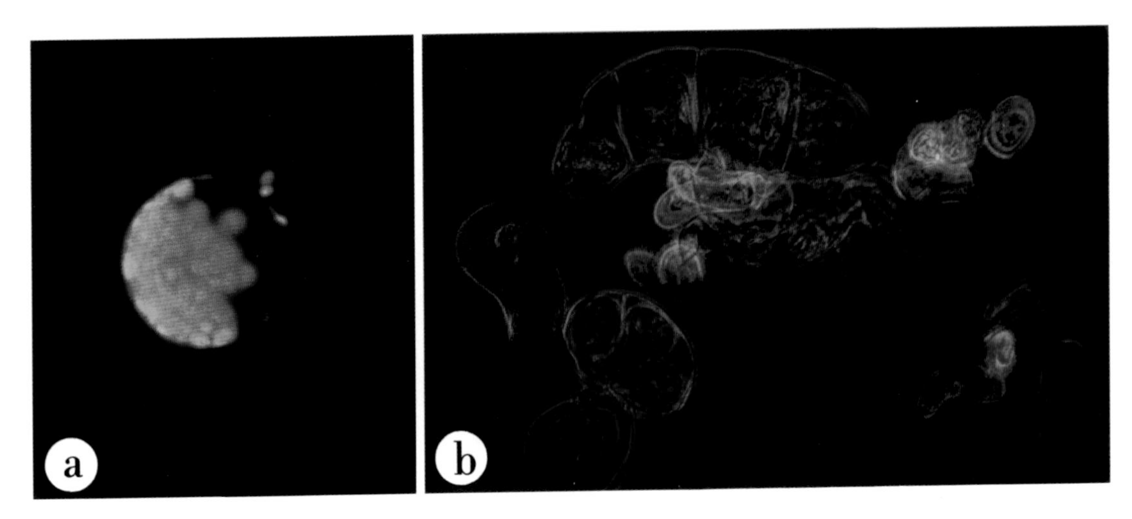

Chapter 9, Fig. 3 Immersion immunofluorescence. An oilseed rape leaf protoplast has been labeled with MAC 207 (a), and some suspension-cultured carrot cells have been labeled with JIM8 (b). The immunofluorescence is green. The AGP epitope recognized by MAC 207 is present at the outer surface of the plasma membrane; without fixation, the MAb has caused patching of the plasma membrane antigen. The epitope recognized by JIM8 is present in the cell walls of some of the cells. ×440.

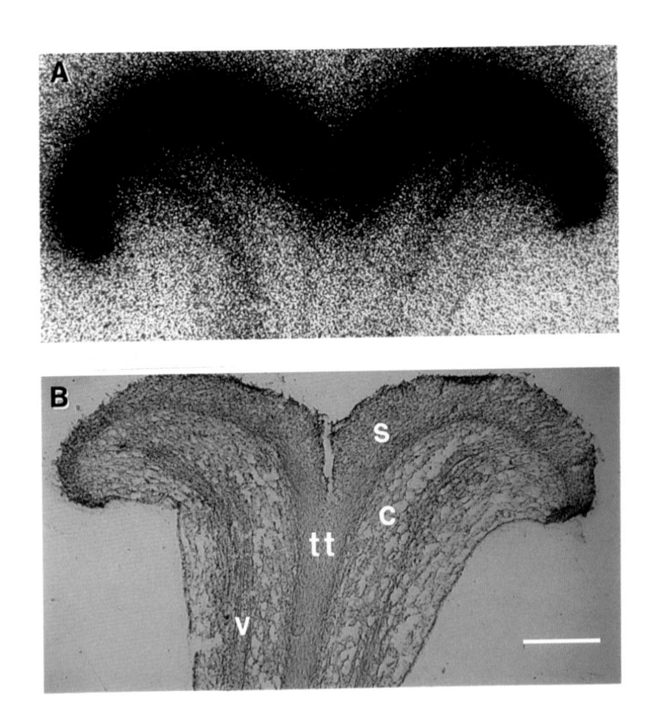

Chapter 12, Fig. 1 Macroscopic localization (Section V, B, 2) of mRNA for a type II proteinase inhibitor in *Nicotiana alata*. (A) X-ray film autoradiograph. (B) Cryosection of pistil stained with toluidine blue. The mRNA is most abundant in the stigmatic tissue (s); the transmitting tract (tt) and cortex (c) are not labeled. A faint signal is present in the vascular bundles (v). The probe was a cDNA labeled with ^{32}P by random priming. Reproduced from Atkinson *et al.* (1993), with permission.

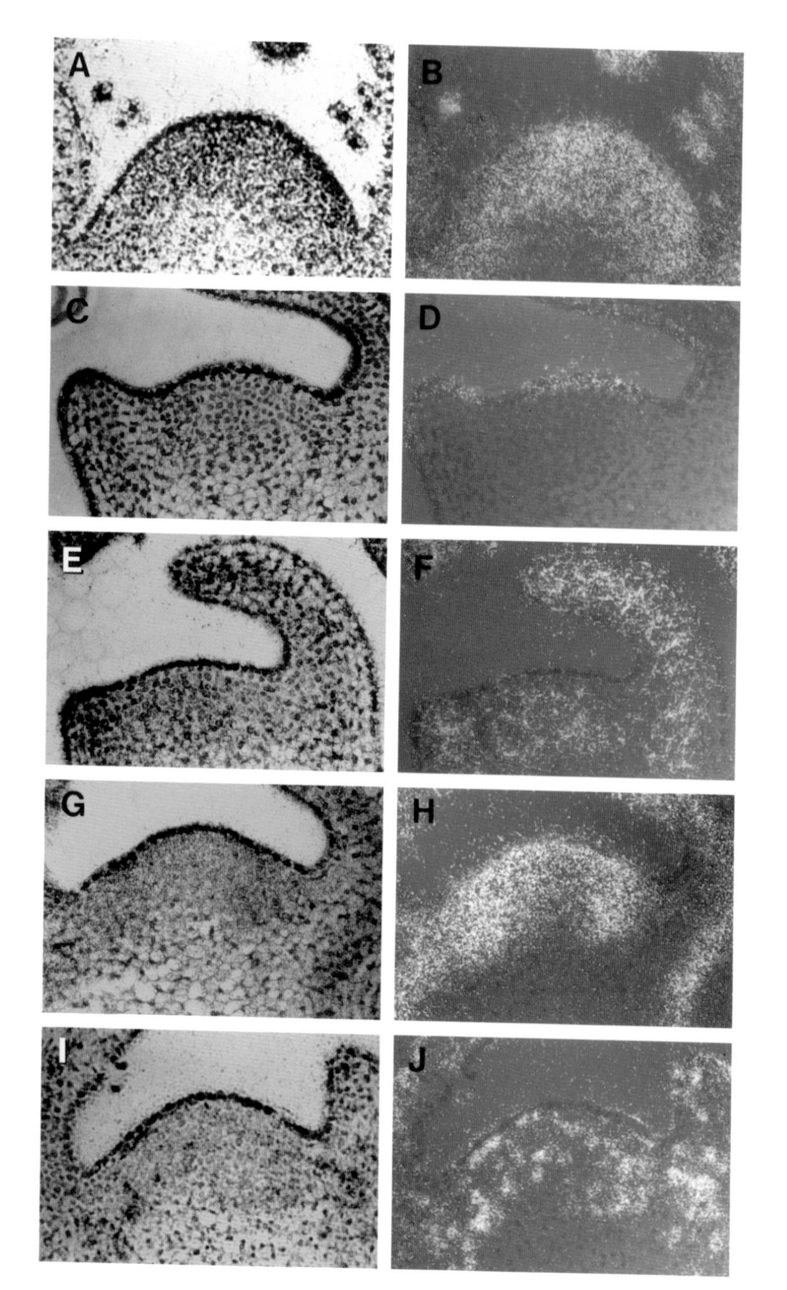

Chapter 12, Fig. 2 Markedly different patterns of gene expression in the apical meristem of tomato detected by microautoradiography (Section V, B,3). The left panels show bright-field micrographs of wax sections each hybridized with a different ^{35}S-labeled RNA probe (A, *rpl*2, a ribosomal protein; C, *Lip*1, lipid transfer protein; E, ADC, arginine decarboxylase; G, *rpl*38, a ribosomal protein; I, *H2A*, a histone). On the right are the corresponding dark-field images in which the silver grains in the emulsion are visible as brilliant white dots. Reproduced from Fleming *et al.* (1993), with permission.

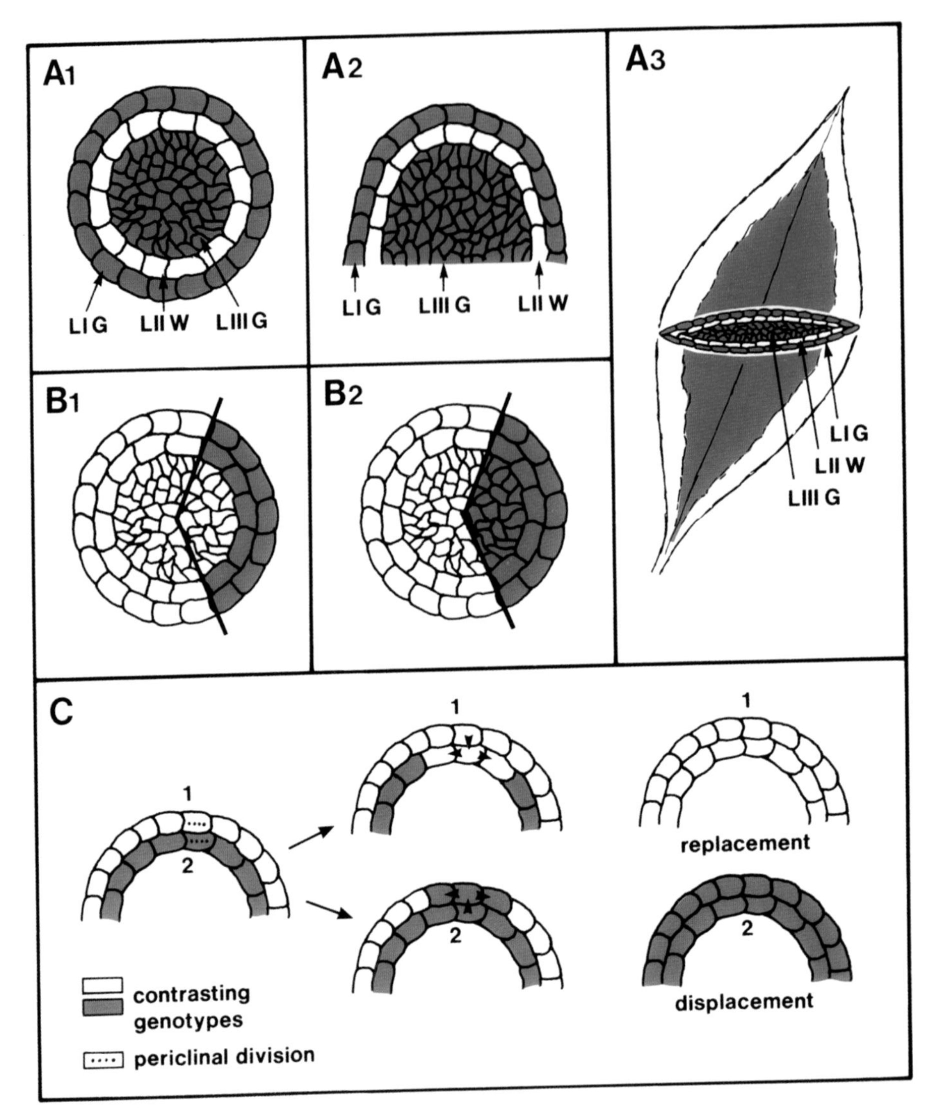

Chapter 23, Fig. 1 (A) Schematic drawings representing the periclinal state in transversal (A1) and longitudinal (A2) sections of a shoot apical meristem of a GWG chimera (LI, Green; LII, White; LIII, Green); (A3) phenotype of a leaf originated from a GWG periclinal chimera. (Note that LI is genetically green. However, in the epidermis, only the guard cells of the stomata develop chloroplasts, so the LI-derived epidermis appears white.) (B) Stem cross sections of mericlinal chimera (B1) and sectorial chimera (B2). (C) Atypical cell divisions cause chimera instabilities by layer replacement (loss of an internal layer, C1), and displacement (loss of an external layer; C2). (D) Pictures of a leaf from a transgenic tobacco chimera with the LIII tagged using two dominant marker: D1, *rolC* phenotypical marker causing a narrowing of the central part of the leaf. The margins of the leaf blade are genotipically wild type (composed only of LI and LII tissue) and appear wrinkled. A wild type leaf is presented at the right. D2, histochemical staining of a petiole cross section showing expression of the *uidA* gene restricted to LIII in the periclinal chimera (indigo color, above), whereas in a nonchimeric 35S rolC/35S-GUS transgenic plant, tissues derived from all three layers are stained (below). Chimerism for the phenotypical marker (*rolC*) was needed to select plants chimeric for the histochemical marker (*uidA*).

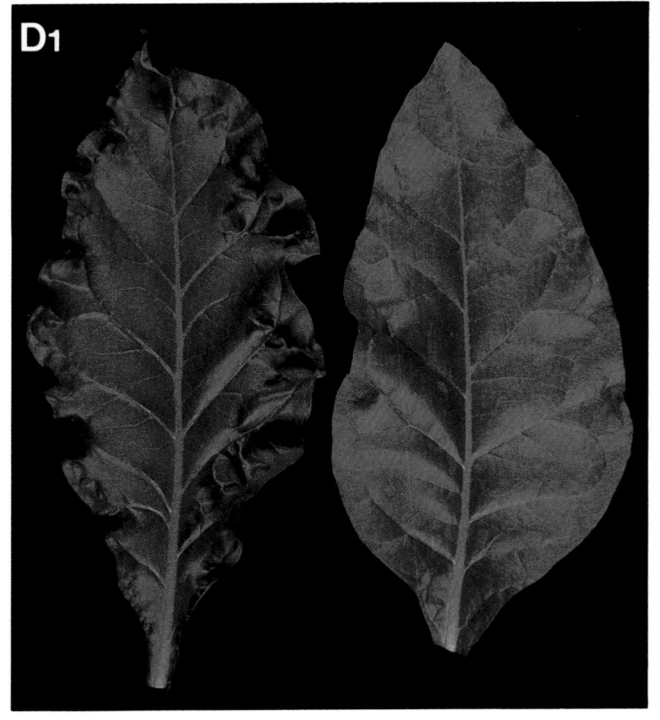

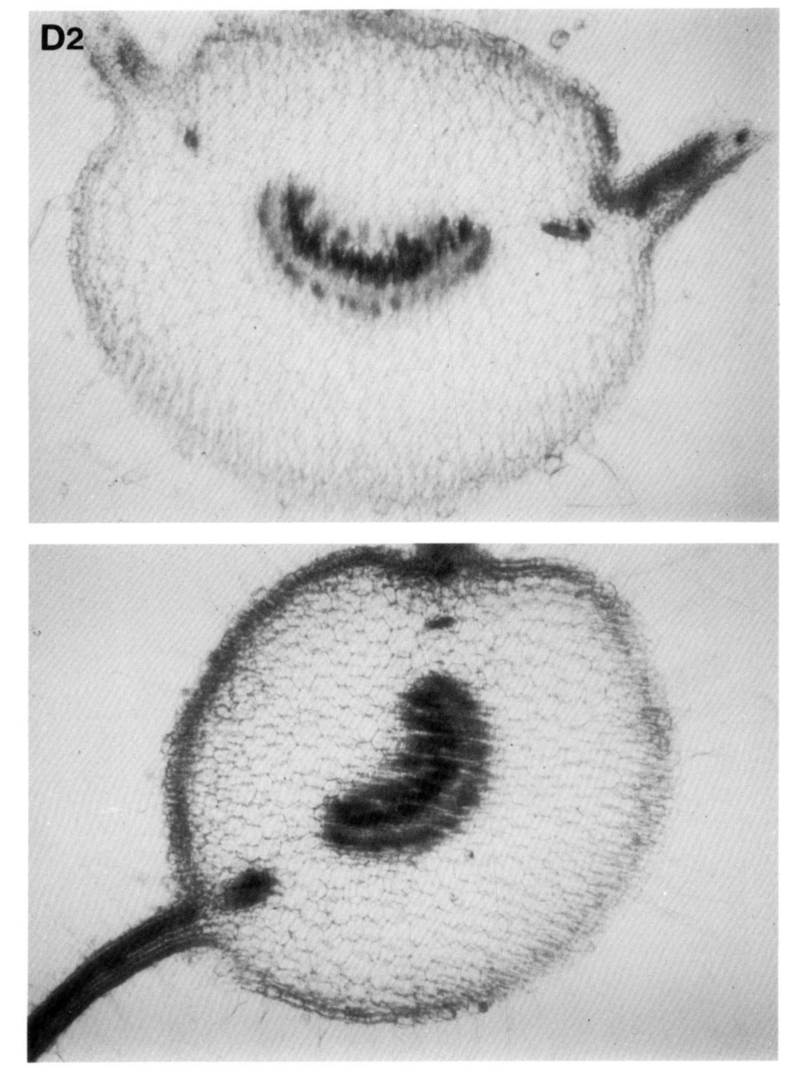

Chapter 23, Fig. 1 *Continued.*

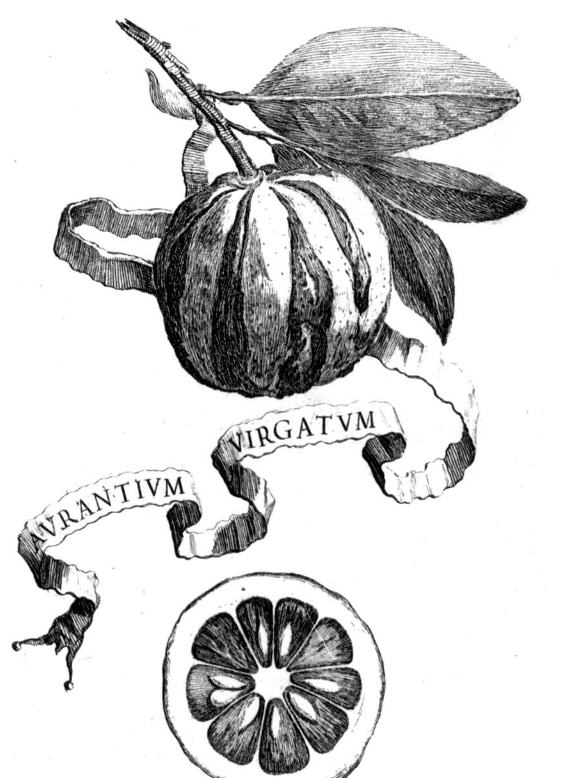

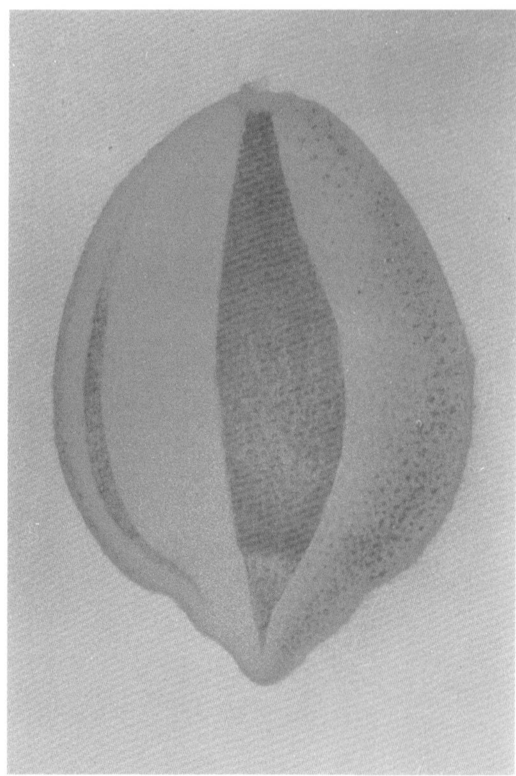

Chapter 23, Fig. 2 (A) *"Virgati nomen aurantio geminus facit, qui cutem variat, color"* (Ferrari, 1646). The *Aurantium Virgatum* is one of the first scientific drawings of a periclinal chimera, and is composed of lemon and orange. The epidermal streaks of lemon tissue are caused by displacement of the LI layer of orange by the underlying lemon layer. (B) "*Limone aranciato*" (Savastano and Parrozzani, 1912) fruit composed of lemon (LI) and orange. The epidermal streaks of orange are caused by layer displacement.

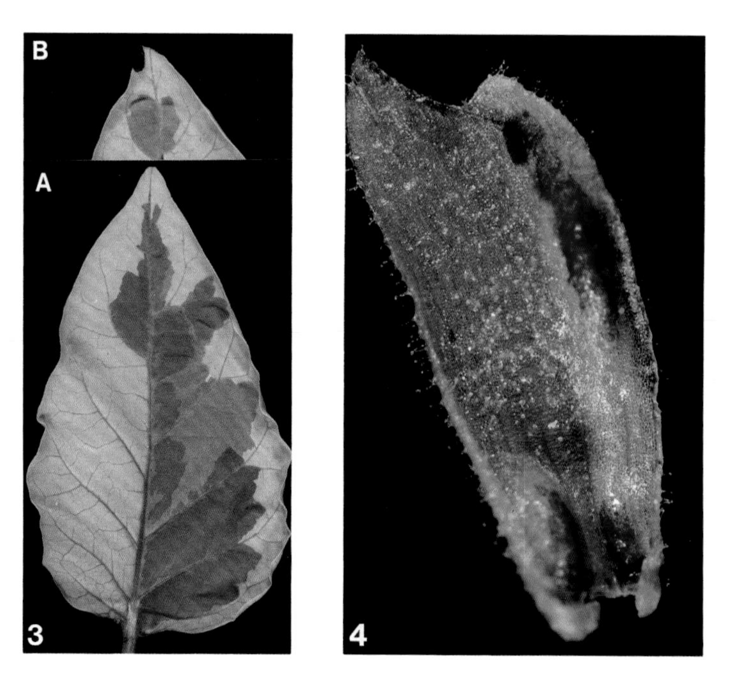

Chapter 23, Fig. 3 Leaves from a GWG periclinal tobacco chimera. (A) Adaxial surface of a leaf showing the differential contribution of the green LIII to the leaf lamina. (B) Periclinal division of the LI generating a green sector at the leaf tip.

Chapter 23, Fig. 4 Somatic mosaic generated in *Anthirriman majus* by the excision of the TAm3 and Tam7 transposable elements. Due to the inactivation of the *Deficiens* gene, the petals are transformed into sepals. However, excision of Tam7 from the *Deficiens* gene causes petaloid sectors to appear surrounded by sepal tissue. The subsequent excision of Tam3 from the *Nivea* locus causes pigmented patches within the petaloid sector (courtesy of Susanna Schwartz-Sommer).

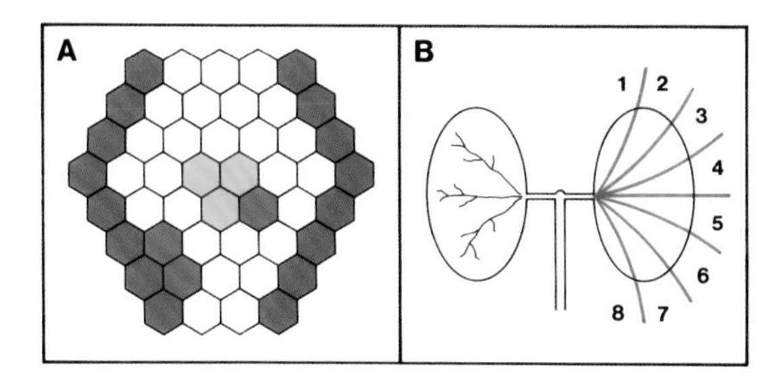

Chapter 23, Fig. 7 (A) Schematic representation of the nascent apex of cotton at the stage of transition from proembryo to embryo. The structure proposed is derived from the analysis of 44 chimeric seedlings generated in semigamic cotton. The proembryo surface is represented by a hexagonal pack of cells. The cotyledonary compartments are eight-celled (green). The compartments for the first and second leaves consists of two and one cells, respectively (red). The compartment for the apical initials is composed of three cells (yellow). (B) Diagram of a young cotton seedling. The right-hand part shows the cotyledon areas that mutant clones of cells tended to fill; this pattern was recorded for each seedling using the midvein and two other prominent veins as points of reference. Boundaries (red lines) between virescent and green tissues corresponded either to the three main ribs of rather precisely bisected the area between two of them (from Christianson, 1986).

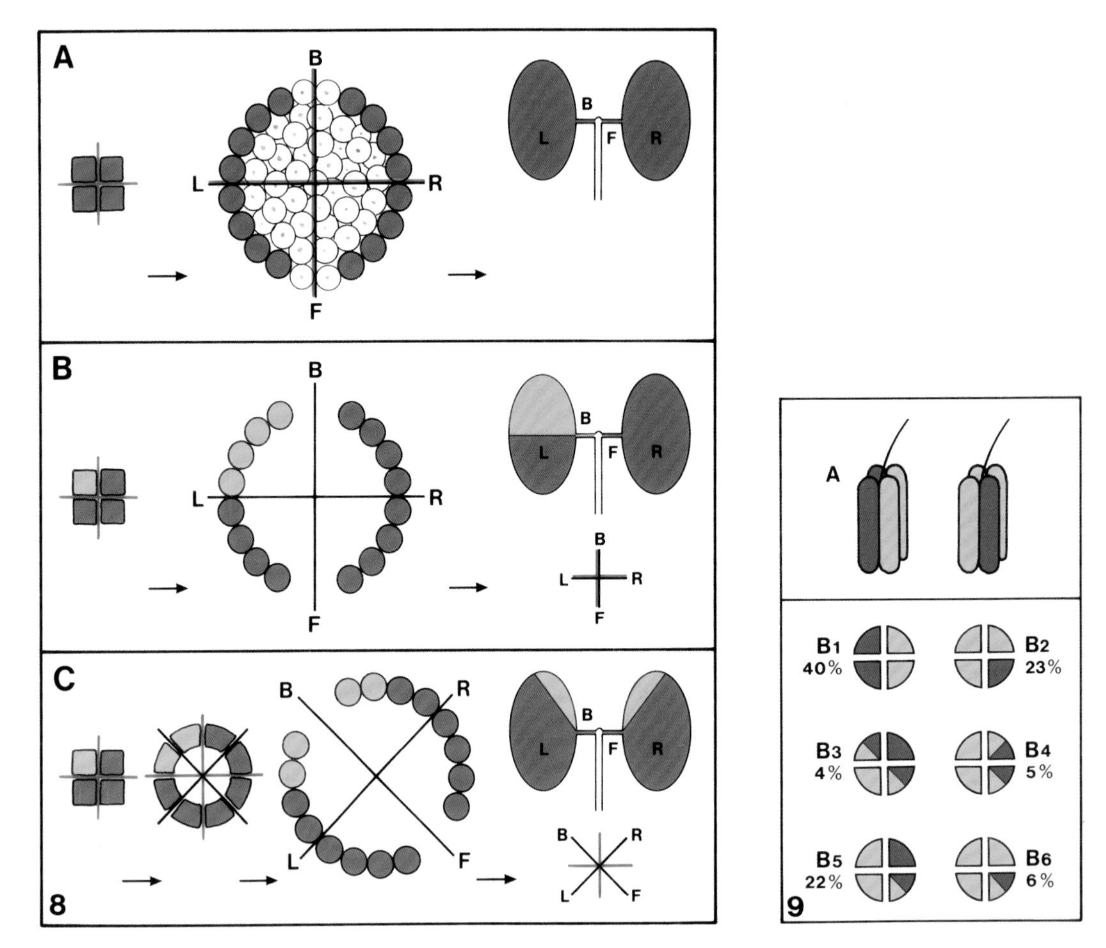

Chapter 23, Fig. 8 Pattern determination of the main planes (black) of symmetry of the cotton seedling based on the planes (red) of the quartet of proembryo cells that generate the adult aerial structures of the seedling (from Christianson, 1986). (A) Cotton seedling as derived from the proembryo quartet of cells (L, left; R, right; B, back; F, front). The four cells divide until the cotyledonary compartments (cells with bold walls) acquire identity. Later, the cotyledons will develop with planes of symmetry corresponding to those of the quartet. (B) Type of sectoring used by Christianson to establish that the planes of symmetry of the seedling were coincident with those of the quartet of cells. (C) The seedling planes of symmetry (black) are shifted 45° from those of the quartet of cells. In our view this shifting is possible if pattern determination takes place at a hypothetical eight-celled stage (second drawing from left in C). The type of sectoring resulting from such a shift would cover a symmetrical area on two cotyledons (2 such cases of variation were observed among the 44 analyzed).

Chapter 23, Fig. 9 Orientation of the four microsporangia of the maize anther based on the planes of the four initial cells generating the anther. This representation illustrates how, in 93 anthers, the boundaries of red sectors intercept the microsporangia boundaries (uncolored areas). (A) Anther sectors corresponding, respectively, to drawings B1 and B2. (B) Sector types B1 and B2 appeared with a frequency of 63% and are the expected classes assuming the orientation of the four initial cells corresponds to the subsequent orientation of the microsporangia. Sector types B3 and B4 indicate that the orientation of the four primordial cells deviated by 45° with respect to B1 and B2. These last two types of sectors together with those represented in B5 and B6 can interpreted by a mechanism similar to that reproduced in Fig. 8C (from Dawe and Freeling, 1991).

(AGPs) at the plasma membrane surface (Pennell *et al.,* 1989; reviewed by Fincher *et al.,* 1983) and the HRGPs termed extensins (Smallwood *et al.,* 1994; reviewed by Showalter, 1993) and the pectic polysaccharides (Liners *et al.,* 1989) in the cell wall. At present, no MAbs have been described that are directed against other classes of cell wall proteins and polysaccharides known from gene expression patterns to be developmentally regulated, for example, the glycine-rich proteins (Keller *et al.,* 1989; Condit, 1993) or the hemicelluloses (Rodkiewicz, 1970). The MAbs that are currently available to cell-specific cell surface carbohydrate epitopes are (*a*) *Directed against AGPs:* PCBC3 (Anderson *et al.,* 1984), PN 16.4B4 (Norman *et al.,* 1986), MAC 64 (Bradley *et al.,* 1988), MAC 207 (Bradley *et al.,* 1988; Pennell *et al.,* 1989), JIM4 (Knox *et al.,* 1989), JIM8 (Pennell *et al.,* 1991), JIM14, JIM15 and JIM16 (Knox *et al.,* 1991), FB8 (Q. C. B. Cronk, unpublished), and LM2 (J. P. Knox, unpublished); (*b*) *Directed against extensin:* 11.D2 (Meyer *et al.,* 1988), JIM11, JIM12, and JIM20 (Smallwood *et al.,* 1994), and LM1 (J. P. Knox, unpublished); (*c*) *Directed against pectins:* 1C7, 2F4, and 7F7 (Liners *et al.,* 1989), JIM5 and JIM7 (Knox *et al.,* 1990), and CCRC-M1 (Puhlman *et al.,* 1994). MAbs raised against *Chlamydomonas* cell wall glycoproteins (Smith *et al.,* 1984a), and MAC 236 (VandenBosch *et al.,* 1989) and MAC 268 (Perotto *et al.,* 1991) also recognize HRGP epitopes (Smith *et al.,* 1984a; Rae *et al.,* 1991; Perotto *et al.,* 1991), as may other MAbs that recognize cell-surface carbohydrate in lower and higher plants (Villanueva *et al.,* 1986; Jones *et al.,* 1990; Perotto *et al.,* 1991; Lynes *et al.,* 1987). At present, the functions of the regulated cell surface carbohydrates to which these MAbs are directed are unknown.

B. Identification of Antigen

Given a partially or fully characterized MAb, the simplest ways to determine presence of antigen involves either an enzyme-linked immunosorbent assay (ELISA) or dot-immunoblotting against antigen (Kieliszewski and Lamport, 1986; Perotto *et al.,* 1991). Since MAbs are monospecific, strong positive results from either technique provide compelling evidence for presence of the antigen, as shown for the pectin in a cell wall extraction series in Fig. 1. The principles of ELISA and dot-immunoblotting are the same, requiring only that the MAb be reacted with an immobilized antigen adsorbed to a plastic plate or dried to a membrane filter, and be sensitively detected by an enzyme reaction that delivers a soluble or insoluble product to the site of antigen–antibody interaction. The advantage of ELISA is that it can be quantified; the advantage of dot-immunoblotting is that it does not require complex apparatus.

Alternatively, ELISA and dot-immunoblotting against defined antigen can be used to screen MAbs and begin MAb characterization (Smith *et al.,* 1984b; Meyer *et al.,* 1987; Lynes, 1992). For example, binding to gum arabic shows that the MAb recognizes AGP, and binding to apple pectin shows that it recognizes pectin (Pennell *et al.,* 1989; 1991). Low concentrations of secondary Ab show up

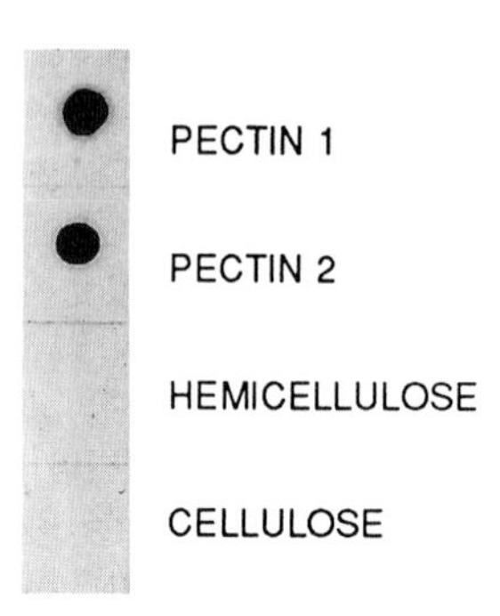

Fig. 1 JIM7 dot immunoblots of cell wall polysaccharides extracted from onion using EDTA. The dots show that the JIM7-reactive epitope, which contains a sequence of galacturonic acid residues, is present in only some of the cell wall polysaccharides, which are judged to be pectins accordingly. Courtesy of Nicola Stacey.

on ELISA plates, so when using ELISA for initial MAb characterization it is essential to determine background interactions through the use of control lanes in which antigen or MAb are omitted.

C. Localization of Antigen

Tissue immunoprinting (TIP) extends the principle of dot-immunoblotting through providing two-dimensional spatial resolution. TIP involves pressing the freshly cut surface of a plant organ or organ system onto a nylon or nitrocellulose membrane filter, removing it, and processing the print in the same manner as a dot-immunoblot (Cassab and Varner, 1987). Fragments of cells, including pieces of membrane and cell wall, adhere nonspecifically onto the membrane during the printing process. These are subsequently labeled with Abs, and can be examined and photographed after staining, using a low-power light microscope. Although a freshly sliced organ can be dabbed onto several membrane filters, the strength of the signal decreases in proportion to the number of times that this is done; this limits the usefulness of replicas. In addition to demonstrating the presence of antigen, TIP reveals in outline patterns of developmental regulation, as is shown in Fig. 2 for four carbohydrate AGP epitopes. Details of all aspects of TIP manipulation can be found in Reid and Pont-Lezica (1991).

Identification of epitopes present at the plasma membrane surface can also be approached by using the technique of protoplast immunoagglutination. This requires that the cell wall be fully degraded by the polysaccharide hydrolases that are used to make the protoplasts (see, for example, Evans and Bravo, 1983). It also requires that the epitopes be resistant to the mixtures of cellulases, hemicellulases, and pectinases that are employed; we have shown that none of these hydrolases degrade AGP carbohydrate epitopes (Fitter *et al.*, 1987; Pennell

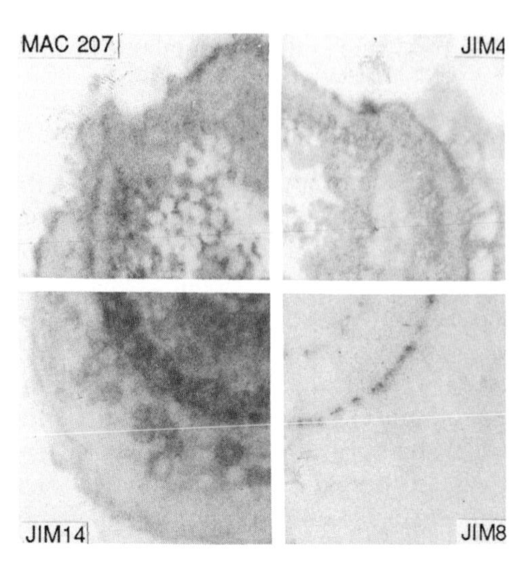

Fig. 2 Quadrant tissue immunoprints of a tomato petiole. The TIP demonstrates that the three carbohydrate epitopes recognized by MAC 207, JIM4, and JIM14 are widespread in the petiole, but that the carbohydrate epitope recognized by JIM8 is associated only with the petiole vasculature. All the carbohydrate epitopes are components of plasma membrane AGPs. ×35. Courtesy of Quentin Cronk.

et al., 1989; 1991). The protoplasts should be prepared from suspension-cultured cells or plant organs grown in optimum conditions of light and water, and should be used immediately after preparation to avoid complications due to resynthesis of cell walls. Epitope saturation points can be established through simple MAb titration, accompanied by observation of agglutination under the light microscope.

Identification of epitopes that are present on the surfaces of protoplasts or single cells can also be done via immersion immunofluorescence labeling. In this case, the MAb is tagged either directly, using a fluorochrome such as fluorescein isothiocyanate (FITC), or indirectly, using a second, fluorochrome-conjugated antibody, and is visualized using epifluorescence microscopy. A protoplast and some suspension-cultured cells prepared in this way are shown in Fig. 3 (see Color Plates). We use immersion immunofluorescence as a definitive test for epitopes that are present at the plasma membrane surface (Pennell *et al.,* 1989; Knox *et al.,* 1989), and for cell-specific carbohydrate epitopes at the plasma membrane and in the cell wall. Patching or capping of plasma membrane epitopes can be employed to illustrate antigen mobility within the phospholipid bilayer (Metcalf *et al.,* 1987); this is seen for the AGPs visualized in Fig. 3a. Concerning the cell wall, only single cells in cell suspension cultures (Pennell *et al.,* 1993), or pollen grains (Li *et al.*, 1992), permit the ready access of MAb to antigen. Cell viability and cell development in culture are unaffected by MAb labeling.

D. Patterns of Epitope Expression

There are many applications for MAbs that are directed against developmentally-regulated carbohydrate epitopes at the plant cell surface, including antigen characterization and antigen and cell manipulation. TIP can provide useful information about plant organ development, especially when the MAb signal is improved by the immunogold silver enhancement (IGS) technique (Springall *et al.,* 1984; Cassab and Varner, 1987). Far greater resolution, however, is offered by thin sectioning of fixed plant organs, followed by MAb-based immunolocalization techniques. Wherever possible, we employ cryostat sections that are about 10 μm thick for detailed developmental studies. These are fast and easy to prepare, offer no physical obstacle to penetration of the MAbs, and allow single-cell resolution (Pennell and Roberts, 1990; Knox *et al.,* 1990). Ultracryostat sections less than 1 μm thick provide better cellular detail, and can easily resolve plasma membrane from cell wall epitopes (Pennell *et al.,* 1989; Knox *et al.,* 1989). Alternatively, and for all electron microscopy, resin-embedded material provides excellent results for MAb localization studies (Pennell *et al.,* 1989; Liners and Van Custem, 1992) when the resin is hydrophilic, and infiltration and polymerization are performed at −20°C (Wells, 1985). We typically employ FITC as a secondary Ab reporter for immunofluorescence microscopy (Pennell *et al.,* 1989), but IGS can also be used for visualizing information within resin-embedded sections (VandenBosch *et al.,* 1989; Perotto *et al.,* 1991). We have also employed colloidal gold particles to visualize the secondary Abs bound to electron microscope grids (Pennell *et al.,* 1989). Examples of cryostat and electron microscope resin section immunolabeling of a cell-specific AGP epitope are shown in Fig. 4.

E. Antigen and Epitope Analysis

When MAbs have identified cell-specific carbohydrate antigens, large volumes of MAb hybridoma culture supernatants or ascites fluids can be produced for antigen immunopurification. The effects of solvents, oxidants, and enzymes on antigen–MAb interactions, quantified in ELISA or Western analysis, readily define the components of plant cell surface antigens (Conrad *et al.,* 1987; Perotto *et al.,* 1991). For example, an effect on MAb binding of sodium metaperiodate, which oxidizes glycosidic bonds, demonstrates antigen glycosylation (VandenBosh *et al.,* 1989; Perotto *et al.,* 1991), and an effect of a specific endo- or exoglycanase indicates the presence of specific internal or terminal sugar residues. ELISA-based inhibition assays, involving competition for MAb–antigen interactions by mono- or oligosaccharides, also can point to the presence of a specific sugar residue in the MAb epitope (Pennell *et al.,* 1989; 1991). In this procedure,

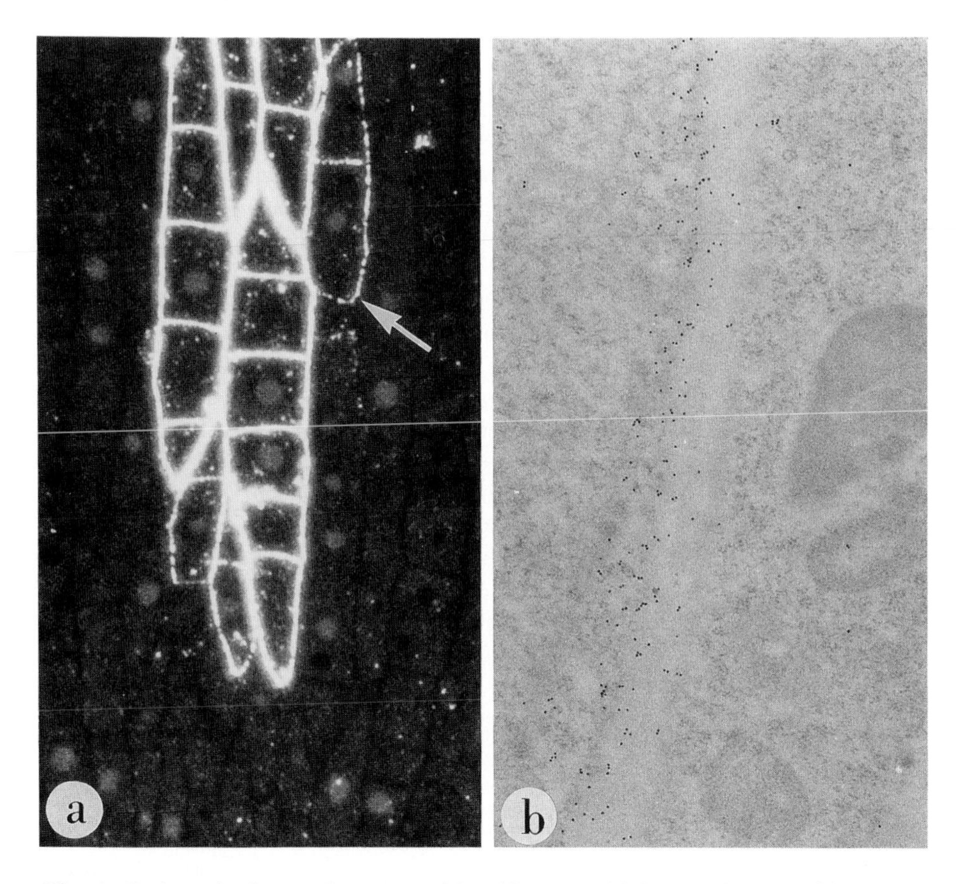

Fig. 4 Resin section immunofluorescence (a) and immunogold electron microscopy (b) with JIM8. The sections are longitudinal, cut from an *Arabidopsis* root close to the root apex. In *Arabidopsis* tissues, JIM8 recognizes a plasma membrane AGP epitope, which signifies specific cell collectives. In roots, the positions of the cell collectives are related to the positions of the developing xylem poles. The arrow in (a) points to the part of the junction between the two cells shown in (b), in which the JIM8-reactive epitope is present only at the plasma membrane on the left. ×440 (a) and ×18,500 (b). Courtesy of Paul Linstead.

the point at which binding becomes inhibited by 50% relative to controls accurately measures the affinity of the MAb for the inhibitor and, therefore, for an equivalent chemical structure in the antigen. Differences in the inhibitory effects of different monosaccharides and different isomers of the same monosaccharide have shown that several AGP-directed MAbs recognize arabinose residues together with other sugars (Pennell *et al.,* 1989; Perotto *et al.,* 1991). Although hapten inhibition itself does not reveal anything about epitope structures, some information about the structures and the relative organization of the epitopes in complex carbohydrate antigens can be deduced from correlated chemical studies (Pennell *et al.,* 1989), as is shown in Fig. 5 for the relative positions of two AGP epitopes.

We also use MAbs for the purification of carbohydrate antigens through immunoaffinity chromatography. This approach can be employed for all water-soluble antigens that are able to freely penetrate the column matrix and which can be recovered in pure form for protein and carbohydrate analysis (Baldwin *et al.,* 1993); heterogeneous populations of large polysaccharides can sometimes cause clogging.

For immunoaffinity chromatography, the MAb fraction of the hybridoma culture supernatant is linked covalently to a support matrix, loaded with antigen, washed, and eluted by pH shock or by hapten competition. If elution is by pH shock, the antigen solution should be neutralized as quickly as possible to prevent hydrolysis of glycosidic linkages. If elution is done with hapten saccharides, the antigen can be dialyzed to remove them. The utility of immunoaffinity columns as means to purify antigen for chemical characterization has limitations; for example, antigens cannot be eluted using complex carbohydrates as competitors, since these would contaminate the antigen. Again, cell-specific carbohydrate epitopes in plants are frequently found within several different cell surface glycoproteins and polysaccharides. This means that purification schemes involving

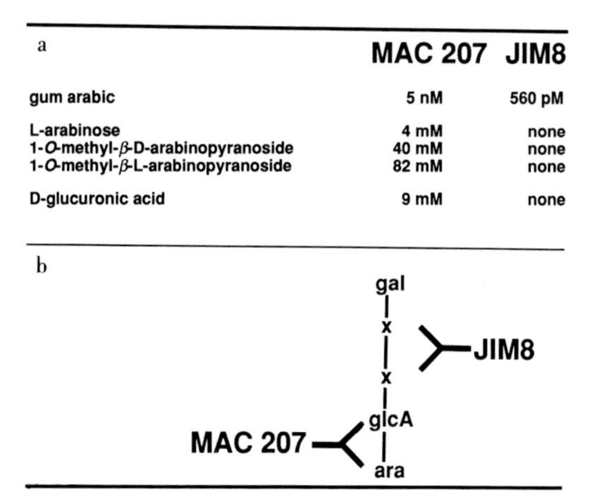

a	MAC 207	JIM8
gum arabic	5 nM	560 pM
L-arabinose	4 mM	none
1-*O*-methyl-β-D-arabinopyranoside	40 mM	none
1-*O*-methyl-β-L-arabinopyranoside	82 mM	none
D-glucuronic acid	9 mM	none

Fig. 5 Monosaccharide components of carbohydrate epitopes. The binding inhibition was determined by ELISA. The inhibition by gum arabic (a), an AGP, shows that MAC 207 and JIM8 recognize AGP epitopes. Further, the different patterns of inhibition by hapten monosaccharides (a) show that the MAC 207 and JIM8 epitopes are different, and that the MAC 207-reactive epitope probably contains arabinose and glucuronic acid. Chemical analysis of AGP carbohydrates suggests that the arabinose is a terminal, so it is likely that the MAC 207-reactive epitope is terminal as well (b). The composition of the JIM8 epitope is unknown but, as shown in (b), it is probably subterminal. The AGP backbone is composed of 1,6-linked galactosyl residues. The numbers in the table refer to the inhibitor concentration required for 50% dimunition in ELISA signal (I_{50}). From Pennell *et al.,* 1989, 1991. Reproduced by permission of The Rockefeller University Press.

immunoaffinity chromatography produce heterogeneous mixtures of epitope-related antigens, which are useless for chemical analysis or protein sequencing. This is a particular problem for cell surface HRGPs (Meyer *et al.*, 1987; Kieliszewski *et al.*, 1992). To purify individual carbohydrate antigens such as individual plasma membrane AGPs, we use MAbs to track the antigen during classical biochemical purification. ELISA or dot-immunblotting of the column fractions from reversed-phase, size-exclusion, and ion-exchange purifications, which for extracellular AGPs at least effectively resolves different molecular species (Chen *et al.*, 1994), allows antigen purification to be easily monitored.

For some types of antigens containing cell-specific carbohydrate epitopes (for example, the plasma membrane AGPs) even classical purifications are inadequate. We have therefore used sodium dodecyl sulfate–polyacrylamide gel electrophoresis (SDS–PAGE) of purified and Triton-X114-fractionated plasma membranes (Kjellbom and Larsson, 1984; Kjellbom *et al.*, 1989) for AGP purification, and MAbs to identify the positions of the antigen bands in Western immunoblots, which are then excised for analysis (Weitzhandler *et al.*, 1993). For this procedure, the sample is loaded into a broad well in an acrylamide "curtain" gel, resolved by SDS–PAGE, and transferred to high-load nylon membranes such polyvinylidene fluoride (PVDF) membranes. The positions of the antigens are determined in marker lanes by immunoblotting. Agarose gels and nitrocellulose membranes should be avoided if carbohydrate analyses are to be done, since these types of gel release galactosyl and glucosyl residues during processing. The blot-slicing technique is limited to carbohydrate antigens containing core proteins that bind SDS (i.e., they cannot be used for pectic polysaccharides), and by the intrinsic resolution of SDS–PAGE. Resolution can be improved by gradient SDS–PAGE, as shown for the 16-kDa-different plasma membrane AGPs in Fig. 6.

McCann *et al.* (1992) have isolated cell wall polysaccharides using MAbs to pectin, and have gone on to map some of the epitopes recognized by these MAbs by molecular immunogold electron microscopy, as shown in Fig. 7. Once the purified antigen is adsorbed onto a coated electron microscope grid, it is treated with an ammonium acetate solution, reacted with a MAb, washed, reacted with a secondary Ab conjugated with colloidal gold particles, and then negative-stained with uranyl acetate so that the antigen and the gold can both be seen.

F. Manipulation of Cell Development

Once MAbs have been obtained and their target antigens characterized, MAb technology can shift from descriptive applications to the more important applications involving functional analysis. In one approach, cell-specific cell surface carbohydrate epitopes can be used as ligands for cell sorting. The effects of cellular context on the early stages of plant development can be studied when single cells from embryogenic plant cell suspension cultures are sorted according to cell wall carbohydrate epitopes such as AGP epitopes (Pennell *et al.*, 1992),

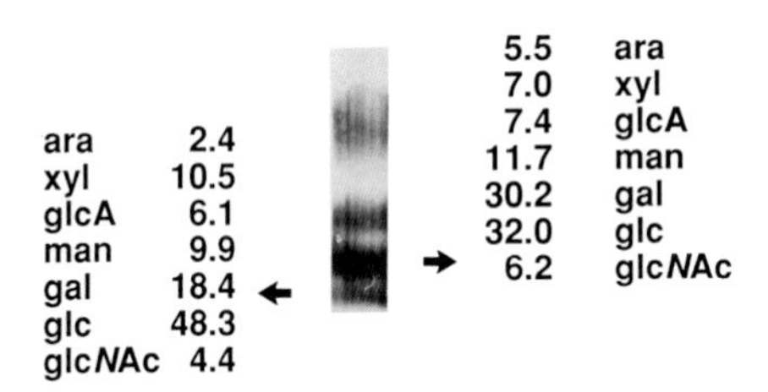

Fig. 6 Sugar analysis from a "curtain" immunoblot of sugar beet plasma membrane antigens. Sugar beet plasma membranes were purified and by aqueous polymer 2-phase partitioning, fractionated with Triton X-114, and resolved by gradient SDS–PAGE. The positions of the MAC 207 antigens were resolved by Western immunoblotting of marker lanes, and the antigen was cut from the curtain for carbohydrate analysis. Examples of the sugar composition that can be determined, in mole%, are shown for the two smallest MAC 207 antigens termed pg 68 and pg 84, which were effectively resolved despite the high degree of glycosylation. Courtesy of Per Kjellbom.

and somatic embryogenesis induced from them (Nomura and Komamine, 1985). In principle, protoplasts can be subjected to fluorescence-activated cell sorting (FACS), following immunofluorescence labeling with MAbs, although FACS is not generally suitable for intact cells or cell clusters. However, immunomagnetic cell sorting (ICS) has also recently become possible for plant cells (Fig. 8). For ICS, single cells are labeled with MAbs to cell-specific cell wall epitopes, washed, and then tagged with a secondary Ab that is conjugated with a paramagnetic bead. Cells are sorted by being placed within a strong magnetic field. Advantages of ICS include that it does not require production of protoplasts, it only takes a few seconds, the sorted cell collectives are pure, and cell viability is unaffected. This means that developmental programs, such as somatic embryogenesis, begin to take place rapidly and efficiently. Magnetically sorted cells can be relabeled with different MAbs and reselected, so that various subsets of these cell collectives can be obtained for further analysis of somatic embryogenesis.

In principle, protoplasts prepared form plant cell suspension cultures (Stacey *et al.,* 1990) or from plant organs (Knox *et al.,* 1989; Pennell *et al.,* 1991) that express cell-specific plasma membrane epitopes can also be separated by immunomagnetic protoplast sorting (IPS), although this has not yet been achieved. However, essentially the same principle has been successfully applied to plastid sorting (Kausch and Bruce, 1994).

G. Genetic Analysis

At present, the functions of cell-specific cell surface carbohydrate epitopes are unknown. Although mutations that affect single sugar (Reiter *et al.,* 1993) or multiple N-linked residues (von Schaewen *et al.,* 1993) have been produced by biochemical screening, carbohydrate epitope mutants cannot be obtained in this way, and at present none have been produced. Plants carrying epitope mutations

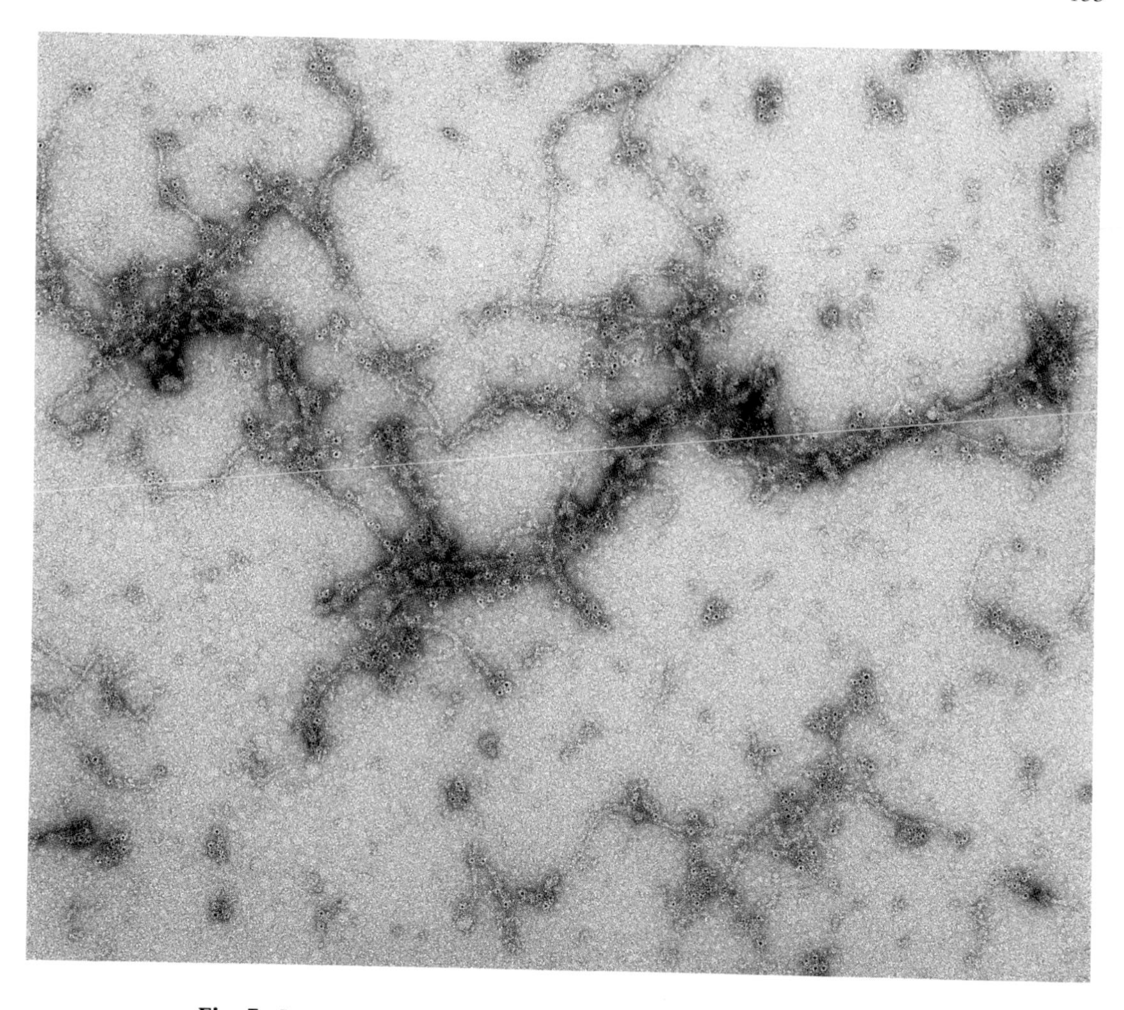

Fig. 7 Immunogold labeling of pectic polysaccharides isolated from onion cell walls using CDTA. The polysaccharides have been adsorbed to a plastic-coated electron microscope grid, and the homogalacturonan polysaccharides tagged with JIM5 and 1-nm gold particles. Both the homogalacturonan molecules and the gold particles are visible against the negative uranyl acetate stain. ×70,000. Courtesy of Maureen McCann.

can only be produced using respective MAbs, by either screening or selection following large-scale ethylmethyl sulfonate mutagenesis (Durand, 1990; Negrutiu, 1990). For screening, the easiest approach is TIP of M2 generation plants (von Schaewen *et al.,* 1993). For selection, the only plausible approach at present is to use ICS or IPS to obtain epitope-defective cells and protoplasts, using MAbs such as the several directed against AGP carbohydrate that recognize either all or none of the wild-type targets (Pennell and Roberts, 1990). From these cells, whole plants can then be regenerated (Collin and Dix, 1990). Although demanding, an equivalent approach with lectins has identified concanavalin A knockouts at the cell surface in mammalian cells (reviewed by Stanley, 1987).

Single cells and protoplasts can in principle be subjected to MAb-based cell killing, but this has not yet been achieved.

II. Methods

A. Enzyme-Linked Immunosorbent Assay

Antigen solution, prepared at 50 μg/ml in phosphate-buffered saline (PBS), is added to each of the wells in a microtiter plate (Dynatech Labs, Chantilly) to saturate the charged sites on the plastic. For example, we use 50 μl of gum arabic solution for each well and allow it to adsorb for about 12 h. Then we block residual charges by adding 100 μl per well of PBS containing 0.2% (w/v) dried milk for 10 min, followed by 50 μl per well of the same solution containing 1% (v/v) of the specific MAb for 1 h. The wells are then washed using a fast jet of PBS, and 50 μl per well of 0.05% (v/v) secondary Ab solution is added. We typically use horseradish peroxidase (HRP) as the catalyst for a colorimetric reaction and develop the reaction after washing the plate, by adding 50 μl per well of a solution comprising 5 ml H_2O, 0.5 ml 50 mg/ml tetramethyl benzidine (TMB) in dimethyl sulfoxide (DMSO), and 30 μl of 30% (v/v) H_2O_2. These reagents are available in kit form (Kiregaard and Perry Labs, Gaithersberg). The HRP reaction is stopped by addition of 20 μl sulfuric acid, and the OD_{450} determined with a plate-reader.

B. Dot-Immunoblotting

Antigen solution is applied as series of 1-μl dots to a nitrocellulose or nylon membrane. We dry the dots and process them with MAbs and secondary ABs in the same way as the ELISA, except that the HRP then catalyzes the formation of an insoluble product that is scored by eye. The developing solution, which should be made fresh, contains 30 ml H_2O, 5 ml 5 mg/ml 4-chloro-1-naphthol dissolved in methanol, and 30 μl of 30 (v/v) H_2O_2.

C. Immunoprinting and Immunoagglutination

TIP blots are processed exactly as dot-immunoblots, using the chloranaphthol solution to develop the reaction *in situ*. For immunoagglutination, we suspend freshly prepared protoplasts to a density of about 10^4/ml in the medium used for protoplast production lacking enzymes but supplemented with 0.2 (w/v) dried milk. The protoplasts are transferred as 1-ml aliquots into a series of Eppendorf tubes; MAb is then added as a series of 10-fold dilutions covering the titration range 0.0001–1% (v/v), and the tube is gently rotated for 20 min. If the MAb recognizes a plasma membrane epitope common to all protoplasts, the protoplasts rapidly agglutinate into large clusters in all but the most dilute MAb solutions. A subset of the protoplasts agglutinate when the MAb is directed against epitopes that are cell-specific, leaving others free in suspension. These should be compared to controls to be certain of the MAb effects, and can be recorded by light microscopy.

D. Immersion Immunofluorescence

Protoplasts and cells should be employed fresh. Labeling of protoplasts is done in microfuge tubes using W5 medium (see Chapter 29, Volume 50), with 0.2% (w/v) dried milk as the blocking agent. Intact cells are labeled in PBS containing 2% (v/v) calf serum. For immunofluorescence, it is important to use saturating amounts of MAb and secondary Ab. Thus, for every 10,000 protoplasts or cells, we add 2% (v/v) of the MAb and 1% (v/v) of the secondary Ab. The protoplasts and cells should be rotated in each of the Ab solutions for 1 h, collected by centrifugation at 600 × *g*, washed, and labeled with secondary Ab for 1 h. Following a final wash using W5 or PBS, they are mounted on glass microscope slides and the FITC signal is viewed under epifluorescence illumination. In our experience, weak FITC signals are due to subsaturating levels of either or both of the Abs, and can be remedied by using fewer protoplasts or cells. We use Fujichrome 1600D color film (Fuji Photo Co., Tokyo), pushed to ASA 3200, for most immunofluorescence photography.

E. Immunodetection on Sections

We employ cryostat and L. R. White resin (London Resin Co., Basingstoke, Hants) sections for immunodetection using sections. For light microscopy, the sections are dried onto glass slides precharged with a 0.05% (w/v) solution of poly-L-lysine; incubation with the MAb and FITC-conjugated secondary Ab is done horizontally within a humid box. We use PBS containing 2% (v/v) calf serum and 2 (v/v) MAb or 1 (v/v) secondary Ab for the labeling; the sections are washed by draining the liquid from the slides in a vertical position. After final washing, semipermanent mounts can be prepared using Citifluor (Citifluor Ltd, London). For electron microscopy, we collect ultrathin sections on plastic-coated gold grids (Agar Scientific Ltd., Stansted, Essex); again, incubation with the MAb and a secondary Ab conjugated with EM grade gold particles (Serotec, Oxford) is done horizontally inside a humid box. To saturate the epitopes that are exposed at the section surface, we float the grids section-side-down on 50-μl drops of TBS containing 5% (v/v) of the calf serum and 5% (v/v) of the MAb for 3 h, and to detect the bound MAb we float the grids for 1 h on the calf serum solution containing 1% (v/v) of the secondary Ab. The grids can be washed with a slow jet of TBS or by repeated immersion in a TBS bath. For mild contrast, we impregnate the immunolabeled sections using a 2% (v/v) solution of uranyl acetate in water for 2 min, prior to examination. For routine purposes, the secondary Abs should be conjugated to 10-nm gold particles. Second MAbs can be biotinylated, applied to the same surface of the sections, and detected with avidin conjugated with gold particles with different sizes, or second MAbs can be applied to the other surface of the sections (using uncoated grids) and detected with secondary Abs conjugated with other gold particles.

F. Inhibition Immunoanalysis

Inhibition analysis is performed by ELISA. We adsorb 50 μl of antigen solution onto 96-well microtiter plates and block residual charges with 63 μl of PBS containing 0.2% (w/v) dried milk. Aliquots (63 μl) of the PBS solution containing 1 m*M* of a hapten saccharide are then added to pairs of wells in column 1, and 50 μl of the PBS solution is added to all the other wells in the microtiter plate. Using a multichannel micropipette, we then transfer 13 μl from well-to-well across the plate, mixing the solutions each time. At lane 12, we remove 13 μl and discard it, thereby leaving 50 μl within each well, and a serial five-fold titration of each competing substance in duplicate, from 1 m*M* on the left of the plate to approximately 5 p*M* on the right. We leave one pair of wells free from hapten as negative controls. Primary Ab is then added to each ELISA well and allowed to bind to the absorbed antigen, and the ELISA completed and read.

G. Immunoaffinity Chromatography

Preconjugated anti-MAb agarose matrices for immunoaffinity chromatography (Sigma Chemical Co., Poole, Dorset) are saturated with MAbs to complex cell surface carbohydrate by mixing the matrices with aliquots of hybridoma culture supernatant. After 1 h, an aliquot is tested by dot-immunoblotting with secondary Ab for the presence of MAb free in solution. Normally, 1 ml of the matrix saturates with about 50 ml of the supernatant. The matrix is then loaded into a column, and thoroughly washed with 10 nm Tris buffer, pH 7.2, containing 0.5 *M* NaCl (TBS). The antigen should be fully soluble in water, for example, the antigen contained in the water phase derived from the detergent-partitioning of plasma membranes. This is diluted to about 1 mg ml^{-1} protein in TBS, and sufficient sample is loaded onto the column until traces of antigen appear in the wash-through. The column is then throughly washed using TBS, then is eluted with a single volume of 10 m*M* Tris buffer, pH 2.5, or pH 11, or of 15 m*M* hapten monosaccharide (if known). Fractions are collected and tested for the presence of the epitope recognized by the MAb; controls are included to detect leaching of MAb from the matrix. Serial dialysis against distilled water and lyophilization produces antigen suitable for subsequent carbohydrate and protein analysis.

H. Western Immunoblotting

Nongradient or gradient slab gels such as ExcelGels (Pharmacia LKB Biotechnology Uppsala) can be used for SDS–PAGE and Western immunoblotting. For chemical analysis of the resolved antigens, we load the gels as a single well up to 20 cm across, and blot onto high-load nylon membranes such as ProBlott membranes (Applied Biosystems, Foster City). These membranes are superior to nitrocellulose, which has a lower capacity and releases glucose on acid hydrolysis. To detect resolved antigens, 5-mm strips are cut from each edge and from the center of the membrane, and processed with MAbs and secondary Abs as described for dot-immunoblotting and TIP. The developed strips are then dried and realigned in their original positions with the remainder of the membrane, and the antigen bands, which extend between them, are cut out using a scalpel.

I. Molecular Immunolabeling

Cell suface macromolecules that have been isolated by conventional procedures can be labeled with MAbs and gold particles and visualized with an electron microscope, to see the disposition of epitopes. Plastic-coated electron microscope grids should be prewashed with a 0.06 *M* sodium phosphate buffer solution (pH 6.5) and floated for 5 min on the solution of target molecules. For the immunogold labeling, we transfer the grids to 3 μl of a 0.05 *M* sodium acetate solution for 1 min, PBS containing 2% calf serum for 30 min, and 3 μl of the MAb and secondary Ab in the PBS solution also for 30 min each (prepared as described for immunogold labeling of sections). Each step is preceded by washing with water. The gold particles should be 1 μm in diameter. The antigen molecules and the attached gold particles are then visualized by negative staining with a 2% (w/v) uranyl acetate solution for 2 min and examined at high magnification under the electron microscope.

J. Immunomagnetic Cell Separation

To perform ICS with cell-specific cell wall epitopes, we obtain single cells from plant cell suspension cultures by sieving the cultures using 22- and 10-μm nylon meshes. The cells falling within this size range are then labeled by immersion. For ICS, all the labeling is performed in fresh cell culture medium containing 0.2% (v/v) calf serum. We use secondary Ab that is conjugated with Dynabeads [Dynal (UK) Ltd., New Ferry, Wirral]. The labeled cells are then placed into a magnetic particle concentrator such as the MPC-1 (Dynal), from which nontarget cells can be removed after a few moments, followed by the target cells, according to the manufacturers instructions. Micromolar concentrations of hapten competitors are then used to remove the Abs and beads from the walls of the target cells (see Fig. 8).

III. Perspectives

The essential advantage of MAbs over antisera for plant cell biology research is the opportunity to generate highly specific molecular probes from simple

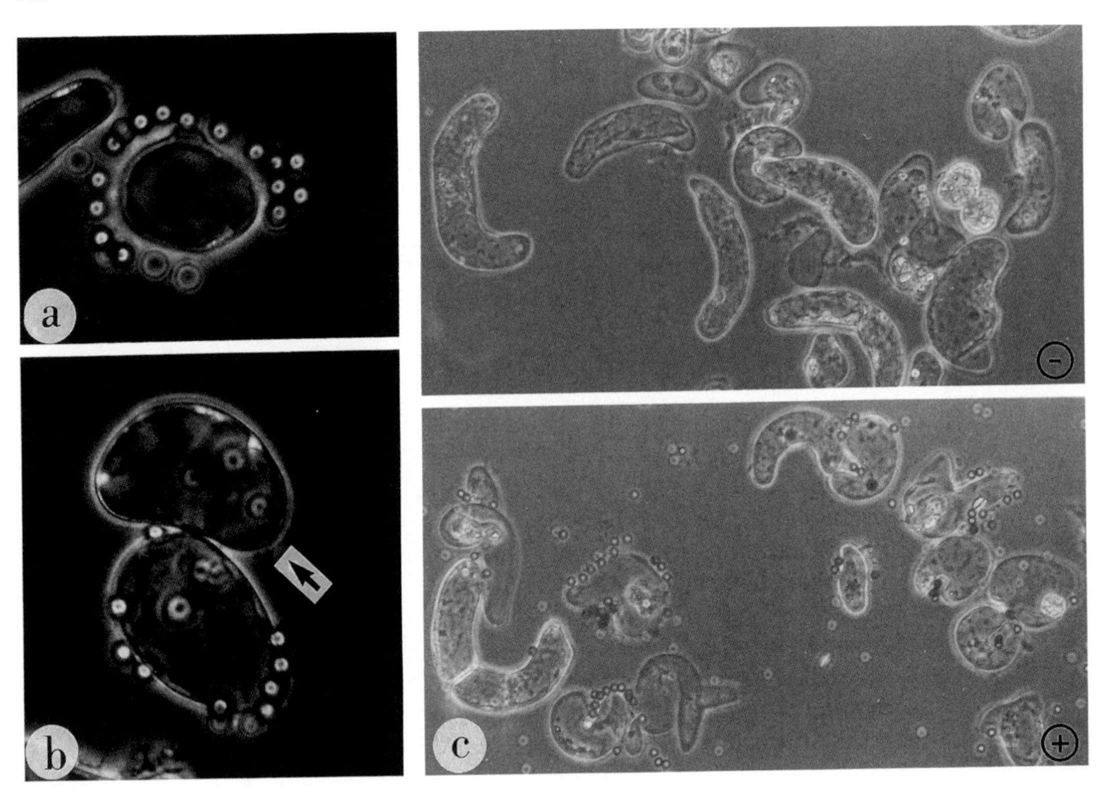

Fig. 8 Single carrot cells sieved from an embryogenic cell suspension culture, labeled at the cell wall by immersion in solutions of JIM8 and paramagnetic beads (a,b) and subjected to immunomagnetic cell sorting (c). The secondary Ab effectively magnetizes JIM8-reactive single cells (a). Because the JIM8 cell wall carbohydrate epitope is cell-specific (b), JIM8-ICS produces two JIM8-defined cell collectives designated (−) and (+). ×1350 (a,b) and ×340 (c). Courtesy of Paul McCabe.

immunizations with impure antigen mixtures, and then to be able to use the MAbs in versatile techniques for the purification, characterization, and manipulation of antigens and the cells that carry them. MAbs used in approaches of this kind have in the past driven the biology of the regulated AGPs at the plasma membrane surface. Since AGPs appear to be present in all green plants, MAbs are now revealing conserved patterns of evolution in the AGP carbohydrate, an entirely novel concept. Weak bonds hold MAbs to epitopes, and to the conjugated ABs used for the localization. These bonds can be broken biochemically, freeing the MAbs from the targets, which, if they are living cells or protoplasts, can subsequently be cultured. Thus, ICS and IPS offer the possibility of isolating cells according to surface criteria signifying developmental phenomena; the possibility also exists for regenerating whole plants. The related application of epitope mutant screening and selection, directed toward an analysis of the influence of cell surface carbohydrates on cellular differentiation in plants, may also open the field of carbohydrates to genetic and molecular dissection. It is also possible to envisage the use of microinjection of MAbs or MAb antigen-binding fragments into the apoplast for MAb-based cell ablation, a powerful tool for studies of cell lineages and of the function of cell–cell interactions in plants. In line with somatic cell genetics and tissues culture, MAbs will turn out to be powerful manipulative tools for the cell biological and molecular study of plant development.

References

Anderson, M. A., Sandrin, M. S., and Clarke, A. E. (1984). A high proportion of hybridomas raised to a plant extract secrete antibody to arabinose or galactose. *Plant Physiol.* **75,** 1013–1016.

Baldwin, T. C., McCann, M. C., and Roberts, K. (1993). A novel hydroxyproline-deficient arabinogalactan-protein secreted by suspension-cultured cells of *Daucus carota. Plant Physiol.* **103,** 115–123.

Cassab, G. I., and Varner, J. E. (1987). Immunocytolocalization of extensin in developing soybean seed coats by immunogold-silver staining and by tissue printing on nitrocellulose paper. *J. Cell Biol.* **105,** 2581–2588.

Chen, C.-G., Pu, Z.-Y., Moritz, R. L., Simpson, R. J., Bacic, A., Clarke, A. E., and Mau, S.-L. (1994). Molecular cloning of a gene encoding an arabinogalactan-protein from pear (*Pyrus communis*) cell suspension culture. *Proc. Natl. Acad. Sci. U.S.A.,* **91,** 10305–10309.

Collin, H. A., and Dix, P. J. (1990). Culture systems and selection procedures. *In* "Plant Cell Line Selection" (P. J. Dix, ed.), pp. 3–18. New York: VCH Publishers.

Condit, C. M. (1993). Developmental expression and localization of petunia glycine-rich protein 1. *Plant Cell* **5,** 277–288.

Conrad, T. A., Lamport, D. T. A., and Hammerschmidt, M. R. (1987). Detection of glycosylated and deglycosylated extension precursors by indirect competitive ELISA. *Plant Physiol.* **83,** 1–3.

Durand, J. L. (1990). Mutagenesis: EMS treatment of cell suspensions of Nicotiana sylvestris. *In* "Methods in Molecular Biology, Volume 6: Plant Cell and Tissue Culture" (J. W. Pollard and J. M. Walker, eds.), pp. 431–441. Clifton: Humana Press.

Evans, D. A., and Bravo, J. E. (1983). Protoplast isolation and culture. *In* "Handbook of Plant Cell Culture, Volume 1: Techniques for Propagation and Breeding" (D. E. Evans, W. R. Sharp P. V. Ammirator, and Y. Yamada, eds.), pp. 124–176. New York: Macmillan Co.

Fincher, G. B., Stone, B. A., and Clarke, A. E. (1983). Arabinogalactan-proteins: Structure, biosynthesis and function. *Ann. Rev. Plant Physiol.* **34,** 47–70.

Fitter, M. S., Norman, P. M., Hahn, M. G., Wingate, V. P. M., and Lamb, C. J. (1987). Identification of somatic hybrids in plant protoplast fusion with monoclonal antibodies to plasma-membrane antigens. *Planta* **170,** 49–54.

Goding, J. W. (1986). "Monoclonal Antibodies: Principles and Practice." London: Academic Press.

Harlow, E., and Lane, L. (1988). "Antibodies: A Laboratory Manual." Cold Spring Harbor, NY: Cold Spring Harbor Laboratory Press.

Jones, J. L., Callow, J. A., and Green, J. R. (1990). The molecular nature of *Fucus serratus* sperm surface antigens recognized by monoclonal antibodies FS1 to FS12. *Planta* **182,** 64–71.

Kausch, A. P., and Bruce, B. D. (1994). Isolation and immobilization of various plastid subtypes by magnetic immunoabsorption. *Plant J.* **6,** 767–779.

Keller, B., Templeton, M. D., and Lamb, C. J. (1989). Specific localization of a plant cell wall glycine-rich protein in protoxylem cells of the vascular system. *Proc. Natl. Acad. Sci. U.S.A.* **86,** 1529–1533.

Kieliszewski, M., and Lamport, D. T. A. (1986). Cross-reactivities of polyclonal antibodies against extension precursors determined vial ELISA techniques. *Phytochemistry* **25,** 673–677.

Kieliszewski, M., Kamyab, A., Leykam, J. F., and Lamport, D. T. A. (1992). A histidine-rich extension from *Zea mays* is an arabinogalactan protein. *Plant Physiol.* **99,** 538–547.

Kjellbom, P., and Larsson, C. (1984). Preparation and polypeptide composition of chlorophyll-free plasma membranes from leaves of light-grown spinach and barley. *Physiol. Plant* **62,** 501–509.

Kjellbom, P., Larsson, C., Rochester, C. P., and Andersson, B. (1989). Integral and peripheral proteins of the spinach leaf plasma membrane. *Plant Physiol. Biochem.* **27,** 169–174.

Knox, J. P., Day, S., and Roberts, K. (1989). A set of cell surface glycoproteins forms an early marker of cell position but not cell fate in the root apical meristem of *Daucus carota* L. *Development* **106,** 47–56.

Knox, J. P., Linstead, P. J., King, J., Cooper, C., and Roberts, K. (1990). Pectin esterification is spatically regulated both within cell walls and between developing tissues of root apices. *Planta* **181,** 512–521.

Knox, J. P., Linstead, P. J., Peart, J., Cooper, C., and Roberts, K. (1991). Developmentally-regulated epitopes of cell surface arabinogalactan proteins and their relation to root tissue pattern formation. *Plant J.* **1,** 317–326.

Li, Y.-Q., Brunn, L, Pierson, E. S., and Cresti, M. (1992). Periodic disposition of arabinogalactan epitopes in the cell wall of pollen tubes of *Nicotiana tabacum. Planta* **188,** 532–538.

Liners, F., Letesson, J.-J., Didemborg, C., and van Custem, P. (1989). Monoclonal antibodies against pectin. *Plant Physiol.* **91,** 1419–1424.

Liners, F., and van Custem, P. (1992). Distribution of pectic polysaccharides throughout walls of suspension-cultured carrot cells. *Protoplasma* **170,** 10–21.

Lynes, M. A., Lamb, C. A., Napolitano, A., and Stout, R. G. (1987). Antibodies to cell-surface antigens of plant protoplasts. *Plant Sci.* **50,** 225–232.

Lynes, M. A. (1992). Immunochemical analysis of the temporal and tissue-specific expression of an *Avena sativa* plasma membrane determinant. *Plant Physiol.* **98,** 24–33.

McCann, M. C., Wells, B., and Roberts, K. (1992). Complexity in the spatial localization and length distribution of plant cell-wall matrix polysaccharides. *J. Microsc.* **166,** 123–136.

Metcalf, T. M., III, Villanueva, M. A., Schindler, M., and Wang, J. L. (1987). Monoclonal antibodies directed against protoplasts of soybean cells: Analysis of the lateral mobility of plasma membrane-bound antibody MVS-1. *J. Cell Biol.* **102,** 1350–1357.

Meyer, D. J., Afonso, C. L., and Galbraith, D. W. (1988). Isolation and characterization of monoclonal antibodies directed against plant plasma membrane and cell wall epitopes: Identification of a monoclonal antibody that recognizes extensin and analysis of the process of epitope biosynthesis in plant tissues and cell cultures. *J. Cell Biol.* **107,** 163–175.

Moore, P. J., Darvill, A. G., Albersheim, P., and Staehelin, J. A. (1986). Immunogold localization of xyloglucan and rhamnogalacturonan I in the cell walls of suspension-cultured sycamore cells. *Plant Physiol.* **82,** 787–794.

Negrutiu, I. (1990). *In vitro* mutagenesis. *In* "Plant Cell Line Selection" (P. J. Dix, ed.). pp. 19–38. New York: VCH Publishers.

Nomura, K., and Komamine, A. (1985). Identification and isolation of single cells that produce somatic embryos at a high frequency in a carrot suspension culture. *Plant Physiol.* **79,** 988–991.

Pennell, R. I., Knox, J. P., Scofield, G., N., Selvendran, R. R., and Roberts, K. (1989). A family of abundant plasma membrane-associated glycoproteins related to the arabinogalactan proteins is unique to flowering plants. *J. Cell Biol.* **108,** 1967–1977.

Pennell, R. I., and Roberts, K. (1990). Sexual development in the pea is presaged by altered expression of arabinogalactan protein. *Nature* **344,** 547–549.

Pennell, R. I., Janniche, L., Kjellbom, P., Scofield, G. N., Peart, J. M., and Roberts, K. (1991). Developmental regulation of a plasma membrane arabinogalactan protein epitope in oilseed rape flowers. *Plant Cell* **3,** 1317–1326.

Pennell, R. I., Janniche, L., Scofield, G. N., Booij, H., de Vries, S. C., and Roberts, K. (1992). Identification of a transitional cell state in the developmental pathway to carrot somatic embryogenesis. *J. Cell Biol.* **119,** 1371–1380.

Perotto, S., VendenBosch, K. A., Butcher, G. W., and Brewin, J. J. (1991). Molecular composition and development of the plant glycocalyx associated with the peribacteroid membrane of pea root nodules. *Development* **112,** 763–773.

Puhlmann, J., Bucheli, E., Swain, M. J., Dunning, N., Albersheim, P., Darvill, A. G., and Hahn, M. G. (1994). Generation of monoclonal antibodies against plant cell wall polysaccharides. I. Characterization of a monoclonal antibody to a terminal α-(1 $\rightarrow$ 2)-linked fucosyl-containing epitope. *Plant Physiol.* **104,** 699–710.

Rae, A. L., Perotto, S., Know, J. P., Kannenberg, E. L., and Brewin, N. J. (1991). Expression of extracellular glycoproteins in the uninfected cells of developing pea root nodules. *Mol. Plant-Microbe Interact.* **4,** 563–570.

Roberts, K. (1989). The plant extracellular matrix. *Curr. Opin. Cell Biol.* **1,** 1020–1027.

Roberts, K. (1990). Structures at the plant cell surface. *Curr. Opin. Cell Biol.* **2,** 920–928.

Rodkiewicz, B. (1970). Callose in cell walls during megasporogeneis in angiosperms. *Planta* **93,** 39–47.

Reid, P. D., and Pont-Lezica, R. F. (1991). "Tissue Printing" San Diego: Academic Press.

Reiter, W.-D., Chapple, C. C. S., and Sommerville, C. R. (1993). Altered growth and cell walls in a fucose-deficient mutant of *Arabidopsis. Science* **261,** 1032–1035.

Ryser, U., and Keller, B. (1992). Ultrastructural localization of a bean glycine-rich protein in unlignified primary walls of protoxylem cells. *Plant Cell* **4,** 773–783.

Showalter, A. M. (1993). Structure and function of plant cell wall proteins. *Plant Cell* **5,** 9–23.

Smallwood, M., Beven, A., Donovan, N., Neil, S. J., Peart, J., Roberts, K., and Knox, J. P. (1994). Localization of cell wall proteins in relation to the developmental anatomy of the carrot root apex. *Plant J.* **5,** 237–246.

Smith, E., Roberts, K., Hutchings, A., and Galfré, G. (1984a). Monoclonal antibodies to the major structural glycoprotein of the *Chlamydomonas* cell wall. *Planta* **161,** 330–338.

Smith, E., Roberts, K., Butcher, G. W., and Galfré, G. (1984b). Monoclonal antibody screening: Two methods using antigens immobilized on nitrocellulose. *Anal. Biochem.* **138,** 119—124.

Springall, D. R., Hacker, G. H., Grimelius, L., and Polak, J. M. (1984). The potential of the immunogold-silver staining method for paraffin sections. *Histochem.* **81,** 603–608.

Stacey, N. J., Roberts, K., and Knox, J. P. (1990). Patterns of expression of the JIM4 arabinogalactan-protein epitope in cell cultures and during somatic embryogenesis in *Daucus carota* L. *Planta* **180,** 285–292.

Stafstrom, J. P., and Staehelin, L. A. (1988). Antibody localization of extension in cell walls of carrot storage roots. *Planta* **174,** 321–332.

Stanley, P. (1987). Glycosylation mutants and the functions of mammalian carbohydrates. *Trends Genet.* **3,** 77–79.

Swords, K. M. M., and Staehelin, A. L. (1993). Complimentary immunolocalization patterns of cell wall hydroxyproline-rich glycoproteins studies with the use of antibodies directed against different carbohydrate epitopes. *Plant Physiol.* **102,** 891–901.

VandenBosch, K. A., Bradley, D. J., Know, J. P., Perotto, S., Butcher, G. W., and Brewin, N. J. (1989). Common components of the infection thred matrix and the intercellular space identified by immunocytochemical analysis of pea root nodules. *EMBO J.* **8,** 335–342.

Villanueva, M. A., Metcalf, T. N., III, and Wang, J. L. (1986). Monoclonal antibodies directed against protoplasts of soybean cells. *Planta* **168,** 503–511.

von Schaewen, A., Sturm, A., O'Neill, J., and Chrispeels, M. J. (1993). Isolation of a mutant *Arabidopsis* plant that lacks N-acetyl glucosaminyl transferase 1 and is unable to synthesis Golgi-modified complex N-linked glycans. *Plant Physiol.* **102,** 1109–1118.

Weitzhandler, M., Kadlecek, D., Avdalovic, N., Forte, J. G., Chow, D., and Townsend, R. R. (1993). Monosaccharide and oligosaccharide analysis of proteins transferred to polyvinylidene fluoride membranes after sodium dodecyl sulfate-polyacrylamide gel electrophoresis. *J. Biol. Chem.* **268,** 5121–5130.

Wells, B. (1985). Low temperature box and tissue handling device for embedding biological tissue and immunostaining in electron microscopy. *Micron Microsc. Acta* **16,** 49–53.

CHAPTER 10

Epitope Tagging for the Detection of Fusion Protein Expression in Transgenic Plants

Mark J. Guiltinan and Lauren McHenry

Department of Horticulture and The Biotechnology Institute
The Center for Gene Expression
Pennsylvania State University
University Park, Pennsylvania 16802

I. Introduction

Methods for the genetic transformation of plants have made possible new experimental approaches, revolutionizing the science of plant biology. This technology is also the basis for the production of genetically engineered plants with enhanced or novel genetic traits (Gasser and Fraley, 1992). When conducting genetic transformation studies, it is necessary to have available molecular probes to enable the detection of the transgene and its RNA and protein products (trans-message and trans-protein) via nucleic acid hybridization, antibody local-

METHODS IN CELL BIOLOGY, VOL. 49

ization and/or various functional assays. In some cases, it may also be necessary to distinguish the trans-molecules from any similar cross-reactive endogenous factors.

When existing molecular probes are not available or when endogenous factors interfere with detection, it may be advantageous to engineer into a transgene a short DNA sequence specifying a known polypeptide epitope (an epitope tag). A monoclonal antibody with strong binding specificity for the epitope tag can then be used to detect sensitively the expression of a trans-protein using standard techniques (Western blot analysis, ELISA, or *in situ* immunolocalization). Although larger molecular fusions have also been used for detection, one advantage of an epitope tag is its small size, minimizing the potential for disruption of the proper folding and/or activity of the trans-protein.

One well-characterized epitope is a 10-amino acid sequence derived from the human c-*myc* gene (containing sequences specifying amino acids 410–419). This polypeptide is specifically recognized by the monoclonal antibody Mycl-9E10 (Evan *et al.,* 1985). This epitope has been used to detect the expression of fusion protein in transformed animal and yeast cells. (Ellison and Hochstrasser, 1991; Fowlkes *et al.,* 1992; Munro *et al.,* 1986; Peculis and Gall, 1992). A similar approach utilizing an 8-amino acid epitope tag derived from the human tenascin gene has been used for detecting recombinant RNA binding protein in transfected protoplasts of *Nicotiana plumbaginifolia* (Mieszczak *et al.,* 1992). We describe here the development of the c-*myc* epitope tag system for the detection of trans-protein expression in transgenic tobacco plants. An expression vector for plant c-*myc* epitope tagging was constructed and introduced into tobacco plants via *Agrobacterium*-mediated transformation. Our results show that c-*myc* epitope tagged trans-protein can be detected in extracts from as little as 5 mg of leaf tissue. The Mycl-9E10 monoclonal antibody shows no cross-reactivity to endogenous tobacco or *Arabidopsis thaliana* proteins. Furthermore, the antibody can be used to localize expression in various tissues using the tissue print method (Cassab and Varner, 1987).

II. Methods

A. c-*myc* Epitope Tag Vector Construction

A plant expression vector was designed for the fusion of the c-*myc* epitope tag to any coding sequence, and for expression of the tagged fusion protein in transgenic plants. The vector was derived from pMON881, with the incorporation of an ATG start codon in frame with DNA sequences specifying 10 amino acids of the human c-*myc* protein flanked by the cauliflower mosaic virus 35S promoter and the nopaline synthase 3′ untranslated region. pLM1 (Fig. 1) carries a fusion gene consisting of the c-*myc* epitope tag and the DNA binding domain (λGC19) of the wheat EmBP-1 gene (Guiltinan *et al.,* 1990). Additional experimental results using the c-*myc*/GC19 transgenic plants will be presented elsewhere.

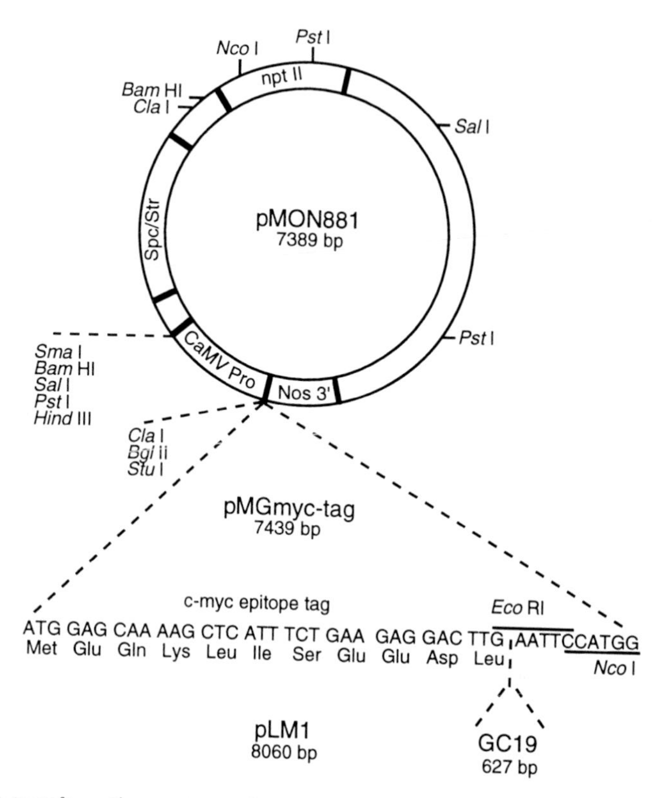

Fig. 1 Plant transformation vector and sequence of c-*myc* epitope tag. Sequences encoding a 30-bp portion of the human c-*myc* gene were inserted into the plant transformation vector, pMON881 (Monsanto; St. Louis, MO), to create pMGmyc-tag. An ATG start codon is present just 5′ to sequences encoding the epitope tag and there is a unique *Eco*RI cloning site directly following the epitope tag. The plant cell selectable marker gene (kanamycin resistance, npt II) is indicated. The DNA binding and dimerization domain (GC19) of the EmBP-1 protein (Guiltinan *et al.,* 1990) was cloned into the *Eco*RI site of pMGmyc tag to produce pLM1 used in the production of transgenic tobacco plants.

Standard protocols were used for DNA isolation and manipulation (Sambrook *et al.,* 1989), and for transformation of *Nicotiana tabacum,* SR1 (Horsch *et al.,* 1988). The *Hind*III/*Spe*I fragment of pMG99.23, containing sequences specifying amino acids 410–419 of the human c-*myc* gene fused to EmBP-1 sequences from the *Eco*RI insert of λGC19 (Guiltinan *et al.,* 1990), was rendered blunt with T4 polymerase and subcloned into the similarly blunt-ended *Eco*RI site of the plant expression vector pMON881 (Monsanto, St. Louis, MO), to yield pLM1 (Fig. 1).

pMG99.23 was constructed by inserting the Klenow filled *Eco*RI insert of λGC19 (Guiltinan *et al.,* 1990) into the *Bam*HI cut and filled vector pAU1 to form pAU2. pAU1 was derived from pBSKSc-*myc* (Peculis and Gall, 1992), which contains a 30-bp synthetic oligonucleotide, representing a portion of the human c-*myc* coding region (Fig. 1), inserted into the *Hin*dIII/*Eco*RI site of pBluescript KS+ (Promega, Madison, WI). Stop codons in all three reading frames were introduced downstream of the unique *Spe*I site of pBSKSc-*myc* to form pAU1 by cutting, filling, and religating at the *Xba*I site. This change and other critical features of the construct were verified by DNA sequencing. The *Sac*I/*Xho*I fragment of pAU2, containing the short c-*myc* fragment fused to the 5′ end of the GC19 sequences, was subcloned into *Sac*I/*Xho*I-digested pRT101 (Topfer *et al.*, 1987) to create pMG99.23.

B. Plant Transformation

pLM1 was introduced into the *Agrobacterium tumefaciens* strain ABI via triparental mating (Van Haute *et al.*, 1983) utilizing pRK2013 as helper plasmid. Tobacco (*N. tabacum* Petite Havana cv. SR1) leaf discs were transformed with the resulting *A. tumefaciens* strain, and regenerated shoots (R_0) were selected for their ability to root on MSO media (MS salts, Gamborg's vitamins, 1% sucrose, 0.3% phytagel) containing 100 μg/ml kanamycin monosulfate. Stable transformation of nine individual lines was confirmed by segregational analysis of the *npt*II selectable marker in seed lots (F1) from self-fertilized primary transformants plated on germination media (MS salts, Gamborg's vitamins, 0.7% glucose, 0.3% sucrose, 0.3% phytagel) containing 100 μg/ml kanamycin.

C. Protein Extraction, Electrophoresis, and Blotting

Primary transformants (R_0) were self-fertilized and the resulting kanamycin-resistant offspring (F1) were tested for expression of the c-*myc*/GC19 fusion protein by extracting total SDS-soluble protein from 3-week-old seedlings and subjecting it to Western blot analysis (Fig. 2). After 3 weeks of growth on germination media supplemented with 100 μg/ml kanamycin, 10 kanamycin-resistant seedlings of each transgenic line were randomly selected and pooled. Each pool was homogenized with a mini-mortar in a 1.5-ml microcentrifuge tube with a small volume of 2× Laemmli buffer (Laemmli, 1970). The samples were placed in a boiling water bath for 10 min and then microfuged for 10 min at 4°C to remove debris. The volume of each sample was adjusted to a final concentration of 1 mg fresh weight per microliter with the addition of 10× loading dye (0.1% bromphenol blue in 80% glycerol) and water. Protein from roots and leaves of mature soil-grown *Arabidopsis* was prepared in the same manner.

Approximately equal amounts of each sample, including a wild-type SR1 control protein extract, were electrophoresed through a 10% SDS–polyacrylamide gel using a discontinuous buffer system. Separated proteins were electroblotted onto an Immobilon-P transfer membrane (Millipore Corp., Bedford, MA) using a submerged mini trans-blot electrophoretic transfer cell (BioRad; Richmond, CA) according to the manufacturer's instructions by applying 100 V for

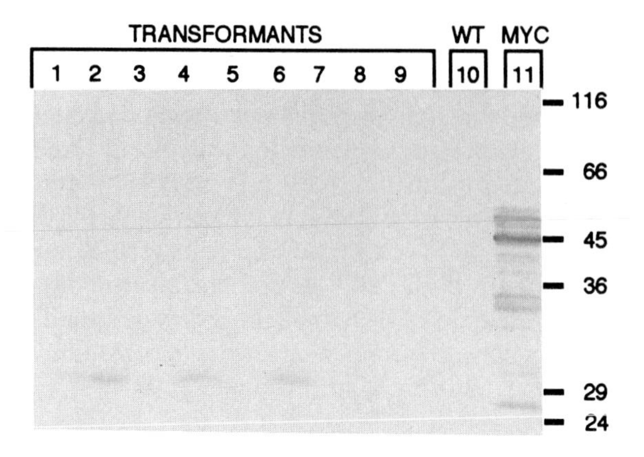

Fig. 2 Western blot analysis of protein extracted from c-*myc*/GC19 transgenic tobacco plants reacted with an antibody directed against the c-*myc* epitope. Total SDS-soluble protein from pools of kanamycin-resistant seedlings from self-crossed primary transformants were separated by polyacrylamide gel electrophoresis and transferred to Immobilon-P. The filter was reacted with a monoclonal antibody (Mycl-9E10) directed against the human c-*myc* protein. Each lane contains an extract equivalent to approximately 5 to 10 mg of fresh weight-seedling tissue. Lanes 1–9, nine independent transformants; Lane 10, wild-type SRI tobacco; Lane 11, c-*myc*-tagged protein derived from expression of the *Ste7* gene of *Saccharomyces cerevisiae* in *Escherichia coli.*

1 h in a transfer buffer composed of 25 m*M* Tris [hydroxymethyl]aminomethane, 192 m*M* glycine, 20% (v/v) methanol.

D. Tissue Printing and Protein Staining

Transgenic F2 seedlings propagated on MSr plates containing 100 μg/ml kanamycin, and control SR1 seedlings on MSr plates without kanamycin, were rinsed with sterile distilled water and blotted onto nitrocellulose (0.45 μm S&S NC, Schleicher & Schuell, Keene, NH) as previously described (Cassab and Varner, 1987). Blots were then stained to confirm protein transfer by a 1-min soak in 0.5% Ponceau-S in 1% acetic acid and destained by several subsequent rinses in distilled water. Immunodetection was performed as described below. After color development, nitrocellulose blots were rinsed in full strength Clorox bleach for 2 min to reduce residual chlorophyll.

E. Antibody Incubations and Immunodetection

The membranes with affixed proteins were equilibrated in TBS (Tris-buffered saline: 20 m*M* Tris, pH 7.5, and 500 m*M* sodium chloride) and then blocked with 5% Carnation instant nonfat dry milk in TBS for 1 h at room temperature. The primary antibody, Mycl-9E10, was a monoclonal antibody raised against the human c-*myc* protein in mouse cells (Evan *et al.,* 1985) that were grown to confluency in Dulbecco's medium (GIBCO). The membrane was saturated with antibody medium supernatant after it had been blocked as described and rinsed twice with TBS supplemented with 0.05% Tween-20 (TTBS). Two rinses in TTBS preceded incubation for 1 h in TTBS, 5% nonfat dry milk, and 1:7500 dilution of 1 mg/ml anti-mouse IgG AP conjugate (Promega, Madison, WI). The incubation was followed by two rinses in TTBS, one rinse in TBS, and one rinse in carbonate buffer (0.1 *M* sodium bicarbonate, pH 9.8, and 1 m*M* magnesium chloride). Color development proceeded until full color of reacting proteins was achieved with 0.3 mg/ml nitro blue tetrazolium and 0.15 mg/ml 5-bromo-4-chloro-3-indoyl phosphate in carbonate buffer.

III. Results and Discussion

A fusion gene was constructed consisting of the c-*myc* epitope tag and a portion of the wheat EmBP-1 gene under the control of the CaMV 35S promoter (Fig. 1). Transgenic tobacco lines with the tagged gene were generated via Agrobacterium-mediated gene transfer. Protein extracts from nine transgenic and one normal plant were analyzed for the presence of the fusion protein by Western blot analysis (Fig. 2). An antibody directed against the c-*myc* epitope (Mycl-9E10) allowed detection of the c-*myc*/GC19 protein with the expected apparent molecular mass of 30 kDa in crude extracts from four of nine transformants (Fig. 2, lanes 1, 2, 4, and 6). Expression level variation among independent transgenic lines is the most likely explanation for why no fusion protein was detected in five of the plants. No c-*myc* reactive protein was detected, even after prolonged color development, in SR1 wild-type tobacco plants (Fig. 2, lane 10), or in protein extracts from roots or leaves of *Arabidopsis thaliana* (data not shown). Although we have not yet determined the sensitivity of this detection system, we were capable of detecting protein from as little as 5 mg of fresh weight leaf tissue.

Tissue printing allows the simple detection of the amounts of protein or mRNA present at the whole organism level. To test the suitability of the c-*myc*-tag system to tissue printing, whole seedling prints were prepared and reacted with the c-*myc* antibody. The antibody strongly detected expression of the fusion protein in the leaves, roots, and cotyledons of transgenic F1 seedlings (Fig. 3), consistent with the known expression pattern of the CaMV35S promoter. A stronger signal was seen on the periphery of the tissue, perhaps due to more efficient extraction of protein around the edges. No cross-reactivity of the antibody to tissue prints of control, nontransformed tobacco plants was detectable.

IV. Conclusions and Perspectives

The ability of the Mycl-9E10 antibody to detect the 10-amino acid c-*myc* epitope on Westerns blots and tissue prints and the absence of antibody cross-

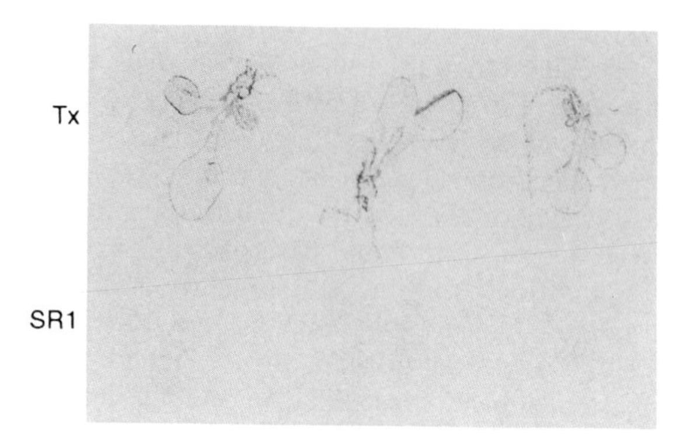

Fig. 3 Tissue prints of c-myc/GC19-transformed tobacco plants reacted with an antibody directed against the c-*myc* epitope. Whole seedlings of either c-*myc*-tagged GC19-transformed (Tx) or wild-type (SR1) lines were blotted onto nitrocellulose and reacted with a monoclonal antibody (Mycl-9E10) directed against the human c-*myc* protein.

reactivity to endogenous tobacco and *Arabidopsis* proteins make this epitope–antibody pair an excellent choice as a general marker for protein expression in transgenic plants. In cases where no enzymatic activity has been demonstrated for a protein, or in which no antibody specific to the encoded protein is availabile, epitope-tagging provides a simple alternative to monitoring protein expression of introduced genes.

Tissue prints of excised leaves can also be used to detect rapidly the expression of the c-*myc* tagged trans-protein in a large population of segregating progeny (data not shown). This is particularly advantageous in the cosegregational analysis of a trans-protein and its presumptive phenotypic effects. Leaf disks taken from transgenic seedlings can be arrayed in a grid and rapidly tested for trans-protein expression. This allows for hundreds of samples to be processed in a single day, thus enabling the screening of sufficient numbers of progeny to confidently test for cosegregation with a phenotypic character scored separately for each seedling.

Epitope tagging is not without its potential pitfalls. The most important consideration is the theoretical possibility that the epitope tag might in some way destabilize a fusion protein, alter or eliminate its biological function, or change its subcellular localization pattern. Functional inactivation is frequently observed in the production of bacterial fusion proteins when large affinity purification tags are used such as β-galactosidase, maltose binding protein, or glutathione S-transferase. In cases where an N-terminal fusion is a problem, it would be necessary to attempt C-terminal or internal fusions, which would be difficult with our present vector. The effect of an epitope on the behavior of a fusion protein is likely to be highly variable and dependent on the structure of the protein under study. It is not currently possible to predict accurately protein structure from sequence data, and thus such effects must be tested on a case by case basis.

A. Potential Improvements and Applications of Epitope Tags

In addition to the use of alternative detection systems, improvements in sensitivity might be gained with the use of epitope multimers, four or more tandem arrays of the sequence. In addition to increasing the number of epitope moieties per trans-protein molecule, multimeric epitopes may help ensure that the epitope is located on the exterior of the native protein and thus is available for antibody recognition. This could be especially important for *in situ* immunolocalization applications. Multimeric epitopes should also improve the ability of a monoclonal antibody to immunoprecipitate the trans-protein. This powerful technique can be used to study protein–protein interactions via coprecipitation experiments. One possible adverse effect of multimerization is that longer fusions have inherently higher probability of causing structural perturbation to the protein and thus increased potential to reduce or eliminate its functional activity.

An additional potential of the epitope tag system is the possibility of using the DNA sequence encoding the c-*myc*-tag as a hybridization probe to detect the transgene or its message in DNA and RNA isolated from transgenic plants. This would be advantageous when endogenous genes or mRNAs interfere with the specific detection of a transgene and/or its message by cross-hybridization to the engineered gene probe. Nucleic acid probes shorter than 30 nucleotides have been successfully used in similar hybridization experiments, so there is no a priori reason this should not be possible. It may also be possible to use such probes to localize the trans-message at a cellular level using *in situ* hybridization. However, the small size of such a probe may reduce the detection sensitivity below acceptable levels or cause high background hybridization. These limitations might be avoided by the use of short primers to amplify the tagged messages *in situ* using PCR. If possible, this would allow for the sensitive detection of the tissue, cellular, and subcellular distribution patterns of trans-gene expression levels at the level of mRNA.

The c-*myc* epitope-tag system provides a sensitive and specific tool for the analysis of gene expression in transgenic plants. The relative ease by which such constructions can be generated, the availability and high specificity of the Mycl-9E10 monoclonal antibody, and the various well-developed immunodetection techniques available make epitope tagging a powerful tool in the study of plant molecular biology.

B. Vector and Antibody Availability

The plant expression vector pMGmyc-tag (Fig. 1), containing the c-*myc* epitope tag, is available from the authors after first obtaining permission for use of the parental plasmid pMON881 from the Monsanto Co. (Dr. Harry Klee, 700 Chesterfield Village Parkway, St. Louis, MO 63198). The c-*myc* antibody cell line (Mycl-9E10.2; ATCC CRL 1729) is available from the American Type Culture Collection c/o Sales and Marketing Department, 12301 Parklawn Drive, Rockville, MD 20852, 1-800-638-6597.

Acknowledgments

We thank Dr. Beverly Erredy (University of North Carolina at Chapel Hill) for supplying c-*myc* tagged *Ste*7 protein, Dr. Richard Cyr and Debra Fisher (Penn State University) for producing the Mycl-9E10 antibody supernatant, and Dr. Harry Klee and the Monsanto Co. for providing the pMON881 vector. This work was supported in part by grants to M.J.G. from the NSF (MCB 920 6095) and from Penn State University College of Agricultural Sciences (CRIS 3278).

References

Cassab, G. I., and Varner, J. E. (1987). Immunocytolocalization of extensin in developing soybean seed coats by immunogold-silver staining and by tissue printing on nitrocellulose paper. *J. Cell Biol.* **105,** 2581–2588.

Ellison, M. J., and Hochstrasser, M. (1991). Epitope-tagged ubiquitin. *J. Biol. Chem.* **266,** 21150–21157.

Evan, G. I., Lewis, G. K., Ramsay, G., and Bishop, M. J. (1985). Isolation of monoclonal antibodies specific for human c-myc proto-oncogene product. *Mol. Cell Biol.* **5,** 3610–3616.

Fowlkes, D. M., Adams, M. D., Fowler, V. A., and Kay, B. K. (1992). Multi-purpose vectors for peptide expression on the surface of the M13 viral surface. *Biotechniques* **13,** 422–428.

Gasser, C. S., and Fraley, R. T. (1992). Transgenic plants. *Sci. Am.* June, 62–69.

Guiltinan, M. J., Marcotte, W. R., and Quatrano, R. S. (1990). A plant leucine zipper protein that recognizes an abscisic acid response element. *Science* **250,** 267–271.

Horsch, R. B., Fry, J., Hoffmann, N., Neidermeyer, J., Rogers, S. G., and Fraley, R. T. (1988). Leaf disc transformation. *In* "Plant Molecular Biology Manual" (S. B. Gelvin, R. A. Schilperoort, and D. P. S. Verma, eds), pp. A5/1–A5/9. Dordrecht, The Netherlands: Kluwer.

Laemmli, U. K. (1970). Cleavage of structural proteins during the assembly of the head of bacteriophage T4. *Nature* **227,** 680–685.

Mieszczak, M., Klahre, U., Levy, J. H., Goodall, G. J., and Filipowicz, W. (1992). Multiple plant RNA binding proteins identified by PCR: Expression of cDNAs encoding RNA binding proteins targeted to chloroplasts in Nicotiana plumbaginifolia. *Mol. Gen. Genet.* **234,** 390–400.

Munro, S., and Pelham, H. R. B. (1986). An Hsp70-like protein in the ER: Identity with the 78 kd glucose-regulated protein and immunoglobulin heavy chain binding protein. *Cell* **46,** 291–300.

Peculis, A. B., and Gall, J. G. (1992). Localization of the nucleolar protein NO38 in amphibian oocytes. *J. Cell Biol.* **116,** 1–14.

Sambrook, J., Fritsch, E. F., and Maniatis, T. (1989). "Molecular Cloning: A Laboratory Manual." Cold Spring Harbor, NY: Cold Spring Harbor Laboratory Press.

Topfer, R., Matzeit, V., Gronenborn, B., Schell, J., and Steinbiss, H. H. (1987). A set of plant expression vectors for transcriptional and translational fusions. *Nucl. Acids Res.* **15,** 5890.

Van Haute, E., Joos, H., Maes, M., Warren, G., Van Montagu, M., and Schell, J. (1983). Intergeneric transfer and exchange recombination of restriction fragment cloned in pBR322: A novel strategy for reversed genetics of the Ti plasmids of Agrobacterium tumefaciens. *EMBO J.* **2,** 411–417.

CHAPTER 11

In Situ Enzyme Histochemistry on Plastic-Embedded Plant Material

Marc De Block

Plant Genetic Systems N.V.
Jozef Plateaustraat 22
B-9000 Gent, Belgium

I. Introduction

In situ enzyme histochemistry is a powerful method to help unravel the biochemical complexity of a plant. It permits the study of the biochemical functions of a single cell type without removing those cells from their normal biological context. In this way, the activity patterns of specific enzymes can be studied. To obtain a better understanding into the cell and developmental biology of plants, much recent research has focused on the regulation of gene expression. A strategy often used in these studies is the fusion of isolated plant promoters to a reporter gene. These chimeric genes are introduced into the plant genome, and their expression is studied in transgenic plants. The most widely used reporter gene

METHODS IN CELL BIOLOGY, VOL. 49

for higher plants is the β-glucuronidase (*uidA*) gene of *Escherichia coli* (Jefferson, 1987).

Several requirements must be fulfilled in order to obtain, at the enzyme histochemical level, as much information as possible. First, tissue and cell structure, as well as the enzymatic activity of the marker, must be preserved during embedding, sectioning, and further processing of the sections. Second, the deposition of the (colored) end product of the histochemical reaction must occur at the site of activity. Low-temperature processing and embedding in a water-miscible glycol methacrylate resin has been used for histochemical localization of a variety of enzymes in embedded tissue (De Block and DeBrouwer, 1993; 1992; Murray *et al.*, 1988; Pretlow *et al.*, 1987; Ashford *et al.*, 1986; Soufleris *et al.*, 1983; Namba *et al.*, 1983). Embedding in this resin has various advantages over wax embedding and cryostat sectioning. There is superior preservation of tissue morphology with enhanced resolution of cellular detail. Since the resin can be infiltrated and polymerized at low temperature, there is minimal loss of enzymatic activity. However, to avoid fixation of the material to which many enzymes are sensitive, previous methods have involved freeze-substitution or freeze-drying (Murray and Ewen, 1990; Murray *et al.*, 1989). These techniques are cumbersome and often give poor results with plant material, which has a higher water content and is composed of cells with very large vacuoles.

In this chapter, a modification of the enzyme histochemical methods, as originally described by De Block and Debrouwer (1992), is outlined. This method is based on the following principles: processing of the tissue on crushed ice, no fixation but, instead, a pretreatment with spermidine, partial dehydration with acetone, and final embedding in water-miscible glycol methacrylate at 5°C.

II. Methods

A. Processing of the Plant Material

Plant tissue should be maximum of 2 mm in diameter and 5 mm in length. Compact or large structures, or explants with an impermeable surface, must be cut longitudinally or transversely with a razor blade. Trim the tissue in such a way that the solutions used during the processing can reach all parts of the tissue (but do not excessively wound the tissue).

The processing of the material is done in 15-ml disposable glass vials containing 3 ml of solution.

The whole process is done in the cold room (5°C) on crushed ice and under continuous shaking, unless otherwise indicated.

Vacuum infiltration is done by means of a water aspirator.

B. Pretreatment

Incubate for 15 min in plant medium (for example, Murashige and Skoog medium, or Gamborg B5 medium, or other appropriate medium.) containing 1 mM spermidine.

Vacuum infiltrate for 10 to 15 min.

C. Dehydration

Dehydration must be done with acetone. The acetone dilutions are made with 0.85% NaCl.

The dehydration scheme is as follows: 1 h in 50% acetone, wash with 70% acetone, overnight in 70% acetone, 2 h in 80% acetone, 1 h in 90% acetone, 1 h in 90% acetone.

D. Embedding

Embedding is done in Historesin. The Reichert-Jung 7O-2218-500 Historesin embedding kit is a three-component resin: component 1, basic resin (glycol methacrylate monomer, polyethylene glycol 400, hydroquinone); component 2, activator (benzoyl peroxide with 50% plasticizer); component 3, hardener (derivative of barbituric acid in DMSO).

To preserve enzyme activities, the hydroquinone present in the basic resin must be removed. This is done by shaking 100 ml of Historesin with 4 g of activated charcoal (100–400 mesh) for 1 h. The Historesin is separated from the activated charcoal by filtering through a fine-mesh paper filter (Schleicher and Schuell 602H). The treated Historesin is stored at 4°C. The embedding is done as follows:

4 h in 50% acetone (90%)/50% basic resin.

Overnight in 30% acetone (90%)/70% basic resin.

4 h in 100% basic resin.

Replace the 100% basic resin, and vacuum infiltrate for 20 min. Incubate for about 20 h.

Wash specimen for 5 min with basic resin + activator (0.6%) + hardener (1 ml for 15 ml basic resin), called the embedding medium.

Place specimens in BEEM embedding capsules (polythene capsules with a truncated cone). Use capsules that are 6 mm in diameter (BEEM 3 capsules, about 300 μl volume), containing at the bottom 50 μl of polymerized embedding medium (about 30 min at 55°C). Should the specimens be too large, capsules of 8 mm in diameter (BEEM 00 capsules, about 1000 μl volume) can also be used; these then should be prefilled with 100 μl of polymerized embedding medium at the bottom. Orient the specimen on the sticky surface of the polymerized embedding medium. Fill the capsules to the top with fresh nonpolymerized embedding medium. Close the capsules tightly (the polymerization of Historesin at 5°C is oxygen-sensitive). We use TAAB capsule racks made from aluminium, which facilitate cooling of the capsules during polymerization. Allow polymerization to proceed for 1 to 2 days at 5°C in darkness. Store the polymerized historesin blocks containing the plant material in the polythene capsules at 5°C or −20°C. The embedded tissue can be stored in this way for several months without significant loss of enzyme activities.

E. Sectioning

Bring the BEEM capsule with the polymerized Historesin to room temperature (use a vacuum desiccator to prevent water condensation, which can soften the Historesin block).

Remove the polythene capsule from the polymerized Historesin. Be sure that the material is at room temperature, otherwise the hydrophilic Historesin will take up water due to condensation.

File the Historesin block to obtain one flat side. Glue the Historesin block by its flat side onto a 1-cm^3 plexiglass (Perspex) block.

Trim the Historesin block squarely around the specimen. Never put high pressure on the Historesin block; when polymerized, Historesin is a soft plastic and deforms easily. It is almost impossible to obtain good sections from a deformed Historesin block.

Mount on the microtome.

5- to 30-μm sections are easily cut on a dry ralph glass knife.

The ralph glass knife is made on −1 position of the "histoknifemaker" of Reichert-Jung (using 6-mm-thick glass rods). The cutting angle is about 10° for small specimens and up to 14° for large specimens.

F. Enzyme Reaction

1. On Slides

Use Vectabond-treated slides (Vector Laboratories, Burlingame).

Float 5- to 10-μm sections on 400 μl of cold water.

Remove most of the water.

Air-dry the sections at 4°C for 1 to a maximum of 2 h (sections must be dry, otherwise they will detach during the enzyme reaction).

Put 400 μl of the enzyme reaction mixture onto the sections and incubate in a humidified box, or put the slides in a verticle staining dish (suited for eight slides) filled with 30 ml of reaction mixture.

After the enzyme rection, the sections are washed three times 5 to 10 min with distilled water in horizontal staining jars (shake gently).

The slides are then dried and mounted with Eukitt (O. Kindler).

2. In Petri Dishes

This method is about 10 times more sensitive than the previous method. Moreover, sections up to 30 μm in thickness can be used. If complex structures have to be studied (e.g., whole flower buds) thicker sections often give a better morphological resolution.

The reactions are done in small (about 3.5 cm) *glass* (not plastic) petri dishes containing about 2.5 ml of reaction buffer.

Sections of 10-30 μm are put in the reaction buffer, on the bottom of the petri dish.

The reactions are stopped by washing the sections in demineralized water. This is done in the following way.

Fill the petri dish carefully to the top with water.

Place the petri dish in a pyrex baking dish filled with water.

Pick up the sections with a fine pincet and place the sections on a Vectabond-treated slide. This is done in the water. Never remove the sections out of the water with the pincet.

Take the slide with the attached sections out of the water.

The slides can be dried immediately or can be washed further in a horizontal staining dish (shake gently). When sections of 20–30 μm in thickness are dried, they often detach partly from the slide. However, when enough mounting medium is used and light pressure is applied on the cover glass after the mounting medium has spread over the sections, most of the sections will be in one plane.

G. Enzyme Assays

Histochemical methods have been described for many enzymes. The reader is refered to the review of Van Noorden and Frederiks (1992). Only the *β-glucuronidase* assay (of which the modifications are not described yet) and a few other examples are given here.

1. β-Glucuronidase

Three Buffers Can Be Used

Buffer 1: 10% polyvinylalcohol (70K–100K) in 100 m*M* Tris, pH 7 (dissolve PVA by heating at 90°C), 50 m*M* NaCl, 2 m*M* 5-bromo-4-chloro-3-indolyl-β-D-glucuronic acid cyclohexylammonium salt (X-Gluc) (100 mg/ml stock in dimethylformamide), 1 m*M* potassium ferricyanide.

Buffer 2: 10% polyvinylalcohol (70K–100K) in 100 m*M* Tris, pH 7.5 (dissolve PVA by heating at 90°C), 50 m*M* NaCl, 0.4 m*M* X-Gluc (100 mg/ml stock in dimethylformamide), 0.4 m*M* nitro-blue tetrazolium (NBT) (80 mg/ml stock in 70% dimethylformamide). Add first X-Gluc and afterward in two parts, NBT.

Buffer 3: As buffer 1 but without the addition of PVA.

If the reactions are done on slides, buffer 1 or 2 has to be used. The best results are obtained with buffer 2, especially when the explants (cells) are very small or contain refractive structures or if the expression of the *uidA* gene is very low. Buffer 3 is used when the reactions are done in petri dishes.

Incubate for 1 h to overnight at 32°C (if the reactions are done on slides) to 37°C (if the reactions are done in petri dishes). If the reactions are done with buffer 1 or 3, sections can be counterstained for 5 min with 0.1% acid fuchsin. Wash afterwards for 5 min with running tap water and rinse a few times with demineralized water.

2. Succinate Dehydrogenase

Buffer: 100 m*M* Tris, pH 7.8, 50 m*M* NaCl, 100 m*M* Na-succinate, 1 m*M* NBT (80 mg/ml stock in 70% dimethylformamide), 1.5 m*M* NAD.

Negative control: omit Na-succinate.

Incubate at 24°C for 4 h (to overnight) in darkness.

3. Peroxidases and Catalases

Buffer: 0.05 *M* Tris–HCl, pH 7.6, 0.01 *M* imidazole, 0.05% 3,3-diaminobenzidine-tetrahydrochloride, 0.05% H_2O_2.

Negative control: omit H_2O_2.

Incubate at 24°C for 5 to 15 min in darkness.

Peroxidases can be distinguished from catalases. Peroxidases are inhibited by 1% H_2O_2, whereas catalases are inhibited by 0.1 *M* 3-amino-1,2,4-triazole.

4. Alcohol Dehydrogenase

Buffer: 0.1 *M* Tris–HCl, pH 8, 1.15 m*M* NAD, 2.3 m*M* NBT, 10% ethanol.

Negative control: omit ethanol.

Incubate overnight at 24°C in darkness.

III. Results and Discussion

When the method described above is applied to different kinds of plant material, enzymatic activities can be localized with high accuracy, as is demonstrated with a few examples (Fig. 1 and 2). Much of the success of the method depends on how the material is processed and pretreated. To allow efficient penetration of the acetone and Historesin, the air within intercellular spaces must be removed by vacuum infiltration. However, to prevent collapse of the tissues and cells during this process, the specimen must be prewetted. During this period, membranes should be stabilized, and protease activity must be minimized. Spermidine

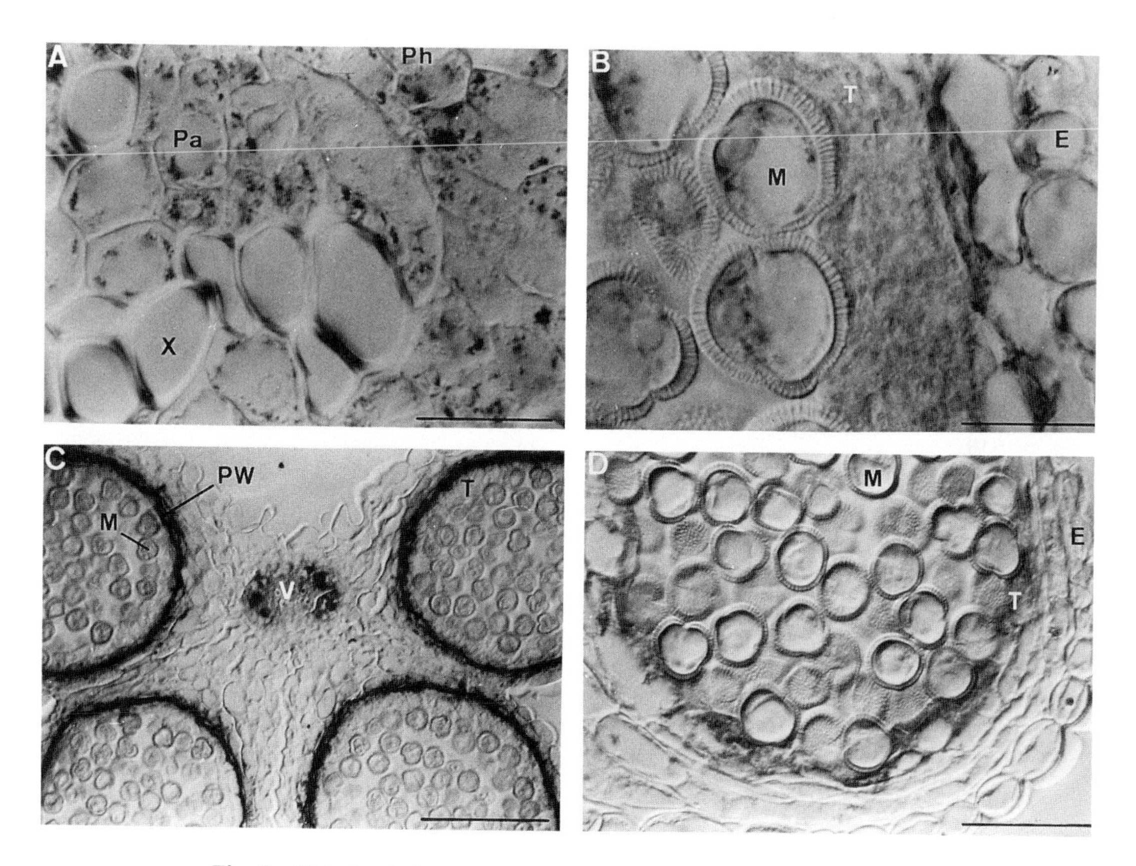

Fig. 1 Histochemical enzyme assays done on 10-μm sections of Historesin-embedded plant material. (A) Cross section of a vascular bundle from a rice node stained for succinate dehydrogenase; the parenchyma cells contain high succinate dehydrogenase activity. (B) Cross section of a flower bud from *Brassica napus* stained for succinate dehydrogenase; the activity is mainly localized in the microspores and the cells of the endothecium. The tapetum starts to degenerate at this developmental stage. (C) Cross section of a flower bud from *B. napus* stained for peroxidase; the highest peroxidase activities are found in the peritapetal wall and the vascular tissue. (D) Cross section of a flower bud from *B. napus* stained for alcohol dehydrogenase; the activity at this developmental stage is exclusively localized in the tapetum. Bars, 20 μm (A and B); 50 μm (D); 100 μm (C). C, connectivum; E, endothecium; M, microspore; Pa, parenchyma cell; Ph, phloem; PW, peritapetal wall; T, tapetum; V, vascular tissue.

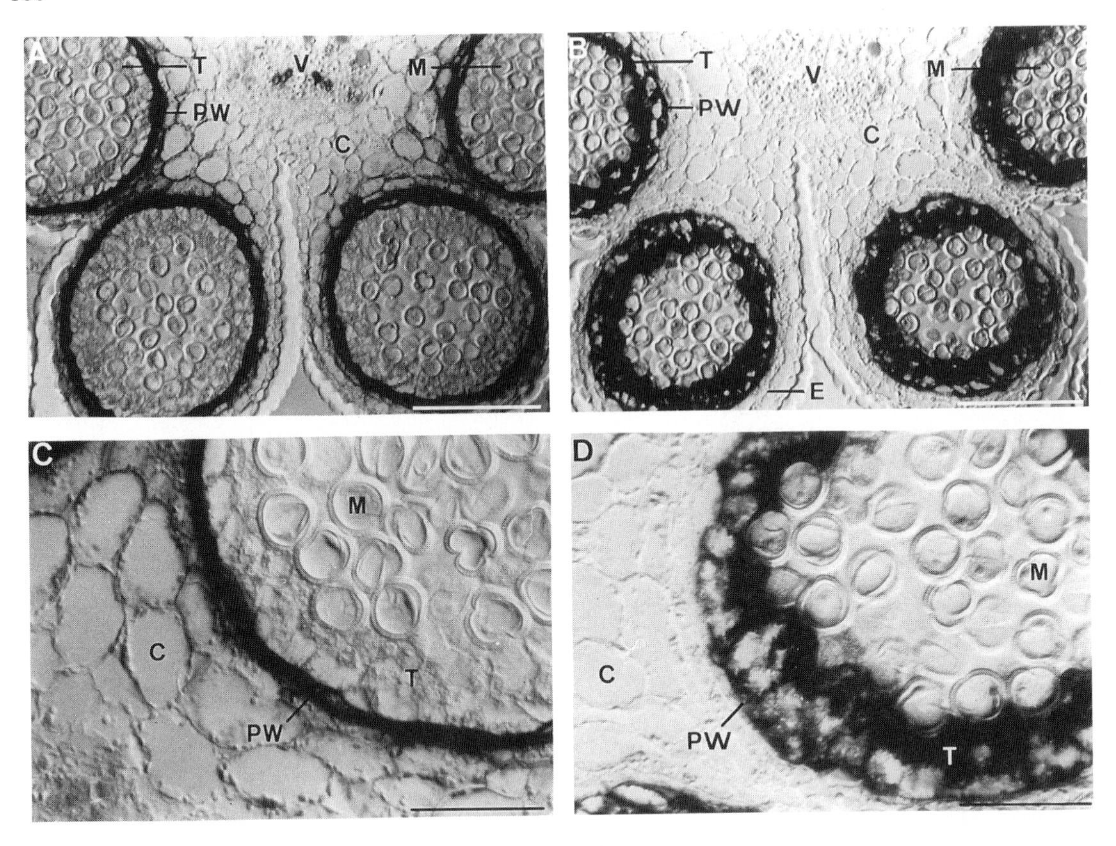

Fig. 2 The influence of ferric ions on the deposition of indigo blue in the β-glucuronidase (GUS) assay. The GUS assays were carried out on 10-μm cross sections of flower buds from transgenic *Brassica napus* plants containing the *uidA* gene under the control of a tapetum specific promoter. (A, and C) No ferric ions were added to the reaction buffer. The indigo blue is deposited at places with high peroxidase activity, in this case the peritapetal wall and vascular tissue (see Fig. 1C). (B, and D) 2 m*M* potassium ferricyanide was added to the GUS reaction buffer; the GUS activity is localized in the tapetum. Bars, 50 μm (C and D); 100 μm (A and B). C, connectivum; E, endothecium; M, microspore; PW, peritapetal wall; T, tapetum; V, vascular tissue.

is known to stabilize membranes and to inhibit proteases and RNases. A short pretreatment of the tissue with an aqueous solution containing 1 m*M* spermidine, followed by vacuum infiltration, results in excellent preservation both of tissue structure and of enzymatic activities. Spermidine pretreatment is preferred to fixation because many enzymes are sensitive to even the lowest levels of fixation. In the original protocol (De Block and Debrouwer, 1992), the spermidine was dissolved in a sodium-phosphate buffer. However, we have since observed that if plant tissue is treated with sodium-phosphate buffer, (stress) genes are induced, which in particular cases might result in artifacts. These artifacts can be avoided by replacing the phosphate buffer with plant tissue culture medium.

Although glycol methacrylate has a very low viscosity, it does not penetrate all cells and tissues equally well. Homogeneous infiltration of the entire specimen is of the utmost importance, not only to obtain a good structural preservation, but also to retain the enzymes in the sections during the histochemical reaction, and to allow an equal diffusion of the enzyme substrates and color reagents in the section. Complete infiltration can be obtained by correct processing of the tissue, by modification of the infiltration time, and by using (low) vacuum.

The final embedding is done in polyethylene capsules. Because the polymerization of the Historesin is incomplete at the bottom and edges of the capsule, a small amount of Historesin is prepolymerized at the bottom of the capsule. The specimen is placed on the sticky surface of the polymerized Historesin and is oriented in such a way that no contact is made with the edges of the capsule. Small polythene capsules should be used, because larger volumes of Historesin produce excessive heat during the polymerization process, and this can be disastrous for many enzymes.

Although the principles of most histochemical enzyme assays are simple, the biochemical complexity of the background in which these reactions occur can create artifacts. Before any specific histochemical reaction is done, it is of importance to check the metabolic activity of the different tissues and cell types of the "embedded" specimen. Metabolic activity can differ greatly among different tissue and cell types. Before any enzyme activity pattern can be termed cell- or tissue-specific, a correlation (i.e., a calibration) should be made with the metabolic activity pattern. High enzyme activities are often found in metabolically active cells, whereas only low or no (i.e., below the detection level) enzyme activities are found in metabolically inactive cells. Moreover, different cell types can have different sensitivities to embedding. For example, cytoplasmatically rich cells are less sensitive to embedding than highly vacuolated cells. To check survival and metabolic activity, we use the succinate dehydrogenase assay. As an enzyme of the Krebs' cycle, succinate dehydrogenase is present in every living cell and, furthermore, the metabolic activity of a cell is reflected in the Krebs cycle. In practice, serial sections are placed on two slides or in two petri dishes, one being used for the succinate dehydrogenase assay, the other for the assay of the enzyme under study.

Because the sensitivity of an enzyme to embedding cannot be predicted (all enzymes will be affected to a certain degree), it is advisable to first determine the activity of the enzyme in crude extracts. If activity is found in extracts and not in sections, this suggests the enzyme may be destroyed during embedding. In this case other, more sophisticated, histochemical techniques such as snap-freezing and cryosectioning must be applied (Van Noorden and Frederiks, 1992).

The colored end product of the histochemical reaction does not necessarily precipitate at the site of the enzyme activity. The diffusion of reaction intermediates and enzymes can interfere with correct localization. Whereas enzymes are more or less immobilized by the resin, the low-molecular-weight reaction intermediates can diffuse freely. An example of a false localization caused by a diffusion of the reaction intermediates is described for the β-glucuronidase assay using

X-Gluc as substrate (De Block and Debrouwer, 1992). The slow dimerization of the indoxyls, formed by the hydrolysation of X-Gluc by β-glucuronidase, results in the precipitation of the dimerized product, indigo blue, at oxidative sites (peroxidase activity) and not at the site of the β-glucuronidase activity. This artifact can be avoided by using an oxidant, such as potassium ferricyanide or nitroblue tetrazolium, in the reaction mixture (Fig. 2).

Other enzymes or chemical compounds present in the section may interfere with the method of detection. Phenazine methosulfate (PMS) or (1-methoxy)-phenazine methosulfate (MPMS), which are used as exogenous electron carriers in the indoxyl-tetrazolium salt methods, can be reduced nonspecifically by other systems. The reduced forms, PMSH and MPMSH, in turn can reduce the tetrazolium salt to the purple precipitate formazan. This will result in a false detection of activity. Figure 3 shows a transverse section of a rice flower that was incubated with PMS and NBT, and in the absence of indolyl substrate. After overnight incubation, formazan precipitation was found on the pollen wall and in the pollen cytoplasm. With NBT alone in the reaction mixture, no formazan formation occurred.

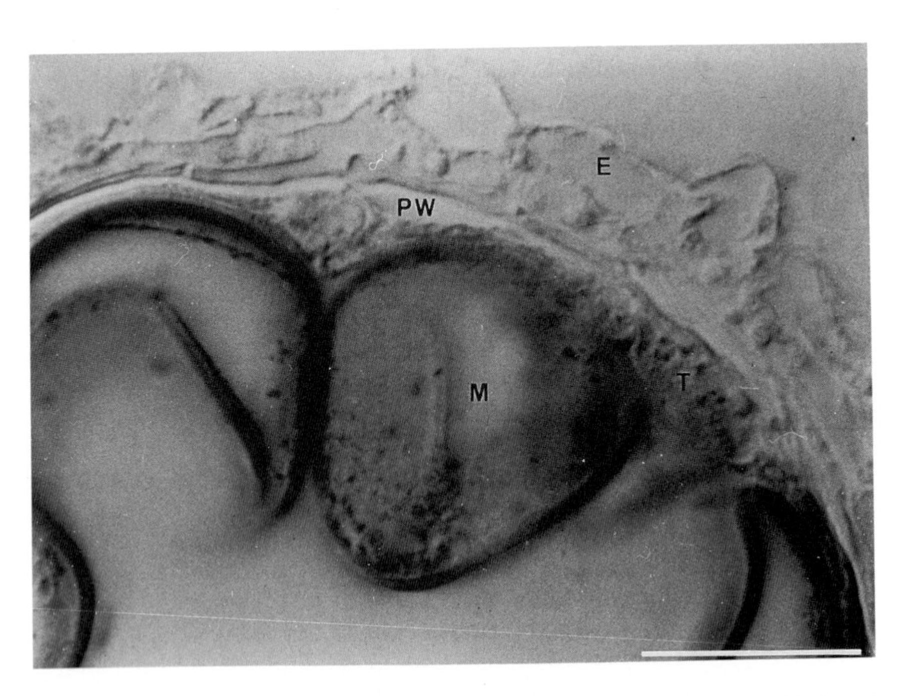

Fig. 3 Artifacts can be created by using nitroblue tetrazolium (NBT) in combination with phenazine methosulphate (PMS). Ten-micrometer cross sections of flower buds of rice were incubated with 0.4 m*M* NBT and 0.05 m*M* PMS. After an overnight incubation, formazan precipitate was found at the pollen wall, in the pollen cytoplasm, and to a lesser extent in the tapetum. Bar, 20 μm. E, endothecium; M, microspore; PW, peritapetal wall; T, tapetum.

IV. Conclusion

In the discipline of plant development biology, *in situ* enzyme histochemistry holds an important place because cell and tissues are studied in their natural context. However, the histochemical data cannot stand on their own and have to be related to data obtained by other techniques such as *in situ* hybridization. It has to be emphasized that although enzyme histochemistry on plastic embedded material allows the localization of many enzymes, sufficient controls must be included to check for homogeneous infiltration and polymerization of the resin in the specimen, for the stability of the enzyme during the embedding, and for the specificity of the histochemical reaction.

Although the method described gives a qualitative impression of the enzyme activities between cell and tissue types, it would be interesting to obtain more quantitative information. Different laboratories are developing quantitative enzyme histochemical techniques, but due to the biochemical and technical complexity many problems must first be solved before these techniques can be applied routinely.

Acknowledgements

I thank Dr. E. Krebbers (Dupont, U.S.A.) for the critical reading of the manuscript.

References

Ashford, A. E., Allaway, W. G., Gubler, F., Lennon, A., and Sleegers, J. (1986). Temperature control in Lowicryl K4M and glycol methacrylate during polymerization: Is there a low-temperature embedding method? *J. Microsc.* **144,** 107–126.

De Block, M., and Debrouwer, D. (1992). *In situ* enzyme histochemistry on plastic-embedded plant material. The development of an artefact-free β-glucuronidase assay. *Plant J.* **2,** 261–266.

De Block, M., and Debrouwer, D. (1993). Engineered fertility control in transgenic *Brassica napus* L.: Histochemical analysis of anther development. *Planta* **189,** 218–225.

Jefferson, R. A. (1987). Assaying chimeric genes in plants: The GUS gene fusion system. *Plant Mol. Biol. Rep.* **5,** 387–405.

Murray, G. I., Burke, M. D., and Ewen, S. W. B. (1989). Enzyme histochemistry on freeze-dried, resin-embedded tissue. *J. Histochem. Cytochem.* **37,** 643–649.

Murray, G. I., Burke, M. D., and Ewen, S. W. B. (1988). Enzyme histochemical demonstration of NADH dehydrogenase on resin-embedded tissue. *J. Histochem. Cytochem.* **36,** 815–819.

Murray, G. I., and Ewen, S. W. B. (1990). Enzyme histochemistry on freeze-substituted glycol methacrylate-embedded tissue. *J. Histochem. Cytochem.* **38,** 95–101.

Namba, M., Dannenberg, A. M., and Tanaka, F. (1983). Improvement in the histochemical demonstration of acid phosphatase, β-galactosidase and non-specific esterase in glycol methacrylate tissue sections by cold temperatures embedding. *Stain Technol.* **58,** 207–213.

Pretlow, T. P., Lapinsky, A. S., Flowers, L. C., Grane, R. W., and Pretlow, T. G. (1987). Enzyme histochemistry of mouse kidney in plastic. *J. Histochem. Cytochem.* **35,** 483–487.

Soufleris, A. J., Pretlow, T. P., Bartolucci, A. A., Pitts, A. M., MacFadyen, A. J., Boohaker, E. A., and Pretlow, T. G. (1983). Cytological characterisation of pulmonary alveolar macrophages by enzyme histochemistry in plastic. *J. Histochem. Cytochem.* **31,** 1412–1418.

Van Noorden, C. J. F., and Frederiks, W. M. (1992). "Enzyme Histochemistry: A Laboratory Manual of Current Methods." London/New York: Oxford Univ. Press, Royal Microscopy Society.

CHAPTER 12

In Situ Hybridization

Geoffrey Ian McFadden

Plant Cell Biology Research Centre
School of Botany
University of Melbourne
Parkville VIC 3052, Australia

I. Introduction

In situ hybridization is a cytochemical technique for localizing specific DNA or RNA sequences within an organism. Like Northern and Southern blots, *in situ* hybridization relies on Watson/Crick base pairing (commonly termed hybridization) between two polynucleotides with complementary sequences. However, unlike Northern and Southern blots, where the nucleic acids are first isolated and then separated by electrophoresis prior to probing, for *in situ* hybridization

METHODS IN CELL BIOLOGY, VOL. 49

the target sequences are left within the tissue. The probe, which is labeled, is sent into the tissue, allowed to hybridize with complementary target sequences, then rendered visible with some form of marker. Applied correctly the *in situ* hybridization technique provides precise information about the location of a specific DNA or RNA sequence. It is an extremely powerful tool for studying tissue-specific expression, and is also becoming an invaluable adjunct in chromosome mapping.

Applications of *in situ* hybridization technology are diverse. The most common usage in plant cell biology is localization of a mRNA at the light microscopic level, and this chapter will focus on methods for this. Exciting new applications, such as localization of DNA elements on isolated chromosomes (Heslop-Harrison *et al.*, 1993), localization of genes or transcripts at the subcellular level by electron microscopy (McFadden, 1991), and *in situ* PCR (Nuovo, 1992) are also introduced briefly.

II. Which Protocol to Use?

Because of the wide range of applications, there is unfortunately no single universal protocol for localizing nucleic acid species. Each worker will have to adopt a protocol suited to their system. This depends on what type of tissue they are working with, and what level of resolution they require. Various claims are made about the relative sensitivity of *in situ* hybridization, but in my experience only those mRNAs readily detected by Northern analysis can be successfully localized by *in situ* hybridization. However, it can occur that a mRNA that is highly localized within a particular cell type is easily detected by *in situ* hybridization but is difficult to detect by Northern blot analysis. This is due to the dilution effect of nonexpressing cells included in the tissue sample from which the RNA is extracted. Conversely, a mRNA present in low levels throughout all cell types may be readily detected by Northern analysis, but could be difficult to detect by *in situ* hybridization.

A problem somewhat peculiar to *in situ* hybridization analyses using plant tissues is the presence of vacuoles and cells of differing size. These features result in very different amounts of cytoplasm per unit section area in different tissues, and this should be taken into account when interpreting the relative levels of signal in a section. Tissues with small vacuoles in the cells (such as the tapetum, vascular bundles or apical meristems) will be most heavily labeled, even though the gene may not be most highly expressed in these tissues. A useful way to test this is to use a rRNA probe as a positive control to get an overview of cytoplasmic density in comparison with expression of the gene of interest (e.g., Fig. 5 in McFadden *et al.*, 1991).

Greatest success in localizing mRNAs in plant tissues has been achieved using ^{35}S-labeled RNA probes on wax sections. This approach was pioneered by Angerer and Angerer (1989) and adapted to plant systems by Cox and Goldberg

(1988). Improved protocols for ^{35}S-labeled RNA probes on wax sections are presented in detail here. Protocols for nonisotopic labeling and production of resin or cryosections can be found elsewhere (McFadden, 1994; Boehringer Mannheim, 1992; Brunning *et al.*, 1993).

A. Preparing Wax Sections of Plant Tissue

Embedding tissue in wax requires fixation and dehydration prior to infiltration with the embedding medium. Aldehyde fixation is optimal, and a combination of 4% paraformaldehyde and 0.5% glutaraldehyde suits most plant material. The fixative should be prepared fresh in a buffer isotonic to the growing conditions. Do not use Tris in conjunction with aldehyde fixatives; phosphate or "Good" buffers such as Hepes or Pipes are best. Fixation of plant tissues with extensive waxy cuticles can be improved by use of the phase-partition fixation technique (McFadden *et al.*, 1988a, and see section II,A,3).

1. Solutions and Materials

Plastic slide staining boxes holding 25 slides from Vit-Labs/Vitri Friedrich-Ebert Str 33-35, D-6104 Seeheim-Jugenheim, Germany

1% (v/v) solution of Decon 90 detergent (Rhone Poulenc)

poly-L-lysine (0.1 mg/ml)

distilled water

100 m*M* Pipes (pH 7.3)

20% formaldehyde (Ladd Research Industries)

8% glutaraldehyde (Serva GmbH, Carl Benz Str 7, D-6900 Heidelburg, Germany)

10% ethanol, 20% ethanol, 30% ethanol, 40% ethanol, 50% ethanol, 60% ethanol, 70% ethanol, 90% ethanol, 100% ethanol

4% paraformaldehyde (v/v), 0.5% glutaraldehyde (v/v) in 50 m*M* Pipes (pH 7.3)

n- heptane

Clearene (less-toxic alternative to xylene, Surgipath Medical Industries, Inc., P.O. Box 769, Ziegler Drive, Graylake, IL 60030)

Paraplast embedding wax chips (BDH Chemicals Ltd., Poole BH12 4NN, UK)

embedding molds (Tissue Tek, No. 4566, Miles, Inc., Elkhart, IN 46515)

pronase (0.1 mg/ml in Tris–HCl, pH 7.6)

glycine/histidine (2 mg/ml each in PBS)

2. Coating Slides

Fit slides into rack of Vitri box and immerse in detergent for 5 min. Rinse slides well with water and air dry. Dip slides in poly-L-lysine for 5 min. Drain and air dry away from dust.

3. Fixing Tissue

Prepare fresh paraformaldehyde (4%) and glutaraldehyde (0.5%) in 50 m*M* Pipes (pH 7.3). Combine fixative with equal volume of *n*-heptane and shake for 1 min. Allow phases to separate, then decant heptane (upper) phase. Retain aqueous phase for subsequent step. Immerse small pieces of tissue (about 2 × 2 × 2 mm) in fixative-loaded heptane for 10 min at room temperature. Transfer tissue pieces to aqueous paraformaldehyde (4%) and glutaraldehyde (0.5%) in 50 m*M* Pipes (pH 7.3) and fix for further 2 h at room temperature. Wash in buffer three times and proceed to wax embedding.

4. Wax Embedding

Dehydrate fixed tissue through ethanol series (10, 20, 30, 40, 50, 60, 70, 90, 100%) allowing at least 15 min for each step. Transfer tissue into a glass tube containing a mixture of 3 parts ethanol and 1 part Clearene for 60 min. Transfer tissue to a mixture of 1 part ethanol and 1 part Clearene for 60 min. Transfer tissue to a mixture of 1 part ethanol and 3 parts Clearene for 60 min. Transfer tissue to straight Clearene for 60 min. Add several chips of Paraplast embedding wax to each sample in Clearene and leave overnight at room temperature. Add several more chips of Paraplast and transfer tube to 42°C waterbath for 3 h. Place several Paraplast chips in an embedding mold and melt wax in oven at 60°C. Using warmed forceps, transfer tissue pieces from tubes to embedding molds. Incubate for 24 h at 62°C. Remove and store at room temperature.

5. Preparing Wax Sections

Cut sections of desired thickness (3–6 μm) on suitable microtome. Transfer sections to droplet of water on poly-L-lysine-coated slides. Dry down on 42°C hotplate for 2 h. Only perfectly flat sections should be retained. Using a diamond pencil, scratch a circle around the section on the back of the slide. Dewax sections by soaking slides in Clearene for 10 min followed by two washes in ethanol for 5 min each. Rehydrate sections by transferring through graded ethanol series (95, 80, 60, 30%) allowing at least 5 min in each step. Transfer to distilled water. Air dry and store at 4°C. Digest sections with pronase (0.1 mg/ml in Tris–HCl, pH 7.6) for 10 min at room temperature. The amount of digestion may need to be varied with different tissue types. Monitor nucleic acid retention by acridine orange staining (McFadden *et al.*, 1988b). Deactivate pronase by dunking slides in glycine/histidine (2 mg/ml in PBS). Wash twice in water and air dry.

III. Labels, Tags, and Detection Systems

There are two major categories of labels and detection systems for *in situ* hybridization: isotopic and nonisotopic. Both have relative merits, depending on the system used. Isotopic labeling is familiar to most molecular biologists, and standard probe production techniques (nick-translation or random priming) can be used. However, microautoradiography (the method used to visualize the bound probe) is an exacting procedure, and not always easily mastered. Nonisotopic systems are safer, have potentially higher resolution and sensitivity, and produce probes with longevity.

A. Isotopic Labels

Isotopic labels are detected by autoradiography. Latent silver grains produced by β particles colliding with silver halide in an emulsion are chemically developed (Pardue, 1986). Macroscopic autoradiography can be performed by apposing fine-grain, single-coated X-ray film directly to the labeled sections. Microautoradiography involves coating the sections with a very thin layer of melted emulsion. After a suitable exposure period, silver grains in the emulsion are chemically developed.

Three isotopes emitting β particles commonly used for *in situ* hybridization are ^{32}P, ^{35}S, and ^{3}H. The β particles from ^{32}P have the highest energy and spread of the particles results in low resolution. However, ^{32}P has the highest specific activity and this isotope gives maximum sensitivity in low-resolution systems (Fig. 1). Although seldom used, ^{33}P is potentially well suited to *in situ* hybridization applications because it combines a high specific activity with a relatively low β particle energy (Evans and Read, 1992). ^{35}S β particles have a lower emission energy and provide better resolution. The longer half-life of ^{35}S extends probe longevity slightly. ^{35}S-labeling is most useful for applications localizing mRNAs to tissues or cell layers in sections (Fig. 2). Very fine resolution is achieved with ^{3}H, which has the lowest emission energy of the three. Subcellular localization can be achieved using ^{3}H-labeled probes for electron microscopy (Penschow *et al.*, 1991). The specific activity of ^{3}H-labeled probes is relatively low and prolonged exposures can be necessary, but the probes do have the advantage of being extremely long-lived.

B. Nonisotopic Labels

Various nonisotopic labels or tags are now in use, and they can be separated into two categories: direct and indirect. Direct refers to labels that are themselves intrinsically visible. Indirect refers to labels that must be rendered visible by subsequent manipulation. The most common direct labels are fluorochromes. Fluorochromes emit visible light when excited by UV radiation in the light microscope. Direct fluorochrome labeling is relatively simple (Boehringer Mannheim, 1992; Brunning *et al.*, 1993), and the bound probe is immediately detectable by fluorescence microscopy after post-hybridization washing.

Indirect methods involve initial incorporation of a tag molecule (the label) into the probe. Tags on the bound probe are then detected with an antibody or affinity reagent to which is coupled a visible marker (such as a fluorochrome or a gold bead) or an enzyme (such as alkaline phosphatase), which can be supplied with a substrate that it converts to an insoluble, visible product. Indirect methods are more complex than direct methods, but they offer greater flexibility in detection methods and the potential to amplify signals (McFadden, 1994).

Nonisotopic labeling is best done by enzymatic incorporation of tagged nucleotides into a probe molecule produced from a cloned template (Langer *et al.*, 1981). The tag or label is usually attached at the C5 position on a pyrimidine. The C5 position is not involved in base pairing during hybridization, and modifications do not adversely affect recognition of the nucleotide substrate by commonly used nucleic acid modifying enzymes. The tag is attached to the base by an allylamine spacer arm that keeps the tag accessible to the detection reagents, even though the probe is duplexed with the target. An 11- or 14-atom spacer arm is most effective. Labeling of RNA probes is normally done by incorporating tagged rUTP. Oligos and double-stranded DNA probes are labeled using tagged dUTP as a dTTP analogue.

Biotin (vitamin H) was the first tag employed for *in situ* hybridization. It was originally chosen because of the extraordinary affinity of the egg white protein avidin for biotin (Wilchek and Bayer, 1989). Avidin and also the bacterial cell wall protein streptavidin bind to biotin with dissociation constants in the order of K_{dis},10^{-15}. When these proteins are coupled to indicator molecules, an excellent affinity detection system can be devised.

Virtually any moiety can be used as a tag, providing a suitable means for detecting the tag is available and that the tag's presence does not disrupt hybridization. Digoxygenin, the aglycone of the plant cardiac glycoside digoxin, has recently been introduced as an alternative to biotin, which was sometimes found to be unsuitable as a tag in animal tissues with high levels of endogenous biotin. Digoxygenin (DIG) is incorporated into probes in the same ways as biotin (Boehringer Mannheim, 1992). Detection is via an anti-digoxygenin antibody. The only other tag commonly used for *in situ* hybridization is dinitrophenol (Narayanswami and Hamkalo, 1991).

IV. Probe Types

Three types of probes can be used for *in situ* hybridization: synthetic oligodeoxyribonucleotides (oligos), double-stranded DNA probes (i.e., cDNAs or genomic clones), and single-stranded RNA probes (i.e., antisense/sense RNAs, cRNAs, or "riboprobes"). Each of these probe types has advantages and disadvantages.

A. Oligonucleotides

Oligonucleotides (which are usually between 15 and 50 nucleotides in length) are now readily available to most workers and can be produced relatively quickly.

Working with oligos requires no cloning expertise and probes can be produced by any worker from published sequence data. A notable advantage of oligos is that they can be directed to particular portions of the target species. Several different oligos directed at the coding region, introns, or untranslated regions can be used to localize the same target and provide information about target processing in different tissues.

Various labeling and detection strategies are possible with oligos. Isotopic labeling can be achieved by kinasing with T4 polynucleotide kinase using $\gamma[^{32}P]$NTP, $\gamma[^{3}H]$NTP, or $\gamma[^{35}S]$NTP (McFadden, 1994) or by tailing with terminal transferase to add tagged dNTPs at the 3′ end (Boehringer Mannheim, 1992).

Nonenzymatic attachment of tags or labels to oligos is also possible using the "amino-link" system (Applied Biosystems User Bulletin No. 49, 1988). An amine group is incorporated at the 5′ end of the oligo during synthesis. When the amine-bearing oligo is mixed with an *N*-hydroxysuccinimide ester of a fluorochrome, biotin, or DIG at alkaline pH, the unprotonated amine attacks the ester linkage in the NHS–tag complex, resulting in an amide bond between the oligo and the tag molecule. The NHS tag esters have allylamine linker arms.

Recently, biotin (Misiura *et al.,* 1990) or fluorescein amidites (Applied Biosystems Product Bulletin, 1993) have become available, allowing biotin or fluorescein to be incorporated directly into the oligonucleotide during synthesis. The amidites are usually incorporated at the 5′ prime end during the last synthesis cycle but can be incorporated at any chosen site in the oligonucleotide.

B. Double-Stranded DNA Probes

These probes are produced from cDNA or genomic clones that have been amplified in a cloning vector supported by a suitable bacterial host (Ausubel *et al.,* 1988). Double-stranded probes can be labeled with isotopes or nonistopic labels by either of two methods: nick-translation or, preferably, random priming (Feinberg and Vogelstein, 1983; McFadden, 1994). Double-stranded refers to the fact that both the coding strand and the noncoding strand are included in the probe. Although they are reasonably satisfactory for localization of DNA, double-stranded probes suffer from some major disadvantages when localizing RNA targets. Only the coding strand hybridizes with RNA targets. The labeled noncoding strand is not only superfluous, it actually hybridizes back to the coding strand, thereby competing against the target. Moreover, because the unlabeled template remains with the probe, it competes with the labeled probe to hybridize with targets, severely reducing the signal. Additionally, the low yield of probe produced (typically less than 100 ng) is only sufficient for a small number of *in situ* hybridization experiments.

C. Single-Stranded RNA Probes

RNA probes complementary to cellular RNA can be produced by *in vitro* transcription. The antisense RNA of cRNA (complementary RNA) is produced from a vector in which the noncoding strand is sited downstream of a bacteriophage RNA polymerase promotor. Discrete length "run off" transcripts incorporating either isotopically or nonisotopically labeled nucleotides are made from a linearized plasmid template using phage RNA polymerase. Large quantities of probe can be produced in this manner. The unlabeled DNA template is relatively insignificant as a competitor to the probe but can be removed by DNase digestion. Another advantage of RNA probes is the stronger hybrids formed between two strands of RNA, allowing a higher stringency (see Section V).

1. False Binding with RNA Probes

A potentially serious drawback with RNA probes is a tendency to bind nonspecifically to rRNAs. Recently, it was demonstrated that very short G/C-rich motifs in riboprobes can hybridize to complementary sequences in the rRNAs of human tissue (Witkiewicz *et al.*, 1993). Several 9-base pair motifs comprising the *Not*I, *Sma*I, and *Sac*I sites in the polylinker of the transcription vector pBluescript KS II (Stratagene, Inc.) were found to have complements in the human large subunit rRNA (Witkiewicz *et al.*, 1993). Somewhat surprisingly, these 9-base pair motifs cross-hybridize with rRNA at standard stringency (50% formamide, 1× SSC, 50°C), probably because RNA/RNA duplexes are particularly stable. (Witkiewicz *et al.*, 1993). Transcripts of the polylinker without insert gave the same signal as those with the insert, and Northern blotting revealed that the majority of hybridization was to the large subunit rRNA (Witkiewicz *et al.*, 1993).

I have examined the potential for similar problems in plant systems and found that commonly employed transcription vectors (pBluescript, pBluescript II, and several of the pGEM series) contain motifs with complements in a number of different plant rRNAs. For instance, the T7 transcript through the *Sma*I site of pBluescript SK ($^{5'}$CCCCCGGGCT$^{3'}$) has a complement in the large subunit rRNA of *Oryza sativa,* and the T3 transcript through the *Not*I site of the same vector ($^{5'}$GCGGCCGCC$^{3'}$) also has a complement in the same rice rRNA. Similarly, the T7 transcript through the *Apa*I site of pBluescript KS ($^{5'}$CGGGCCCCCC$^{3'}$) has a complement in the rice chloroplast large subunit rRNA. These and other motifs represent a possible source of spurious hybridization, and serious consideration should be given to the design of an *in situ* hybridization experiment employing RNA probes. Depending on the site and orientation of the insert within the transcription vector, either the sense or the antisense RNA probe strand could cross-hybridize with plant rRNA.

There are a number of precautions that should be followed to avoid being misled by such spurious hybridization. Best practice would be to perform a Northern blot with the same RNA probe to determine that the probe is actually detecting your mRNA and not a rRNA. This blot should be done at an equivalent or slightly lower stringency (see Section V) than the *in situ* hybridization. Another useful control would be to run a parallel *in situ* hybridization using runoff transcripts of the same polylinker without any insert to check for spurious signal in either the sense or the antisense. Where practical it would be prudent to eliminate G/C-rich motifs from your *in vitro* transcript system by linearizing the vector upstream of these regions. Some of the pGEM series (e.g., pGEM3z, pGEM3zf, pGEM4z, and pGEM7zf, Promega Corp.) lack G/C-rich motifs in their polylinkers, and it might be worthwhile using these vectors where possible, but there is no guarantee that these polylinkers, or even your own insert, do not contain other motifs that could cross-hybridize to nontarget RNAs in your tissue. Good controls will be essential in establishing a *bona fide* signal. It should also be possible to minimize problems by using higher stringency. I routinely perform hybridization with short RNA probes (ca. 100 bp) at 65°C in 50% formamide, and up to 70°C for longer probes (800–2000 bp). The sense strand should no longer be considered an adequate control, because it is possible to have a false positive with the antisense but still get a satisfactory negative control with the sense strand because it does not contain the same motif.

D. Making ^{35}S-Labeled RNA Probes

This method produces single-stranded RNA probes complementary to the target. The cloned sequence must be subcloned into an *in vitro* transcription vector such that the noncoding strand is downstream of a bacteriophage RNA polymerase promoter engineered into the vector. The polymerase then transcribes a complementary or antisense RNA from the template. Most commercially available vectors have a different RNA polymerase promoter on either side of the multiple cloning site so that the sense RNA can be transcribed from the same construct simply by using a different polymerase. By cutting the vector with a restriction endonuclease downstream of the insert, it is possible to limit the transcription to discrete length runoffs and produce labeled probe molecules of defined length. The pBluescript II vectors (Stratagene, La Jolla, CA) have restriction sites for *Bss*HII flanking the RNA polymerase promoters allowing a transcription cassette, suitable for both sense and antisense transcriptions, to be released with a single enzyme digestion.

A typical *in vitro* transcription will produce several micrograms of labeled RNA probe. RNA is easily destroyed by ribonucleases. These enzymes are extremely resilient and are easily transferred from our skin to reaction tubes and pipette tips. Always wear gloves while preparing RNA probes, autoclave all tubes and tips, and treat water for all buffers with DEPC (Ausubel *et al.*, 1988).

1. Materials and Reagents

template DNA

5× transcription buffer (200 m*M* TRIS, pH 7.5, 30 m*M* $MgCl_2$, 10 m*M* spermidine, 50 m*M* NaCl)

100 m*M* DTT

RNasin (20 U/μl, Promega Corp, 2800 Woods Hollow Rd, Madison, WI 35711-5399)
10 m*M* ATP, 10 m*M* GTP, 10 mM UTP
phage RNA polymerase (20 U)
DEPC-treated water
RQ1 RNase-free DNase (1 U/μl, Promega)
phenol/chloroform saturated with TE
chloroform : isoamyl alcohol (24 : 1)
BioSpin 30 column (Bio-Rad, 3300 Regatta Blvd, Richmond CA 94804)
1 liter TBE (0.1 *M* Tris-borate, 2m*M* EDTA, 0.1 *M* boric acid)
agarose
1% ethidium bromide (w/v)
loading dye [0.25% (w/v) bromphenol blue, 40% (v/v) glycerol]
agarose gel electrophoresis unit
distilled water
RNA ladder (Bethesda Research Labs/GIBCO, MD)
0.2 *M* Na_2CO_3
0.2 *M* $NaHCO_3$
3 *M* NaOAc (pH 6)
10% glacial acetic acid
4 *M* LiCl
ethanol
hybridization buffer (50 m*M* piperazine ethane sulfonic acid (pH 7.2), 0.15 *M* NaCl, 5 m*M* Na_2-ethylenediaminetetraacetic acid (EDTA), 100 μg ml^{-1} powdered herring sperm DNA (Type D-3159, Sigma), 0.1% Ficoll 400 (Pharmacia, Sweden), 0.1% polyvinyl pyrrolidine 40, 0.1% BSA, 50% deionized formamide. Aliquots of buffer should be stored frozen.

2. *In Vitro* Transcription

Linearize template and determine concentration (Ausubel *et al.*, 1988). Avoid using enzymes that generate 3′ overhangs, as these allow the polymerase to turn back and continue transcribing off the other strand producing a hairpin probe. If an enzyme generating 3′ overhangs must be used to linearize, blunt the ends with T4 polymerase (Ausubel *et al.*, 1988).

At room temperature add these reagents in this order: 4 μl of 5× transcription buffer, 2 μl of 100 m*M* DTT, 1 μl of RNasin, 1 μl of 10 m*M* ATP, 1 μl of 10 m*M* GTP, 1 μl of 10 m*M* UTP, 5 μl of α[^{35}S]CTP (10 mCi/ml), 1 μl of template DNA (0.5–2.0 μg), 1 μl (20 units) of appropriate RNA polymerase (T7, T3, or SP6, depending on which promoter is upstream of the insert), sufficient DEPC-treated water to make a final reaction volume of 20 μl. Mix components. Incubate at 37°C for 1 h. Remove a 3-μl aliquot and set aside for electrophoretic analysis (Section IV,D,3) if required.

3. Gel Electrophoresis of Labeled Probe

When preparing RNA probes it is advisable to check the transcripts by electrophoresis. A simple nondenaturing gel is adequate for this purpose. Dissolve 0.5 g of agarose in 50 ml of TBE in microwave oven. Add 2 μl of 1% (w/v) ethidium bromide (ethidium bromide is toxic). Pour agarose solution into "minigel" casting mold and insert comb (see Ausubel *et al.,* 1988, for more detail). Allow gel to set before removing comb. Add 1 μl of loading dye and 7 μl of water to the 3 μl set aside from the transcription reaction. A useful standard is 3 μg of "RNA ladder" 9.5–0.24 knt. Add the dye and water as above. Load the samples and electrophorese at 5 V/cm for 1 h. View the gel using UV 300-mn transilluminator. The apparent molecular weight of the labeled transcripts will not be exactly correct due to the nondenaturing conditions. An approximate estimate of the yield can be made by comparing the fluorescent intensity of the transcript band with that of one of the bands in the RNA ladder standard. It is also possible (but not optimal) to run a gel using a portion of the probe after it has been precipitated and resuspended in hybridization buffer. The buffer and electrophoretic apparatus will need to be decontaminated for radioactivity.

4. Removal of Template and Unincorporated Nucleotides

Add 2 μl of RQ1 RNase-free DNase to transcription mix and incubate 15 min at 37°C. Add 180 μl of DEPC-treated water. Extract with phenol/chloroform followed by chloroform : isoamyl alcohol (24 : 1). Pass the aqueous phase through a spin column to remove unicorporated nucleotides by exclusion chromatography.

5. Probe Size

If the probe is less than 600 nt, I recommend using the full-length probe. Longer probes should be cut into shorter fragments by limited alkaline hydrolysis as follows. The optimal size is between 150 and 400 nt, depending on the porosity of the tissue. Estimate the volume of the spin column eluate. For each 100 μl of eluate add 60 μl of 0.2 *M* Na_2CO_3 and 40 μl of 0.2 *M* $NaHCO_3$. Calculate the appropriate hydrolysis time from the equation

$$t = (L_o - L_f)/(KL_oL_f),$$

where L_o = length in knt of your runoff transcript, L_f = desired length of hydrolysis products, $K = 0.11$, and t = time in minutes. For instance, if the runoff transcript is 2 knt, and it is decided to cut the probe down to pieces with an average length of 0.5 knt, 14 min hydrolysis is required. Stop the hydrolysis by adding 3 *M* NaOAc to a final concentration of approximately 0.1 *M* then add 10% glacial acetic acid to a final concentration of 0.5%. The size of the hydrolysis fragments can be checked by electrophoresis as described in Section IV,D,3.

6. Precipitation of Probe

Once the unincorporated nucleotides have been removed using the spin column and size reduction has been accomplished, it is necessary to precipitate the probe and resuspend it in hybridization buffer. Estimate the volume of the spin column eluate or the terminated hydrolysis mix if size reduction was undertaken. Add 0.1 vol of 4 *M* LiCl. Add 2.5 vol of ethanol. Stand in freezer for at least 1 h. Spin in microfuge at 4°C for 15 min. Pour off supernatant and stand tube upside down to drain for 15 min. Resuspend the pellet in suitable volume[1] of hybridization buffer.

V. Hybridization Conditions

Hybridization of the probe to the target is governed by a range of physical parameters. The hybridization occurs through base pairing to create hydrogen bonds linking the probe to the target. The number of hydrogen bonds determines the strength of the hybrid. Shorter probes form less stable hybrids. Probes that do not have a perfectly complementary sequence (often known as heterologous probes) also form less stable hybrids. For a successful *in situ* hybridization experiment, conditions maximizing specific annealment of the probe to the target must be determined. The conditions under which hybridization is attempted are known as the "stringency," where low stringency allows weaker hybrids to remain as hybrids and high stringency is less permissive. The stability of the hybrid is represented by the melting temperature (T_m), the temperature at which half the population of hybrids become dissociated or "melted." A guide to stringency conditions can be obtained from the following relationship, which predicts Tm for two RNA molecules:

$$T_m = 79.8°C + 18.5 \log M + 0.584(\%G/C) - 300 + 200M/L - 0.35(\%F) - 1.4(\%\text{mismatch}),$$

where M = ionic strength (mol liter^{-1}), %G/C = mole percentage of guanine/cytosine pairs in the probe/target hybrid; L = length of the probe in nucleotides;

[1] The volume of buffer used to resuspend the probe is dependent on the amount of probe synthesized and the concentration at which the probe is to be used. Probe concentrations in the order of 1 μg/ml are usually suitable. It is better to maintain consistent probe concentration than to vary the amount of probe in order to apply equivalent counts in each experiment. Resuspend probe in a minimal volume and test a dilution series to establish which dilution produces the optimal signal-to-noise ratio in your system. Remember, excess probe will increase the nonspecific hybridization and create noise. Store probe in hybridization buffer at −20°C or use immediately.

%F = percentage (v/v) of formamide in the hybridization buffer; and %mismatch = the percentage of noncomplementary base pairs between the hybridizing strands. Thus, by increasing the salt concentration, or decreasing the formamide concentration, or decreasing the hybridization temperature, the stringency can be lowered, allowing short probes or probes with a small degree of sequence mismatch to be used. Conversely, higher stringency can be attained by increasing the formamide concentration, or lowering salt concentration or by increasing temperature. Formamide increases the solubility of the bases and is a duplex destabilizing agent; it is usually used at 50% concentration. This allows lower temperatures to be used, minimizing damge to the tissue sample. Standard hybridization buffer includes 50% formamide and 0.15 *M* NaCl, and it is usually best to keep this constant and adjust stringency by varying the temperature. The simplest way to optimize an *in situ* hybridization system is to run a series of experiments using the standard buffer at different temperatures and monitor the signal-to-noise ratio. As a guide, DNA/DNA hybridization should be done at 37–42°C, DNA/RNA hybrids at 42°C, and RNA/RNA hybrids at 50–70°C. When working with oligos, decrease the formamide concentration to 40%.

Posthybridization washes are done at a temperature equivalent to or higher than the hybridization temperature. Salt concentration can be reduced in the wash buffer to increase stringency, but best results are obtained by optimizing the hybridization conditions rather than trying to reduce noise with stringent posthybridization washing; once probe has annealed *in situ* it is hard to dislodge.

A. Hybridization Protocol

1. Materials

hybridization buffer (Section IV,D,1)

SSC—Prepare a stock of 20× SSC (3 *M* NaCl, 0.3 *M* Na citrate) and store at room temperature

ethanol (technical grade)

ethanol (AR grade)

0.1 *M* triethanolamine–HCl, pH 8.

acetic anhydride

circular coverslips (12 mm diameter)

chloroform

probe in hybridization buffer

plastic meat defrosting container with draining rack for hybridization box

2. Prehybridization

Dip slides with sections in hybridization buffer at room temperature for 5 min. Transfer to hybridization buffer at 38–42°C for 1 h. Rinse in 1× SSC. Dehydrate in ethanol (technical grade) followed by ethanol (AR grade). Drain and store up to 4 weeks at 4°C in a closed staining box containing about 4 ml of ethanol.

3. Acetylation of Slides

Slides coated with poly-L-lysine should be acetylated to prevent probe from adhering to the coating. Dip slides in 0.1 *M* triethanolamine–HCl, pH 8. While stirring vigorously, add acetic anhydride to concentration of 5 ml/liter. Wash slides in 2× SSC for 5 min. Drain and air dry.

4. Hybridization and Washing

Wash circular coverslips in chloroform and dry. Place coverslips on small, dark platform (e.g., the lid of the Vitri staining box) and dispense 5 μl of probe onto each slip. Invert slide onto coverslip so that the section contacts the probe solution and picks up the coverslip. The circle scratched on the back of the slide around the section (II,A,5) acts as a useful guide at this stage. The droplet of probe should spread over the entire coverslip with no bubbles. If the section is thick, you may have to add a few extra microliters of probe at one edge of the coverslip with a Gilson-type pipette. Lay slides in hybridization box that contains about 50 ml of hybridization buffer beneath the support rack. If the lid seals well, a vapor of buffer will prevent the probe under the coverslips from drying out and it will not be necessary to seal the edges of the coverslips with mineral oil, as is sometimes recommended (Angerer and Angerer, 1989). Hybridize at selected temperature overnight. To remove coverslips, stand slides in beaker of 4× SSC. Gently agitate slides until coverslips fall off. This may take 10–20 min. Never pry off the coverslips, as this dislodges the sections. Transfer slides to rack and wash in 2× SSC. Wash in 1× SSC at hybridization temperature. Wash in <1× SSC at selected temperature if higher stringency is required. Dehydrate in ethanol (technical grade). Dehydrate in ethanol (AR grade).

B. Autoradiography

1. Materials

X-ray film cassette
Kodak XAR X-ray film
Kodak Liquid X-ray Film Developer Type 2
DuPont Cromex MRF 32 single-coated film
distilled water
Kodak NTB-2 emulsion
Large, airtight, light-proof container (instant coffee tins are ideal) with silica gel
Kodak D19 developer

Kodak unifix
0.25% (w/v) toluidine blue
Merckoglass mounting medium (Merck, D-6100 Darmstadt, Germany)
lead weights (5 g fishing sinkers)

2. X-Ray Film Autoradiography—[^{32}P] and [^{35}S] Probes Only

This type of autoradiography is very simple and gives a useful overview of labeling at a macroscopic level (Fig. 1, see Color Plates). Tape slides, section upward, onto a sheet of stiff paper in X-ray film cassette. Tape additional new slides around your probed slides to form a flat surface. In the darkroom under a red safelight (Kodak Wratten No. 2), place a sheet of Kodak XAR X-ray film over the slides. Expose at room temperature without an intensifying screen for 4–12 h [^{32}P] or 24–72 h [^{35}S]. Develop film at 20°C for 2 min, wash, fix, and rinse under running water. Finer resolution can be achieved with DuPont Cromex MRF 32 single-coated film. Expose for four times the suitable exposure determined with XAR film.

3. Liquid Emulsion Microautoradiography

Microautoradiography provides finer resolution and is useful at the tissue or cell level (Fig. 2, see Color Plates). This procedure can be done after the X-ray film autoradiography has been completed. Liquid emulsion can only be handled under the prescribed safelight (Kodak Wratten No. 2). Since long drying periods are necessary, it is convenient to have a darkroom with double doors or a large light-proof box in which to store slides while they dry. The unused emulsion should be stored in 4-ml aliquots in scintillation vials away from extraneous radiation. Prolonged storage of emulsion increases background. Blank slides should always be included to check the status of the emulsion. Good resolution requires a thin emulsion layer.

Add 2 vol of distilled water to aliquot of Kodak NTB 2 emulsion. Stand in 40°C waterbath for 1 h. Warm a pasteur pipette by gently squirting emulsion in and out several times. Hold slide on slight angle and slowly squirt a small stream of emulsion over the section. Stand the slide on a piece of absorbent paper and allow to dry for 1 h. I find this method more reliable than dipping for obtaining a thin layer. Repeat for all slides. Transfer slides to tray and place in light-proof, airtight container containing silica gel. Expose for suitable period.[2] Develop in Kodak D19 for 2 min at 15°C. Wash gently in water for 2 min at 15°C. Fix in Kodak Unifix at 15°C for 2 min. Wash at 15°C for 30 min in gently running water. Maintenance of constant temperature minimizes wrinkling and cracking of the emulsion. Air-dry at room temperature.

[2] Exposure periods range from about 1 day up to several weeks, depending on the isotope used and the abundance of target. It is best to have several duplicate slides that can be taken out and developed at intervals to check for adequate exposure.

Stain section under a drop of 0.25% toluidine blue for 1 min. Rinse well with water and air dry. Make a permanent mount by placing about 20 μl of Merckoglass on the section, cover with coverslip and weight down with small piece of lead. Allow to harden overnight. Silver grains can be viewed by standard bright field microscopy, under which they appear as small black spots. The silver particles can also be viewed by dark-field optics[3] in which they appear as brilliant white points (see Fig. 2).

VI. Controls

A number of different control experiments can be used to verify the authenticity of the signal. Some very convincing false positives can occur with *in situ* hybridization, so good controls are essential. Controls peculiar to RNA probes are outlined in Section IV,C. When localizing RNAs, it is useful to predigest some sections with RNase, which should remove most of the signal [digest with 1 mg/ml pancreatic RNase (Boehringer Mannheim, Germany) in 2 m*M* $MgCl_2$, 0.1 *M* Tris–HCl, pH 7.5, at 37°C for 1 h, then wash extensively with 5 m*M* EDTA, 0.1 *M* Tris–HCl, pH 7, before air-drying). Similarly, DNase digestion can be used to eliminate DNA targets. An irrelevant probe (i.e., one for which there is no target) can be used in parallel to detect nonspecific binding. When using indirect nonisotopic systems, it is recommended to process several sections in which one of the detection reagents is omitted in order to demonstrate that no spurious signal is being generated. A positive control is very useful for optimizing a new *in situ* hybridization experiment. Using a probe for an abundant target such as rRNA, or a highly expressed housekeeping gene, can help in optimizing parameters. Checking retention of nucleic acids in your preparations by acridine orange staining (McFadden *et al.*, 1988b) is also recommended.

VII. New Techniques

Recent innovations have opened new avenues for *in situ* hybridization. Finer resolution and increased sensitivity now allow us to approach new questions. Techniques for *in situ* hybridization at the EM level are answering questions about endosymbiosis (McFadden *et al.*, 1994) and virology (Bonfiglioli *et al.*, 1994). The use of fluorochromes as labels offers two novel advantages: high resolution and the ability of label different probes with different colors and use them simultaneously (Titus, 1991). The key application of fluorochromes has been in mapping genes on metaphase chromosomes. Sometimes known as chromosome painting, or alternatively as FISH (fluroescent *in situ* hybridization), this technique now allows visualization of the position of a DNA sequence on

[3] Consult reference O'Brien and McCully (1986) for setting up dark-field optics.

its carrier plant chromosome (Heslop-Harrison *et al.*, 1993; Heslop-Harrison and Bennett, 1990). By using three different colors (i.e., fluorescein, rhodamine, and coumarin) it is possible to map three different DNA elements to a single metaphase spread by triple-label *in situ* hybridization (Heslop-Harrison *et al.*, 1993). Currently it is possible to detect a 10kb target on a chromosome.

The principle source of noise in *in situ* hybridization experiments is nonspecific binding of probe to the tissue. The labeled probe provides a signal even though it has not hybridized with a target. One approach to avoid such noise is PRINS (primed *in situ* labeling). The principal behind this technique is to incorporate the label into a newly formed DNA strand *in situ* (Koch *et al.*, 1991). The first step involves annealing a primer to the target sequence. The primer is then extended by a polymerase, and the labeled nucleotides are incorporated into the new strand (Koch *et al.*, 1991). In theory, label is only incorporated at sites where the primer has successfully annealed to the target, thereby providing particularly high signal-to-noise ratios from a very rapid procedure (Koch, 1992).

The PRINS technique represents the first footsteps in the development of the latest innovation to *in situ* hybridization technology—the *in situ* PCR. The power of the PCR is its ability to turn vanishingly small quantities of DNA into visible amounts. To be able to do an amplification *in situ* will be an invaluable aid in detecting particularly rare target sequences. A number of papers describing *in situ* PCRs have now appeared (Nuovo, 1992) and the protocols are relatively simple. Slide griddles—on which the denaturation, annealment, and extension cycles can be performed on the slide—are now available for several brands of thermal cyclers. Like the *in vitro* PCR, *in situ* PCRs make use of a thermostable polymerase so that repeated cycles can be undertaken. Two approaches to visualizing the amplification product have been tried. The first involves an initial amplification protocol, then a standard *in situ* hybridization protocol with a labeled probe designed to detect the PCR products. The second approach is to incorporate a tagged nucleotide into the new strands during the PCR. The tags are then detected with antibodies and visible markers. Increased sensitivity allows detection of single-copy sequences, but like *in vitro* PCRs the *in situ* PCR can be tricky to optimize and good controls are essential (Nuovo, 1992).

Acknowledgments

Ms. Ingrid Bönig provided excellent assistance in the development of the protocols presented here. I thank Prof Adrienne Clarke for supporting this work and making the facilities of the Plant Cell Biology Research Centre available. A Senior-Research Fellowship from the Australian Research Council is gratefully acknowledged.

References

Angerer, L. M., and Angerer, R. C. (1989). *In situ* hybridization with ^{35}S-labelled RNA probes. *DuPont Biotechnol. Update* **4** (5), 1–6.

Applied Biosystems (1988). "User Bulletin No. 49," August 1988. Foster City, CA: ABI.

Applied Biosystems (1993). "6-FAM and HEX amidites for fluorescent dye labelling of oligonucleotides." User Bulletin number 73, March 1993. Foster City, CA: ABI.

Atkinson, A. H., Heath, R. L., Simpson, R. J., Clarke, A. E., and Anderson, M. A. (1993). Proteinase-inhibitors in *Nicotiana alata* stigmas are derived from a precursor protein which is processed into five homologous inhibitors. *Plant Cell* **5,** 203–213.

Ausubel, F. M., Brant, R., Kingston, R. E., Moore, D. D., Seidman, J. G., Smith, J. A., and Struhl, K. (1988). "Current Protocols in Molecular Biology." New York: Wiley–Interscience.

Boehringer Mannehim (1992). "Nonradioactive *In situ* Hybridization: Application Manual." Boehringer Mannheim, GmbH–Biochemica, PO Box 310120, D-6800 Mannheim 31, Germany.

Bonfiglioli, R. G., McFadden, G. I., and Symons, R. H. (1994). *In situ* hybridization localizes avocado sunblotch viroid on chloroplast thylakoid membranes and coconut cadang cadang viroid in the nucleus. *Plant J.* **6,** 99–103.

Brunning, S., Cresswell, L., Durrant, I., and Eccleston, L. (1993). Direct peroxidase labeling of hybridization probes and chemiluminescence detection. *In "In situ* Hybridization: A Guide to Radioactive and Non Radioactive *in situ* Hybridization Systems." Amersham Place, Buckinghamshire HP7 9NA, England: Amersham International.

Cox, K. H., and Goldberg, R. B. (1988). Analysis of plant gene expression. *In* "Plant Molecular Biology: A Practical Approach" (C. H. Shaw, ed.), pp. 1–35. Oxford: IRL Press.

Evans, M. R., and Read, C. A. (1992). ^{32}P, ^{33}P, and ^{35}S—Selecting a label for nucleic acid analysis. *Nature (London)* **358,** 520–521.

Feinberg, A. P., and Vogelstein, B. (1983). A technique for radiolabeling DNA restriction endonuclease fragments to high specific activity. *Anal. Biochem.* **132,** 6–13.

Fleming, A. J., Mandel, T., Roth, I., and Kuhlemeier, C. (1993). The patterns of gene-expression in the tomato shoot apical meristem. *Plant Cell* **5,** 297–309.

Heslop-Harrison, J. S., and Bennett, M. D. (1990). Nuclear architecture in plants. *Trends Genet.* **6,** 401–405.

Heslop-Harrison, J. S., Schwarzacher, T., Leitch, A. R., and Heslop-Harrison, J. S. (1993). DNA-DNA *in situ* hybridization—Methods for light microscopy. *In* "Plant Cell Biology: A Practical Approach" (N. Harris and K. J. Oparka, eds.), pp. 127–137. Oxford: IRL Press.

Koch, J. (1992). Nonradioactive labelling and detection of nucleic acids *in situ* by "primed *in situ* labelling" ("PRINS"). *In* "Nonradioactive *In situ* Hybridization: Application Manual." pp. 31–33. Boehringer Mannheim, GmbH–Biochemica, PO Box 310120, D-6800 Mannheim 31, Germany.

Koch, J., Hindkjaer, J., Morgensen, J., and Kolfvraa, S. (1991). Nonradioactive, sequence-specific detection of RNA *in situ* by using denatured double-stranded DNA probes as primers in a primed *in situ* labeling. *GATA* **8,** 171–178.

Langer, P. R., Waldrop, A. A., and Ward, D. C. (1981). Enzymatic synthesis of biotin-labeled polynucleotides: Novel nucleic acid affinity probes. *Proc. Natl. Acad. Sci. U.S.A.* **78,** 6633–6637.

McFadden, G. I. (1991). *In situ* hybridization techniques: Molecular cytology goes ultrastructural. *In* "Electron Microscopy of Plant Cells" (J. L. Hall and C. R. Hawes, eds.), pp. 219–255. London: Academic Press.

McFadden, G. I. (1994). *In situ* hybridization of RNA. *In* "Plant Cell Biology: A Practical Approach" (N. Harris and K. J. Oparka, eds.), pp. 97–124. Oxford: IRL Press.

McFadden, G. I., Bönig, I., Cornish, E., and Clarke, A. E. (1988a). A simple fixation and embedding method for use in hybridization histochemistry on plant tissues. *Histochem J.* **20,** 575–586.

McFadden, G. I., Ahluwalia, B., Clarke, A. E., and Fincher, G. B. (1988b). Expression sites and developmental regulation by genes encoding (1-3, 1-4)-β-glucanases in germinated barley. *Planta* **173,** 500–508.

McFadden, G. I., Anderson, M. A., Bönig I., and Clarke, A. E. (1991). Self-incompatibility: Insights through microscopy. *J. Microsc.* **166,** 137–148.

McFadden, G. I., Gilson, P. R., Hofmann, C. J. B., Adcock, G. J., and Maier, U.-G. (1994). Evidence that an amoeba acquired a chloroplast by retaining parts of an engulfed eukaryotic alga. *Proc. Natl. Acad. Sci. U.S.A.* **91,** 3690–3694.

Misiura, C., Durrant, E., Evans, M. R., and Gait, M. J. (1990). Biotinyl and photyrosinyl phosphoramidite derivatives useful in incorporation of multiple reporter groups on synthetic nucleotides. *Nucl. Acids Res.* **18,** 4345–4354.

Narayanswami, S., and Hamkalo, B. A. (1991). DNA sequence mapping using electron microscopy. *GATA* **8,** 14–23.

Nuovo, G. J. (1992). "PCR *In situ* Hybridisation: Protocols and Applications." New York: Raven Press.

O'Brien, T. P., and McCully, M. E. (1986). "The Study of Plant Structure. Principles and Selected Methods." Melbourne: Termacaphi Pty Ltd.

Pardue, M. L. (1986). *In situ* hybridization to DNA of chromosomes and nuclei. *In* "Drosophila. A Practical Approach" (R. B. Robertson, ed.), pp. 111–137. Oxford, UK: IRL Press.

Penschow, J. D., Haralambidis, J., and Coghlan, J. P. (1991). Location of glandular kallikrein mRNA in mouse submandibular gland at the cellular and ultrastructural level by hybridization histochemistry using ^{32}P and ^{3}H labeled oligodeoxyribonucleotide probes. *J. Histochem. Cytochem.* **39,** 835–842.

Titus, D. E. (1991). "Promega Protocols and Applications Guide." Promega Corp., 2800 Woods Hollow Rd., Madison, WI 53711-5399, USA.

Wilchek, M., and Bayer, E. A. (1989). Avidin-biotin technology ten years on: Has it lived up to its expectations? *Trends Biochem. Sci.* **14,** 408–412.

Witkiewicz, H., Bolander, M. E., and Edward, D. R. (1993). Improved design of riboprobes from pBluescript and related vectors for *in situ* hybridization. *BioTechniques* **14,** 458–463.

CHAPTER 13

Localization of RNA by High Resolution *in Situ* Hybridization

Xingxiang Li and Thomas W. Okita
Institute of Biological Chemistry
Washington State University
Pullman, Washington 99164-6340

I. Introduction

Histological localization of RNA involves *in situ* hybridization techniques. At the light microscopy (LM) level, this method yields sufficient resolution to visualize the cellular distribution of RNA species and has been especially useful in determining whether a transcript is present uniformly throughout a tissue or concentrated in a few cell types. LM *in situ* hybridization techniques have also allowed localization of mRNAs to specific regions of the cell. In these instances, the subcellular distributions of the mRNAs were nonrandom and localized to discrete cytosolic regions in which their encoded proteins were enriched (reviewed in Kislauski and Singer, 1992; Wilhelm and Vale, 1993). This phenomenon is easily observed in large cells such as oocytes, eggs, and the developing blastoderm, or in cells exhibiting cytological polarity such as muscle and neuron cells, and fibroblasts. This intracellular localization may provide an important mechanism in targeting proteins to specific subcellular compartments. Asymmetric distribution of mRNAs is likely to occur in many, if not all, cell types.

Current views on the mechanism of intracellular RNA localization suggest a two-step process: transport from the perinuclear region and then anchoring of the RNA to a specific subcellular location (Kislauski and Singer, 1992; Wilhelm and Vale, 1993). Transport processes involve assembly of the RNA with cellular factors and movement of the complex along microfilaments and/or microtubules. In contrast little is known about the anchoring process. To identify the cellular structures that provide RNA anchoring sites, high resolution *in situ* hybridization techniques at the electron microscopy (EM) level are required. Moreover, the high resolution of EM may reveal details and intricacies of RNA distribution patterns that will facilitate our understanding of this phenomenon.

Earlier EM *in situ* hybridization techniques employed radioactive probes that provided limited resolution. Subsequent methods used nonradioactive DNA probes that offered substantially improved resolution but were of limited sensitivity. Introduction of efficient *in vitro* transcription systems, use of digoxigenin, and indirect labeling procedures with biotin, however, all provided marked improvements in the resolution and sensitivity of *in situ* hybridization (Li *et al.*, 1993). We describe here our protocol for detecting the nonrandom distribution of rice storage protein mRNAs on the endoplasmic reticulum (ER) using nonradioactive RNA probes.

II. Principles of *in Situ* Hybridization Technique at the Electron Microscopy Level

Since ultrathin sections (50–100 nm) are used for *in situ* hybridization detected by EM, the amount of RNA under study is limited. These sections have a thickness equivalent to a length of about 140 to 280 bases of fully extended mRNA (3.6 Å between bases). Thinner sections offer better resolution and yield higher cellular detail but contain less mRNA within the section. Thus, there is a tradeoff between optimal cytological resolution and quantity of hybridizable RNA needed to obtain a hybridization signal. The success of EM *in situ* hybridization therefore relies on experimental conditions for production of high specific activity nonisotopic probes, saturated hybridization kinetics, and efficient detection of the hybridization signal. The procedures employed here are designed to achieve these goals.

Like other *in situ* hybridization techniques, the first step of EM *in situ* hybridization is the preparation of the tissue sample. Several parameters should be considered at this stage. The resulting specimens should allow good preservation of cellular morphology and sectioning. In addition, cellular RNAs must be retained on the sections and yet remain accessible for subsequent hybridization. The use of acrylate–methacrylate-based resin, Lowicryl K4M, appears to fulfill all these requirements primarily because of its highly cross-linked and hydrophilic nature (Binder *et al.,* 1986).

The detection of RNAs by EM is accomplished through hybridization using specific probes that are labeled with nonisotopic nucleotide derivatives. Earlier methods used biotinylated DNA probes, as biotin-derivatized dNTPs are readily incorporated to high specific activity by nick-translation. A significant disadvantage of nick-translated probes, however, is their relatively small size (a model size of about 250 bases), which limits the capacity to detect the hybridization event. Moreover, hybridization of immobilized nucleic acid with nick-translated probes is not very efficient due to the fact that annealing of the complementary strands in solution is favored over immobilized sequences (Sambrook *et al.,* 1989).

These limitations of nick-translated probes have been overcome by the introduction of cloning vectors containing bacteriophage promoters that allow the synthesis of single-stranded RNA probes. Although biotinylated nucleotide are relatively poor substrates for RNA polymerase, the introduction of new biotinylation labeling techniques as well as the nonisotopic label digoxigenin enables the synthesis of nonradioactive RNA probes to high specific activity. Besides the elimination of the complementary strand, which can interfere with hybridization, RNA probes offer a number of advantages over DNA probes (Sambrook *et al.,* 1989). RNA hybrids are more stable than those containing DNA. Both sense and antisense RNAs can be synthesized thereby providing both test and control nucleic acid probes. Moreover, ample quantities of probe can be synthesized containing, on average, one derivatized nucleotide in about every 20 nucleotides. While the employment of high concentration of single-stranded RNA probes will ensure saturated conditions for hybridization, high specific activity of the probes favors efficient detection. Moreover, the large size of a probe provides an effective means for signal enhancement. For example, if 50 bases of a cellular RNA molecule are exposed and hybridized to a RNA probe of 1000 bases, a potential 20-fold signal enhancement may be attained compared to a small probe of 50 bases.

The detection of hybridized probes employs antibodies that specifically recognize these nonisotopic labels. In the case of biotinylated probes one can also use streptavidin. Thus, the detection protocol is essentially one involving immunocytochemistry, a well-established electron microscopic (Krishnan *et al.,* 1986) technique where the hybridization event is represented by electron-dense gold particles.

III. Materials

A. Chemicals

Pipes and Tris buffers were obtained from U.S. Biochemical and NTP solutions (100 n*M*) and RNase inhibitor (placental) were purchased from Pharmacia. [α^{32}-P]ATP was from DuPont/NEN. Digoxigenin-11-UTP and mouse anti-digoxigenin were from Boehringer-Mannheim. N^6-amino-hexyl-ATP, ε-caproylamidobiotin-*N*-hydroxysuccinimide (CAB-NHS ester), nitroblue tetrazolium (NBT), and 5-bromo-4-chloro-3-indolyphosphate *p*-toluidine (BCIP) are available from Bethesda Research Laboratories, Inc. T3 RNA polymerase and T7 RNA polymerase were purchased from Promega or Epicentre Technologies. Spermidine, polyethylene glycol 8000 (PEG 8000), bovine serum albumin, polyvinylpyrrolidone 40,000, Ficoll, salmon sperm DNA, streptavidin–gold, anti-digoxin, goat anti-mouse and goat anti-rabbit immunoglobulin G conjugated with alkaline phosphate, rabbit anti-biotin conjugated with alkaline phosphatase, and Sephadex G-50 were obtained from Sigma Chemical. Protein A–gold particle (5 and 15 nm) were from Amersham and nitrocellulose (0.2 μm) was from Costar. SDS and formamide were from Accurate Biochemicals and Fluka, respectively. Glutaraldehyde, Lowicryl K4M, osmium tetroxide, paraformaldehyde, and uranyl acetate were purchased from Polysciences, Inc.

B. Equipment

EM *in situ* hybridization requires a transmission electron microscope. Major equipment also includes a microtome such as DuPont MT5000 for preparing ultrathin sections. In addition, one also needs nickel grids (Polysciene, Inc.) and a UV lamp (Philips TLAD 15W/05 fluorescent tube) for polymerization of the embedding material.

IV. Methods

A. Specimen Preparation

Fixative Solution (Li and Franceschi, 1990):
- 10 m*M* Pipes (pH 7.2)
- 2.5% paraformaldehyde
- 1.25% glutaraldehyde

10 m*M* Pipes–KOH, pH 7.2

Ethanol Series:
- 30% ethanol
- 50% ethanol
- 70% ethanol
- 95% ethanol
- 100% ethanol

Lowicryl K4M Mixture (Hayat, 1986):

K4M monomer	26 g
K4M crosslinker	4 g
Initiator	150 mg

1. Using a razor blade, dissect the plant tissue into 5-mm sections and place them in fixative solution at 4°C overnight.
2. Wash the samples thoroughly (4–5 times, 10 min each) at room temperature with 10 m*M* Pipes, pH 7.2.
3. Dehydrate the tissue in the series of ethanol solutions (15 min at each step).
4. When the samples are ready for infiltration, degas the Lowicryl resin solution under a vacuum, as oxygen inhibits polymerization (Hayat, 1986).
5. Infiltrate the tissue at 4°C using the following schedule (Hayat, 1986):

i. 1:1 mixture of 100% K4M and 90% ethanol	1 h
ii. 2:1 mixture of 100% K4M and 90% ethanol	1 h
iii. 100% K4M mixture	1 h
iv. 100% K4M mixture	12 h

6. Transfer the tissue sections in gelatin capsules, fill the capsules with pure resin, and then cap them.
7. Polymerize the resin by UV-irradiating the capsules. Allow polymerization to occur overnight at 4°C in a walk-in cold room.
8. Continue UV irradiation for another 2–3 days at room temperature. UV radiation can generate a considerable amount of heat and, therefore, should be carried out in a well-ventilated area.
9. Store the polymerized resin blocks under partial vacuum and over desiccant, as these conditions improve their sectioning properties.

B. Sectioning

Due to the hydrophilic nature of Lowicryl K4M resin, 50- 60-nm sections of the specimen are best obtained using a diamond knife. Alternatively, one may find it easier to prepare satisfactory slightly thicker sections with a glass knife ("gold" color sections, about 100 nm). The sections are then transferred to carbon–Formvar-coated grids (200–300 mesh) and stored up to several months before use. Nickel grids are favored over copper ones, as the latter may be oxidized during hybridization in high salt solutions above ambient temperatures.

C. Preparation of Single-Stranded RNA Probes

1. Overview

Assuming that the relevant DNA sequence has been cloned into multicopy cloning vectors, e.g., Bluescript, pGEM, containing the promoter sequences for T3 RNA polymerase, T7 RNA polymerase, and/or SP6 RNA polymerase, antisense (and sense) RNA probes can be prepared by *in vitro* transcription. To prepare the template for transcription, the plasmid DNA should be linearized by digestion with a restriction enzyme whose site is downstream of the 3′ end of the complementary RNA sequences.

With present technology, two nonisotopic labels can be incorporated into synthetic RNA, digoxigenin and biotin. Digoxigenin-11-UTP is readily incorporated into RNA by RNA polymerase. According to Boehringer-Mannheim, RNA polymerases incorporates digoxigenin-11-UTP on average about once every 25 bases under the reaction conditions outlined below. In contrast, the biotin couterpart, biotin-11-UTP, is a relatively poor substrate for RNA polymerase. More efficient biotinylation of RNA molecules can be achieved by a two-step process. First, during *in vitro* RNA transcription, the reaction contains N^6-aminohexyl-ATP, which is efficiently incorporated into RNA about once every 12 bases under the recommended conditions (Folsom *et al.*, 1989). The synthetic RNA is then modified with biotin using the acylating agent biotin *N*-hydroxysuccinimide, which reacts with the primary amine in the hexyl chain. About 80% of the primary amines are modified with biotin, resulting in about one biotin label for every 15 nucleotides. Methods for the preparation of probes containing either nonisotopic label are described below.

2. Synthesis of Digoxigenin-Labeled Probes

Assemble the reaction mixture at room temperature in a 0.5-ml microcentrifuge tube as follows:

12 μl sterile water

1 μl (1 mg/ml) linerazed template DNA

2 μl 10× transcription buffer (400 m*M* Tris–HCl, pH 8, 60 m*M* $MgCl_2$, 100 m*M* NaCl, 20 m*M* spermidine, 100 m*M* DTT)

2 μl NTP mix (10 m*M* each of ATP, GTP, CTP, 6.5 m*M* UTP, and 3.5 m*M* digoxigenin-11-UTP; the solution is neutralized with Tris base)

1 μl [α-P^{32}]-ATP (1 μCi/μl)

1 μl (20 units/μl) RNase inhibitor

1 μl (40 units/μl) T3 RNA polymerase or T7 RNA polymerase

1. Incubate the reaction at 37°C for 2 h.

2. Terminate the reaction by the addition of 2 μl of 200 m*M* EDTA (pH 8).

3. Estimate the yield of RNA synthesis by removing 1 μl of the reaction and adding it to 50 μl of 100 μg/ml of yeast tRNA. Precipitate the RNA by the addition of 100 μl of 10% TCA and placing the solution on ice for 10 min. The precipitate is then collected on glass fiber filters (GF/C), washed twice with about 3 ml of 5% TCA, and then washed twice with 3 ml of 95% ethanol. The filter is dried and then the amount of radioactivity measured by liquid scintillation counting. Assuming a liquid scintillation counting efficiency of 80%, the yield of RNA synthesis (in micrograms) is estimated by the following equation (No. of CPM $\times$ 20/1.76 $\times$ 10^5) $\times$ 26.4.

4. Dilute the rest of the reaction mixture to 200 μl with TE (10 m*M* Tris–HCl, pH 8, 1 m*M* EDTA). Add 200 μl of phenol and vortex for 30 s. Add 200 μl of chloroform and shake the tube contents for another 30 s. Spin in a microcentrifuge for 1 min.

5. Collect the upper phase and add 20 μl of 3 *M* sodium acetate, pH 4.8, and 500 μl of ethanol. Place the tube at −20°C for 30 min and then centrifuge for 30 min.

6. Remove the supernatant. Wash the pellet by adding 500 μl of cold 70% ethanol, centrifuging for 1 min, and removing the supernatant. Dry the RNA pellet under vacuum. The resulting RNA probe can be dissolved directly in hybridization solution (see below) at a concentration of 40–50 μg/ml. Supplement with yeast tRNA to 0.5 mg/ml.

3. Synthesis of Biotin-Labeled RNA Probes

1. Prepare an *in vitro* transcription assay as described above except (i) restore UTP level to 10 m*M* and eliminate digoxigenin-11-UTP and (ii) reduce ATP to 5 m*M* and add 5 m*M* N^6-aminohexyl-ATP.

2. Add RNA polymerase and incubate at 37°C for 2 h.

3. Terminate the reaction by the addition of 2 μl of 200 m*M* EDTA and the dilute to 200 μl with TE.

4. Extract with phenol and chloroform followed by ethanol precipitation as described above. The RNA is then suspended in sterile H_2O at a concentration of 80 μg/ml.

5. The synthetic RNA is biotinylated by the following reaction:

   50 μl synthetic RNA (about 4 μg) containing N^6-aminohexyl-AMP

   50 μl freshly prepared 0.4 *M* sodium bicarbonate (about pH 8.2)

   20 μl CAB–NHS ester (freshly prepared in dimethylformamide at 10 mg/ml).

6. After incubating for 2 h at room temperature, terminate the reaction by adding 100 μl of 1 *M* Tris–HCl, pH 7.6

7. Resolve the RNA from the unicorporated biotin ester by gel filtration chromatography. A 5-ml disposable plastic pipette is plugged with siliconized glass wool at the end and packed with about 6 ml of swollen Sephadex G-50 (this is conveniently done by autoclaving) equilibrated with sterile 1× SSC (0.015 *M* sodium citrate, 0.15 *M* NaCl) containing 0.05% SDS. The RNA solution is diluted with 200 μl of 1×SSC, 0.5% SDS, and then passed through a 6-ml Sephadex G-50 column. The RNA in the void volume is pooled and precipitated in the presence of 50 μg of tRNA, 30 m*M* sodium acetate, pH 4.8, and 70% ethanol. The RNA pellet is directly dissolved in 100 μl of hybridization solution.

D. Estimation of Specific Activity of the Nonisotopically Labeled RNA Probes

The specific activity of the incorporated nonisotiopc labels can be estimated using specific antibodies conjugated to alkaline phosphatase and colorometric methods as described below. Alternatively, nonisotopic nucleic acid detection kits are available for both biotinylated and digoxigenin-labeled nucleic acids from several commercial sources and are optimized to detect picrogram amounts of nucleic acid.

1. Serial dilute (1 to 1000 pg) the nonisotopically labeled RNAs in 200 μl of sterile 10× SSPE and then immobilize the RNAs on a nitrocellulose membrane using a dot blot apparatus.
2. Wash the nitrocellulose membrane in sterile 3× SSPE, allow it to air dry for 15 min, and then place it in a vacuum oven set at 80°C for 2 h.
3. Incubate the nitrocellulose membrane in 3% acetylated BSA (Zimmerman and Sandeen, 1966) made in PBS (Sambrook *et al.*, 1989) for 30–60 min.
4. Dilute the antibodies (anti-digoxigenin or anti-biotin) conjugated with alkaline phosphatase in blocking solution according to the manufacturers' recommendations and incubate the filter for 1 h.
5. Rinse the filter twice with washing buffer for 15 min each, followed by two 5-min rinses with alkaline phosphatase buffer.
6. Incubate the filter in NBT–BCIP solution. A minimum of 10 pg of RNA should be detected within 30 min. Smaller concentrations of RNA can be detected with longer incubation times.

E. Hybridization of Thin Sections with RNA Probes

Hybridization Solution
- 50% formamide
- 7.5% polyethylene glycol
- 1% BSA
- 10 mg/ml Ficoll

10 mg/ml polyvinylprrolidone
1 m*M* EDTA
0.25 *M* NaCl
0.25 *M* sodium phosphate (pH 7.2)
4× SSPE (prepared without SDS; see Sambrook *et al.*, 1989)
2× SSPE
1× SSPE

1. Prehybridize the EM specimen sections by floating the grids on a droplet of hybridization solution placed on parafilm. Incubate for 15–30 min at room temperature.

2. Heat the probe (4–5 μg/100 μl of hybridization solution) at 65°C for 15 min and then quench on ice.

3. Place two or three grids on a 50-μl droplet of probe solution and incubate in a moist and sealed container at 42°C for at least 5 h.

4. Wash the grids sequentially in 5 ml of 4× SSPE (5 min), 2× SSPE (5 min), and twice in 1× SSPE (30 min each) at room temperature.

5. If detection is to be performed immediately, transfer the grids to TBST–BSA buffer (see below). If the grids are to be stored, they should be washed again with 1× SSPE for 30–60 min. After the grids are briefly rinsed in distilled water, they are air-dried.

1. General Comments

a. SDS is not included in the hybridization solution, since proteins and RNA appear to be dissolved from the tissue sections during hybridizations, resulting in the reduction of probe detection and poor EM images.

b. Treatment of the ultrathin sections with proteases is not recommended since several studies have shown that it can have a detrimental effect on hybridization presumably due to loss of RNA (Lawrence and Singer, 1985; Binder, 1986). However, protease treatment may improve the detection of DNA sequence (Puvion-Dutilleul and Puvion, 1989).

c. The minimal amount of probe needed for saturated kinetics of hybridization has not been determined. However, the amount (4–5 μg/100 μl hybridization solution) of probe recommended in this study is sufficient for saturated hybridization conditions while minimizing background labeling.

d. Although several studies have indicated that hybridization on ultrathin sections is completed within 5–6 h (Lawrene and Singer, 1985; Binder *et al.*, 1986), an overnight (10–16 h) incubation is more convenient and does not appear to increase the extent of background labeling.

e. Earlier methods recommended buffers containing formamide (50%) for washing the grids. Although it is effective in reducing background, this procedure also removes hybridized probes. We found that extensive washing with saline buffer can achieve a minimal background while retaining the hybridized probe.

f. Grids should not be allowed to dry during the washing steps. Otherwise background labeling becomes quite significant.

F. Detection of Hybridized RNA Probes

To detect digoxigenin-labeled RNA, we used a polyclonal antiserum against digoxin, which reacts with digoxigenin at excellent efficiency. Since the development of our method, an anti-digoxigenin is now commercially available from Boehringer-Mannheim. Antiserum with the highest titer should be purchased and checked by blot colorometric method as described above, since batch-to-batch difference may occur. The optimal concentration of the antibodies is dependent on the titer and should be determined empirically. To detect biotinylated probes, streptavidin–gold is a convenient choice, although one can also use gold-conjugated antibodies that recognize biotin. Prior to carrying out the reaction, prepare the following solutions:

1. TBST

   50 m*M* Tris–HCl, pH 7.2
   250 m*M* NaCl
   1% Tween 20

2. TBST–BSA

   TBST supplemented with 1% bovine serum albumin

1. Float the grids on TBST–BSA for 15 min and then transfer them to the same buffer containing either anti-digoxin or streptavidin–gold (about 1:100) dilution) for digoxigenin or biotin labeled probes, respectively.

2. Incubate for 3–4 h and then wash the grids four times with TBST–BSA for 10-min a wash.

3. Incubate the sections hybridized with digoxigenin-labeled probes with protein A–gold (1:100 dilution in TBST–BSA) for two h. For sections hybridized with biotinylated probes proceed to step 5.

4. Wash the grids as in step 2.

5. Wash for 10 min with TBST followed with sterile water, and then air-dried.

6. Poststain the sections with 1% uranyl acetate and 1% lead citrate as follows. Float the grids on a drop of 1% lead citrate on a piece of parafilm in a petri dish. After 4 min the grids are transferred to distilled water, rinsed for 2 to 3 min with distilled water, and then transferred to 1% uranyl acetate. After

5 min the grids are washed as before followed by air-drying. The grids can now be examined under electron microscopy.

3. General Comments

a. Sense RNA probes are appropriate controls. The control probes are labeled, hybridized, and detected as for the antisense RNAs. Alternatively, sections may be treated with RNase prior to hybridization. Both controls should give little background labeling.

b. Although detection of the digoxigenin-labeled RNA probes requires an additional step (incubation with protein A–gold), compared to biotinylated probes, both nonisotope labels yield similar labeling densities.

c. The ability to generate RNAs with two different nonisotopic labels with different but compatible detection methods allows double *in situ* hybridization approaches where two different RNAs can be probed simultaneously. This method has been successfully used to localize the transcripts for two storage proteins on the ER in rice endosperm cells (Li *et al.,* 1993).

V. Results and Discussion

Previous studies by Kim and Okita (1993) have demonstrated that glutelin mRNAs were in twofold excess over prolamine transcripts in the polysomal fraction isolated from a microsomal membrane fraction enriched in cisternal ER. By RNA blot quantitative analysis, Li *et al.* (1993) confirmed this initial observation and also showed that prolamine transcripts were enriched in protein body fraction, suggesting that glutelin and prolamine transcripts are not randomly distributed on the ER membranes. To obtain unequivocal evidence that indeed these storage proteins were localized on specific ER types, the distribution of these storage protein mRNAs were analyzed by high resolution *in situ* hybridization using methods described here. We initially tested both digoxigenin-labeled and biotinylated RNA probes. Figure 1 shows micrographs of EM *in situ* hybridization using antisense glutelin RNA probes labeled either with digoxigenin (Fig. 1A) or biotin (Fig. 1B). In either case, glutelin mRNAs as visualized by the distribution of protein A–gold (Fig. 1A) or streptavidin–gold conjugates were restricted to the cisternal ER (C–ER). In contrast, glutelin-specific probes were rarely associated with the ER (PB–ER) that delimits the prolamine protein bodies.

Because the hybridization was conducted under saturating conditions, the density of gold particles (No. of gold particles/μm ER membrane cross section) should be indicative of the relative mRNA levels associated with these ER membranes. This correlation was substantiated by analysis of representative endosperm sections probed with either glutelin or prolamine sense and antisense

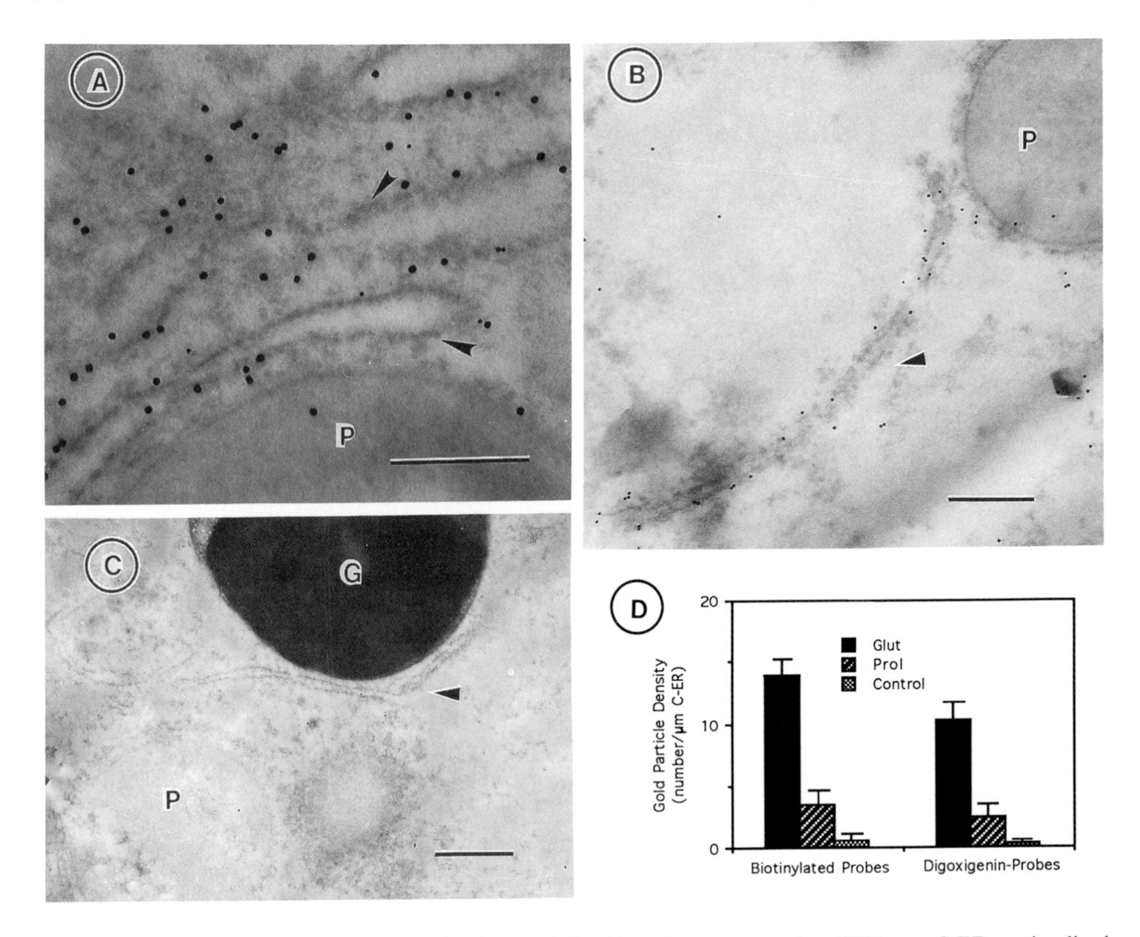

Fig. 1 The spatial distributions and densities of storage protein mRNAs on C-ER as visualized by single *in situ* hybridization analysis. Labeling of C-ER is readily evident when probed with antisense glutelin RNA labeled with digoxigenin and visualized with 15 nm gold particles (A) or labeled with biotin and visualized with 10-nm gold particles (B). The extent of background labeling with sense glutelin RNA is shown in (C). Similar analysis was conducted with prolamine probes (not shown). (D) Gold particle densities representing glutelin and prolamine transcripts on the C-ER. Note that the relative proportion of these storage protein mRNAs is the same irrespective of the nonisotopic labeled employed. Differences in the gold particles densities is due to the use of different size gold particles. Bars, 0.5 μm. (Reprinted from Li *et al.*, 1993, with permission from *Cell*).

probes. Under saturating hybridization conditions, the relative density of glutelin transcripts exceeded those of prolamine species by 4.7-fold on C-ER (Fig. 1D). When corrected for the size difference between glutelin (1.8 kb) and prolamine (0.9 kb) RNA probes, the relative densities of glutelin and prolamine transcripts on the C-ER was about 2.3 : 1, a value almost identical to the relative distribution of the transcripts estimated by blot hybridization analysis of RNA extracted from an enriched C-ER membrane fraction.

In Fig. 1D, the absolute gold particle densities obtained with RNA probes labeled with digoxigenin were somewhat less than values obtained with biotinylated probes. These differences in observed gold particle densities were not due to the different detection methods but rather to the use of different size gold particles. The digoxigenin-labeled probes were visualized with 15-nm gold particles, whereas the biotinylated probes were detected with 10-nm particles. Other studies (Li and Okita, unpublished) have shown that 5-nm gold particles yielded a twofold greater density labeling pattern than 15-nm gold particles. Therefore, the use of larger gold particles results in lower gold particle densities probably due to steric effects of binding or the propensity of larger gold particles to be removed during the posthybridization washing steps.

With the different nonisotopic labeling and detection methods, two different mRNAs can be simultaneously detected in the same EM section. Figures 2A and 2B illustrate a double *in situ* hybridization experiment where glutelin and prolamine mRNA probes were labeled with digoxigenin (15-nm gold particles) and biotin (5-nm gold particles), respectively. The labeling pattern indicates that glutelin mRNAs are enriched on the cisternal ER, whereas prolamine transcripts predominate on the ER that delimits the prolamine protein bodies (Fig. 2C). Under these experimental parameters, the twofold enhancement of detection gained by the differences in probe lengths is offset by the 2-fold reduction of detection mediated by differences in gold particle sizes. Therefore, the observed gold particle densities directly reflect the relative concentrations of these transcripts on these ER membranes.

The apparent differences in efficiency of detection of these nonisotopic labels can be negated by reversing the nonisotope label–gold particle combination. In this case, glutelin RNA probes were labeled with biotin and detected with 5-nm gold particles, whereas prolamines were labeled and detected with digoxigenin and 15-nm gold particles, respectively. By averaging the gold particle densities obtained by both combinations of the *in situ* hybridization, as well as taking into account the effect of probe sizes, the relative distribution of these storage protein mRNAs can be directly assessed. In this example, glutelin transcripts were 2.2-fold excess compared to prolamines on C-ER, whereas prolamine transcripts predominated on the PB-ER by 7-fold (see Li *et al.*, 1993).

VI. Perspectives

Because of the excellent ultrastructural resolution, EM *in situ* hybridization is the technique of choice when the exact subcellular location of a nucleic acid needs to be resolved. Moreover, the ability to conduct double *in situ* hybridization analysis at saturated hybridization kinetics enables one to evaluate the relative abundance levels of two mRNAs under study and whether these messages differ

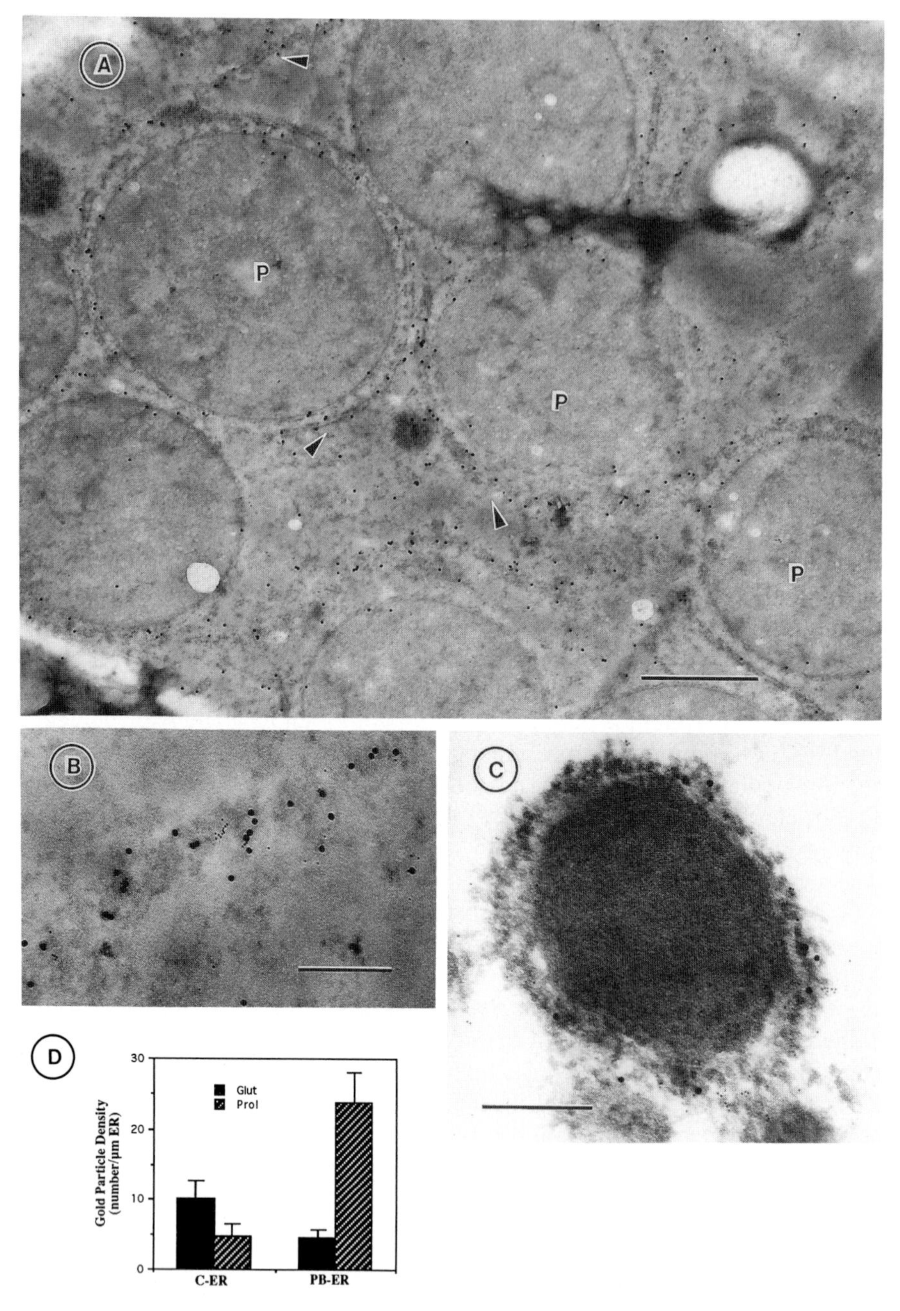

Fig. 2 Double *in situ* hybridization analysis of glutelin and prolamine mRNAs on C-ER and PB-ER membranes. Hybridized digoxigenin-labeled antisense glutelin probe was visualized with 15-nm gold particles, whereas biotinylated-labeled antisense prolamine probe was detected with 5-nm gold particles. (A) Micrograph at low magnification where the 5-nm gold particles are barely visible. (B) and (C) Distribution and densities of glutelin and prolamine mRNAs on C-ER and PB-ER, respectively. (D) Relative distribution of these storage protein mRNAs on these ER membranes are reflected by the densities of their gold particles. P, prolamine protein body. Bar in (A), 1 μm; bars in (B) and (C), 0.25 μm. (Reprinted from Li *et al.*, 1993, with permission from *Cell*).

in their cellular location. The degree of success of this technique will depend on the overall abundance of the transcripts in the cells. In the example used here, prolamine and glutelin transcripts each constitute about 3–5% of the total mRNAs in middeveloping endosperm cells. Moreover, these mRNAs are associated with the ER membranes, thereby increasing the effective intracellular concentration of these RNAs. For detecting less abundant mRNAs, several experimental parameters should be explored to improve efficiency of this technique. Increasing the length of the RNA probe (for instance, by transcribing intron sequences together with antisense sequences) and the use of smaller gold particles would enhance the sensitivity of detection. Using thicker specimen sections would increase the amount of available hybridizable nucleic acid although possibly at the expense of ultrastructural definition. Moreover, RNase-free conditions more stringent than the ones described here could be implemented during the hybridization and washing steps, thereby maintaining the integrity of the RNA probe and hybrid.

Acknowledgments

This work was supported in part by Project 0590, College of Agriculture and Home Economics, Washington State University.

References

Binder, M., Tourmente, S., Roth, J., Renaud, M., and Gethring, W. J. (1986). *In situ* hybridization of ultrathin sections of Lowicryl K4M-embedded tissue using biotinylated probes and protein A-gold complexes. *J. Cell Biol.* **102,** 1646–1653.

Folsom, V., Hunkeler, M. J., Haces, A., and Harding, J. D. (1989). Detection of DNA targets with biotinylated and fluoresceinated RNA probes. *Anal. Biochem.* **182,** 309–314.

Hayat, M. A. (1986). "Basic Techniques for Transmission Electron Microscopy." Orlando: Academic Press.

Kim, W. T., Li, X., and Okita, T. W. (1993). Expression of storage protein multigene families in developing rice endosperm. *Plant Cell Physiol.* **34,** 5954–603.

Kislauski, E. H., and Singer, R. H. (1992). Determinants of mRNA localization. *Curr. Opin. Cell Biol.* **4,** 975–978.

Krishnan, H. B., Franceschi, V. R., and Okita, T. W. (1986). Immunochemical studies on the role of the Golgi complex in protein-body formation in rice seeds. *Planta* **169,** 471–480.

Lawrence, J. B., and Singer, R. H. (1985). Quantitative analysis of *in situ* hybridization methods for the detection of actin gene expression. *Nucleic Acids Res.* **13,** 1777–1799.

Li, X., and Franceschi, V. R. (1990). Distribution of peroxisomes and glycolate metabolism in relation to calcium formation in *Lemna minor. Eur. J. Cell Biol.* **51,** 9–16.

Li, X., Franceschi, V. R., and Okita, T. W. (1993). Segregation of storage protein mRNAs on the rough endoplasmic reticulum membranes of rice endosperm cells. *Cell* **72,** 869–879.

Puvion-Dutilleul, F., and Puvion, E. (1989). Ultrastructural localization of viral DNA in thin sections of herpes simplex virus type 1 infected cells by *in situ* hybridization. *Eur. J. Cell Biol.* **49,** 99–109.

Sambrook, J., Fritsch, E. F., and Maniatis, T. (1989). "Molecular cloning: A laboratory manual." 2nd Ed., Cold Spring Harbor, NY: Cold Spring Harbor Laboratory Press.

Wilhelm, J. E., and Vale, R. D. (1993). RNA on the move: The mRNA localization pathway. *J. Cell Biol.* **123,** 269–274.

Zimmerman, S. B., and Sandeen, G. (1966). The ribonuclease activity of the crystallized deoxyribonuclease. *Anal. Biochem.* **14,** 269–277.

CHAPTER 14

Recombinant Aequorin Methods for Intracellular Calcium Measurement in Plants

Heather Knight and Marc R. Knight
University of Oxford
Department of Plant Sciences
South Parks Road, Oxford OX1 3RB
United Kingdom

I. Introduction

This chapter discusses the use of a novel technique for the measurement of intracellular calcium ($[Ca^{2+}]_i$). The measurement of $[Ca^{2+}]_i$ in plants is becoming increasingly popular as its role as a second messenger is uncovered. There exists already a powerful technology for the measurement of $[Ca^{2+}]_i$, in the form of the calcium-sensitive fluorescent dyes. However, some difficulties have been experienced when attempting to apply this technique to plants (Callaham and Hepler, 1991) and severe problems are encountered in fungi (H. Knight *et al.*, 1993). Recombinant aequorin methods complement these techniques and also provide some new advantages.

A class of naturally occurring photoproteins found in coelenterates (hydroids and jellyfish) emit light in response to calcium ions. These proteins have been characterized and light emission has been shown to relate directly to calcium concentration. Because of this property, such photoproteins can be used to report calcium levels *in vivo* by measuring the amount of light emitted.

The best characterized of these photoproteins are obelin and aequorin, although at least four other similar proteins are known to exist (Campbell, 1988). Aequorin is highly sensitive to calcium and can potentially detect free calcium levels of up to 100 μM (Campbell, 1988); therefore it is a versatile intracellular reporter for this ion. In practice, aequorin measurements of calcium are usually made within the range 10 nM–10 μM. The protein is a single polypeptide chain (ca. 22 kDa) and is synthesized under normal conditions by the jellyfish *Aequorea victoria.* The gene product, apoaequorin, requires a prosthetic group, a luciferin molecule called coelenterazine (MW 432), in order to form functional aequorin. The presence of molecular oxygen is also required. The aequorin molecule itself is similar in structure to the calcium binding protein calmodulin, having three EF hand structures that constitute three calcium binding domains. A fourth domain constitutes the binding site for coelenterazine and oxygen. When calcium is bound, coelenterazine is oxidized to coelenteramide and the protein undergoes a conformational change accompanied by the release of CO_2 and the emission of blue light (Fig. 1).

This reaction, which occurs naturally in the jellyfish, can be made to occur in other organisms *in vivo* and used to measure $[Ca^{2+}]_i$ providing that the following conditions can be met:

1. introduction of apoaequorin into cells
2. introduction of coelenterazine into cells
3. detection of blue light emission, often at low levels

Giant muscle fibers of the corn barnacle (*Balanus nubilis)* were the first single cells to be microinjected with aequorin (Ridgway and Ashley, 1967). Microinjection, however, is not always possible, due to a number of problems. Iontophoretic injection cannot be used, as there is too much salt present in aequorin preparations and pressure injection may not deliver the amount of aequorin required for the subsequent visualization of luminescence. Increasing the amount of aequorin in the cell necessitates either the use of more concentrated solutions of aequorin which are viscous, causing micropipette tips to become easily blocked, or the introduction of unacceptably high volumes into the cell, a particular

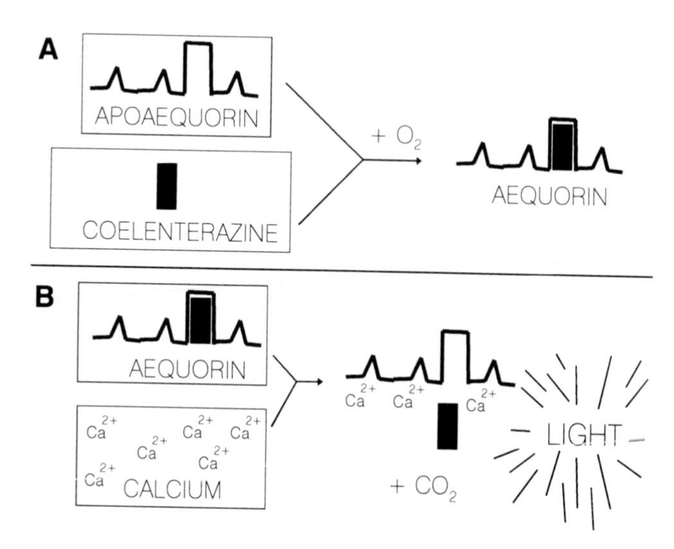

Fig. 1 (A) Reconstitution of functional aequorin from apoaequorin and coelenterazine. (B) Discharge of aequorin upon binding of Ca^{2+}, showing release of coelenterazine and emission of light.

problem with small cells. The highest concentration of aequorin that is practical to use is 2% w/v (Shimomura, 1991). Despite these drawbacks, however, microinjection has been successful in a number of systems including frog cardiac muscle (Allen and Blinks, 1978), mouse oocytes, and rat heart and liver cells (Cobbold and Lee, 1991). Only a few cell types under 50 μm in diameter have been injected (Blinks *et al.*, 1978). The only instance of measurements being made in intact plant cells is in the giant green alga *Chara* (Williamson and Ashley, 1982) but most plant cells are much smaller than this.

Other techniques for loading aequorin into cells have included cell fusion with liposomes or erythrocyte ghosts containing aequorin or its precursors, release of aequorin from internalized micropinocytotic vesicles, intracellular synthesis from mRNA or cDNA, and scrapeloading (Campbell, 1988). Aequorin can also be introduced into cells by a number of methods involving cell permeation (Cobbold and Rink, 1987) including electroporation (Gilroy *et al.*, 1989). Most of these methods, however, are not applicable to intact plant cells.

A method was required, therefore, for introducing sufficient aequorin into plant cells to enable reliable measurements to be made without disruption to the cell. This led to the development of a technique based on the genetic transformation of plants with an apoaequorin gene so that after the addition of coelenterazine, the plants could be used to measure their own calcium levels (Knight *et al.*, 1991b). This method also has the advantage that all cells in one plant can be loaded with the indicator simultaneously and thus calcium changes can be studied in the tissues of intact plants in response to stimuli relevant to the whole plant, such as wind (Knight *et al.*, 1991). This method has also been applied to bacteria (Knight *et al.*, 1991a), yeast (Nakajima-Shimade *et al.*, 1991), and human cells (Sheu *et al.*, 1993).

II. Expression of Recombinant Aequorin in Plants

A. Materials

Escherichia coli JM101 containing plasmid pMAQ2 (Fig. 2), *E. coli* HB101 containing plasmid pRK2013, *Agrobacterium tumefaciens* LBA4404. Luria-broth [10 g/liter bactotryptone (Difco), 10 g/liter sodium chloride (BDH), 5 g/liter bacto yeast extract (Beta Lab); 15 g/liter agar for bacterial plates], antibiotics (Sigma): rifampicin (50mg/ml in DMSO), streptomycin sulfate (300 mg/ml in water), kanamycin sulfate (100 mg/ml in water).

Mature *Nicotiana plumbaginifolia* plants, sodium hypochlorite (BDH), MS medium (Flow labs, Irvine) sucrose (BDH), kinetin (Sigma), 1-naphthylacetic acid (Sigma), bacto-agar (Difco), carbenicillin (disodium salt, 500 mg/ml, Sigma), 11-cm petri dishes (Sterilin), plastic universal tubes (Sterilin), plant pots (Stewart), Levington's compost.

B. Methods

1. Transfer of pMAQ2 Construct to *A. tumefaciens* by Triparental Mating

1. Inoculate a large single colony of LBA4404 from a freshly streaked plate and culture in 5 ml of sterile Luria broth (LB) containing rifampicin

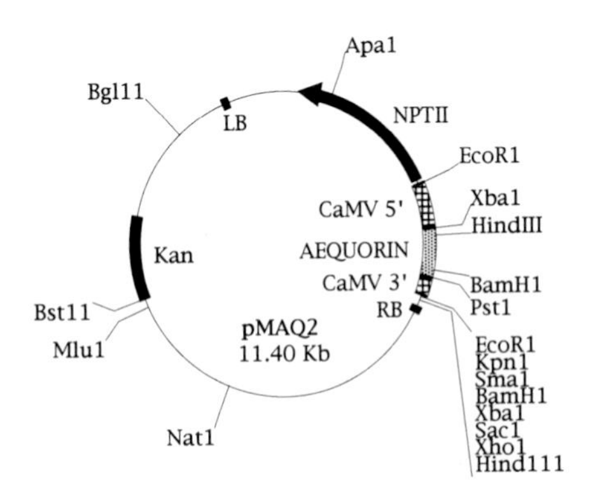

Fig. 2 Plasmid pMAQ2, binary vector for transformation of higher plants with the 35S apoaequorin gene. CaMV 5′, cauliflower mosaic virus (CaMV) 35S promoter; CaMV 3′, CaMV 35S transcriptional terminator; AEQUORIN, apoaequorin coding region from cDNA clone; LB and RB, T-DNA left- and right-hand borders, respectively; NPTII, neomycin phosphotransferase gene (kanamycin resistance in plants); Kan, bacterial kanamycin resistance gene. Important restriction endonuclease sites are also shown.

(100 mg/liter) and streptomycin (300 mg/liter) for 24 h at 29–30°C, shaking vigorously (ca. 250 rpm).

2. Take single colonies of HB101, and JM101 containing pMAQ2, and inoculate each separately into 5 ml LB containing kanamycin (100 mg/liter); incubate overnight at 37°C with shaking. The timing of the inoculations should be arranged so that all bacterial cultures reach stationary phase simultaneously.

3. When cultures have reached stationary phase, combine 100 μl of each of the three cultures and spread on an LB agar plate containing no antibiotics. Incubate overnight at 29–30°C.

4. The plates should now be covered with a bacterial lawn. Take a streak from the plate and add to 0.5 ml sterile LB in a 1.5-ml microfuge tube. Vortex well.

5. Take 2 aliquots of 250 μl and spread on agar plates containing rifampicin, streptomycin, and kanamycin (RSK plates) at the concentrations given in steps 1 and 2. Incubate for 2–3 days at 29–30°C.

6. Distinct colonies should become apparent. Streak these colonies on RSK plates. There may be a background of very small colonies.

7. Screen colonies for transformants by analyzing a mini-prep of agrobacterium plasmid DNA (An *et al.*, 1988).

2. Genetic Transformation of *N. plumbaginifolia*

All manipulation of plant tissue is carried out in a laminar-flow cabinet to prevent contamination.

1. Grow *A. tumefaciens* LBA4404 containing pMAQ2 in L-broth containing 100 mg/liter kanamycin at 28°C for 24 h or until stationary phase is achieved.

2. Harvest well-expanded *N. plumbaginifolia* leaves. Sterilize leaves by washing in 70% ethanol for 30 s followed by 10% sodium hypochlorite for 15 min. Wash leaves 6 times in sterile water.

3. Cut leaves into 8- to 10-mm squares, avoiding major veins, and place these explants in 4.7 g/liter MS salts, 10 g/liter sucrose (pH 5.8; using 0.1 *M* KOH).

4. Add bacterial culture to make a 1:50 dilution. Incubate explant/bacterial mixture for 15 min agitating intermittently.

5. Transfer explants to plates containing 4.7 g/liter MS medium, 10 g/liter sucrose, 2 mg/liter kinetin, 0.2 mg/liter 1-naphthylacetic acid, 8 g/liter bacto-agar (pH 5.8). Seal plates with parafilm but cut slots to allow gas exchange.

6. Culture plates at 25°C in the light (100–150 $\mu E/m^2/s$) for 48 h.

7. Transfer explants to fresh plate of the same medium containing 200 mg/liter kanamycin sulfate and 500 mg/liter carbenicillin.

8. After shoot formation on the cut edges of the leaf explants (approx. 6 weeks), transfer shoots to plates containing 2.35 g/liter MS medium, 5 g/liter sucrose, 250 mg/liter carbenicillin and 200 mg/liter kanamycin sulfate, and 8 g/liter bacto-agar (pH 5.8). Culture in same conditions as before for 1 week.

9. Remove shoots and dissect off any callus material and lower leaves. Make a fresh cut at the bottom of the stem of these shoots before transferring them singly to universal tubes containing 10 ml 2.35 g/liter MS medium, 100 mg/liter kanamycin sulfate, 100 mg/liter carbenicillin, and 0.8% bacto-agar. Ensure that the bottom of the plantlet is inserted into the solid medium.

10. After root induction (1–3 weeks) transfer plants to pots containing organic compost (Levington's), covering them with a polythene bag secured with an elastic band. Grow at same conditions as before but with an 18-h photoperiod. After 1 week remove elastic band and loosen polythene bag. After a further week remove bag completely and grow as normal.

11. Check transformants by Southern and Western blots as described (Knight *et al.*, 1991b).

III. Reconstitution of Aequorin

A. Materials

N. plumbaginifolia seeds from plants transformed with pMAQ2 (Section II,B,2), coelenterazine (Molecular Probes), sodium chloride (BDH), β-mercaptoethanol (Aldrich), EDTA (BCL), Tris (BCL), gelatin (BDH). Solutions should be stored in plastic containers to avoid leaching of calcium from glass.

B. Methods

Reconstitution of aequorin requires the entry of coelenterazine into the plant tissues. Fortunately, as it is a relatively hydrophobic molecule, coelenterazine can pass easily through plant membranes and thus into cells.

1. For *in vivo* reconstitution float 7- to 8-day-old *N. plumbaginifolia* seedlings on water. Add 0.01 vol of 250 μM coelenterazine in methanol and mix well. Reconstitution reaches a maximum after about 6 h so an overnight reconstitution is often convenient.

2. For *in vitro* reconstitutions homogenize 1–5 mg (fresh weight) of tissue in 500 μl of reconstitution medium [0.5 M NaCl, 5 mM β-mercaptoethanol, 5 mM EDTA, 0.1% gelatin (w/v) and 10 mM Tris–HCl, pH 7.4; Campbell *et al.*, 1988]. Sediment debris by microfuging for 10 min at high speed (16,000 g) and retaining the supernatant. To 50 μl of supernatant add 50 μl of fresh reconstitution medium. Add 1 μl of 100 μM coelenterazine in methanol and mix. Reconstitution *in vitro* is usually maximal after 3 h.

C. Controls

The time taken for functional aequorin to reconstitute in plant tissues is estimated by measuring Ca^{2+}-dependent luminescence at various time points. In 7-

day-old *Nicotiana* seedlings maximum reconstitution is observed after 6 h in coelenterazine and levels remain high for at least 24 h (Knight *et al.*, 1991b). Other semisynthetic aequorins (Section V,4) are stable for shorter periods. To be sure of achieving maximum reconstitution of aequorin in plants of other species or age, it is useful to conduct a preliminary time course study of reconstitution. This is done by homogenizing tissue in calcium-free buffer after various lengths of time in coelenterazine and discharging the reconstituted aequorin with calcium, (as described in Section IV,A,2). The amount of aequorin reconstituted increases with the concentration of coelenterazine up to a coelenterazine concentration of at least 10 μM (Knight *et al.*, 1991b).

IV. Measurement of Light

The level of light emission from recombinant aequorin is 4.30–5.16 $\times 10^{15}$ photons/mg of aequorin (Shimomura, 1991). At present the actual levels of aequorin that can be expressed in plant tissues are relatively low (a few pg protein/mg fresh weight of tissue) and therefore detection of the blue light emitted in response to calcium requires the use of very sensitive light counting equipment. A luminescence detector needs to be able to detect light signals over a wide range varying by several orders of magnitude of intensity; from only a few photons per second to several tens of thousands. It is also important that the speed of the detector be much greater than the rate of the fastest response to be measured (Campbell, 1988).

Light emission is most commonly recorded by photographic film, photodiodes, or photomultiplier tubes (PMTs). All methods of measuring light record the amount of light emitted over a set period of time. Light pulses may be measured every 10 ms, for instance, for samples emitting higher levels of light, whereas low light emission, for instance, during imaging of wounding in plants (M.R. Knight *et al.*, 1993), may need to be integrated over periods of tens of seconds (see Fig. 3).

Luminescence from whole plants transformed with the aequorin gene can be measured by one of two means:

1. luminometry
2. low-level light imaging

The setting up and operation of light counting devices is covered in great detail by Campbell (1988), so the following descriptions will be restricted to a brief outline of the equipment. Stanley (1992) has published a survey of a great number of luminometers and imaging devices and the reader may wish to refer to this to aid in the selection of a suitable device. The following sections describe the basic functions of the most useful devices for aequorin luminescence measurement, accompanied by details of the equipment we have used in our own laboratory.

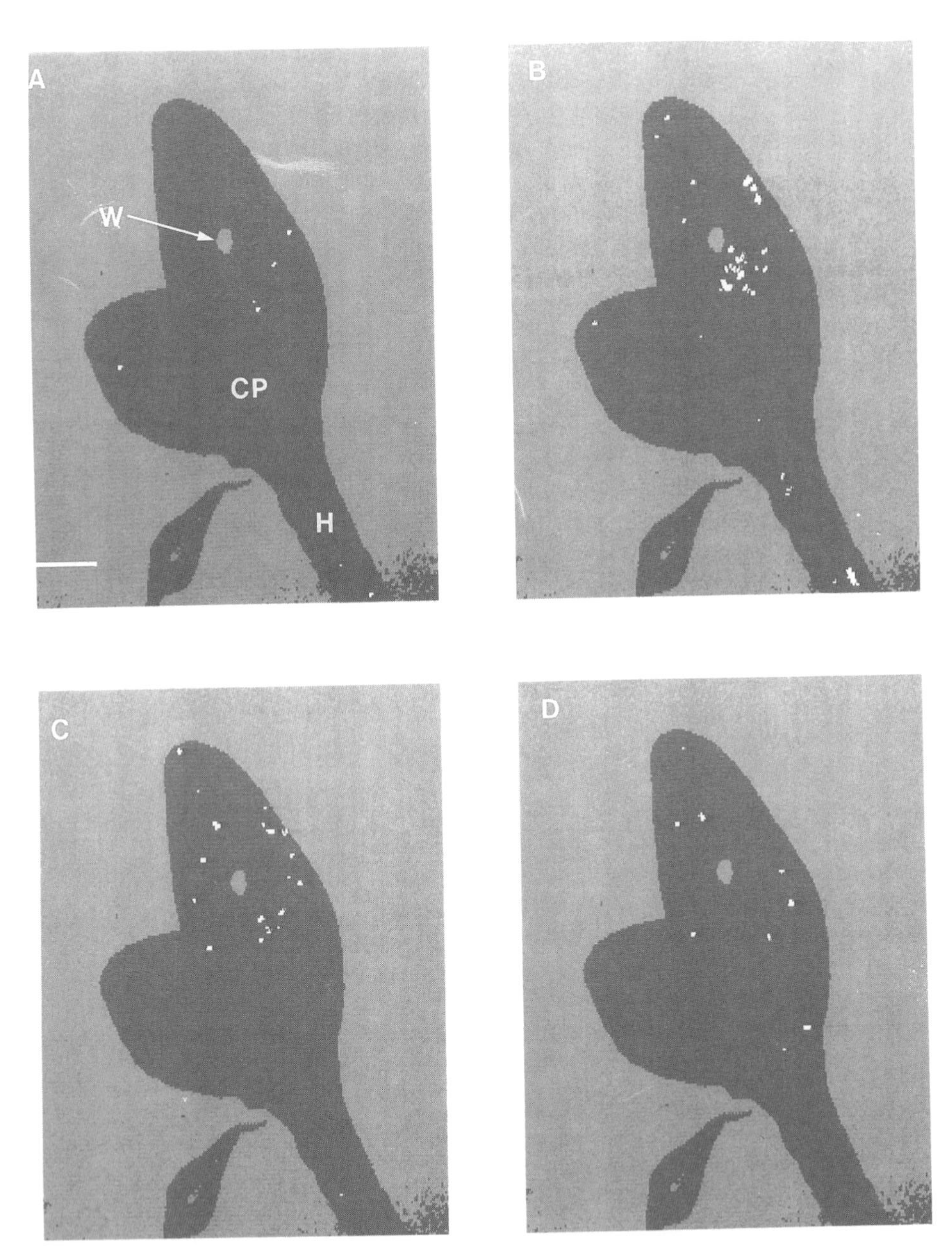

Fig. 3 Time course experiment showing changes in $[Ca^{2+}]_i$ in a tobacco seedling cotyledon pair (CP) in response to a wound (W) applied to the cotyledon tissue by piercing with a fine syringe needle. Light emission is shown by the white pixels superimposed on the black silhouette of the seedling. H indicates the position of the hypocotyl. This response has been imaged using h-coelenterazine. (A) 0 s after wounding. (B) 30 s. (C) 60 s. (D) 90 s. Each image is an integration of photon counts made over a 25-s period. Scale bar represents 500 μm.

A. Luminometry

A luminometer is a simpler and by far the cheaper of the two options. The device can be designed to hold whole plants within a sample cuvette (Knight *et al.,* 1991b). Luminometry experiments provide information on the changes in total luminescence (and therefore $[Ca^{2+}]_i$) from the whole plant but no spatial information. Imaging is required to produce this type of data and involves more complex and expensive equipment.

There are a number of commercially available luminometers but purpose-built models allow greater flexibility, for instance, in the design of the sample chamber.

The basis of a luminometer is a light-tight sample housing containing a sample cuvette adjacent to a PMT connected to a signal processor and to an output device, which can be a chart recorder or a computer. The PMT is a photosensitive device that generates electrons in response to photons striking a photocathode. The electrons leave the cathode and cross a vacuum in the tube in which they are focused and amplified a number of times before striking the anode at the opposite end of the PMT. A PMT can be described as, for instance, 11-stage, and this refers to the number of electron amplification stages.

Measurement of aequorin luminescence requires a PMT with a low "dark current" or "thermal noise" (the background signal registered by the detector even in the absence of a luminous sample); choose one with a dark current of <0.1 nA for an 11-stage PMT or <1 nA for a 13-stage device (Campbell, 1988). The signal : noise ratio refers to the balance between the photon counts attributable to the luminescent sample and those produced as background noise by the PMT, and the tube should have the highest signal : noise ratio obtainable. The signal : noise ratio can be improved by cooling the tube. All photomultiplier tubes are more sensitive in the blue regions of the spectrum than in the red, and bialkali PMTs provide better sensitivity to blue light than do tri-alkali tubes, making them the best choice for aequorin work. (The peak of aequorin light emission is at a wavelength of 468 nm.)

A discriminator is used to select light pulses of above a certain energy level for subsequent amplification and thereby avoids, as far as is possible, the amplification and registration of background noise. The discriminator level can be set by the experimenter when the level of background noise has been determined.

The electrical signal produced by the PMT is amplified by sending it to a signal processor. The signal may be analogue or digital and at high light fluxes each are equally favorable. However, at low light levels, such as those frequently encountered in recombinant aequorin luminometry, digital luminometers are slightly more sensitive (and therefore preferable) due to their more stable instrument noise and better signal : noise ratio (Campbell, 1988).

The following are some considerations to bear in mind when choosing or designing a luminometer. First, the experiment may require temperature regulation within the cuvette and this can be brought about by using a peltier cooler and heater thermostat or by having the sample housing in a jacket connected to a regulated bath. Second, the luminometer should also have some means of introducing solutions to the cuvette during experiments, and this can be achieved using a syringe held in the sample housing and capable of injecting into the sample cuvette. Before interpretation of data, consider the time it may take for the injected solution to mix thoroughly in the cuvette. Although magnetic stirrers speed up mixing, their use should be avoided, as they generate electrical noise in the photon detector (Campbell, 1988). Third, it is important to avoid the use of materials such as paints, silicon grease, silica gel, and certain glass or plastic tubes, which luminesce themselves, in the system. Fourth, as the levels of aequorin luminescence are low, it is necessary to maximize the proportion of emitted light that actually reaches the detector. This means that the distance between the sample and the detector should be as short as possible; the sample cuvette being adjacent to the PMT. Mirrors, white paint, or silvering inside the sample housing may help reflect the light from the sample out of the sample chamber and onto the detector (Campbell, 1988).

1. Materials

The luminometer configuration that we favor is a 2-inch EMI 9235B photomultiplier tube (with dark current of 0.06 nA) contained within an EMI cooled photomultiplier housing. Connected to this is the electronic control unit (Nashcourt Ltd., Cardiff, Wales, UK), which comprises a variable EHT supply of 500–1500 V at 1 mA, an 8-digit counter/display with a maximum counting rate of 80 MHz, microprocessor-based multirange delay and integration timer, an adjustable amplifier/discriminator mounted on the photomultiplier housing, multirange analogue meter with a chart recorder output, electrical contact for initiating automatic injectors, etc., and a port providing data for input to an external computer. We use a purpose-built brass sample tube housing to hold luminometer cuvettes in front of the PMT, which has a temperature controller (all from Nashcourt Ltd.). This housing has a port at the top for any additions required to the cuvette. Cuvettes are 12-mm-diameter Röhren tubes (Sarstedt). Additionally a chart recorder and/or personal computer is required to collect and process output.

2. Methods

1. To estimate the amount of reconstitution *in vitro* add 10 μl of the reconstitution reaction described in Section III,B to 500 μl of 200 m*M* Tris–HCl, 0.5 m*M* EDTA, pH 7, in a luminometer cuvette.

2. Load cuvette into sample housing and turn dial to bring tube in line with PMT.

3. Take up 500 μl of 50 m*M* calcium chloride into a 1-ml syringe and insert needle into port at top of sample housing. Prior to insertion, ensure that the needle is wiped clean to prevent premature discharge of aequorin.

4. Ensure that chart recorder and/or computer are active and the range of sensitivity is appropriate for the luminescence counts expected.

5. Take a 10-s reading prior to addition of calcium chloride as background.

6. Activate counter (and hence chart recorder and/or computer) *just before* injecting calcium chloride. Subtract background counts from total.

7. To estimate the amount of reconstitution *in vivo* homogenize 1–5 mg (fresh weight) of plant tissue treated with coelenterazine (Section III,A) in 500 μl of 200 m*M* Tris–HCl, 0.5 m*M* EDTA, pH 7, and then measure luminescence counts as described above.

8. Once *in vivo* reconstitution has been demonstrated, whole seedlings (7–12 days old) can be loaded in front of the PMT and $[Ca^{2+}]_i$ changes measured in response to different stimuli.

B. Low-Level Light Imaging

Low-level light imaging cameras can be purchased separately and built into an imaging system, but there are now a growing number of "off-the-shelf" complete imaging systems (see Stanley, 1992). The image is sent from the camera to a computer loaded with software for processing and analysis. Copies of the stored image can be printed using a color video copy processor.

Most imaging systems are based around the charge-coupled device (CCD). CCDs are made up of an array of light sensors in which each acts as an individual light detector (Aikens, 1990). Incoming photons break bonds between the silicon atoms in the semiconductors, and generate electron hole pairs. The conversion of photon to electron is a linear process, allowing the measurement of light to be quantifiable. The electrons produced in this way are collected in a potential well, each well corresponding to a pixel on the screen of the imaging device. Exposure to light during imaging causes the CCD to acquire a pattern of electronic charge in the wells. This pattern of information is transmitted through a parallel register (of the same layout as the array) onto a serial register that transmits the information row by row to the output circuit. An image is then reconstructed by the computer. "Blooming" occurs when there is too much charge for one well to hold (i.e., too much light has been allowed to enter the imaging device) and charge spills over to the adjacent wells.

All imaging devices are subject to noise. There are several components to this noise; some are random and can be eliminated by signal processing, others arise due to the quantum nature of light and cannot be avoided. Dark current (thermal noise) arises due to thermal agitation in the silicon lattice producing electrons. This occurs at room temperature and can be reduced by cooling the camera.

The two types of CCD cameras available can be classified by the method employed to improve the sensitivity of the camera. They are the cooled CCD and the image-intensified CCD. In the cooled CCD, sensitivity is increased by reducing the background noise by cooling the camera, allowing lower levels of light to be detected. The coolants may be water, forced air, or others. Improvement of the signal : noise ratio is thus achieved by lowering the noise component. The disadvantage of this kind of camera is that a slow scan speed is needed and therefore rapid changes in light emission (typical of plant calcium responses) cannot be recorded. In the image-intensified CCD, the signal from the light sensors is intensified (using microchannel plates or a phosphor–cathode sandwich) before detection and so the signal : noise ratio is improved by increasing the strength of the signal. This is a more sensitive device than the cooled CCD at the low levels of light expected from this type of experiment. We have used a Hamamatsue intensified CCD camera for our imaging work and we describe its use below.

1. Materials

Nikon Diaphot inverted microscope, ×4 and ×10 plan-apo objectives, Hamamatsu intensified CCD camera Model C2400-20 and Argus-50 image processor (Hamamatsu Photonics (UK) Ltd., Enfield.), IBM-compatible PC with 80486 processor and 16 Mb RAM (Compaq), silicon grease, microscope coverslips.

2. Methods

1. Fix a *N. plumbaginifolia* transgenic seedling (Section II,B,2) treated with coelenterazine (Section III,B) to a coverslip with silicon grease.
2. View under microscope and bring into focus. With the gain of the Argus-50 controller turned down to minimum, obtain a bright field image for later superimposition with luminescence image.
3. Block out all light to the sample and turn the discriminator setting down to 100. Just prior to recording images set the Argus-50 controller gain to maximum (10).
4. Set integration times for collection of data and initiate data collection sequence.
5. Use the Argus-50 image analysis software to superimpose luminescence images on bright field image thereby obtaining spatial information on the luminescence response. This software can also be used to calculate absolute photon counts and their distribution for a given image.

3. The Cold-Shock Control

The cold-shock response occurs when plant tissues come into contact with water at a temperature of 0–5°C, producing an immediate and large increase in $[Ca^{2+}]_i$. By demonstrating this response, the worker can be sure that functional aequorin has been reconstituted in the plant cells and that the luminometer or imaging equipment is capable of measuring Ca^{2+}-induced changes in luminescence. This is effected by placing a small piece of ice next to the seedling on the microscope stage. When the ice melts, cold water reaches and stimulates the seedling. When using the luminometer, the cold-shock response can be caused by injecting ice-cold water into the luminometer cuvette containing the plant.

V. Perspectives

Modification of aequorin to change its properties can be effected by

1. Use of synthetically produced coelenterazine analogues which have altered properties e.g. altered sensitivity to calcium.

2. Modification of the apoaequorin by protein engineering (Shimomura and Shimomura 1985), e.g., color of emitted light (Ohmiya *et al.*, 1992).

A. Semisynthetic Aequorins

Semisynthetic aequorins are molecules made up of natural apoaequorin coupled with a chemically synthesized analogue of coelenterazine (Shimomura *et al.*, 1988). Of the 40 semisynthetic aequorins that have been described, there is a very wide range of sensitivities to Ca^{2+} ranging from ca. 0.01 to 200 times that of natural aequorin (Shimomura, 1991). It should be noted, however, that semisynthetic aequorins have significantly lower stability and a marked reduction in half-life compared with natural aequorins; therefore measurement of luminescence must be carried out within a few hours of reconstitution. Semisynthetic aequorins may be reconstituted *in vitro,* for subsequent loading by traditional methods (Lliñas *et al.*, 1992) but can also be reconstituted in whole plants combining chemical analogues of coelenterazine with the recombinant apoaequorin expressed in the plant tissues, (M. R. Knight *et al.*, 1993).

Semisynthetic aequorins can be used to measure Ca^{2+} levels over a wider range than normal cytoplasmic Ca^{2+} concentrations. For instance, *n*-aequorin with a low sensitivity to calcium has been used in neuron cells to report very high Ca^{2+} levels (Lliñas *et al.*, 1992), whereas *h*-aequorin, which is very sensitive to calcium, has been used to demonstrate very small changes in $[Ca^{2+}]_i$ that occur during the wounding response in plants (M. R. Knight *et al.*, 1993).

Fast response aequorins are among the semisynthetics available and these may have a luminescence half-rise period of less than 3 ms, compared with 12 ms for natural aequorin. These can be used in studying very rapid changes in $[Ca^{2+}]_i$ provided that an equally responsive light measuring device is used, but are probably not usually necessary for the study of plant calcium responses.

A variant of coelenterazine known as *e*-type coelenterazine confers on aequorin a bimodal emission peak. Light emission can be measured at 2 wavelengths (approx. 405 and 465 nm) and the ratio of the amounts of light is directly proportional to the calcium concentration but independent of the concentration of aequorin in the tissues, making this method the most reliable way of quantifying calcium concentrations measured by aequorin bioluminescence (Shimomura *et al.*, 1988).

B. Engineered Aequorins

Ten different isoforms of apoaequorin exist naturally and their sensitivities to calcium vary such that the most sensitive is about 10 times more sensitive than the least (Shimomura, 1991). Other modifications in the protein structure can affect the calcium-binding properties of aequorin. Aequorin has three cysteine residues that appear to have a role in the bioluminescence reaction, either in a catalytic function or in the regeneration of active aequorin. Replacing these residues causes a reduction in the amount of luminescence produced by the protein, except when all three are replaced by serine, in which case luminescence increases (Kurose *et al.*, 1989). Single amino acid substitutions in the EF hand regions of apoaequorin produce a protein with a reduced affinity for calcium (Kendall *et al.*, 1992). This type of aequorin can be used for making measurements in cellular locations where Ca^{2+} levels are expected to be orders of magnitude higher than in the cytosol, e.g., the mitochondria, and provides an alternative to the use of *n*-aequorin, with the advantage of avoiding the use of the less stable *n*-coelenterazine.

Engineered aequorins can now be produced with different emission spectra (Ohmiya *et al.*, 1992) and these aequorins that emit different colors of light may be of use in future developments (see below).

C. Conclusions and Future Developments

A major improvement in the recombinant aequorin method of calcium measurement in plants is that the response can now be quantified using the dual wavelength coelenterazines (M. R. Knight *et al.*, 1993). The future of the method will involve refinement of the technique to localize calcium signaling to a subcellular level. This will be achieved by targeting expression of apoaequorin to organelles and subcellular locations using known target sequences or by producing gene constructs that are expressed as apoaequorin attached to a cellular protein normally present at a particular location in the plant cell.

If apoaequorin is to be expressed as a fusion protein it is necessary to be aware of the features of the protein essential for maintaining its activity as a calcium reporter. The C-terminal proline residue of apoaequorin is essential for the long-term stability of reconstituted aequorin (Watkins and Campbell, 1993). Even if this amino acid is present but linked to the N-terminal amino acid of another protein, the resulting fusion protein is likely to be very unstable. Therefore, all fusion proteins must be designed to have apoaequorin as the C-terminal part of the protein and the other polypeptide as the N-terminal part of the protein. Activity comparable to that of normal aequorin has been observed in fusion with even large proteins in this orientation (Casadei *et al.*, 1990). Aequorin has been targeted in this way to the mitochondria and chloroplasts (M. R. Knight, A. K. Campbell, and A. J. Trewavas, unpublished results) and work is under way to target aequorin to the nucleus and the endoplasmic reticulum. By targeting engineered aequorins with different emission spectra to different parts of the cell, it may one day be possible to image calcium in two or more subcellular domains simultaneously by dual- or multi-wavelength imaging.

References

Aikens, R. S. (1990). CCD Cameras for video microscopy. *In* "Optical Microscopy for Biology" (B. Herman and K. Jacobson, eds.), pp. 207–218. New York: Wiley-Liss, Inc.

Allen, D. G., and Blinks, J. R. (1978). Calcium transients in aequorin-injected frog cardiac muscle. *Nature* (*London*) **273,** 509–513.

An, G., Ebert, P. R., Mitra, A., and Ha, S. B. (1988). Binary vectors. *In* "Plant Molecular Biology Manual" (S. B. Gelvin and R. A. Schilperoort, eds.), pp. A3:1–19. Dordrecht, The Netherlands: Kluwer.

Blinks, J. R., Mattingly, P. H., Jewell, B. R., van Leeuven, M., Harrer, G. C., and Allen, D. G. (1978). Practical aspects of the use of aequorin as a calcium indicator: Assay, preparation, microinjection and interpretation of signals. *Methods Enzymol.* **57,** 292–328.

Callaham, D. A., and Hepler, P. K. (1991). Measurement of free calcium in plant cells. *In* "Cellular Calcium. A Practical Approach" (J. G. McCormack and P. H. Cobbold, eds.), pp 383–412. Oxford, England: Oxford Univ. Press.

Campbell, A. K. (1988). "Chemiluminescence Principles and Applications in Biology and Medicine." Chichester, England: Ellis Horwood Ltd.

Campbell, A. K., Patel, A. K., Razavi, Z. S., and McCapra, F. (1988). Formation of the Ca^{2+}-activated photoprotein from apo-obelin and mRNA inside human neutrophils. *Biochem. J.* **252,** 143–149.

Casadei, J., Powell, M. J., and Kenten, J. H. (1990). Expression and secretion of aequorin as a chimeric antibody by means of a mammalian expression vector. *Proc. Natl. Acad. Sci. U.S.A.* **87,** 2047–2051.

Cobbold, P. H., and Lee, J. A. C. (1991). Aequorin measurements of cytoplasmic free calcium. *In* "Cellular Calcium. A Practical Approach" (J. G. McCormack and P. H. Cobbold, eds.), pp. 54–81. Oxford, England: Oxford Univ. Press.

Cobbold, P. H., and Rink, T. J. (1987). Fluorescence and bioluminescence measurement of cytoplasmic free calcium. *Biochem. J.* **248,** 313–328.

Gilroy, S., Hughes, W. A., and Trewavas, A. J. (1989). A comparison between quin-2 and aequorin as indicators of cytoplasmic calcium levels in higher plant cell protoplasts. *Plant Physiol.* **90,** 482–491.

Kendall, J. M., Sala-Newby, Ghalaut, V., Dormer, R. L., and Campbell, A. K. (1992). *Biochem. Biophys. Res. Commun.* **187,** 1091–1097.

Knight, H., Trewavas, A. J., and Read, N. D. (1993). Confocal microscopy of living fungal hyphae microinjected with Ca^{2+}-sensitive fluorescent dyes. *Mycol. Res.* **97,** 1505–1515.

Knight, M. R., Campbell, A. K., Smith, S. M., and Trewavas, A. J. (1991a). Recombinant aequorin as a probe for cytosolic free Ca^{2+} in *Escherichia coli*. *FEBS Lett.* **282,** 405–408.

Knight, M. R., Campbell, A. K., Smith, S. M., and Trewavas, A. J. (1991b). Transgenic plant aequorin reports the effects of touch and cold-shock and elicitors on cytoplasmic calcium. *Nature* (*London*) **352,** 524–526.

Knight, M. R., Smith, S. M., and Trewavas, A. J. (1992). Wind-induced plant motion immediately increases cytosolic calcium. *Proc. Natl. Acad. Sci. U.S.A.* **89,** 4967–4971.

Knight, M. R., Read, N. D., Campbell, A. K., and Trewavas, A. J. (1993). Imaging calcium dynamics in living plants using semi-synthetic recombinant aequorins. *J. Cell Biol.* **121,** 83–90.

Kurose, K., Inouye, S., Sakaki, Y., and Tsuji, F. I. (1989). Bioluminescence of the Ca^{2+}-binding photoprotein aequorin after cysteine modification. *Proc. Natl. Acad. Sci. U.S.A.* **86,** 80–84.

Lliñas, R., Sugimori, M., and Silver R. B. (1992). Microdomains of high calcium concentration in a presynaptic terminal. *Science* (*Washington, DC*) **256,** 677–679.

Nakajima-Shimada, J., Iida, H., Tsuji, F. I., and Anraku, Y. (1991). Galactose-dependent expression of the recombinant Ca^{2+}-binding photoprotein aequorin in yeast. *Biochem. Biophys. Res. Commun.* **174,** 115–122.

Ohmiya, Y., Ohashi, M., and Tsuji, F. I. (1992). Two excited states in aequorin bioluminescence induced by tryptophan modification. *FEBS Lett.* **301,** 197–201.

Ridgway, E. B., and Ashley, C. C. (1967). Intracellular injection of the Ca^{2+}-sensitive bioluminescent protein aequorin into giant single muscle fibers of the corn barnacle *Balanus nubilis. Biochem. Biophys. Res. Commun.* **29,** 229–234.

Sheu, Y.-A., Kricka, L. J., and Pritchett, D. B. (1993). Measurement of intracellular calcium using bioluminescent aequorin expressed in human cells. *Anal. Biochem.* **209,** 343–347.

Shimomura, O. (1991). Preparation and handling of aequorin solutions for the measurement of cellular Ca^{2+}. *Cell Calcium* **12,** 635–643.

Shimomura and Shimomura (1985). Halistaurin, phialidin and modified forms of aequorin as Ca^{2+} indicators in biological systems. *Biochem. J.* **228,** 745–749.

Shimomura, O., Musicki, B., and Kishi, Y. (1988). Semi-synthetic aequorin. *Biochem. J.* **251,** 405–410.

Stanley, P. E. (1992). A survey of more than 90 commercially available luminometers and imaging devices for low-light measurements of chemiluminescence and bioluminescence, including instruments for manual, automatic and specialised operation, for HPLC, LC, GLC and microtitre plates. Part 1: Descriptions. *J. Biolumin. Chemilumin.* **7,** 77–108.

Watkins, N J., and Campbell, A. K. (1993). Requirement of the C-terminal proline residue for stability of the Ca^{2+}-activated photoprotein aequorin. *Biochem. J.* **293,** 181–185.

Williamson, R. E., and Ashley, C. C. (1982). Free Ca^{2+} and cytoplasmic streaming in the alga *Chara. Nature* (*London*) **296,** 647–650.

CHAPTER 15

Confocal Microscopy of the Shoot Apex

Mark P. Running, Steven E. Clark, and Elliot M. Meyerowitz
Division of Biology
California Institute of Technology
Pasadena, California 91125

I. Introduction

Recent advances in computer technology have led to the widespread use of increasingly sophisticated imaging techniques. One of the most significant of these techniques is confocal laser scanning microscopy (CLSM), a specialized type of fluorescence microscopy. In CLSM, a sample is treated with a fluorescent dye, and a laser beam is focused on a point in the sample, causing the emission

METHODS IN CELL BIOLOGY, VOL. 49

of fluorescent light. This light emitted from the illuminated point is focused on an aperture placed in front of a photodetector. Fluorescent light emanating from above or below the plane of focus falls outside the aperture itself and is largely eliminated, resulting in greatly increased contrast, as well as a small gain in resolution, compared to conventional fluorescent microscopic techniques. A two-dimensional image is obtained by scanning the exciting beam over the sample in raster fashion. The resulting image is an optical section through the sample, and is stored on a computer in digital form. To obtain three-dimensional images, accessory software assembles a series of images acquired at user-defined intervals along the z axis.

The use of CLSM in the study of plant development has many advantages over conventional histological techniques. Because CLSM data are stored digitally, the data can not only be reconstructed in three dimensions, but also animated or displayed as stereo images, to aid in visual interpretation. Once the sample is reconstructed on a computer, virtual sections can be made from any orientation. Specimen preparation for CLSM is also much less labor intensive compared to serial sectioning, and avoids problems such as recovering and mounting individual sections, a time-consuming and error-prone task. The integrity of the sample is preserved in CLSM, allowing rescanning using different parameters.

Scanning electron microscopy (SEM) can also be used to examine whole-mounted samples, but in SEM only surface cells are visible. CLSM, on the other hand, allows the examination of the number and pattern of interior cells. CLSM also has great advantages over SEM in the study of tissues that are hidden from view or difficult to dissect, such as the late embryonic apical meristem, access to which is blocked by the cotyledons, or the early floral meristem, which is covered by the sepals.

Here we describe our method of examining plant tissue using CLSM, particularly in studies of the structure, cell number, and cell pattern of shoot apical meristems and floral meristems. The development of this technique is particularly timely due to the recent explosion of interest in developmental mutants that affect apical and floral meristem structure (Leyser and Furner, 1992; Medford *et al.*, 1992; Sung *et al.*, 1992; Clark *et al.*, 1993, Tsukaya *et al.*, 1993). We developed the technique for use with *Arabidopsis thaliana,* which, owing to its small size, is particularly amenable to whole-mount preparation and study. Still, the methods outlined here should be generally applicable to the study of other plant species.

II. Materials

A. Chemicals (available from Sigma except where noted)

1. Formalin (formaldehyde solution)
2. Propionic acid
3. High grade 100% ethanol

4. Xylene
5. Propidium iodide (store at 4°C)
6. L-Arginine (free base)
7. Immersion Oil type A (Fisher Catalog No. 12368A)
8. Fingernail polish (from any drug store)
9. Acetone

B. Equipment

1. Vacuum desiccator (VWR Catalog No. 24987-004)
2. Glass scintillation vials (VWR Catalog No. 66021-553) or similar container
3. Fine forceps (Biomedical Research Instruments Catalog No. 10-1425)
4. Standard microscope slides and coverslips
5. Depression slides (VWR Catalog No. 48324-001)
6. High-powered dissecting scope (80× magnification is suitable)

C. Instrumentation

1. Confocal laser scanning microscope with helium/neon and/or argon laser and corresponding filter set.
2. High-capacity storage device (e.g., Magneto optical drive)
3. Image manipulation software (e.g., VoxelView)

III. Methods

A. Overview

We have developed a technique that allows staining of plant tissue with the nuclear stain propidium iodide (PI). PI has several advantages as a fluorescent marker: it is excitable in the visible range (whereas the use of UV-excitable dyes, such as DAPI, requires expensive quartz optics), it is quite resistant to bleaching, and it binds fairly specifically to DNA. Its use in animal tissue is quite common, and the staining procedure in animals is for the most part straightforward. Plant tissue is more difficult to stain, possibly because the cuticle and cell wall present a barrier to staining, and because most of the plant tissues that we wish to examine are thicker than most animal tissues studied. We obtain the best results by staining the tissue for a lengthy period in low concentrations of PI, followed by a series of washing steps to eliminate nonspecific staining. In most cases fixing the tissue before staining gives us the best results. After staining and rinsing, treatment in xylene is required to clear the plant tissue.

B. Fixing

Fixation is usually necessary for maintaining the integrity of the tissue during the subsequent staining, rinsing, and dissection steps. Underfixed tissue tends to fall apart if kept in aqueous solution too long, and is harder to manipulate during dissection and mounting. On the other hand, we have found that overfixing, by using glutaraldehyde, or using formaldehyde under strong conditions, hinders staining. We also add a fairly high concentration of ethanol in the fixative solution in order to eliminate chlorophyll, which may absorb the fluorescent light emitted by PI, and which is itself highly autofluorescent. Applying a vacuum, as is traditional in the fixation of plant tissue, allows full and rapid penetration of the fixative. The fixing solution we use is a variation of the classical acid fixing mixture containing formaldehyde, acetic acid (in this case substituted with propionic acid), and ethanol (Sass, 1958).

1. Prepare fixation solution (make up fresh for each use):

Formalin (37% formaldehyde solution)	10% by volume
Propionic acid	5%
100% ethanol	70%
Distilled Water	15%

2. Put 10–15 ml of fixing solution into each glass scintillation vial or similar container.

3. Clip off desired plant tissue and immediately place into fixing solution. Do not put too much tissue into each vial; tissue should not be tightly packed, and all pieces should be submerged.

4. Place vials into vacuum desiccator. Using an aspirator, apply full vacuum, then release slowly; 15 min under vacuum is ideal.

5. Remove vials and stir to make tissue sink. If tissue does not sink, reapply vacuum until it does.

6. Fix for 4 h to overnight (overnight is recommended), at room temperature.

7. Pour off fixing solution. During all pouring steps, we use a fine mesh screen to keep the samples in the vial. Replace with 70% ethanol.

8. Bring the sample through an ethanol series (85, 95, 100%), with about 30 min or more between ethanol changes. (Small changes in ethanol concentration are necessary to prevent tissue damage.) Leave overnight in a tightly capped vial in 100% ethanol, to remove the remaining chlorophyll and complete the fixation process. If pressed for time, a few hours in 100% ethanol should be adequate to remove chlorophyll from most tissues. Thicker tissue samples may require more time for complete chlorophyll elimination.

C. Staining

It is difficult to get adequate and uniform penetration of PI in whole plant tissue. Staining for a long period of time allows full penetration, whereas using a low concentration reduces nonspecific staining.

1. Bring the sample through a decreasing ethanol series (95, 85, 70, 50, 30, 15) to distilled water, 30 min or more for each change.

2. Make a stock solution of propidium iodide. A convenient stock solution is 100 μg/ml in 0.1 *M* L-arginine free base, with the pH adjusted to 12.4 by the addition of 5 *M* sodium hydroxide. Keep the stock solution refrigerated, wrapped in aluminum foil. This stock lasts about 4–6 months at 4°C. The solution is no longer usable when it turns a dull, dark orange color.

3. Stain in 5 μg/ml PI in a solution of 0.1 *M* L-arginine, pH 12.4. The volume of staining solution used is critical; use increasing volumes for more tissue. For Arabidopsis apices, add about 500 μl staining solution per apex in the vial.

4. Leave in stain at 4°C out of direct light for at least 1 day. For Arabidopsis apices, 4 days works well, as long as the tissue has been fixed overnight. Larger samples may require longer staining times. After the staining procedure, the tissue may appear slightly orange.

D. Rinsing

For best viewing of the nuclei, a rinsing step is necessary to remove background staining. If the tissue is not rinsed well, the nuclei will be more difficult to differentiate from the cytoplasm under the confocal microscope.

1. Rinse with 0.1 *M* L-arginine buffer, with the pH adjusted to 8 with HCl.

2. Leave in arginine buffer at 4°C for 4 days without agitation, changing the rinsing solution once every day.

E. Clearing

One of the most critical steps in the procedure is the clearing of the sample, that is, changing the refractive index of the sample to match that of glass, approximately 1.5. This gives the sample a clear, glassy appearance, allowing good penetration of the confocal laser and the excitation of PI.

There are many solvents that have been used for clearing biological tissue. The one that we have found to be most advantageous is xylene. Xylene penetrates and clears the sample reasonably rapidly, without destroying the tissue. In fact, the tissue can be stored in xylene indefinitely, since PI is not soluble in xylene. Xylene is also inexpensive and readily available. Tissue cleared in xylene becomes hardened, simplifying certain dissection procedures, especially the removal of leaves and flowers from the apex. One disadvantage is its high toxicity, so, as with most organic solvents, care should be taken in its handling (use of a fume hood, proper disposal of waste). Another disadvantage is that it forms a white emulsion in the presence of water, so the tissue must be completely dehydrated before xylene is added.

1. Bring the sample through an ethanol series (15, 30, 50, 70, 85, 95, 100, 100, 100), 30 min or more per change. The last two 100% ethanol changes should be

made with either a fresh bottle of high-quality ethanol (e.g., Gold Seal) or 100% bulk ethanol that has been treated with molecular sieves (Sigma M-6141), in order to completely dehydrate the sample.

2. Bring the sample through a xylene series (75:25 ethanol:xylene, 50:50, 25:75) to 100% xylene, with at least 2 h between changes. Shorter changes result in incomplete clearing. Change the 100% xylene solution three times (2 h between changes), and leave the tissue overnight in the last change. Leaving the tissue longer than 2 h in any of the xylene series solutions does not harm the sample.

F. Dissection

For viewing the shoot apex or young flowers, some dissection is necessary in order to remove the larger primordia. Dissecting in xylene is inconvenient because of its toxicity and its low vapor pressure, so we dissect in immersion oil, which we also use as the mounting medium. Xylene is completely miscible with immersion oil. In order to remove all the xylene, we transfer the sample through several drops of immersion oil.

1. Place a series of 4 individual drops of immersion oil on a clear standard microscope slide. The first drop should be large enough to contain the entire sample.

2. Using fine forceps, place the tissue sample in the first drop, and begin dissection under a dissecting scope. In the case of the shoot apex, hold the stem with one forceps, and break off the older flowers by pushing them toward the base of the stem. Because the sample is dissected in solution, direct overhead lighting, which results in glare, is unsuitable. One solution is to use strong indirect lighting, such as fiber optic light sources.

3. Dissect until the first drop of oil becomes too cluttered, then transfer the apex to the next drop of immersion oil for further dissection, increasing the magnification if necessary.

4. Continue dissection and transferring to a new drop of immersion oil until dissection is complete and the sample is in the final drop of immersion oil. For the study of the shoot apex, most of the visible floral primordia should be removed. This requires a magnification of 80× or more to be accomplished easily.

G. Mounting

With well-cleared samples, the working distance of the lens is the limiting factor in determining the depth at which the sample can be sectioned. Therefore, it is important to mount most samples in such a way that the area of interest is close to the coverslip surface. This is facilitated if the size of the sample is minimized after dissection. In the case of the shoot apex, we cut off as much of the stem as possible. The sample is secured to the coverslip by the surface tension of the immersion oil.

1. After removing as much tissue as possible from the sample, transfer the sample onto the center of a clean coverslip, using fine forceps. In many cases multiple samples can be placed on the same coverslip.
2. Add a small amount of immersion oil to the sample. This can be accomplished by dipping the forceps in a drop of oil, and transferring some to the sample. There should be enough immersion oil so that no part of the sample is dry, but there should not be so much that the sample is not secure in place.
3. For thick samples, adjust the position of the sample such that the area of interest is close to the surface of the coverslip. Shoot apices should be abutting the coverslip surface.
4. Turn over the coverslip, and place the coverslip on the slide. For flat samples, such as mature leaves, sepals, or petals, one can use conventional microscope slides, but for thick samples, such as the shoot apex, depression slides are more useful. In this case place the coverslip over the depression, with the sample attached to and below the coverslip but not touching the slide. Also, none of the immersion oil should touch the slide.
5. Seal the coverslip with nail polish. Other sealing methods can be used, but nail polish is easily removed with acetone, which allows the removal and reorientation of samples, and the reuse of depression slides.

H. Viewing the Sample

Propidium iodide has a maximum absorption near 520 nm. Fluorescence can thus be excited by either a helium/neon laser, which emits at 543 nm, or an argon laser emitting at 514 nm. We use the argon laser, since in our instrument it is more powerful. In most cases the laser can be attenuated to 10% of full power, thus reducing the bleaching of the dye. The emission maximum of PI is at 610 nm, so we use a long pass barrier filter allowing passage of light at wavelengths greater than 590 nm. The lens we use for viewing is a Zeiss Neofluar 40× oil immersion lens with a numerical aperture of 1.30.

Most confocal microscopes are equipped with a computer-controlled z motor, which can be used to control the number of optical sections and the distance between sections. An image can be obtained at each focal plane, and each image can be stored on whatever storage device the computer uses. Image quality can be enhanced by averaging a defined number of images in a line or a frame; in this way background is greatly reduced.

I. Image Analysis

Once the images are obtained, several options are available for manipulating and viewing them. Some confocal microscopes have built-in image processing software; in addition, the images can also be transferred to other computers, such as those specialized in handling three-dimensional graphics processing. With a suitable combination of software and hardware, a series of images can be rendered in three dimensions, rotated in any direction, and adjusted and enhanced. Individual images can be transferred to high-end personal computers equipped with professional image manipulation software, such as Adobe Photoshop, for brightness and contrast adjustment, image enhancement, cropping, and intensity coloring. Hard copies of the images can be obtained by taking a picture directly off the confocal screen, by printing using high-resolution printers, or by using slide-making machines.

J. A Special Case—The Mature Embryo Shoot Apex

The above protocol is general and should work for most plant tissues with adjustments in dissection methods. One special case worth noting is the mature embryo or seed stage. This stage is useful in studies of mutants, such as *emf* (Sung *et al.*, 1992), that affect the shoot apex very early. The advantage of looking at the mature embryo stage, as opposed to later or earlier stages, is that a large number of samples at the same stage can be studied, making comparisons easier. In order to stain and clear the tissue, however, the seed coat must be removed.

1. Imbibe the seeds in a petri dish on Whatman No. 3 filter paper in 15% ethanol at 4°C for several hours to overnight. The ethanol and cold temperature serve to prevent growth of the seeds during imbibition and subsequent steps.

2. Pick up the seeds, along with some filter paper fibers (see below), with forceps and transfer them to a scintillation vial containing 15% ethanol.

3. Using a micropipet, transfer some seeds to a standard microscope slide.

4. Under the dissecting scope, hold the seed with one forceps, and gently scrape off part of the seed coat with the other. Then gently squeeze the first forceps and pop out the embryo. This is difficult at first, and requires some practice. One technique is to grab the seed while it is associated with some filter paper fibers, so that it will be easier to handle. If the microscope slide dries, add more 15% ethanol.

5. Once the seed coat is removed, use the pipet to place the embryo in a new vial.

6. Stain, rinse, and clear the sample as normal. Fixing is not necessary.

7. No further dissection is necessary. For mounting, transfer the cleared embryos (using a micropipet) onto a standard microscope slides with a drop of immersion oil on it. Using forceps, transfer the embryos through several additional drops of immersion oil to remove the xylene. Mount the embryo on a coverslip and place on a depression slide, as above. The embryo should be placed on its side, with the root and both cotyledons resting against the coverslip. In this orientation the embryonic shoot apical meristem is easily visualized under the confocal microscope.

IV. Results and Discussion

Confocal microscopy has several advantages in the study of plant structure and development, especially in allowing the rapid analysis of a large number of samples, and the ability to analyze directly data via computers. One example of its use is in the study of wild-type and mutant shoot apex structure in Arabidopsis.

In the wild-type shoot apex (Fig. 1A), the central zone and the peripheral zones, which have been defined histologically by differential cytoplasmic and nuclear staining of plastic sections in certain plant species (Steeves and Sussex, 1989), are not readily distinguished, although the areas of more rapidly dividing cells, such as in the epidermal layer, show up clearly as being more intensely stained, and in some cases many mitoses are seen.

By taking a series of optical sections throughout the entire apex, it is possible to determine cell number in the apical meristem. The issue of cell number is complicated, however, by the question of whether a cell is part of the apical meristem, or whether it should be considered part of the nascent lateral primordium. The positional definition (Medford, 1992) holds that the shoot apical meristem includes all the cells distal and centric to the last formed primordium. This definition is problematic in that it excludes cells that may be meristematic but fall below the emerging primordia without contributing cells to that primordium. It is especially true for the apical meristem of the mature embryo (seed) stage (Fig. 2A), where the apical dome is relatively flat, and few of the cells in the meristem are above the cotyledons. We prefer a definition of the shoot apical meristem as the area containing mitotically active cells that have not been incorporated into lateral primordium. The determination of whether a cell is part of a newly emerging primordia or the shoot apical meristem may be facilitated by examining 3D reconstructions of confocal images; making such an assignment with serial sections alone is more difficult. Cells of the apical meristem are smaller and more densely stained, which is most clearly seen in the mature embryo (Fig. 2A). Irish and Sussex (1992) also used these criteria for determining which cells of the mature embryo are part of the shoot apical meristem.

The effect of meristem mutants on apical meristem cell pattern can also be rapidly assessed using confocal microscopy. The *clavata1-1* mutation (Leyser and Furner, 1992; Clark *et al.,* 1993) leads to disrupted phyllotaxy, enlargement of the apical dome (Fig. 1B), and sometimes fasciation (Fig. 1C). Confocal analysis shows that the overall L1, L2, and L3 cell layers are still intact in the mutant, even in the fasciated meristem, but that the lateral meristems emerge much lower on the apical dome. Using either the positional or the functional definition of the shoot apical meristem, the number of cells, and not the size of the cells, is increased in the mutants. In some samples the central zone and the peripheral zone can be identified based on differential staining, the peripheral zone staining more densely (Fig. 1B). In fasciated meristems, the meristem grows as a line instead of a point, and the apical dome is not apparent (Fig. 1C). Again, the

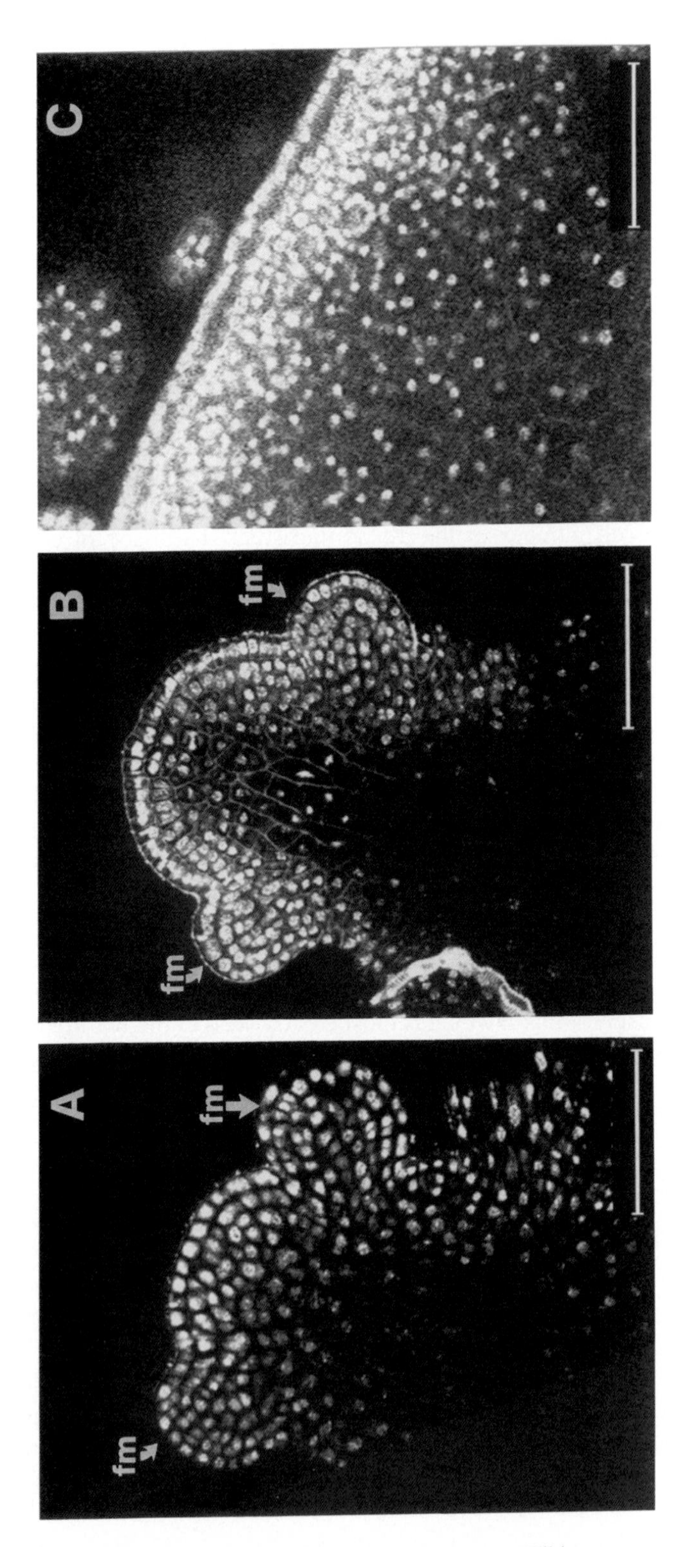

Fig. 1 Optical section through the center of the mature shoot apex. Wild-type, ecotype Landsberg erecta (A), and *clavata1-1* (B and C) shoot apexes are shown. The *clavata1-1* shoot apex in (B) is enlarged in height and width compared to wild type, and the *clavata1-1* shoot apex in (C) has become fasciated. fm, floral meristem. Bar, 50 μm.

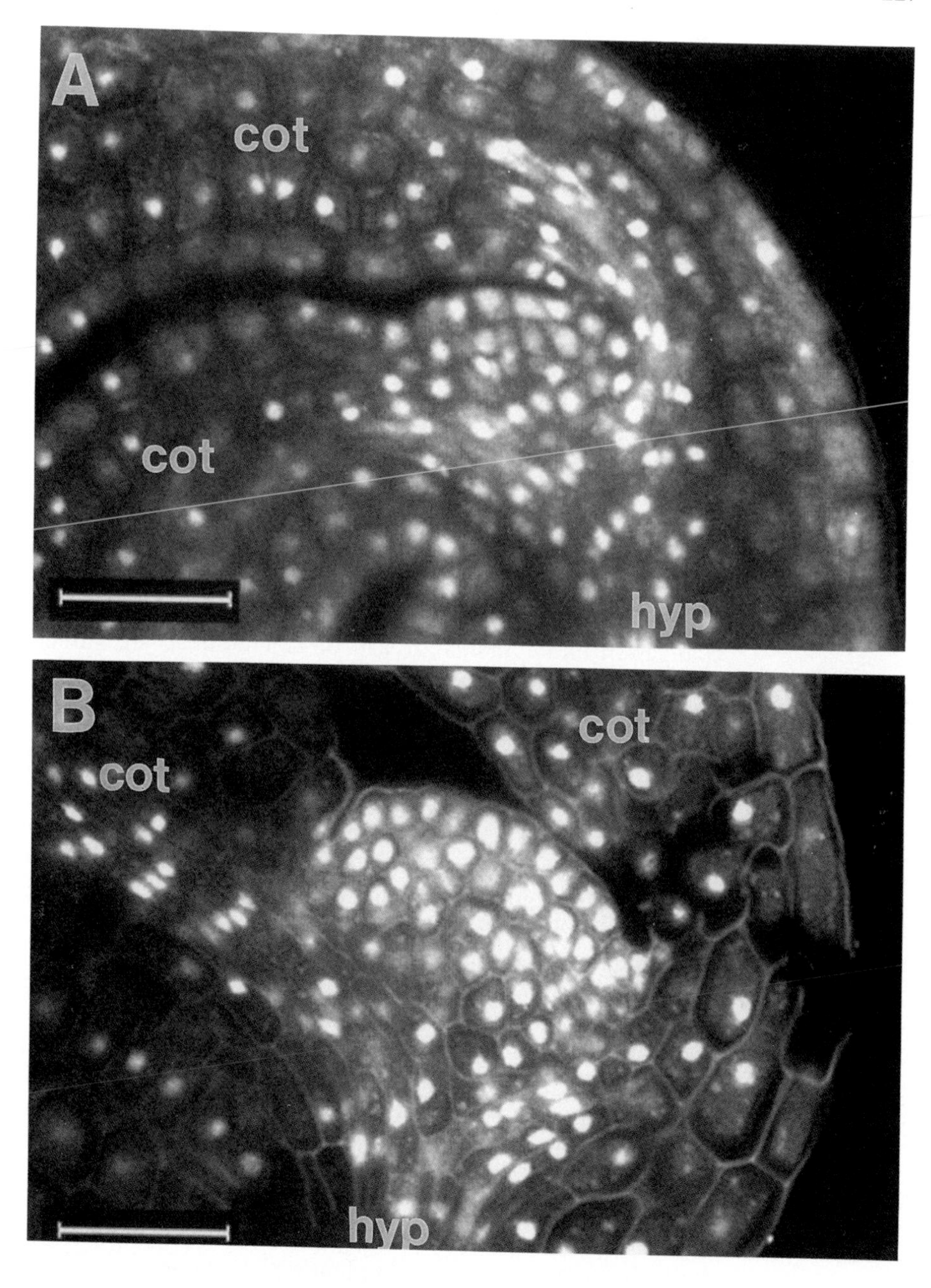

Fig. 2 Optical section through the mature embryo shoot apical meristem. Wild-type, ecotype Landsberg erecta (A) and *clavata1-4* (B) embryos are shown. The base of both cotyledons (cot) are visible, as is the top of the hypocotyl (hyp). Cells of the apical meristem are identified by their smaller size and more intense nuclear staining. Even at this stage, the apical meristem of *clavata1* mutants is much larger than wild type. Bar, 25 μm.

size increase of the apical meristem is in the number, and not the size, of cells. Lateral meristems emerge on either side of the fasciated meristem.

Defects in *clavata1* mutant plants can be traced back to the mature embryo stage (Fig. 2B). Examination of the shoot apex reveals a larger number of cells in the *clavata1-4* embryo shoot apex, and that the meristem is taller and deeper than wild-type. Again, confocal microscopy is very useful here, because the size change in the shoot apical meristem of *clavata1-4* mature embryos is subtle when looking at a two-dimensional section and could be missed if comparing a small sample size.

V. Conclusions and Perspectives

The use of confocal microscopy should allow more rapid comparative studies of mutants affecting cell patterns, as well as interspecies comparisons. The results obtainable by CLSM will be useful for reexamining several issues in plant development. For example, from the study of *clavata1,* we can infer some aspects about how phyllotaxy is determined. Increasing both the size of the meristem and the number of cells in the meristem disrupts phyllotaxy, even though the overall structure (cell size and cell layering) does not change, suggesting that changes in either meristem size or cell number are sufficient to disrupt the pattern of lateral shoot initiation. The study of other mutants disrupting meristem structure using confocal analysis may lead to further insights into the factors important for proper phyllotaxy. CLSM will also be useful for looking at closely related species, which may vary in shoot apical meristem size, cell number, or both, while conserving phyllotaxy.

Confocal microscopy has the tremendous advantage of allowing the visualization of every cell in its three-dimensional orientation with respect to the surrounding tissue. This aids in the visualization of three-dimensional cell patterns that may not be easy to notice in serial sections. It will also be useful in the analysis of mutants that disrupt normal cell patterning, such as *tso,* which causes abnormal organization in floral meristem cell layers (Z. Liu, M.P.R., and E.M.M., unpublished).

With continuing advances in image analysis software, it will soon be possible to gain even more information from confocal microscopic data. For instance, the computer will be able to determine the number of nuclei, and thus the number of cells, in a given structure, and compare it to mutants that may affect the development of various pattern elements in the plant. It will also help in determining nuclear DNA content in intact tissues, and give clues into cell division patterns in three dimensions. These advances will help answer some of the long-standing questions in plant development.

Acknowledgments

We thank C. Chang, S. Jacobsen, Z. Liu, J.-L. Riechmann, H. Sakai, L. Sieberth, and B. Williams for review of the manuscript, and A. Readhead for help with tissue preparation. We especially thank

Dr. Jean-Paul Revel for advice and help with using the CLSM instrument, advice and suggestions for sample preparation, and review of the manuscript. This work was supported by U.S. National Science Foundation (NSF) Grant MCB-9204839 to E.M.M. M.P.R. was a Howard Hughes Predoctoral Fellow, and S.E.C. was supported by an NSF Postdoctoral Fellowship in Plant Biology.

References

Clark, S. E., Running, M. P., and Meyerowitz, E. M. (1993). CLAVATA1, a regulator of meristem and flower development in *Arabidopsis. Development* **119,** 397–418.

Irish, V. F., and Sussex, I. M. (1992). A fate map of the *Arabidopsis* embryonic shoot apical meristem. *Development* **115,** 745–753.

Leyser, H. M. O., and Furner, I. J. (1992). Characterization of 3 shoot apical meristem mutants of *Arabidopsis thaliana. Development* **116,** 397–403.

Medford, J. I. (1992). Vegetative apical meristems. *Plant Cell* **4,** 1029–1039.

Medford, J. I., Behringer, F. J., Callos, J. D., and Feldmann, K. A. (1992). Normal and abnormal development in the *Arabidopsis* vegetative shoot apex. *Plant Cell* **4,** 631–643.

Sass, J. E. (1958). "Botanical Microtechnique." The Iowa State College Press, Ames, Iowa.

Steeves, T. A., and Sussex, I. M. (1989). "Patterns in Plant Development." Cambridge: Cambridge Univ. Press.

Sung, Z. R., Belachew, A., Shunong, B., and Bertrand-Garcia, R. (1992). EMF, an *Arabidopsis* gene required for vegetative shoot development. *Science* **258,** 1645–1647.

Tsukaya, H., Naito, S., Rédei, G. P., and Komeda, Y. (1992). A new class of mutations in *Arabidopsis thaliana, acaulis1,* affecting the development of both inflorescences and leaves. *Development* **118,** 751–764.

CHAPTER 16

Measurements of Wall Stress Relaxation in Growing Plant Cells

Daniel J. Cosgrove
Department of Biology
Pennsylvania State University
University Park, Pennsylvania 16802

I. Introduction

The wall of a typical growing plant cell is a thin polymeric network that possesses two crucial, but opposing, properties: the wall must have sufficient mechanical integrity to withstand the large tensile stresses generated by cell turgor, and at the same time it must maintain sufficient pliancy to permit the tension-bearing polymers to slip, shear, wiggle, or slide past one another to generate the surface area needed for cell enlargement. Physical considerations dictate that cells with rigid walls must regulate their growth (enlargement) by regulating the yielding properties of their walls. Yielding properties refer to the ability of the wall to expand irreversibly. Contrary to the common view, wall yielding is not simply due to wall viscoelasticity. Rather, wall yielding is a physical consequence of one or more biochemical processes that modify or rearrange the tension-bearing bonds between the polymers of the wall. This process has been described as a *chemorheological* one, because the flow properties (rheology) of the wall polymers depend on chemical processes in the wall. The direct result of wall yielding is that wall stress is reduced, and this creates the necessary reduction in cell turgor and water potential that enables the cell to take up water, thereby enlarging the cell volume and expanding the cell wall. This subject is treated in recent reviews (Tomos *et al.,* 1989; Cosgrove, 1993a,b).

Numerous methods have been used in attempts to measure the yielding properties of growing cell walls. Many of these methods suffer from the faulty assumption that wall yielding is simply the result of viscoelastic deformations in the wall. Cosgrove (1993a) has critically assessed the theory behind many of these methods and the interpretation of the resulting data. Although there is no ideal method for measuring wall yielding properties, *in vivo* stress relaxation is probably the best method at present for analysis of wall yielding properties because it can be quantitatively related to the biophysical theory for cell expansion and because it can be used on living cells, which actively participate in the regulation of wall loosening.

This chapter describes the pressure-block technique for stress relaxation *in vivo*. The method requires some specialized equipment, but is currently the most informative and most useful method for analyzing the wall yielding properties that govern plant cell growth. Once the apparatus is set up, this method is relatively easy to use and is suitable for measurements on a range of multicellular organs. The pressure-block technique is readily applied to intact plants, which means that it can be used to study many growth responses that are lost or attenuated upon excision of the growing tissue. Moreover, it appears to provide the most reliable assessment of the yielding properties of the growing cell wall (Cosgrove, 1987; 1993a).

II. Theory Underlying the Method

When a nongrowing cell takes up water, its walls become distended and an elastic restoring force is generated as the wall polymers are distorted from their relaxed state. The result is that wall stress and turgor pressure increase as water is taken up, until an equilibrium is reached. At this point, turgor pressure and cell size remain stationary. In a growing cell, equilibrium is never quite reached because wall loosening processes continuously break, shift, or otherwise rearrange the load-bearing polymers of the wall, so that wall stress is reduced. The consequence is that cell turgor pressure and water potential are reduced, and the cell takes up water in a steady fashion (that is, it enlarges at a constant rate). Under such steady-state growth conditions, stress relaxation because of wall loosening is exactly matched by the increase of wall stress of water uptake, with the result that turgor and wall remain constant as the cell increases in size.

To measure wall stress relaxation in growing cells, one needs to prevent water uptake (that is, hold cell size constant). Then wall loosening results in a measurable decrease in wall stress and turgor pressure, rather than an increase in size. In earlier procedures for *in vivo* wall relaxation, we prevented cell water uptake by excising the growing tissue and depriving it of a water source; relaxation was then observed as a decrease in turgor pressure, measured directly with the pressure probe or with a psychrometer (Cosgrove, 1985; 1987). These procedures are conceptually simple, but suffer from technical limitations in the measurements, as well from the need for tissue excision, which can produce various artifacts. These limitations are largely avoided with the pressure-block technique.

In the pressure-block technique, the growing part of the plant is sealed into a pressure chamber (Fig. 1) and growth is monitored at high temporal resolution, typically with an electronic position transducer attached to the plant inside the chamber. Stress relaxation is started by applying the minimum pressure needed to stop the plant from growing. As the walls are loosened by biochemical processes, wall stress and turgor pressure fall. Normally, this would draw water into the cell, but in the pressure-block method this is prevented by controlled increases in chamber pressure, finely adjusted to keep the size of the plant exactly constant—neither growing nor shrinking. When used in this fashion, the chamber pressure provides both the *means* for keeping size constant (a necessary condition for observing wall relaxation) and the *measure* of the relaxation process.

III. Materials

A. Suitable Plant Materials

In preparation for the standard pressure-block method, one must first identify the growing region of the plant organ, usually by detailed marking experiments (Silk, 1984). The plant needs to be manipulated so that one end of the growing region is sealed into the chamber, the other end of the growing zone is attached to the position transducer, and the water source for growth is outside the chamber. For most stems and leaves, this is easily arranged by setting up the plant as shown in Fig. 1.

We have worked mostly with growing stems, in which the growing zone is readily accessible and the growth rates range from 0.1 to 3 mm h^{-1}. With more slowly growing organs, the measurement of growth with adequate temporal resolution is a problem. (Questions arise such as, is the plant growing at pressure X? Should the pressure be increased? Decreased? The slower the growth rate, the longer one must wait to be sure of these answers, and therefore the poorer the temporal measurement of wall relaxation.)

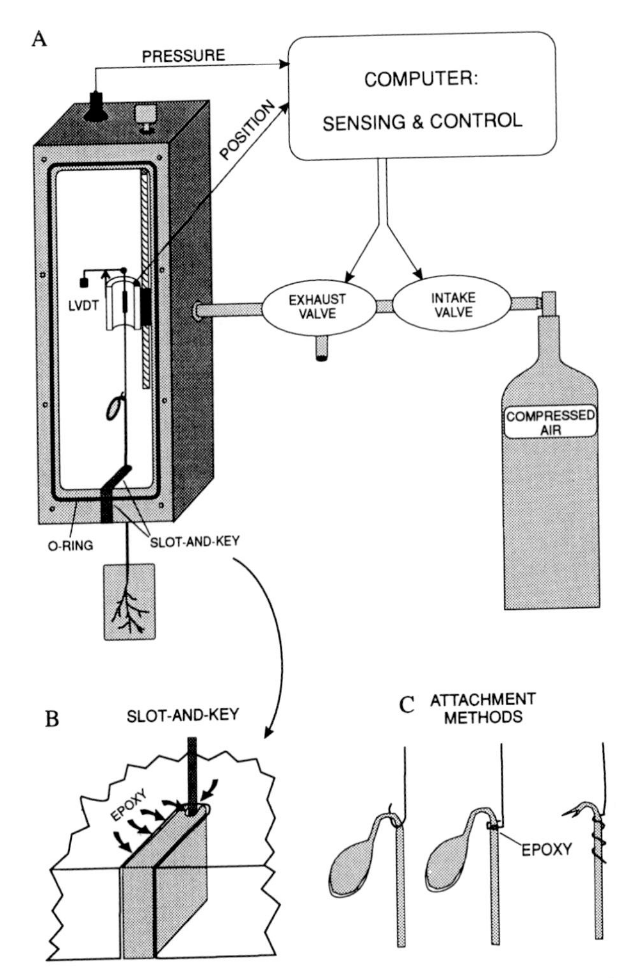

Fig. 1 (A) Diagram of the pressure-block apparatus. The instrument consists of a custom-made pressure chamber with electronic growth and pressure sensors connected to a microcomputer that regulates chamber pressure via electronic valves. Plant growth is monitored by a position transducer (LVDT) attached to the growing stem and mounted on a movable worm-screw slider. The slider extends outside the chamber via a Teflon sleeve that provides a pressure-tight seal. The growth transducer is an LVDT type (HR-050 with GMP108 signal conditioner, Schaevitz, Pennsauken, NJ) and the moveable core is attached to the plant by a thin wire and is counter-weighted as shown to provide a slight upward tension (equivalent to 10–110 mg of force). A 12-mm-thick Plexiglas plate (not shown) is attached to the face of the chamber by bolts (high tensile strength) and sealed with a rubber O-ring. The pressure sensor (type 22-100G; ICSensors, Sunnyvale, CA) is glued to a port in the aluminum block and continuously reports chamber pressure to the computer. The valves (type SV-24 12DB13, Valcor; Springfield, NJ) are electronically actuated to lower chamber pressure by venting the chamber to the outside or to raise chamber pressure by allowing entry of compressed air. A standard gas regulator (not shown) attached to the compressed air cylinder is used to provide a constant pressure source (about 6 bar) to the intake valve. The rate of gas flow through each electronic valve is limited with an adjustable needle valve. (B) Close up of the slot-and-key arrangement for sealing growing organs into the pressure chamber. The key is machined out of brass stock to fit the slot and to have a deep groove to accommodate the stem of the seedling. Alternatively, the key can be molded in place using thermoplastic (e.g., hot melt glue sticks). A thin film of epoxy (arrows) on top of the junctions between plant, slot, and key is applied to provide a pressure-tight seal. (C) Ways of attaching growing organs to the position transducer. The wire of the LVDT core assembly may be bent to form a loose-fitting hook (left). Alternatively, the wire may be bent into a tighter hook and secured to the stem with a small drop of epoxy (center). Another arrangement uses a corkscrew-shaped wire to catch the stem. Slight upward force on the wire keeps the core moving upward as the stem elongates.

Roots present a particular problem because of their delicacy and because they ordinarily obtain water for cell enlargement from their surroundings. We have had some success in measuring relaxation in robust roots by turning the chamber upside down (so the roots enter from the top of the chamber and grow downward) and by designing a split root system, wherein the root inside the chamber obtains its water via the xylem from parts of the plant outside the pressure chamber (J. Kigel and D. J. Cosgrove, unpublished).

B. Construction of the Apparatus

1. Pressure-Block Chamber

Our standard chamber was designed for measuring growth and wall relaxation in the stems of young seedlings and small plants (Fig. 1). The bulk of the chamber is made from an aluminum block in which a cavity was bored to hold the plant and the position transducer. The plant is sealed into the chamber with a small amount of fast-setting epoxy (1-min or 5-min epoxy, from Devcon Corp, Wood Dale, IL, or GC Electronics, Rockford, IL) and is attached to the position transducer with a piece of wire or string, sometimes with the aid of a bit of glue to keep the attachment from shifting. The transducer is mounted on a mechanical drive (a worm slide), with the adjustment knob extending outside the chamber through a pressure-tight seal. This arrangement allows one to raise or lower the transducer without opening the chamber. The front plate of the chamber is made of clear Plexiglas (12 mm thick), which allows one to inspect the plant and transducer setup, as well as control the lighting on the plant. The plate is made air tight with a large rubber O-ring that sits in a groove machined into the inside face of the plate. High tensile-strength steel bolts are used to tighten the face plate onto the chamber. Care in construction and assembly of the chamber is important to avoid accidental rupture of the pressurized chamber, a situation that could present hazards from impact with exploding pieces of the chamber (this has never happened to us, but suitable precautions should be taken by any users of this pressure chamber).

2. Pressure Sensing and Control

An electronic pressure sensor is sealed into a port in the chamber and is used to monitor chamber pressure, either on a strip chart recorder or by sampling with a microcomputer. Pressure is increased by injecting air from a compressed air cylinder into the chamber via an intake port. The same port is used to decrease pressure by exhausting gas from the chamber. In our original instrument, we controlled chamber pressure manually by turning the adjustment knob on a standard pressure regulator whenever the stem length began to increase. This method works fine, but soon becomes tedious.

Our current instrument reduces the tedium by use of a computer, which monitors the signal from the electronic position transducer and raises the chamber pressure whenever the plant begins to grow. The computer program has two control loops. One loop senses the signal from the pressure transducer and compares this value with the pressure setpoint—the pressure at which the chamber is supposed to be. If the actual pressure is outside the tolerance window of the setpoint, intake or exhaust valves are opened to raise or lower the chamber pressure to bring it within tolerance. A second control loop monitors the growth of the plant and raises the setpoint if the plant is growing and lowers the setpoint if the plant is shrinking. The program can be adjusted to change the pressure quickly for rapidly growing plants or more slowly for more lethargic plants. Whenever the setpoint is changed, the program records the time and the new setpoint. These data are stored on disk for subsequent analysis.

IV. Methods

The following section describes a step-by-step protocol for measuring wall relaxation in the epicotyl of a young, etiolated pea seedling. For other plant materials some modification of the procedures may be necessary, as dictated by experience and by the morphology of the tissue.

1. Select the plant and the growth region to be measured. Avoid sickly, damaged, or crooked tissues, as these might respond in an atypical manner (e.g., by collapsing or bending in response to the chamber pressure).
2. Seal the lower part of the growth zone into the base of the pressure chamber. This entails placing the stem into the slot in the bottom of the chamber, sliding the key into the slot, and applying a thin film of epoxy to the junctions between the chamber, the key, and the stem (see Fig. 1B). We have found it important to handle the plant very carefully at this stage to avoid bruising the cuticular surface or the epidermal cells; such damage can dramatically impair the growth and relaxation abilities of the tissue (see notes below).
3. Attach the upper part of the growth zone to the position transducer. In the case of a seedling with a well-formed apical hook, this may be done simply by counter weighting the transducer core assembly so that it spontaneously moves upward, and then forming a hook or loop in the wire to catch hold of the seedling hook (see Fig. 1C). Then, as the stem elongates the transducer core moves upward. This arrangement is easy, but presents some danger in misinterpreting the transducer signals if the apical hook begins to open or close during the relaxation measurement. Figure 1C shows some other attachment methods that have worked well in our lab.
4. Attach the face plate and monitor the growth rate until it stabilizes. Usually we wait at least 30 min after applying the epoxy before sealing the chamber. This allows time for the glue to harden and the epoxy vapors to disperse. Before sealing the chamber, we usually put a wet paper towel in the chamber to raise humidity and reduce transpiration by the plant.

Some experience is needed to know how to tighten down that bolts sealing the face plate. If they are tightened unevenly or insufficiently, then the chamber will leak air as the pressure reaches high levels. Over tightening should be avoided, as it may lead to crushing of the plant tissue or even damage to the chamber or the face plate. Once the face plate is attached, we usually monitor growth for about 30 min to verify that the plant is growing straight and at a reasonable, steady rate.

5. Start wall relaxation by raising chamber pressure to the point where stem elongation is momentarily prevented. If the plant is growing slowly (say, 0.1–0.5 mm h^{-1}), then a small initial pressure increase (e.g., 0.02 to 0.1 bar) is usually sufficient to stop growth, at least momentarily. As the cells in the growth zone continue to loosen their walls, the chamber pressure must be gradually increased to prevent growth. It is critical to have rapid and highly sensitive measurements of the growth of the plant, to be able to apply just the right chamber pressure to keep size constant. Shrinkage because of over pressuring should be avoided, as this gives a false representation of wall relaxation.

If the plant is growing very fast (say, 3 mm h^{-1}), it is sometimes difficult at first to "capture" the growing organ, that is, to apply just the right increase in pressure to keep it from growing. This difficulty arises in part from the need to increase the chamber pressure quickly and smoothly to values of 0.5 to 1 bar, and in part from the delay in water flow that occurs upon changes in the chamber pressure (the delay is caused by the hydraulic resistances and capacitances in the growing tissue). As a result, in fast-growing tissues there is sometimes a period of a minute or two after the initial step-up in chamber pressure during which growth rate is not zero but gradually approaches zero. A few preliminary trials with the plant material is usually sufficient to enable the investigator to judge the best rate of pressure increase to bring the plant to zero growth without overshoots, oscillations, or shrinkage. During this transient period, the internal water potential gradient that supported water uptake and cell expansion in the growing organ collapses (Cosgrove, 1987). Note that this initial pressure needed to halt growth provides an estimate of the size of this gradient, and only subsequent increases in pressure are due to continued wall relaxation.

6. Continue adjusting chamber pressure to keep the stem at constant length. If all works ideally, the pressure will increase gradually and monotonically, eventually to stabilize. This may take as little as 20–30 min (as etiolated cucumber hypocotyls), 60 min (etiolated pea epicotyls), or much longer for slowly growing tissues. The maximum pressure may be as little as 0.5 bar to more than 6 bar.

7. When relaxation has gone to completion, end the procedure by exhausting the chamber to bring chamber pressure to ambient level and to permit the plant to grow again. It is useful to monitor the recovery in growth to verify that the plant is undamaged; the growth recovery may also contain information that is pertinent to the growth treatments in question (e.g., timing, magnitude, and form of the response).

8. Open the chamber and examine the plant for signs of physical damage, bending, or other artifact.

V. Critical Aspects of the Procedure

A. Safety

Because of the high gas pressures that might be used in this method, it is essential to construct the pressure chamber and face plate with conservative engineering practices. Accidental breakage of the face plate or other pieces of a pressurized chamber could injure nearby people or damage equipment. This has never happened to us, but be sure to take appropriate cautions. In particular, there should be fail-proof limits to the maximum pressure allowed in the chamber.

B. Chamber Leakage

The tendency for the chamber to leak increases as the pressure increases. In our experience, leaks show up in only two places: around the epoxy that seals the plant into the base of the chamber, and around the rubber seal of the face plate. We find that close attention to detail, i.e., cleanliness of the rubber seals and careful application of epoxy, eliminates most of these problems. Judicious application of a pliant putty-like material (e.g., Blue Bostic) to trouble spots—before sealing the chamber—sometimes helps curb leaks in worn areas of the seal. Leaks in the epoxy–plant seal may arise if the surfaces are poorly prepared or if the epoxy is applied too late (after it has started to thicken). Sometimes such leaks can be remedied by applying a fresh layer of epoxy and starting again. Leaks around the face plate during a pressure-block procedure can sometimes be remedied by use of a C-clamp to tighten the plate in the area of the leak.

C. Plant Damage

Damage to the plant can arise from rough handling, from adverse reactions to the epoxy, from crushing when the face plate is tightened, and from mechanical damage when the chamber pressure reaches high values. Such damage, when it occurs, usually diminishes the growth of the plant and its ability to relax its walls. It also sometimes shows up later as visible alterations of the tissue (they become translucent, collapsed, or wilted). Such appearance is prima facie evidence for mechanical or chemical damage, and the relaxation results should be viewed with appropriate suspicion. These problems can usually be overcome be careful attention to detail during installation of the plant and by trying different brands of epoxy cements.

D. Nutations, Tropisms, Bending

Such bending can be confused with growth or shrinkage, and therefore should be avoided (e.g., watch where you locate your light source, and do not turn the plant sideways while installing it in the chamber). If it is very small, nutation will just add an artifactual oscillation to the record of stress relaxation. Large nutations must be dampened or eliminated before this technique will work.

VI. Results and Interpretation

A. Ideal Relaxations

The time courses for ideal pressure-block experiments are shown in Fig. 2A. The chamber pressure should increase rapidly at first, then gradually approach an asymptotic value in an exponential fashion. In general terms, the pressure-block relaxation gives information on the total magnitude of wall relaxation and the rate of relaxation.

Ideal kinetics for wall relaxation can be predicted from the growth model $r = \phi(P - Y)$, in which r is the growth rate, ϕ is the wall yielding coefficient ("extensibility"), P is the cell turgor pressure, and Y is the minimum turgor, or yield threshold, required for cell enlargement (Cosgrove, 1985). This growth model can be related to the relaxation results in the following ways: The asymptotic value attained by the chamber pressure is an estimate of $(P - Y)$. The rate constant for the relaxation decay is given by the product $\phi\varepsilon$, where ε is the volumetric elastic modulus of the cell. The initial rate of relaxation is given by the product $\phi\varepsilon(P - Y)$.

Measurements of wall relaxation are most often used to investigate *changes* in wall yielding properties. Figure 2A illustrates three ways in which wall yielding properties might change, and how they would affect the relaxation time course. In treatment b, the only change is a decrease in the final pressure attained; the rate constant is not affected by the treatment. This result is best interpreted as a decrease in $(P - Y)$, perhaps due to a decrease in P or an increase in Y, or both. Independent measurements of P would be needed to distinguish these possibilities, but in our experience changes in P are rarely causative for changes in growth, so these results would strongly suggest that treatment b led to an increase in the yield threshold.

In treatment a, the final chamber pressure is not different from the control, but the rate constant is reduced, as is the initial rate of relaxation. This result is best interpreted as a change in the quantity $\phi\varepsilon$. Independent estimates of ε would be needed to test whether ε changed. This might be most easily checked by measuring the elastic extensibility of isolated walls in a tensile tester, or by standard pressure probe or pressure bomb methods (Melkonian *et al.*, 1982; Tyree and Jarvis, 1982; Tomos, 1988).

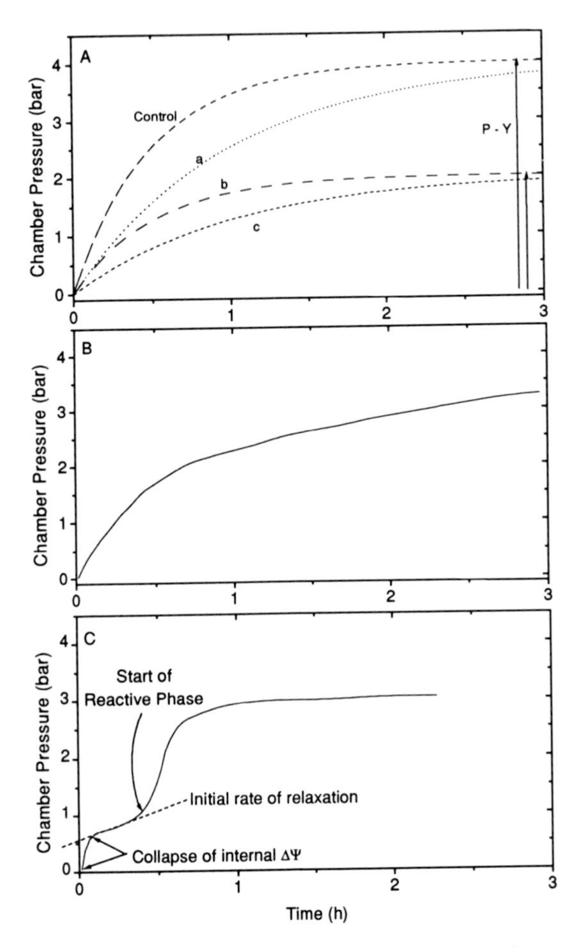

Fig. 2 Time courses for ideal (A) and more realistic (B–C) wall relaxations, measured with the pressure-block method. (A) An ideal relaxation would have the form of an exponential decay in turgor pressure to a constant value (the yield threshold). In a pressure-block relaxation, this would appear as increase in chamber pressure that approached a limiting value with an exponential decay. A change in the wall yield coefficient (extensibility) would appear as a change in the time constant of the exponential, as in treatment a (where ϕ was halved). A change in the yield threshold would appear as a change in the asymptotic pressure, without a change in time constant, as in treatment b (where Y increased by 2 bar, so $P - Y$ deceased by 2 bar). Treatment c shows slower relaxation because of both a decrease in ϕ and an increase in Y. The arrows at right indicate the value of $P - Y$. (B) A pressure-block relaxation in which the chamber pressure does not stabilize but continues to rise slowly after most of the wall relaxation is complete. This type of curve is often seen with slowly growing pea seedlings (Behringer *et al.*, 1991). (C) A complicated relaxation curve with three phases. In the first phase, chamber pressure rises quickly as growth is suppressed and the internal water potential gradient dissipates. Following this is a period of relaxation (dotted line) that is quickly followed by a reactive phase in which wall relaxation is enhanced, evidently as a reaction to the growth blockage. This reactive phase is typical of rapidly growing cucumber stems, but is less pronounced in most other tissues and totally absent in many slowly growing tissues.

In treatment c, final chamber pressure is reduced and the rate constant is also reduced. This would be the case if Y were increased and f were reduced in the treated plants.

B. Realistic Complications

Real plants typically exhibit one or more complications that make their pressure-block relaxations more complicated than the ideals described above. The most important ones are listed below, with some comments on our best interpretations of these complications and how to deal with them.

(a) In some plants, the chamber pressure does not stabilize but shows a slow, steady tendency to increase with time (Fig. 2B). This increase could be the result of continued phloem unloading and solute accumulation into the cells of the growing region. As the cell osmotic pressure increased, the chamber pressure would have to increase to offset this effect. This possibility could be checked by sampling the osmotic pressure at various times after this phase is reached. An alternative possibility is that the yield threshold is gradually reduced during this time, through metabolic modification of the wall. There are several precedents for this type of behavior (Cramer and Bowman, 1991; Hsiao and Jing, 1984; Nakahori *et al.,* 1991; Ortega *et al.,* 1989; Pritchard *et al.,* 1990; Randall and Sinclair, 1988; Schmalstig and Cosgrove, 1988). In cases where we have observed this gradual "creep" of the chamber pressure, we have used a pragmatic approach with minimal theoretical justification: namely, we have taken the chamber pressure at a fixed time point shortly after the relaxation has reached this phase as an estimate of $(P - Y)$. This value gives an estimate of the total relaxation, without overemphasizing the presumed Y-shifting behavior. In principle it is possible to quantify changes in Y (or in cell osmotic pressure, if that is basis for the change in chamber pressure) by monitoring the chamber pressure during this phase of the relaxation measurement.

(b) In plants that have a sizable internal gradient in water potential, one sees at least two phases in the pressure-block relaxation (Fig. 2C). In the first phase, chamber pressure is used to stop growth and to collapse the internal gradient in water potential. This phase goes to completion quickly (1–5 min is typical) and then is followed by wall relaxation. It is possible to estimate the size of the internal water potential gradient by extrapolating the rate of relaxation back to time zero (Fig. 2C, dotted line). It is important not to confuse this initial equilibration phase with the subsequent relaxation phase.

(c) Rapidly growing plants often show signs of reaction or adaptation to growth suppression by the pressure-block method. They react by stimulating the rate of wall relaxation (Fig. 2C), probably by changing the value of Y or of ϕ. Sometimes the reactive phase, when it occurs, starts in 5 to 10 min after the start of the measurement; in other cases it occurs later. There is no easy formula for interpreting the relaxation curves of such plants, except to measure the total relaxation and perhaps the rates of relaxation at the start of relaxation and during the reactive phase. Such data can sometimes be related to the growth behavior of the plants in insightful ways (Behringer *et al.,* 1990; Cosgrove, 1988; Kigel and Cosgrove, 1990).

VII. Conclusion and Perspectives

Ultimately, plant cells enlarge because their walls relax and thereby create the driving forces for water uptake, vacuole enlargement, and cell surface expansion. Conventional tests of wall mechanical properties have not proved successful in characterizing or quantifying the wall yielding processes that underlie the growth process. Methods of *in vivo* wall stress relaxation come much closer toward this goal. This chapter summarized the principles and methods for measuring wall relaxation by the pressure-block technique. The method is adaptable to many plant tissues, it can be used on intact plants, and the results may be related to the biophysical theory for plant growth. Rapidly growing tissues often behave in a way that is more complicated than can be accounted for in such theories. In such cases, the pressure-block method may prove useful not only as a method for quantifying wall relaxation processes but also for analyzing the basis for more complicated growth behaviors.

Acknowledgments

The author's work is supported by grants from the U.S. Department of Energy and from the National Science Foundation. The expert technical assistance of Mr. Daniel M. Durachko is gratefully acknowledged.

References

Behringer, F. J., Cosgrove, D. J., Reid, J. B., and Davies, P. J. (1990). The physical basis for altered stem elongation rates in internode length mutants of *Pisum. Plant Physiol.* **94,** 166–173.

Cosgrove, D. J. (1985). Cell wall yield properties of growing tissues. Evaluation by in-vivo stress relaxation. *Plant Physiol.* **78,** 347–356.

Cosgrove, D. J. (1987). Wall relaxation in growing stems: Comparison of four species and assessment of measurement techniques. *Planta* **171,** 266–278.

Cosgrove, D. J. (1988). Mechanism of rapid suppression of cell expansion in cucumber hypocotyls after blue-light irradiation. *Planta* **176,** 109–116.

Cosgrove, D. J. (1993a). Wall extensibility: Its nature, measurement, and relationship to plant cell growth. *New Phytologist* **124,** 1–23.

Cosgrove, D. J. (1993b). Water uptake by growing cells: An assessment of the controlling roles of wall relaxation, solute uptake and hydraulic conductance. *Int. J. Plant Sci.* **154,** 10–21.

Cramer, G. R., and Bowman, D. C. (1991). Kinetics of maize leaf elongation. I. Increased yield threshold limits short-term, steady-state elongation rates after exposure to salinity. *J. Exp. Bot.* **42,** 1417–1426.

Hsiao, T. C., and Jing, J. (1984). Biophysical parameters underlying slower expansion of water-stressed maize leaves: Shifts in yield threshold counter to osmotic adjustment. *Plant Physiol.* **75,** S174.

Kigel, J., and Cosgrove, D. J. (1990). Photoinhibition of stem elongation by blue and red light: Effects on hydraulic and cell wall properties. *Plant Physiol.* **95,** 1049–1056.

Melkonian, J. J., Wolfe, J., and Steponkus, P. L. (1982). Determination of the volumetric modulus of elasticity of wheat leaves by pressure-volume relations and the effect of drought conditioning. *Crop Sci.* **22,** 116–123.

Nakahori, K., Katou, K., and Okamoto, H. (1991). Auxin changes both the extensibility and the yield threshold of the cell wall of *Vigna* hypocotyls. *Plant Cell Physiol.* **32,** 121–129.

Ortega, J. K. E., Zehr, E. G., and Keanini, R. G. (1989). In vivo creep and stress relaxation experiments to determine the wall extensibility and yield threshold for the sporangiophores of *Phycomyces. Biophys. J.* **56,** 465–475.

Pritchard, J., Wyn Jones, R. G., and Tomos, A. D. (1990). Measurement of yield threshold and cell wall extensibility of intact wheat roots under different ionic, osmotic and temperature treatments. *J. Exp. Bot.* **41,** 669–675.

Randall, H. C., and Sinclair, T. R. (1988). Leaf wall yield threshold of field-grown soybean measured by vapor pressure psychrometry. *Plant Cell Environ.* **12,** 441–448.

Schmalstig, J. G., and Cosgrove, D. J. (1988). Growth inhibition, turgor maintainance, and changes in yield threshold after cessation of solute import in pea epicotyls. *Plant Physiol.* **88,** 1240–1245.

Silk, W. K. (1984). Quantitative descriptions of development. *Ann. Rev. Plant Physiol.* **35,** 479–518.

Tomos, A. D. (1988). Cellular water relations of plants. *Water Sci. Rev.* **3,** 86–277.

Tomos, A. D., Malone, M., and Pritchard, J. (1989). The biophysics of differential growth. *Environ. Exp. Bot.* **29,** 7–23.

Tyree, M. T., and Jarvis, P. G. (1982). Water in tissues and cells. *In* "Physiological Plant Ecology. II. Water Relations and Carbon Assimilation, Encyclopedia of Plant Physiology, Encyclopedia of Plant Physiology, New Series" (O. L. Lange, P. S. Nobel, C. B. Osmond, and H. Ziegler, eds.), pp. 35–77. Berlin: Springer-Verlag.

CHAPTER 17

High-Resolution NMR Methods for Study of Higher Plants

Justin K. M. Roberts and Jian-Hua Xia
Department of Biochemistry
University of California
Riverside, California 92521

I. Introduction

High resolution NMR spectroscopy can provide plant biologists with information on the types of low-molecular-weight metabolites in plant cells, their relative

METHODS IN CELL BIOLOGY, VOL. 49

concentrations, their mobility, and their interactions with other species such as H^+ or paramagnetic ions. The application of NMR spectroscopy to plant biology has been reviewed extensively (Roberts, 1987; Pfeffer and Gerasimowicz, 1989; Ratcliffe and Roberts, 1990), as have some specialized aspects including intracellular pH measurement (Roberts, 1986b) and energy metabolism (Roberts, 1986a). Solid state NMR, and NMR studies of water in plant tissues are not discussed here; the extraordinary recent improvements in biomedical magnetic resonance imaging (MRI) (Crease, 1993) will undoubtedly soon find application in plant research.

This chapter describes the means to obtain high-resolution NMR data from living plant cells and tissues. We focus on one-dimensional NMR (a plot of signal intensity versus frequency). The most important magnetic isotopes in biological NMR are ^1H, ^{13}C, ^{15}N, and ^{31}P. Only one isotope is directly observed, although coupling patterns (seen as multiplets of peaks, e.g., doublets, triplets) reveal attachment of other isotopes, as in molecules containing ^1H-^{13}C or ^{13}C-^{15}N linkages. The term high resolution NMR implies observation of distinct signals in spectra. The distinct signals can reflect different chemical groups; this effect is the chemical shift, and the spectral axis is generally labeled "chemical shift." Distinct signals can also be due to covalent attachments between magnetic nuclei, for example, ^1H-^{13}C or ^{13}C-^{13}C. The spin–spin coupling between attached magnetic nuclei causes splitting of signals. Finally, multiple signals in spectra can reflect heterogeneity in the sample. For example, heterogeneity in pH within the sample will produce multiple chemical shifts of titratable groups, if the pH variations occur within 1–2 pH units of the pK_a of these groups.

II. Materials

A. Plant Material and Nutrients

A great variety of plant material has been inserted into NMR spectrometers over the last two decades, from plant cells cultured *in vitro* to whole plants (Roberts, 1987; Ratcliffe and Roberts, 1990). Use of excised plant tissues, packed near the bottom of the NMR sample tube, is the simplest and most common approach (Roberts, 1986a). Cultured plant cells can be studied using the restraining system of Roby *et al.* (1987), the airlift system of Fox *et al.* (1989), or by imbedding cells in agarose threads (Foxall and Cohen, 1983). The nutrient medium used during NMR experiments can generally be the same as that used for plant culture and physiological experiments. However, plants grown on high levels of nutrients that are paramagnetic (e.g., Mn^{2+}) are generally unsuitable for high-resolution NMR studies, since these ions can broaden or eliminate NMR signals (Pfeffer and Gerasimowicz, 1989; Chang and Roberts, 1989; Gout *et al.*, 1992). Cell culture media generally have paramagnetic trace element levels that complicate NMR spectroscopy, and exceed cell needs for growth and development. An additional constraint is whether the medium will give signals that might obscure or confuse signals from intracellular metabolites, such as P_i in ^{31}P-NMR studies. Finally, control of microbes is essential, through sterile technique and antibiotics.

B. NMR Sample Chambers

NMR sample chambers are generally cylindrical glass tubes that fit in the detection coil of the spectrometer probe. Probe coil diameters are most commonly either 5 mm (generally for *in vitro* chemical analysis) or 10 mm (probes for non-^{1}H nuclei). Spectrometers with wide-bore magnets often have 20-mm-diameter probes for detection of non-^{1}H nuclei. Commercial NMR tubes are thin-walled, to maximize the sample volume in the coil. They are also made with high uniformity (judged by wall thickness, concentricity, and camber) for analytical NMR spectroscopists who spin their samples for improved resolution. Since spinning of living plant material in the NMR is difficult, and because the plant material itself is physically antithetical to a precision-crafted glass cylinder, use of more expensive, precision NMR tubes provides no benefit, compared to cheaper thin-walled tubes.

Sample tubes must permit circulation of liquid medium over the plant material. An NMR tube can be modified, so it is much like a chromatography column, with the perfused tissue supported by a glass–wool or a frit; this arrangement requires a probe that allows exit tubing to pass down through the probe body (Roberts, 1986a). Alternatively, a tube cap and sample support can be constructed to allow flow both into and out of the tube at the top, while the sample is restrained near the bottom of the tube (Lee and Ratcliffe, 1983; Roby *et al.*, 1987; Pfeffer and Gerasimowicz, 1989). The sample tube for observation of roots of intact seedlings is shown in Fig. 1 (Xia and Roberts, 1994).

C. The Perfusion System

The perfusion system consists of a reservoir (in which the perfusion medium can be saturated with the gases of choice), linked to the sample tube by tubing, and a pump capable of flow rates of flow rates up to ~50 ml/min.

D. External References

Solutions of one or more external reference compounds, contained in a sealed capillary and placed coaxially in the sample tube, can provide reference signals that are valuable for measuring chemical shifts of spectral peaks. Chemical shift, δ, is defined as $(\upsilon_s\text{-}\upsilon_{ref})\cdot 10^6/\upsilon_{ref}$, where υ_s and υ_{ref} are the absolute resonance frequencies of a sample and the reference signals, respectively; δ has the dimensionless units of parts per million (ppm). Reference signals are useful to enable quantitation of signals, discussed below. Reference signals also provide a means for simplifying pulse calibration, quantifying spectrometer sensitivity, and checking

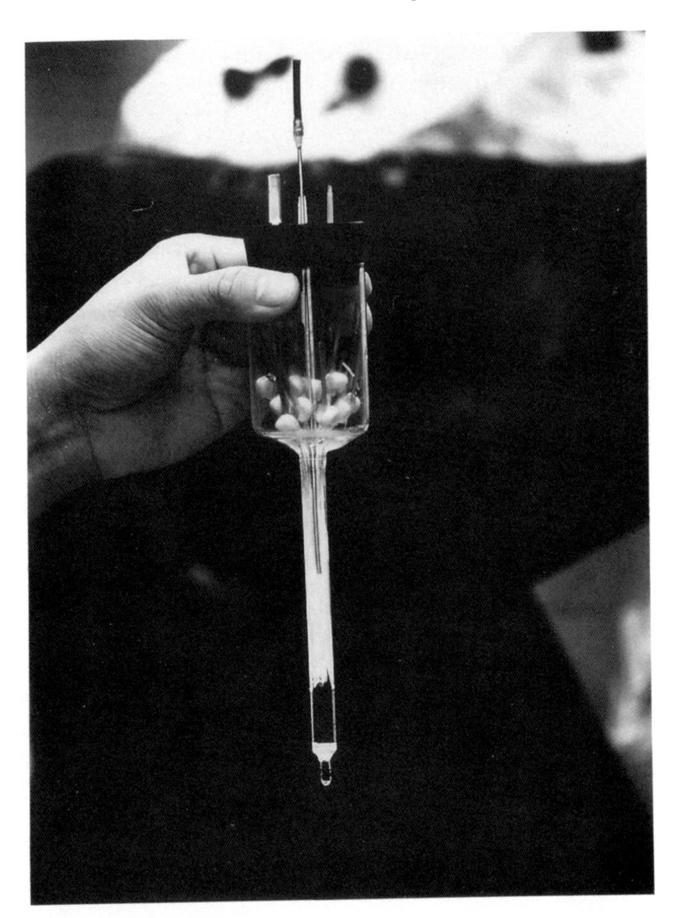

Fig. 1 Intact maize seedlings with root tips ready for analysis by *in vivo* NMR. The seedlings are in a modified NMR tube that fits in the magnet of an 11.75-T magnet (500 MHz ^{1}H frequency). Perfusion medium is pumped into the bottom of the tube. A second pump channel (at a higher flow rate) pulls the medium out through the rubber stopper at the top of the tube; the level of liquid in the tube is determined by the position of the exit tube. Two addition ports through the rubber stopper allow gas to be flushed around the seedlings, above the liquid medium, and also provide a safety exit for perfusion medium. The root tips are positioned so they lie in the middle of the probe's rf coil; hence signals from the apical 5 mm of the roots will be detected. Seedlings were grown as described by Xia and Roberts (1994). Spectra from samples such as this are shown in Figs. 3 and 4.

decoupler effectiveness. Methylene diphosphonate (~0.5 *M* free acid titrated to pH 8.9 with Tris base) is a useful ^{31}P reference. Natural ^{13}C-abundance acetone and chloroform are useful ^{13}C references, as is 2-aminobutyrate (~5% solution), which has distinct signals across the ^{13}C chemical-shift range and is therefore useful for checking uniformity and efficiency of proton decoupling during ^{13}C

acquisition (Xia and Roberts, 1994). For ^{15}N-NMR, ^{15}N-enriched ethanediamine (HCl) can be used (Fig. 2).

E. Fourier Transform NMR Spectrometers

Fourier transform NMR spectrometers operating at proton resonance frequencies of 300, 360, 400, 500, and 600 MHz are suitable for most applications described here. Whereas higher frequency instruments are generally better (more sensitive and higher spectral resolution), the improvements are mostly quantitative, rather than qualitative. The lower sensitivity of lower frequency instruments can be compensated by signal averaging for longer times. Performance and operation of instruments made by Bruker, General Electric, JOEL, and Varian are essentially equivalent. User training for routine operation can be accomplished in a few hours. Acquiring the ability to correct computer hang-ups and to trouble-shoot software and hardware problems can take a lifetime.

F. NMR Probes

NMR probes are aluminum-bodied cylinders inserted into the magnet bore. They contain a coil of copper wire or foil that surrounds the sample tube. The copper is part of an rf circuit tuned and impedance-matched with capacitors to the resonance frequency of interest. Probes are to NMR spectrometers what both the lamp filament and the photomultiplier are to a spectrophotometer. The ability of the probe to excite nuclei and detect induced magnetization is a prime determinant of sensitivity. The best probes are customized/dedicated to a particu-

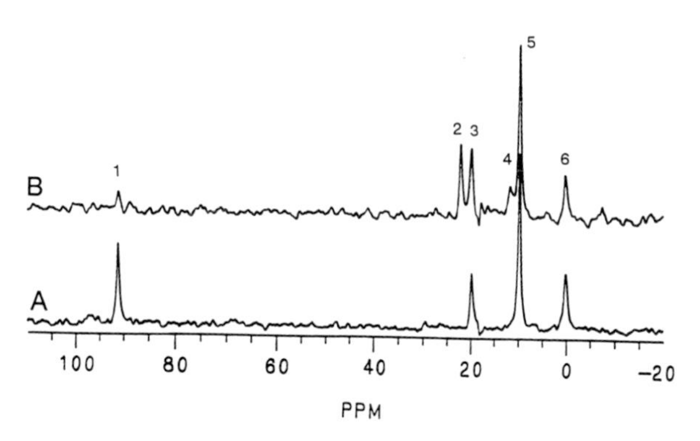

Fig. 2 *In vivo* ^{15}N-NMR spectra of maize root tips. Each spectrum was acquired over 30 min, either during 2.5–3 h of perfusion with O_2-saturated 50 m*M* Glc/0.1 m*M* $CaSO_4$/2.5 m*M* $(^{15}NH_4)_2SO_4$ at 10 ml/min (A) or later, during 1–1.5 h of perfusion with N_2-saturated 0.1 m*M* $CaSO_4$ at 4 ml/min (B). Broad-band proton decoupling was employed. Peak assignments: 1, Gln amide; 2, Ala; 3, Glu + Gln amino; 4, γ-aminobutyric acid; 5, 1,2-ethanediamine (^{15}N-enriched) external reference); 6, ammonium. Chemical shifts are referenced to ammonium at 0 ppm.

lar application, with respect to frequency (single frequency is better than "broad-band"), and with respect to sample configuration (optimized for size, shape, and requirements such as perfusion). Since a probe costs ~$18,000 (<10% that of a spectrometer), attention should be given to the adequacy of available probes, and to the possible beneficial impact that a new, dedicated probe might have on experiments.

In addition to the quality of the rf circuit, the volume of the coil (the "filling factor") contributes to overall probe sensitivity. However, increasing coil width and length can reduce the quality of the rf circuit, the uniformity of rf fields across the sample during irradiation, and the homogeneity of the magnetic field (and so signal linewidths), relative to smaller coils. The use of probes with large coils obviously also requires more plant material and, where employed, more labeled nutrients.

The use of multiply tuned probes, capable of detection of magnetization of more than one isotope, deserves encouragement. On the one hand, such probes have slightly lower sensitivity for each of the detected nuclei, compared to the best, single-tuned dedicated probe. On the other, there can be great advantages gained by simultaneous acquisition of different spectra (e.g., ^{13}C and ^{31}P, or ^{14}N and ^{15}N), if the different spectra contain useful information. First, increased information per experiment can improve reliability and confidence in the results. For example, in studies of carbon metabolism using ^{13}C-NMR, information on intracellular pH and nucleotide status may be useful, both to ensure that replicate samples are physiologically similar and to gain insight into factors that might influence the observed patterns of metabolism. Second, spectra of different isotopes during a given physiological experiment can be obtained using less spectrometer time, compared to that required using single-tuned probes.

G. Isotope-Enriched Chemicals

Isotope-enriched chemicals can be obtained from Isotec (Miamisburg, OH) or Cambridge Isotope Laboratories (Andover, MA).

III. Methods

At the spectrometer, the sample is loaded into the NMR tube, and the tube is connected to the perfusion system. Regarding the positioning of the sample in the NMR tube, physical concerns include the restraint of the tissue within the detection volume, and prevention of gas bubble formation within the sample. Tissues with significant intracellular gas spaces, and non-wetting hairy surfaces, are particularly problematic in that they tend to float on aqueous media, and facilitate bubble formation, which destroys spectral resolution (cf. Roberts, 1986b). Vacuum infiltration and wetting agents may take care of these physical concerns, but not without introducing potential physiological perturbations.

Wounding and other stresses must be evaluated and minimized during sample preparation, and appropriate controls must be performed, in order to provide meaningful data from experiments involving NMR.

A. Tuning of the Probe

When the sample is inserted into the probe, its tuning is usually changed; biological samples, particularly if they contain salts, become a significant part of the rf circuit. Hence, in order to ensure maximum spectrometer sensitivity, tuning and matching of the probe circuits should be checked prior to each experiment. Most spectrometers have built-in capability for probe tuning.

B. Shimming

Shimming is the art of maximizing the homogeneity of the magnetic field across the sample. The more homogeneous the applied magnetic field, the narrower the spectral signals, so that both signal-to-noise and resolution are improved. Field-homogeneity is adjusted by altering the current in about two dozen wires (the "room-temperature shims") inside the magnet's bore, around the head of the probe. The different wires are wrapped in various geometrical orientations. The magnetic fields produced by the wires supplement the field generated by the solenoid of the magnet (and the superconducting shim wires). The signal from H_2O in the sample, measured as the integral of the free-induction decay, can be most easily used to improve field homogeneity, shim currents being adjusted to maximize this signal. Even if a probe does not have an ^{1}H-observe channel, ^{1}H-signals from aqueous samples can be readily detected through the observe channel. Shimming is an iterative procedure, in which shims showing the greatest interactions are adjusted together as a group (e.g., the so-called "spinning-shims" that influence field-strength only along the axis of the magnet's bore), and the various groups are cycled through repetitively. Most spectrometers have computer-driven algorithms for maximizing homogeneity that work well as long as shims are not far off. It is often worthwhile spending an hour or more shimming at the beginning of a series of experiments. Following this initial set up, shimming between similar samples does not require more than 5 min.

C. Data Acquisition

With the sample in the spectrometer, the probe tuned, and shimming complete, several parameters must be defined prior to beginning data acquisition: *(a)* the observed rf pulse length (after calibration); *(b)* the width and position (defined by the central frequency) of the spectral window to be observed; *(c)* number of data points used to define the spectrum; *(d)* the gain of the receiver; *(e)* the delay period after data acquisition and before repetition of the pulse sequence; *(f)* decoupler frequency, modulation, and power levels, where necessary. Proton decoupling is required for ^{13}C- and ^{15}N-NMR, to simplify and enhance spectral signals. For ^{31}P-NMR, proton decoupling is generally useful only for analysis of extracts, because proton splitting of phosphate signals is small relative to *in vivo* peak widths, and because the nuclear Overhauser enhancement is small. Decoupling schemes that avoid heating the sample should be used; for example, high power should be applied only during actual data acquisition. Many spectral scans are added together to obtain sufficient signal, so the number of scans to be signal averaged, corresponding to a specific block of time for accumulation, must be decided upon in directing the spectrometer to begin data acquisition. This decision must weigh sensitivity for observed specific signals against the desired time resolution for observation of changes in signals.

D. Signal Processing

Processing the collected signal involves weighting the free induction decay to favor data points collected earliest in the data acquisition (most commonly using an exponential weighting function, which introduces line broadening—the "price" of enhanced signal to noise). This is followed by Fourier transformation of the signal from the time to the frequency domain and, last, by phase correction leading to a spectrum where all peaks appear as normal absorption signals.

E. Assignment of Spectral Peaks

Assignment of spectral peaks is the first step in interpreting results. Generally more than one line of reasoning must be used to assign convincingly *in vivo* NMR signals. Knowledge of the chemical shifts of biological molecules allows one to assign peaks to general classes of compounds, as in standard organic chemistry. It is important for individual investigators to generate their own chemical-shift tables for different metabolites, prior to definitive assignment, because published chemical-shift values may not apply exactly to the conditions of others. Additionally, titrations of compounds whose chemical shifts are affected by the concentrations of ions, such as H^+ or Mg^{2+}, should be performed (cf. Roberts, 1986b). Once candidate metabolites are identified, it is necessary to demonstrate that the metabolites exist in sufficient concentrations *in vivo* to account for specific peaks. Cell extracts are invaluable in this regard. Extracts can be analyzed by conventional analytical techniques, and NMR spectra of extracts allow determination of how many compounds are contributing to much broader *in vivo* peaks. Extracts may also provide information on isotope enrichment, e.g., $^{12}C/^{13}C$ ratios (e.g., Chang and Roberts, 1992), which is required in order to relate NMR signals to total metabolite concentrations. Perchloric acid extraction (Passonneau and Lowry, 1993) is the most useful general method to obtain a protein-free, aqueous solution of low-molecular-weight metabolites. Some enzymes are resistant to complete removal and inactivation by perchloric acid extraction, notably those capable of hydrolyzing nucleoside triphosphates

(Pradet and Raymond, 1983; Passonneau and Lowry, 1993). Hence, for quantitative analysis of such metabolites, extraction with trichloroacetic acid/ether is best (Pradet and Raymond, 1983). Traces of paramagnetic ions in the extracts can reduce spectral resolution and consequently complicate peak assignment. Chelation with agents such as EDTA is partially effective, but removal with Chelex resin (BioRad, Richmond, CA) is more so. The assignment of spectral peaks to distinct intracellular compartments has been thoroughly discussed elsewhere (Roberts, 1987; Chang and Roberts, 1989).

F. Quantitation

Metabolite concentrations can be determined from areas of peaks in spectra since, for each peak under fixed conditions of data acquisition, area is linearly proportional to the amount of the chemical group giving rise to the peak. The proportionally constant linking area and concentration can differ from peak to peak, and can be altered by changing conditions of data acquisition (e.g., pulse length, pulse interval, use of decoupler). Quantitation is simplest when (*a*) the pulse interval is so long that all nuclei are fully relaxed prior to each pulse and (*b*), if proton decoupling is employed, it is on only during data acquisition, not between acquisition and pulse, so that no nuclear Overhauser effect is apparent (see Roberts, 1987). Under these simplifying, nonsaturating conditions, *in vivo* peak areas are measured relative to a reference peak, and then compared to the area from a standard solution of known concentration, using the same reference. The tissue concentration (or more correctly, perhaps, content) can then be easily determined, if the proportion of sample in the NMR tube in the detection coil is known. More commonly, however, these simplifying conditions do not apply; rapid pulsing and decoupling giving nuclear Overhauser enhancements are used to improve signal-to-noise. Here, corrections must be made for relaxation and Overhauser effects. Correction factors can be determined by comparison of a spectrum collected under normal experimental conditions with a spectrum acquired under nonsaturating conditions with zero nuclear Overhauser effect; the two spectra should be collected in an interleaved manner, to eliminate effect of any change in the sample.

For ^{13}C and ^{15}N experiments, the above procedures lead to concentrations of metabolites containing these isotopes. Measurement of total metabolite concentrations requires knowledge of isotopic enrichment, and is simplest at isotopic steady-state. Isotopic enrichment can be assessed by mass spectrometry (Raven, 1987), or by NMR. Chang and Roberts (1992) determined the ^{13}C-enrichment at Cl of Glc6P by ^{1}H-NMR, and another example is presented below.

IV. Critical Aspects of the Procedures

Scientists employing NMR should at all times be conscious of the potential for harm to persons and equipment. Elimination or restraint of magnetic objects (cardiac pacemakers, credit cards, wrenches, electric motors, etc.), and use of safety measures with liquids and gases in the magnet bore are the prime concerns.

Getting access to a suitable NMR spectrometer with capable spectroscopists is the most obvious obstacle to many plant biologists who may need only a small amount of NMR-derived information, relative to their overall research effort. Fortunately many instruments are available that are administered and staffed so that non-NMR experts can obtain data. The simplest starting point to finding out if a given NMR facility can provide one with particular data is to prepare extracts, which can be used to test both the performance of the instrument at hand and the feasibility of the proposed *in vivo* project. An appreciation of the sensitivity of available instrumentation is required before biological questions can be addressed properly, and specific experimental goals set. Scheduling the running of an extract on NMR spectrometers is generally much easier than for *in vivo* samples. The higher resolution of extract spectra means that if particular NMR signals of interest are not apparent in extracts they will generally not be observable *in vivo*. And where signals are observed, they allow estimation of the time scale for observation *in vivo*. Even for experiments where extraction would lead to loss of specific information of interest, such as resolved signals from cytoplasmic and vacuolar pools of a metabolite, spectra of extracts provide information on the presence of possible compounds that might obscure or complicate observation of any distinct signals arising from metabolite compartmentation.

Inadequate control of experimental conditions may lead to variability, and may limit the biological significance of the results. The separation between the experimenter and the plant sample in NMR experiments, differences in experi-

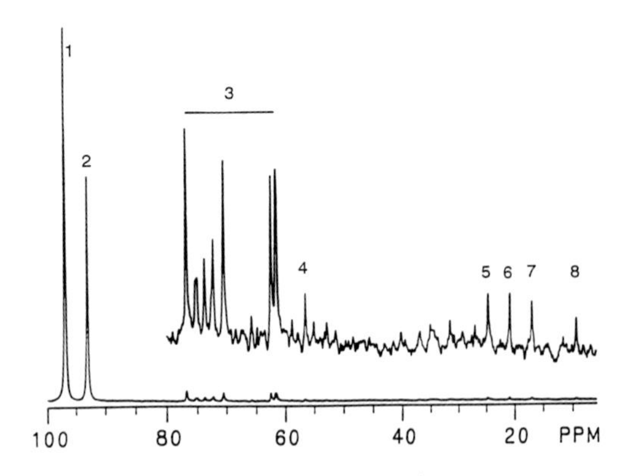

Fig. 3 *In vivo* ^{13}C-NMR spectrum of root tips of whole maize seedlings, perfused with nitrogen-saturated 50 m*M* [1-^{13}C] Glc/0.1 m*M* $CaSO_4$, acquired in 1 h. Roots were prelabeled with oxygenated 50 m*M* [1-^{13}C]Glc for 8 h prior to data acquisition. 2-Aminobutyrate was used as an external reference. Peak assignments: 1, βGlc-C1; 2, αGlc-C1; 3, sugars; 4, 2-aminobutyrate-C2; 5, 2-aminobutyrate-C3; 6, lactate-C3; 7, Ala-C3; 8, 2-aminobutyrate-C4. Chemical shifts are referenced to αGlc-Cl at 93 ppm.

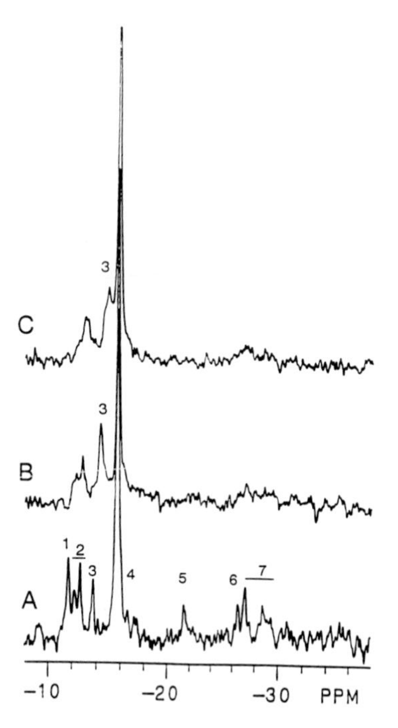

Fig. 4 *In vivo* ^{31}P-NMR spectra of root tips of whole maize seedlings under oxygenated conditions (A), or anoxia (B and C). Peak assignments: 1, Glc-6-P; 2, other monophosphate esters; 3, cytoplasmic P_i; 4, vacuolar P_i; 5, γ-nucleoside triphosphates; 6, α-nucleoside triphosphates; 7, uridinediphosphoglucose and nicotinamide adenine nucleotides. Chemical shifts are referenced to methylene diphosphonate at 0 ppm. Note the increase in the width of peak 3 from spectrum A through spectrum C, indicating increasing heterogeneity of cytoplasmic pH (see Roberts, 1986b). Spectrum C was acquired over the same 1-h time period as the ^{13}C-NMR spectrum in Fig. 3.

mental configuration (and, potentially, conditions) compared to non-NMR experiments, and complexities in harvesting and loading the sample may all present experimental difficulties. This presents particular problems early in an NMR project, when limited data are most likely to be overinterpreted. Replicates, quantitation of effects, and statistical analyses of results are necessary, but not always sufficient. In addition, some independent verification about the physiological state of the plant material under conditions of the NMR experiment allows the NMR results to be more definitively related to other studies. Markers such as growth rate or expression of particular genes provide independent measures of the physiological state in plant cells in the NMR spectrometer, and allow the investigator to be much more confident that the NMR results can be meaningfully related to nonspectroscopic data. Spectroscopic markers such as nucleotide levels or cytoplasmic pH can, of course, be useful indicators of physiological state. And certainly failure to detect nucleoside triphosphates by ^{31}P-NMR in a sample considered to be "unstressed" is cause for concern. But the converse is not true—for example, plant cells starved of sugar, and incapable of normal gene expression, can maintain high ("normal") levels of ATP for long periods (Roby *et al.,* 1987).

V. Results and Discussion

In vivo spectra, such as those in Figs. 2–4, illustrate the diversity of metabolites containing nitrogen, carbon, or phosphorus that can be observed and quantified *in vivo.* Using double-tuned probes, discussed above, it is possible to obtain spectra of different isotopes simultaneously, as in Figs. 3 and 4 (Xia and Roberts, 1994). ^{31}P-NMR is an excellent method for monitoring cytoplasmic pH in plant cells and tissues, through spectra such as those in Fig. 4 (Roberts, 1986b); vacuolar pH is more accurately monitored by ^{13}C-NMR of organic acids (Roberts and Pang, 1992). ^{31}P- and ^{13}C-NMR can also be used to estimate activities of enzymes, when present at high activity *in vivo* (Chang and Roberts, 1992, and references therein).

Spectra of cell extracts can allow investigators to interpret *in vivo* NMR spectra correctly, and may extend the types of information obtainable by NMR. Spectra of extracts (e.g., Fig. 5A) assist in assignment of *in vivo* spectral peaks, discussed under Methods. Extracts can also be used for determination of isotope enrichment, allowing signals in ^{13}C- and ^{15}N-NMR to be related to total metabolite levels. In Fig. 5, ^{1}H- and ^{13}C-NMR spectra of a single cell extract reveals the ^{13}C/^{12}C ratio in carbons 2 and 3 of alanine (cf. Chang and Roberts, 1992).

VI. Conclusions and Perspectives

NMR can be applied to a wide range of biochemical and cell biological problems in plant science. There are a variety of approaches by which plant material can be maintained and examined under defined physiological conditions, such that NMR results can be related to results from non-NMR studies. NMR spectroscopy is most useful when integrated with other approaches to a problem in plant biology. Skepticism of the validity of NMR studies should be held until such time that a particular result leads to predictions of phenomena observed by other methods.

The expense of NMR reflects technological effort aimed at overcoming the inherent insensitivity of the method. NMR signals can readily be obtained from metabolites present at 10^{-3} *M*. The procedures described here should enable the investigator to lower this threshold of detectability by at least an order of magnitude, and thereby extend the utility of the method to research on plants.

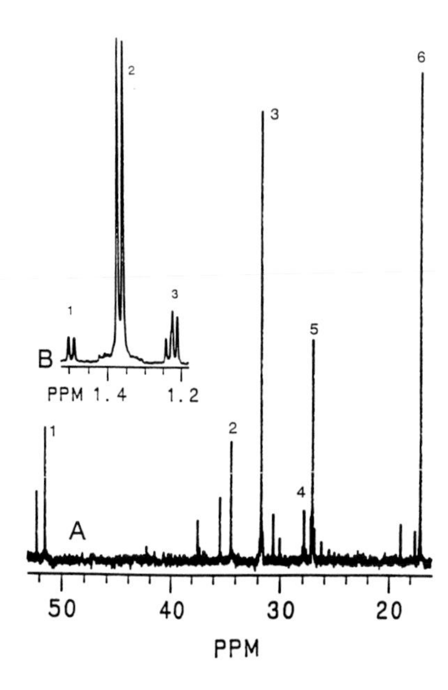

Fig. 5 ^{1}H- and ^{13}C-NMR partial spectra of amino acids extracted from ^{13}C-labeled maize root tips. Both spectra are of the same sample. Amino acids were purified by ion exchange chromatography. (A) Proton-decoupled ^{13}C-NMR spectrum showing signals from Ala-C2 (peak 1); Glu-C4 (peak 2); Gln-C4 (peak 3); Glu-C3 (peak 4); Gln-C3 (peak 5); and Ala-C3 (peak 6). (B) ^{1}H spectrum of the Ala methyl group showing protons attached to ^{13}C (peaks 1 and 3, with peak 3 including a contribution from another compound) and ^{12}C (peak 2); the doublets are due to coupling of the three equivalent methyl protons to the proton at C2. The ^{13}C/^{12}C ratio at Ala C3 is given by the ratio of peak areas: (2 × peak 1)/(peak 2). The ^{13}C/^{12}C ratio at Ala C2 is given by multiplying this ratio by the C2/C3 ratio obtained from spectrum (A).

Acknowledgments

This work was supported in part by USDA Grant 92-37100-7626 and NSF Grant IBN-9310850.

References

Chang, K. J., and Roberts, J. K. M. (1992). Quantitation of rates of transport, metabolic fluxes, and cytoplasmic levels of inorganic carbon in maize root tips during K^+ ion uptake. *Plant Physiol.* **99,** 291–297.

Chang, K. J., and Roberts, J. K. M. (1989). Observation of cytoplasmic and vacuolar malate in maize root tips by ^{13}C-NMR spectroscopy. *Plant Physiol.* **89,** 197–203.

Crease, R. P. (1993). Biomedicine in the age of imaging. *Science* **261,** 521–652.

Fox, G. G., Ratcliffe, R. G., and Southon, T. E. (1989). Airlift systems for in vivo NMR spectroscopy of plant tissues. *J. Magn. Reson.* **82,** 360–366.

Foxall, D. L., and Cohen, J. S. (1983). NMR studies of perfused cells. *J. Magn. Reson.* **52,** 346–349.

Gout, E., Bligny, R., and Douce, R. (1992). Regulation of intracellular pH values in higher plant cells. Carbon-13 and phosphorus-31 nuclear magnetic resonance studies. *J. Biol. Chem.* **267,** 13903–13909.

Lee, R. B., and Ratcliffe, R. G. (1983). Development of an aeration system for use in plant tissue NMR experiments. *J. Exp. Bot.* **34,** 1213–1221.

Passoneau, J. V., and Lowry, O. H. (1993). "Enzymatic Analysis, A Practical Guide." Totowa, New Jersey: Humana Press.

Pfeffer, P. E., and Gerasimowicz, W. V. (1989). "Nuclear Magnetic Resonance in Agriculture." Boca Raton, FL: CRC Press.

Pradet, A., and Raymond, P. (1983). Adenine nucleotide ratios and adenylate energy charge in energy metabolism. *Annu. Rev. Plant Physiol.* **34,** 199–224.

Ratcliffe, R. G., and Roberts, J. K. M. (1990). Recent applications of NMR to higher plants and algae. *Magn. Reson. Med. Biol.* Vol. IV, No. 1, 77–99.

Raven, J. A. (1987). The application of mass spectrometry to biochemical and physiological studies. *In* "The Biochemistry of Plants" (D. D. Davies, ed.), Vol. 13, pp. 127–180. Orlando: Academic Press.

Roberts, J. K. M. (1987). NMR in plant biochemistry. *In* "The Biochemistry of Plants" (D. D. Davies, ed.), Vol. 13, pp. 181–227. Orlando: Academic Press.

Roberts, J. K. M. (1986a). Determination of the energy status of plant cells by ^{31}P-nuclear magnetic resonance spectroscopy. *In* "Modern Methods of Plant Analysis" New series Vol. 2, Nuclear Magnetic Resonance (H. F. Linskens and J. Jackson, eds.), pp. 43–59. Berlin: Springer-Verlag.

Roberts, J. K. M. (1986b). NMR methods for determination of intracellular pH. *In* "Modern Methods of Plant Analysis," New series, Vol. 2, Nuclear Magnetic Resonance (H. F. Linskens and J. Jackson, eds.), pp. 106–126. Berlin: Springer-Verlag.

Roberts, J. K. M., and Pang, M. K. L. (1992). Estimation of ammonium ion distribution between cytoplasm and vacuole using nuclear magnetic resonance spectroscopy. *Plant Physiol.* **100,** 1571–1574.

Roby, C., Martin, J. B., Bligny, R., and Douce, R. (1987). Biochemical changes during sucrose deprivation in higher plant cells. *J. Biol. Chem.* **262,** 5000–5007.

Xia, J. H., and Roberts, J. K. M. (1994). Improved cytoplasmic pH regulation, increased lactate efflux and reduced cytoplasmic lactate levels are biochemical traits expressed in root tips of whole maize seedlings acclimated to a low oxygen environment. *Plant Physiol.* **105,** 651–657.

CHAPTER 18

Electrophysiology

John F. Thain
School of Biological Sciences
University of East Anglia
Norwich NR4 7TJ, United Kingdom

I. Introduction

Electrophysiology has been a part of the plant physiologist's tool kit for over 100 years and in its early years scored some notable successes with the use of surface contact electrodes to elucidate the signaling phenomena involved in the leaf movements of the Venus flytrap (*Dionaea muscipula*) and the sensitive plant (*Mimosa pudica*) (Simons, 1992). However, plant electrophysiology really came of age in the late 1950s with the application of precise electrochemical concepts to the study of ion movements across plant cell membranes (Dainty, 1962) and with the adoption of improved microelectrode techniques for the measurement of electrical potential differences (pd) across plant cell membranes (Walker, 1955; Etherton and Higinbotham, 1960).

Since then, plant electrophysiology has continued to develop, mainly by adapting techniques already used with animal systems, and now four main branches can be identified:

METHODS IN CELL BIOLOGY, VOL. 49

1. Measurements with surface contact electrodes on whole plants or on plant organs
2. Measurements of pds across plant cell membranes with microelectrodes
3. The use of ion-specific microelectrodes to measure intracellular ion activities
4. Patch-clamp methods for the detailed study of ion transport processes at the membrane level

The methods used in patch-clamping and in the construction and use of ion-specific microelectrodes are dealt with in other chapters in this volume. Methods involving microelectrodes to measure transmembrane pds have been extensively reviewed (e.g., Purves, 1981; Blatt, 1991a; Ogden, 1994). This chapter will, therefore, concentrate on the use of surface contact electrodes in measurements on whole plants or plant organs, with some treatment of microelectrode methods, especially in relation to plant cells. The same general principles apply in both cases, but differences of detail arise from the different methods of making contact with the plant.

Despite the early successes mentioned above, and despite the efforts of a few later workers such as Pickard (1973, 1974), the study of electrical events at the level of the whole plant or plant organ has not been a popular approach among Western plant physiologists, although work along those lines did continue in eastern Europe and especially in the former Soviet Union. Partly this has been due to concentration on events at the cell level, but also it has been due to the belief that, apart from a few "special" cases such as *Dionaea* and *Mimosa,* plants do not use long distance electrical signaling. However, some recent observations, such as those on the electrical events accompanying the wound response in tomato seedlings (Wildon *et al.,* 1992), suggest that long distance electrical signaling may be more common in plants than has generally been believed, and have generated renewed interest in the relevant experimental methods.

General references that the interested reader should find useful are the books by Geddes (1972), Hope and Walker (1975), Purves (1981), Ogden (1994), the reviews by Pickard (1973, 1974), Findlay and Hope (1976), Beilby (1989), Blatt (1991a), and Thain and Wildon (1993).

II. Materials and Methods

A. General Aspects

A simple experimental system for making electrical recordings from plants is shown schematically in Fig. 1. The center of the system is the voltmeter (V) which measures the pd between points A and B on the plant. The voltmeter, which is usually called an "amplifier" by electrophysiologists, may itself incorporate an analogue meter or digital readout to allow the measured pd to be read, but it usually also has an output to drive another display device (D). This can be an

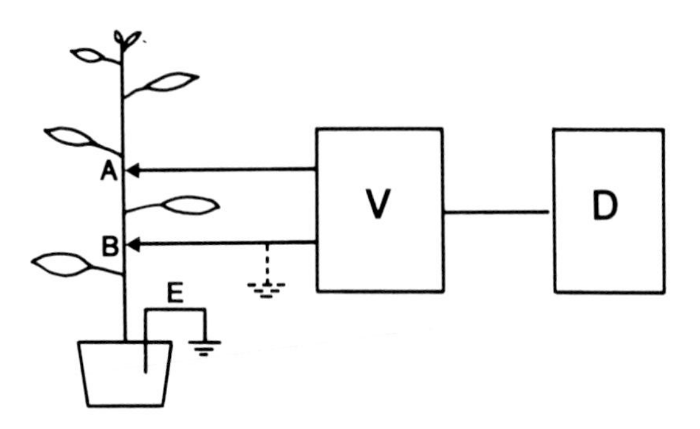

Fig. 1 Basic system for electrophysiological measurements on a plant. (A, B) Surface contact electrodes; V, voltmeter (amplifier); D, display device; E, contact to earth potential; an alternative position for the latter is shown by the dashed lines.

oscilloscope; a chart recorder, if a permanent record of the variation of the pd with time is required; or a computer-based data storage/manipulation/display system.

The voltmeters (V) and display devices (D) used in measurements on plants are in general the same as those used in measurements on animals and are readily available commercially, but the specifications required can, in many cases, be less stringent than those required for work with animal systems. Good electrical contacts (A, B) between the plant and the metal leads to the voltmeter are of crucial importance and usually have to be custom built in the laboratory to suit the particular experimental system.

B. Electrical Contact with the Plant

1. The Nature of the Problem

The experimental problem is how to make a stable and reliable electrical contact between the aqueous apoplast of the plant and the metal wire that connects it to the voltmeter. Measurement of a pd requires the movement of small amounts of electrical charge between the aqueous phase and the metal phase and it is necessary that this movement of charge should be via one dominant, reproducible, and reversible chemical reaction at a metal/solution interface whose properties do not change significantly during the measurement. Such an arrangement is called an electrode and the ones commonly used in measurements of pds in biological systems are the silver/silver chloride electrode and the calomel electrode. The general arrangement is, therefore, that the metal wire from the voltmeter is connected to the electrode which is in contact with a dilute salt solution (e.g., 10 mM KCl), which, in turn, makes contact with the apoplast of the plant:

apoplast/dilute salt solution/electrode/metal wire

The following sections describe, in turn, the electrodes and the way in which contact is maintained between them, the dilute salt solution, and the plant surface.

2. The Silver/Silver Chloride Electrode

If a silver wire coated with silver chloride dips into a solution containing chloride ions, exchange of electric charge across the metal/solution interface is achieved primarily by the reaction:

$$AgCl\ (\text{solid}) + \text{electron} \rightarrow Ag\ (\text{solid}) + Cl^-\ (\text{aqueous})$$

This provides a stable and reliable electrical contact between the silver wire and the solution. As the reaction equation above indicates, the electrical potential measured with a silver/silver chloride electrode will depend on the concentration of Cl^- ions in the solution. It is important, therefore, that this concentration remain constant during an experiment. Silver/silver chloride electrodes can be prepared easily in the laboratory in a variety of shapes and sizes (Purves, 1981, p. 51; Geddes, 1972, p. 32). For wire electrodes, two lengths of silver wire (0.1- to 0.5-mm-diameter, as required) are cleaned by being rubbed with abrasive paper and then wiped with alcohol. The two wires are mounted so that most of their lengths are immersed, without touching each other, in a beaker of 0.1 *M* HCl. One wire is connected to the positive terminal of a 1.5 V battery and the other wire to the negative terminal. Current is allowed to flow for a few minutes during which the wire connected to the positive terminal becomes coated with a layer of silver chloride and bubbles of H_2 gas are liberated at the other wire. The connections of the wires to the battery are then switched over so that the other wire can be chlorided. The silver chloride coating should be uniform over the surface of the wire and of a dark grayish purple color. Silver/silver chloride electrodes can be prepared in this way also from silver foil and silver wire mesh.

Silver/silver chloride electrodes can also be prepared by dipping the silver wire into molten silver chloride. This produces a mechanically stronger coating.

Besides their good electrochemical properties, silver/silver chloride electrodes are popular because they can be made in different shapes and sizes to suit different experimental situations. They are also very suitable for passing electric current.

3. Calomel Electrodes

In a calomel electrode liquid mercury is in contact with a paste of calomel (mercurous chloride, Hg_2Cl_2) that is in contact with an aqueous solution containing Cl^- ions, usually a saturated KCl solution. Charge transfer across the metal/liquid interface is achieved by the reaction:

$$Hg_2Cl_2\ (\text{solid}) + 2\ \text{electrons} \rightarrow 2\ Hg\ (\text{liquid}) + 2Cl^-\ (\text{aqueous})$$

Again, the potential differences observed with this electrode depend on the Cl^- concentration in the solution.

Calomel electrodes are widely used as the reference electrode in pH measurements and are readily obtainable from most suppliers of general laboratory equipment. They are more stable than silver/silver chloride electrodes, but less suitable if current passing is required. They are also more bulky than homemade silver/silver chloride electrodes and, therefore, sometimes more awkward to use.

4. The Salt Bridge

Sometimes it is necessary to make good electrical contact between one aqueous solution and another of different chemical composition. This is usually achieved by means of a salt bridge—a glass or plastic tube filled with agar gel (3% by weight) containing 3 *M* KCl. For present purposes thin-walled flexible plastic tubing of about 2-mm external diameter is convenient. A mixture of 6 g of KCl and 0.6 g of agar powder in 20 ml of water is heated in a small beaker on a water bath until both the KCl and agar are dissolved. A syringe is used to suck the hot solution into the plastic tube, which has also been heated in hot water to avoid the gel solidifying before the tubing has been filled. When not in use, the salt bridges should be stored in 3 *M* KCl solution.

Salts other than KCl can be used in salt bridges, but it is important to use a salt in which the ionic mobilities of the anion and cation are very nearly equal, to minimize the liquid junction potentials (Geddes, 1972, p. 9) that arise at the junction between the salt bridge and a solution of different electrolyte composition.

5. Contact with the Plant

a. Contact via Silver/Silver Chloride Electrodes

A variety of methods have been used to make and maintain electrical contact between the electrode and the surface of the plant, but the details depend on whether silver/silver chloride electrodes or calomel electrodes are to be used.

With silver/silver chloride electrodes the dilute salt solution (e.g., 10 m*M* KCl) that makes contact with the surface of the plant can be the same as that which surrounds the chlorided silver wire. The chlorided silver may be sealed into one end of a glass or plastic tube that contains the dilute salt solution. A wick soaked in the same salt solution protrudes from the other end of the tube and is pressed against the surface of the plant. Wicks have been made from the heads of small paint brushes (Paszewski and Zawadzki, 1973), the tips of felt-tip pens (Zawadzki *et al.,* 1991), cotton thread protruding through a plug of agar gel (Shiina and Tazawa, 1986), and cotton wool (our unpublished results). Contact between the wick and the plant can be maintained by the use of a slotted plastic sleeve that slides over the tube holding the wick and partly encircles the petiole or stem. An arrangement that maintains contact with the plant surface but avoids physical constraint of the plant involves the use of a cotton thread, soaked in 10 m*M* KCl, that is looped around the petiole or stem and dips into a small vial of 10 m*M* KCl; the chlorided silver wire also dips into this vial (Shiina and Tazawa, 1986).

It was mentioned above that the pd observed with silver/silver chloride electrodes varies if the concentration of Cl^- ion in the surrounding solution varies. Possible problems arising in this way can be minimized by arranging that the chlorided silver wire dips into a solution of saturated or 3 *M* KCl; this is connected electrically by a salt bridge to the 10 m*M* KCl solution that makes contact with the plant surface via the wick or thread loop.

b. Contact via Calomel Electrodes

The aqueous phase in commercial calomel electrodes is invariably a 3 *M* or saturated KCl solution. Also, the electrodes themselves usually incorporate their own salt bridge in the form of a small porous section of the outer glass or plastic casing of the electrode. Thus direct contact can be made between the calomel electrode and the dilute salt solution that makes contact with the plant surface via the wick or cotton thread (Paszewski and Zawadzki, 1973; Zawadzki *et al.*, 1991). However, because of the relatively large size of commercial calomel electrodes, this kind of arrangement can be awkward to use in some situations. Currently the system we use most consists of a calomel electrode that dips into a small pot of 3 *M* KCl; this is connected by a salt bridge to a 1.5 ml vial of 10 m*M* KCl from which a cotton thread soaked in 10 m*M* KCl is looped around the petiole or stem. This allows a useful degree of flexibility in the positioning of the electrode with respect to the plant, while retaining the advantage of the electrochemical stability of calomel electrodes.

c. Treatment of the Plant Surface

Given that the aerial surfaces of plants are generally covered with hydrophobic cuticles, it is perhaps surprising that sufficiently good electrical contacts with the apoplast can be achieved by the methods described above. However, this is very often the case. In other cases electrical contact can be improved by gentle abrasion of the surface or by stripping away parts of the surface, but clearly this should be avoided if at all possible.

C. The Voltmeter/Amplifier and Display System

The measuring device or voltmeter is also commonly called an "amplifier," a term which can be misleading because, in many cases, the output from the "amplifier" to the display device is equal in magnitude to the input to the "amplifier." However, the term "amplifier" is so well established among electrophysiologists that it will be used in the rest of this chapter.

Amplifiers may be powered from the mains supply or from batteries. A possible disadvantage of the former is that unwanted mains frequency noise may be introduced into the measured pd and a disadvantage of the latter is that batteries can go flat at inconvenient times.

Amplifiers can also be single-ended or differential. Here it is important to remember that only an electrical potential *difference* between two points can be measured. A single-ended amplifier measures the pd between one contact point on the plant and an internal reference potential in the amplifier, usually earth potential. A second contact point on the plant is necessary to complete the measuring circuit; this contact is connected to the reference (earth) potential either directly or via a second input terminal on the amplifier. A differential amplifier measures the pd between any two contact points on the plant, neither of which need be connected to the reference (earth) potential. As will be discussed below, this means that differential amplifiers are more versatile than single-ended ones and there are some situations where single-ended amplifiers cannot be used. However, differential amplifiers are more expensive than single-ended ones.

Two important aspects of any amplifier used for electrophysiological measurements are its input impedance and its response time. Electrically, the amplifier behaves as a resistance, or more properly an impedance. The proportion of the pd originating in the plant that is detected by the amplifier is equal to the ratio $R_A/(R_A + R_{P+E})$ where R_A is the input impedance (resistance) of the amplifier and R_{P+E} is the total electrical impedance (resistance) of the plant and electrodes. Thus for the recorded pd to be in error by less than 1%, the value of R_A must be more than 100 times greater than R_{P+E}. In measurements with surface contact electrodes the magnitude of R_{P+E} is normally in the range 10^4 to 10^5 Ω, so an amplifier with an input impedance of 10^6 to 10^7 Ω is required.

The response time of the amplifier must be fast enough to record any transient changes in pd arising in the plant. This is not generally a problem because commercially available physiological amplifiers are usually designed to record the much faster electrical transients found in animal systems.

Amplifiers designed for electrophysiological use may have several other useful features. These can include different selectable input ranges, so that small input signals can be measured as accurately as large ones; variable gain (i.e., ratio of output/input), for the same purpose; a back-off control (preferably calibrated) so that attention can be focused on small fluctuations that appear on top of a large constant baseline pd; electrical filters to eliminate unwanted slow signals such as a drift in the pd due to changes in the properties of the electrodes or unwanted fast signals such as rapid transients originating in the mains power supply; an analogue or digital display of the measured pd.

The paper chart recorder has been the display device most commonly used by plant electrophysiologists in the past. Few applications required the fast response time of the oscilloscope. In recent years tape recorders and computer-based systems have become more important especially in applications such as current–voltage analysis and patch-clamping where very fast transient changes in pd or membrane current have to be recorded and the data subjected to further mathematical analysis. Chart recorders remain useful, where records of pd have to be made over longer periods and where little or no further quantitative analysis is required.

D. The Complete System

One way of combining the components described in Sections II,B and II,C for the purpose of using surface contact electrodes to measure the pd between two points in a plant is shown in Fig. 1 where the voltmeter is a differential amplifier. One important point to note is that in any electrophysiological study it is always advisable, and usually necessary, that one, and only one, point on the experimental object be connected to earth potential. Here this has been achieved via a chlorided silver wire inserted into the moist compost in the pot in which the plant is growing. An alternative arrangement would be to connect one of the electrodes A or B to earth potential, as is shown by the dotted lines in the figure.

For the system shown in Fig. 1, the voltmeter could also be a single-ended amplifier. In this case one of the electrodes, A or B, would be connected to earth potential, either directly or via a reference/earth input terminal on the amplifier.

There are some situations where a single-ended amplifier cannot be used. Consider the system shown in Fig. 2, where it is desired to use surface contact electrodes to measure the pd between points A and B on the plant, and also the pd between points C and D. Both voltmeters, V1 and V2, could be differential amplifiers and the plant could be connected to earth potential either via a separate electrode, as E in Fig. 1, or via a connection to one of the electrodes A, B, C, or D. Alternatively one of the voltmeters, e.g., V2, could be a single-ended amplifier, in which case one of the electrodes C or D would be connected to earth either directly or via a reference/earth terminal on the amplifier and no other connection should be made between the plant and earth potential. How-

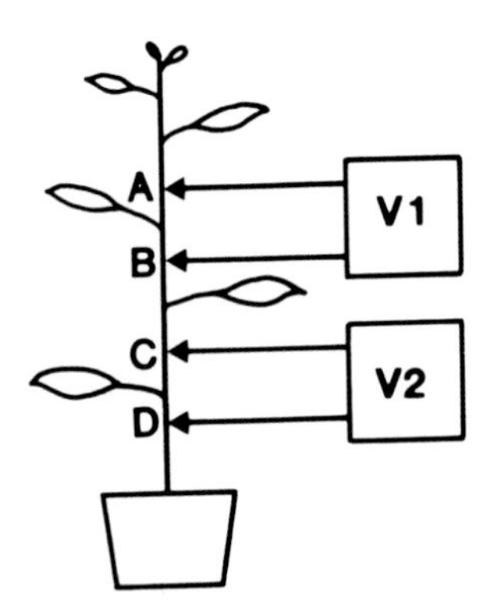

Fig. 2 System for simultaneous measurement of pds at two separate locations (A-B and C-D) on a plant. (A, B, C, D) Surface contact electrodes; V1, V2, voltmeters (amplifiers). See text for discussion.

ever, it is not possible to use single-ended amplifiers for both V1 and V2, as this would require *two* points on the plant [(A or B) and (C or D)] to be connected to earth potential. It is possible to use several single-ended amplifiers in the same experimental system if the requirement is to measure the pds between several different points on the plant and a common reference point (Fig. 3). This arrangement can be seen in the papers of Paszewski and Zawadzki (1973) and of Zawadzki *et al.,* (1991) on the propagation of action potentials in *Lupinus angustifolius* and *Helianthus annuus.*

Returning to Fig. 1, another important factor is the distance between the points of electrical contact (A and B) on the plant. Suppose that a stimulus near the apex of the plant produces a transient change in electrical potential that propagates down the plant. Suppose also that the distance A–B is sufficiently large that the electrical potential at A has returned to its normal value well before the potential at B starts to change. Then the variation in pd between A and B with time would appear on a chart recorder trace as two separate peaks of opposite polarity, the first one representing the transient passing A and the second the transient passing B. If the separation of A and B were decreased the peaks would occur closer together, and if they were too close the transient would appear at B before it had completely passed A so that the two peaks would overlap and be much reduced (Geddes, 1972, Fig. 6.1.). The correct size and shape of the transient would not be observed.

E. Intracellular Recording with Microelectrodes

Measurement of the electrical pd across the plasma membrane of a plant cell requires electrical contact with the cell cytoplasm and with the aqueous medium bathing the cell or tissue. Contact with the cytoplasm requires the use of a

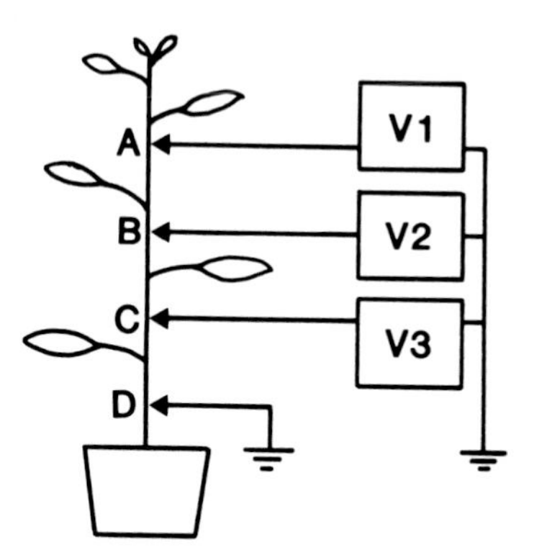

Fig. 3 System for simultaneous measurement of pd between each of three separate positions on a plant (A, B, C) and a common reference D. VI, V2, V3, voltmeters (amplifiers). See text for discussion.

microelectrode—a glass micropipette filled with a conducting electrolyte solution and with a tip diameter of less than 1 μm.

The same general principles apply in the use of microelectrodes as in the use of surface-contact electrodes but the physical characteristics of microelectrodes are such that much greater care is needed to avoid problems arising from electrical interference and mechanical disturbance. The use of microelectrodes has permitted the development of a range of techniques such as current-clamping, voltage-clamping, current-voltage analysis, the measurement of intracellular ion activities, and patch-clamping, some of which involve double- or even multiple-barrelled microelectrodes. Excellent reviews of these techniques already exist (e.g., Purves, 1981; Blatt, 1991a; Ogden, 1994; and other chapters in this volume). Here only a brief review of some of the main aspects of microelectrode use will be given.

Microelectrodes are prepared from glass tubing, generally about 1 to 2 mm in diameter, by stretching it by a controlled pull while a short length of the tube is heated in a controlled micro-furnace. The precise physical characteristics of the micropipette and hence its suitability for a particular purpose depend on a number of factors such as the temperature of the micro-furnace, the length of the heating period, the strength and duration of the pull, and its timing in relation to the heating period. Obtaining the correct settings of the analogue controls available on many electrode pullers is often difficult, and even with the newer digitally controlled ones sharing the puller with other people can be a major test of character.

Filling the microelectrode with the electrolyte solution has become much easier since the introduction of glass tubing containing an internal glass wick. The electrolyte filling solution has commonly been 3 *M* KCl, but more dilute KCl or other salts have been used especially with small cells where leakage of KCl into the cell could be injurious. Electrical contact from the amplifier to the electrolyte solution in the microelectrode can be achieved by several methods: via a chlorided silver wire dipping into the solution in the electrode; via a narrow salt bridge that connects the electrolyte solution to a calomel or chlorided silver electrode; or by holding the microelectrode in a miniature chamber that contains a chlorided silver contact and is filled with the same electrolyte solution as is in the electrode. Because of the small diameter of the electrode tip, the resistance of a microelectrode is generally in the range 10 to 100 MΩ, i.e., much higher than the resistances of surface contact electrodes.

The second, or reference, connection to the amplifier is usually achieved by a salt bridge that connects the medium bathing the tissue to a calomel or silver/silver chloride electrode. A chlorided silver wire dipping directly into the bathing medium can be used, but any change in the Cl^- ion composition of the bathing medium will cause a change in the measured pd.

Electrophysiology with microelectrodes is much more expensive than with surface contact electrodes because of the extra equipment required. This includes a microelectrode puller; a micromanipulator for precise positioning of the microelectrode in the tissue or cell; a microscope to see where the microelectrode tip is going; and equipment to suppress mechanical disturbance due to vibrations in the structure of the laboratory. The latter can range from tables made from heavy steel plates resting on thick rubber pads or motorcycle inner tubes to much more expensive commerical antivibration tables. Also the high resistance of microelectrodes requires more expensive amplifiers with high input impedances (1 to 10 GΩ or more). Techniques such as current clamping, voltage-clamping, patch-clamping, and work with ion-selective microelectrodes require still more complicated and expensive amplifiers and associated electronics.

Because of the small size of the microelectrode tip and the poor optics when using tissues it is usually not possible to see the precise location of the tip in a plant cell. Previously it was believed that most insertions would result in the tip entering the vacuole. More recent observations of the locations of dyes injected through micropipettes suggest rather that the tip is usually located in the cytoplasm, e.g., Oparka and Prior (1992).

Measurements of membrane resistance and its variation in different experimental conditions can, in principle, give useful information about the mechanism of ion transport across the membrane. The fact that in most plant tissues the cells are electrically connected to their neighbors by plasmodesmata produces two problems for measurements of plasma membrane resistance. First, the effective resistance of a number of electrically interconnected cells is small compared with that of a microelectrode. This problem can be overcome by the use of a double-barrelled microelectrode, one barrel being used to pass current pulses of known magnitudes and the other serving to measure the resulting changes in membrane pd. The second problem is that the membrane area, whose resistance is being measured, is unknown. For this reason resistance measurements have been confined to cells that occur naturally as individuals or that can be isolated from their tissues, or to cells such as stomatal guard cells that are not electrically connected to their neighbors.

III. Critical Aspects of the Procedure

Three aspects of procedure that require special care are earthing of equipment, elimination of electrical interference, and elimination of mechanical disturbance or vibrations. Problems arising from lack of care are much more serious with microelectrodes than with surface contact electrodes because of the much higher electrical resistance of the former and for the need to form and maintain an electrically good seal between the microelectrode and the membrane it has penetrated.

The principal function of good earthing is safety. The outer case of each item of equipment powered from the mains supply must be connected to earth, preferably via the earth component of its own mains line. Earth potential also provides a reference potential for amplifiers and other signal processing equipment. Finally, any metal objects such as microscope, micromanipulator, or metal base plate near the experimental system should be earthed to minimize electrostatic interference. Earthing of such objects should be made by leads branching out from one primary earth point.

Electrical interference, i.e., unwanted electrical signals that arise outside the experimental system and that may obscure the electrical events being studied, can arise in several ways. Random spikes or more regular signals can originate in the operation or switching on or off of electrical equipment elsewhere in the vicinity and reach the experimental system via the mains power supply. Often this can be prevented by using mains plugs with appropriate electrical filters. A major source of interference is alternating electrical fields originating in mains power lines in and around the laboratory. The experimental system including the electrodes and the leads running from them to the amplifier can act as a receiving aerial, and pick up a continuous mains-frequency oscillating signal that appears in the recorded pd. The magnitude of this interfering signal depends on the proximity of the mains power lines to the experimental system, and the resistance of the experimental system and electrodes and their physical dimensions. There are several ways of trying to minimize this kind of interference; mains lines running close to the experimental system can be enclosed in earthed braided metal sleeves; leads connecting the electrodes to the amplifier should be kept short—for this reason amplifiers intended for use with microelectrodes usually have a small preamplifier that can be mounted close to, or form part of, the microelectrode holder; the experimental system can be enclosed within a Faraday cage, an earthed enclosure made of metal sheet or mesh and from which mains power lines are excluded; illumination inside the cage can be provided by DC powered lamps or by fiber optic systems; amplifiers can be powered by batteries rather than the mains supply.

Alternating magnetic fields arising in electric motors or transformers can also cause electrical interference by inducing currents in the leads between the amplifier and the experimental system. The frequency of this interference is often two or three times that of the mains frequency and its magnitude is proportional to the area of the "loop" enclosed by the leads from the electrodes to the amplifier. This kind of interference can be minimized by moving motors and transformers away from the amplifier and experimental system and by arranging that the leads from the experimental system to the amplifier follow a common path for as much of their length as possible. Interference of this kind can also arise through interaction of magnetic fields with conducting loops involving both the amplifier leads and various earth connections—earth loops. Such loops can be physically much bigger than those formed by the amplifier leads above and they may, therefore, cause much greater interference. These loops may also be very difficult to identify because they may involve connections inside the amplifier and display device as well as earth connections that do not have any obvious connection with the signal processing circuitry.

An excellent discussion of earthing and interference problems and of measures that can be taken to counter problems caused by vibrations and mechanical disturbance is given by Purves (1981). As a general rule, it is best to assume that, in work with microelectrodes, care should be taken with earthing and the arrangement of leads from electrodes to amplifier, that a Faraday cage should be used, and that some kind of antivibration support will be needed. For measurements involving surface contact electrodes only, the much lower resistance of the experimental system and its lower sensitivity to mechanical disturbance mean that problems due to interference and vibration will be much less. Care should be taken with earthing and the arrangement of leads, and leads from electrodes to amplifier should be made from cable that incorporates an earthed metal braid sleeve. The experimenter can then explore what further precautions are needed in a particular experimental system. A Faraday cage may be necessary, but can be awkward to use in experiments involving whole plants and physiologically appropriate levels of illumination.

Faults can develop in any electrophysiological system and fault tracing should be carried out in a logical manner. Purves (1981) describes a routine for discovering the cause of mains frequency interference. The appearance of instability in the measured pd can indicate the deterioration of an electrical contact resulting in a high resistance somewhere in the experimental system, or can be due to a fault in the amplifier or display device, while inability to obtain a measurement at all can indicate a complete break in electrical continuity in the experimental system (or the fact that the power supply is not switched on!). First, one should check that all obvious electrical contacts are clean and well made. If the fault still persists the various components can be checked one by one, starting with the electrodes that are the most likely source of faults. The electrodes plus plant or tissue can be replaced by electrical resistors of appropriate magnitude (~10 MΩ for a microelectrode, ~10 kΩ for a surface contact electrode), the continuity of the leads from the electrodes to the amplifier can be checked, and the operation of the amplifier and display system can be checked by applying known pds to their inputs. For these simple tests every laboratory should be eqiupped with a good multimeter for measuring resistance, continuity, and voltage, and with a battery-powered calibrated voltage source that can deliver a range of known pds up to about 200 mV.

IV. Results and Discussion

For the past 40 years most electrophysiological studies on plants have involved the use of microelectrode techniques that, in their various forms, have been widely used to study ion transport at the cell and membrane levels. One of the earliest results of this work was the confirmation that a permeability barrier existed between cytoplasm and cell wall, a matter that was still in dispute in the early 1950s. A second important result was the discovery that the pd across the plasma membrane had a large electrogenic component, which is now known to be due to an outward proton pump.

For technical reasons detailed electrophysiological work proceeded more rapidly with studies on giant algal cells (Tazawa *et al.,* 1987; Beilby, 1989) than with higher plant cells but in recent years microelectrode experiments have been important in improving our understanding of the ion transport processes involved in the functioning of stomatal guard cells (e.g., Blatt, 1991b; Thiel *et al.,* 1992). Microelectrode experiments on other higher plant cell types have not yet provided the same level of detailed information about ion transport processes, but they are useful for investigating the changes in ion transport that occur in a wide range of physiological events. These can be studied by other techniques such as the measurement of radioisotope fluxes and chemical analysis but the electrophysiological approach can give continuous monitoring with good time resolution and is nondestructive. The application of patch-clamp techniques to isolated protoplasts and vacuoles is proving to be a very valuable tool for the study of ion transport processes in the plasma membrane and tonoplast and has led to the discovery and characterization of a wide variety of types of ion channels in those membranes.

Experiments with surface contact electrodes measure the pd between two points in the apoplast of the plant. Ionic currents leading to changes in this pd originate in ion movements at the plasma membranes of cells in the tissue but, because of the large distance in cellular dimensions over which the pd is measured, the observed change in pd can have a more complex shape and different magnitude from that occurring at any individual cell in the tissue. It is therefore usually difficult to relate changes in the observed pd to changes in particular ion transports in particular cells. However, it has recently been shown that, in some circumstances, measurements with surface contact electrodes on intact plants can give quite accurate estimates of changes in pd across the plasma membrane of cells in the underlying tissues (references in Thain and Wildon, 1994). The pd changes observed with surface contact electrodes can consist of rapid transients of a few seconds duration, slower changes lasting several minutes, or combinations of these. In some cases (see Thain and Wildon, 1994 for references) evidence obtained with intracellular microelectrodes confirms that the rapid transients represent action potentials propagating through the plant. This is probably true of other cases where microelectrode evidence is lacking and especially where the rapid transients result from electrical stimulation or noninjurious stimulation such as the localized application of ice-cold water. The slower transients, often called "variation potentials," may represent local electrical effects of substances moving through the vascular system of the plant from, e.g., the site of a wound.

The primary use of surface contact electrodes is for monitoring electrical events in the whole plant or in plant organs; the methods are simple and the equipment required is relatively inexpensive. In particular, surface contact electrodes have been used for investigating electrical events that propagate through the plant in response to stimuli such as touch, electrical stimulation, and wounding [reviews by Simons (1992), Thain and Wildon (1993), Thain and Wildon (1994)]. Thus surface contact electrodes can be used to survey the occurrence of electrical events in plants and to investigate their relationships to various stimuli and physiological functions. However, microelectrode experiments are necessary for a more detailed understanding of the cellular events underlying these processes, as is shown by studies aimed at identifying the cells that constitute the electrical signaling pathways of *Mimosa* (Samejima and Sibaoka, 1983) and tomato seedlings (Rhodes, Thain, and Wildon, submitted for publication); in both cases cells in the phloem tissues are involved. An interesting example of the combined use of surface contact electrodes and microelectrodes in the same experiments is provided by the work of Okamoto and colleagues on the relationship between metabolism, ion transport, and plant growth (Ikoma and Okamoto *et al.,* 1988).

V. Conclusion and Perspectives

The range of electrophysiological techniques employed by plant biologists has widened significantly in the past 10 years. Ion-selective microelectrodes and patch-clamping have already added much to our understanding of plant cell biology and it is clear that their contribution will increase greatly in the future. Conventional microelectrode studies will continue to be limited by difficulties due to the electrical interconnectedness of most cells in plant tissues unless some means can be found of blocking plasmodesmata without other undesirable effects taking place, at least in the short term.

Although measurements with surface contact electrodes cannot, in general, give detailed information about events at the cell level, they are useful as a means of uncovering phenomena that can then be studied in detail by microelectrode methods. This will be especially important if long distance electrical signaling is more common in plants than has generally been believed (Wildon *et al.,* 1992).

References

Beilby, M. J. (1989). Electrophysiology of giant algal cells. *In* "Methods of Enzymology" (S. Fleischer and B. Fleischer, eds.), Vol. 174, pp. 403–443. San Diego/London: Academic Press.

Blatt, M. R. (1991a). A primer in plant electrophysiological methods. *In* "Methods in Plant Biochemistry" (K. Hostettmann, ed.), Vol. 6, pp. 281–321. London: Academic Press.

Blatt, M. R. (1991b). Ion channel gating in plants: Physiological implications and integration for stomatal function. *J. Membr. Biol.* **124,** 95–112.

Dainty, J. (1962). Ion transport and electric potentials in plant cells. *Annu. Rev. Plant Physiol.* **13,** 379–402.

Etherton, B., and Higinbotham, N. (1960). Transmembrane potential measurements of cells of higher plants as related to salt uptake. *Science* **131,** 409–410.

Findlay, G. P., and Hope, A. B. (1976). Electrical propterties of plant cells: Methods and findings. *In* "Encyclopaedia of Plant Physiology, Transport in Plants II, Part A: Cells" (U. Lüttge and M. G. Pitman, eds.), pp. 53–92. Heidelberg and New York: Springer.

Geddes, L. A. (1972). Electrodes and the measurement of bioelectric events. New York: Wiley–Interscience.

Hope, A. B., and Walker, N. A. (1975). The physiology of giant algal cells. Cambridge: Cambridge University Press.

Ikoma, S., and Okamoto, H. (1988). The quantitative and chronological relationship between IAA-induced H^+-pump activation and elongation growth studied by means of xylem perfusion. *Plant Cell Physiol.* **29,** 261–267.

Ogden, D. (1994). Microelectrode techniques. Cambridge: The Company of Biologists.

Oparka, K. J., and Prior, D. A. M. (1992). Direct evidence for pressure-generated closure of plasmodesmata. *Plant J.* **2,** 741–750.

Paszewski, A., and Zawadzki, T. (1973). Action potentials in *Lupinus angustifolius* L. shoots. *J. Exp. Bot.* **24,** 804–809.

Pickard, B. G. (1973). Action potentials in higher plants. *Bot. Rev.* **39,** 172–201.

Pickard, B. G. (1974). Electrical signals in higher plants. *Naturwissenschaften* **61,** 60–64.

Purves, R. D. (1981). Microelectrode methods for intracellular recording and ionophoresis. London: Academic Press.

Samejima, M., and Sibaoka, T. (1983). Identification of excitable cells in the petiole of *Mimosa pudica* by intracellular injection of procion yellow. *Plant Cell Physiol.* **24,** 33–39.

Shiina, T., and Tazawa, M. (1986). Action potential in *Luffa cylindlica* and its effects on elongation growth. *Plant Cell Physiol.* **27,** 1081–1089.

Simons, P. (1992). "The Action Plant." Oxford: Blackwell.

Tazawa, M., Shimmen, T., and Mimura, T. (1987). Membrane control in the Characeae. *Annu. Rev. Plant Physiol.* **38,** 95–117.

Thain, J. F., and Wildon, D. C. (1993). Electrical signalling in plants. *In* "Plant signals in Interactions with other Organisms" (J. C. Schultz and I. Raskin, eds.). Rockville, Maryland: Amer. Soc. Plant Physiologists.

Thain, J. F., and Wildon, D. C. (1994). Electrical signalling in plants. *Sci. Prog.* **76,** 553–564.

Thiel, G., MacRobbie, E. A. C., and Blatt, M. R. (1992). Membrane transport in stomatal guard cells: The importance of voltage control. *J. Membr. Biol.* **126,** 1–18.

Walker, N. A. (1955). Microelectrode experiments on Nitella. *Aust. J. Biol. Sci.* **8,** 476–489.

Wildon, D. C., Thain, J. F., Minchin, P. H., Gubb, I. R., Reilly, A. J., Skipper, Y. D., Doherty, H. M., O'Donnell, P. J., and Bowles, D. J. (1992). Electrical signalling and systemic proteinase inhibitor induction in the wounded plant. *Nature* (*London*) **360,** 62–65.

Zawadzki, T., Davies, E., Dziubinska, H., and Trebacz, K. (1991). Characteristics of action potentials in *Helianthus annuus. Physiol. Plant* **83,** 601–604.

CHAPTER 19

Ion-Selective Microelectrodes for Measurement of Intracellular Ion Concentrations

A. J. Miller

Biochemistry and Physiology Department
Rothamsted Experimental Station
Harpenden Hertfordshire AL5 2JQ, United Kingdom

I. Introduction

A. Background

In order to understand how ion uptake and compartmentation are regulated in plants, it is necessary to measure the concentrations of ions in both the cytosol and the vacuole. Several types of single-cell or tissue-based techniques can be used for this purpose. This chapter describes one approach, the use of ion-specific microelectrodes.

Alternatives to microelectrodes include the use of fluorescent probes or dyes (Bush and Jones, 1990), nuclear magnetic resonance (Lee and Ratcliffe, 1991), tracer flux analysis (Pierce and Higinbotham, 1970), X-ray microanalysis (Hajibagheri *et al.,* 1988), and single-cell sap sampling (Malone *et al.,* 1989). The choice of technique depends on the type of information that is required. For higher plants, vacuolar ion concentrations can be estimated by chemical analysis of fully vacuolated tissues because the vacuole dominates such measurements (Jeschke and Stelter, 1976). The single-cell sampling technique removes vacuolar sap from individual cells, with enzymatic or X-ray microanalytical methods then being used to determine the concentrations of a range of ions in the sap (Malone *et al.,* 1989). However, this approach cannot be used to measure cytosolic ion concentrations and, in general, these are more difficult to obtain. Fluorescent probes are often used for probing cytosolic ion concentrations; this technique can also been used to study transport into the vacuole (Oparka, 1991). Various different dye types have been used to measure cytosolic ion concentrations, but calibration of the measurements can be difficult and compartmentalization of the fluorescent probe into the vacuole can complicate interpretation (Bush and Jones, 1990). Fluorescent probes are most appropriate for measurement of rapid changes in ion concentration, such as those occurring during intracellular signalling events. Nuclear magnetic resonance (NMR) can also be used to measure intracellular ion concentrations (Lee and Ratcliffe, 1991), but this technique averages signals from the whole tissue. It should be noted that, in contrast to ion-selective microelectrodes, these techniques either are all destructive or do not allow single cell measurements of both the cytosol and the vacuole.

Ion-selective microelectrodes all conform to the same basic design, in which a hydrophobic ion-selective membrane plugs the tip of a glass micropipette, and the ion-dependent electrical potential is measured across this barrier. Some of the most commonly used sensors for constructing ion-selective electrodes are listed in Table I; in principle, all of these sensors can be used to make microelectrodes suitable for measurements within cells. An aqueous salt solution fills the rest of the pipette behind this membrane and provides a low-resistance path to the half-cell, which is usually a AgCl-coated silver wire or pellet. The ion-selectivity of the membrane plug gives an output voltage dependent upon the activity of the ion bathing the tip. By calibrating this voltage with a series of solutions of the ion, a measurement of ion activity can be obtained when the tip is immersed into solutions containing an unknown concentration of the ion.

One advantage of ion-selective microelectrode measurements is that they enable the calculation of the electrical gradients that exist across membranes *in vivo;* this information is essential for the determination of electrochemical gradients. Furthermore, multibarrelled microelectrodes can be used to measure simultaneously several different ions (Coles and Orkand, 1985), and we have recently used

Table I
Types of Ion-Selective Microelectrode Sensors and Some of Their Properties

Ion	Sensor molecule(s)	Detection limit	Major interfering ions in plant cells
Ammonium	Nonactin[a]	2 μM	K^+
Calcium	ETH 129	10 nM	H^+, K^+, Mg^{2+}
	ETH 1001	40 nM	H^+, K^+, Mg^{2+}
Chloride	Mn(III)TPPC[b]	1–5 mM	Acetate, HCO_3^-, SCN^-, NO_3^- pH >7.6
Proton	Tridodecylamine	>pH 9	K^+
	ETH 1907	pH 9	K^+
Potassium	Valinomycin	100 μM	Ca^{2+}, NH_4^+
Magnesium	ETH 5214	200 μM	Ca^{2+}, K^+
Sodium	ETH 227[a]	3 mM	Ca^{2+}, H^+, K^+
	ETH 157[a]	2 mM	H^+, K^+
Nitrate	MTDDA · NO_3[c]	0.5 mM	Cl^-, NO_2^-, SCN^-

[a] Data from Fluka Chemicals.

[b] Mn(III)TPPC, 5,10,15,20-tetraphenyl-21H,23H-porphin manganese(III) chloride (6).

[c] MTDDA · NO_3, methyl-tridodecylammonium nitrate (Miller and Zhen, 1991). The detection limits quoted are from calibration in solutions approximating to cytoplasmic composition, values will also depend on the tip diameter but the values above are for tips less than 1 μm in diameter. Lower detection limits are possible for extracellular measurements where larger tip diameters can be used. All the sensor molecules (or the precursor for synthesis for MTDDA.NO_3) can be obtained from Fluka Chemicals.

triple-barrelled microelectrodes (Fig. 1) for measuring pH and either K^+ or NO_3^- concentration in barley root cells (D. Walker, S. J. Smith and A. J. Miller, unpublished results). Ion-selective electrodes can also be used to measure ion fluxes at the surfaces of tissues either directly (Henriksen *et al.*, 1990) or when used as vibrating probes (Kühtreiber and Jaffe, 1990).

When impaling a cell, the situation is complicated by the cell membrane potential, because the output from the ion-selective electrode now reports this voltage plus that due to the activity of the ion. In order to obtain the voltage due to the ion alone, the cell membrane voltage must be subtracted from the output. This is done by using an electrode that combines a cell-voltage reporting electrode and one or several ion-selective microelectrodes into a single tip (Fig. 1). Voltage outputs from all barrels are measured against a common reference ground electrode in the external solution. These multibarrelled fluid or liquid membrane electrodes have generally replaced and surpassed the earlier types of ion-selective electrode, which were either solid-state (pH or chloride electrodes, Coster, 1966) or ion-selective glass electrodes with recessed tips (Sanders and Slayman, 1982). The methodology described here is restricted to the manufacture of such fluid or liquid membrane electrodes.

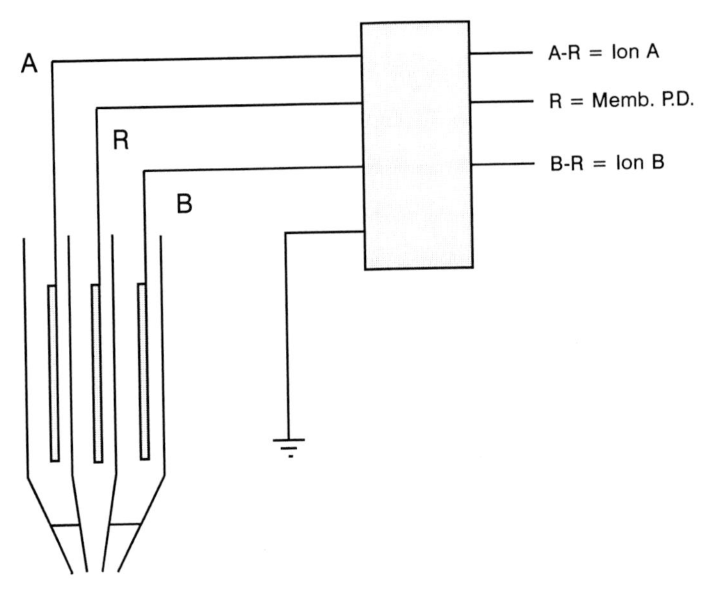

Fig. 1 Diagrammatic representation of a triple-barrelled ion-selective microelectrode. Barrels A and B are ion-selective, whereas barrel R is the KCl-filled reference barrel.

One criticism of intracellular measurements made with microelectrodes is that they report the ion activity at a single point in the cell, resulting in incomplete information if significant ion gradients occur within the cell. Measurements with ion-selective microelectrodes are most appropriate for cells at the surface of tissues or in single cells because impaling does not involve any damage to cells overlying the cell of interest; cells that are found deeper in tissues can only be reached by first damaging outer layers of cells. When measurements are obtained for cells deeper in a tissue, local wound responses may give changes in ion distribution within the cell. Ion-selective microelectrode measurements can also be used to follow the dynamics of changes in cell ion activities. A single electrode can continue to measure ion activity for up to an hour; however, the longer the impalement the less likely it is to recalibrate. This can be overcome by making many individual measurements on different cells of a single tissue following the application of a particular treatment.

B. Theory

An ideal ion-selective microelectrode should show a linear relationship between the electrode voltage and the log of the ion activity. This relationship is described mathematically by the Nernst equation:

$$E_{io} = E' + \frac{RT}{zF} \ln\left[\frac{[A]_o}{[A]_i}\right], \tag{1}$$

where E_{io} is the potential difference in mV between the inside (i) to outside (o) solutions (referenced to the outside), E' is a constant reference potential, z is the valence of ion A, square brackets designate the activity of A, and R, T, and F have their conventional meanings. In an ion-selective microelectrode, the ion activity of the inside represents the backfilling solution and so is maintained constant. So, for an ion-selective electrode, Eq. (1) can be rewritten and simplified to the following form for a monovalent cation at 25°C:

$$E_{io} = E' + 59 \log[A^+]_o. \tag{2}$$

Equation (2) predicts that, for a perfect ion-selective microelectrode calibrated with a range of standard solutions, the resulting output of the electrode should increase linearly with the log of the A ion concentration, with a slope of 59 mV at 25°C. In practice, the situation is more complicated because no ion-selective electrode has ideal selectivity for one particular ion and under most conditions (particularly within cells) there is more than one ion present in the sample solution. These other ions will interfere with the measurements and contribute to the overall voltage output from the electrode and this must be taken into account. This is done by using the Nicolsky–Eisenman equation, a modified Nernst equation:

$$E_{io} = E' + s \log\,[A_o + K_{AB}\,(B)^{zA/zB}], \tag{3}$$

where, K_{AB} is the selectivity coefficient of the electrode for the ion A with respect to ion B. It expresses on a molar basis the relative contributions of ions A and B to the measured output electrical potential difference. The parameter s is the slope of the linear portion of the calibration curve (see Fig. 2) and the parameters

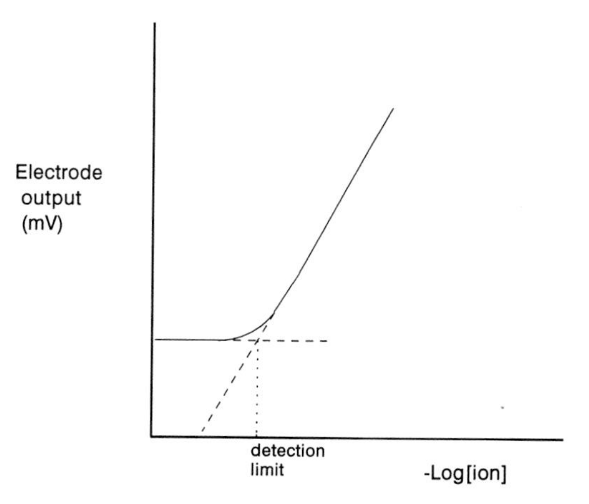

Fig. 2 Electrode output plotted against log ion activity showing the definition of "detection limit."

s and K_{AB} are the two main characteristics defining any type of ion-selective electrode. The selectivity coefficient, K_{AB}, can be determined in several different ways:

1. The fixed interference method involves measuring the electrode response with solutions of constant level of interference (ion B), while varying the activity of the primary ion (A). The voltage output is plotted against the activity of the primary ion and the intersection of the extrapolation of the linear portions of the curve (Fig. 2) will indicate the value of A, which is to be used to calculate K_{AB} from

$$K_{AB} = [A]/[B]^{zA/zB}. \tag{4}$$

2. The fixed primary ion method involves varying the concentration of the interfering ion B at a constant concentration of the primary ion A. This method is the reverse of the fixed interference method but is less commonly used.

3. The separate solution method involves measuring the electrode output with each of two separate solutions, one containing ion A and the other containing ion B at the same activity. The measured output voltages for each single ion solution are E_A and E_B, the value of K_{AB} may be calculated from

$$\log K_{AB} = \frac{E_B - E_A}{2.303RT/z_A} \frac{+}{F} (1\text{-}z_A/z_B)\log A. \tag{5}$$

This method is simple, but unfortunately the selectivity data are often not representative of those for sample solutions containing several ions.

A value of K_{AB} of less than 1 indicates a preference for the measuring ion relative to the interfering ion. However, the value obtained depends both on the method used to determine K_{AB} and on the conditions under which the measurements are made. The fixed interference method is most commonly used to calculate the selectivity coefficient, and it is the method recommended by the International Union of Pure and Applied Chemistry (Ammann, 1986). When stating a selectivity coefficient value, the method of determination should also be quoted.

Two additional parameters defining the properties of an ion-selective microelectrode are the response time and the detection limit. Response time may be important when measuring changes in ion activity. This parameter is dependent on many factors, including tip geometry and the resistance and composition of the ion-selective membrane. Response time can be measured during the calibration as the time taken for the voltage to adjust when ion activity at the tip is altered. The detection limit is the lowest ion activity that can be measured with certainty and it is defined by the intercept of the two extrapolated linear segments of the calibration curve (see Fig. 2), the same point as used in the fixed interference method for the calculation of K_{AB}. The detection limit is determined by the composition of the ion-selective membrane and the tip geometry. Smaller or thinner tips have higher detection limits, and composition alters limits in ways that can only be measured experimentally. The presence of interfering ions changes the detection limit, one example being the effect of chloride on the detection limit of nitrate-selective microelectrodes (Miller and Zhen, 1991). In this case, the detection limit changes from 0.03 to 0.5 m*M* when 100 m*M* chloride ions are added to the calibration solutions. Ion-selective electrodes should be used in the linear portion of the calibration curve. Below the detection limit, the interpretation of measurements is complicated by interfering ions.

II. Materials

A. Equipment

The equipment needed for intracellular measurements with ion-selective microelectrodes is similar to that for normal electrophysiological measurements in plant cells and general details have been described in reviews on electrophysiological methods (e.g. Blatt, 1991). The equipment comprises

1. Microscope with stage-mounted perfusion chamber
2. Electrometer with high input impedance
3. Micromanipulator
4. Faraday cage
5. PC microcomputer with A/D interface
6. Chart recorder
7. Electrode puller

Only a few special features of equipment for ion-selective microelectrode work will be described here and most of these are required because ion-selective microelectrodes have high impedances. The microscope is a fixed-stage type with a fiber-optic light source. The lamp must be located outside the Faraday cage to avoid electrical interference from its power cable. The chamber to hold tissue is mounted on the microscope stage and is designed so that the tissue can be continously perfused with the experimental nutrient solution throughout the measurement. This avoids developing a concentration gradient at the surface of the tissue. A high-impedance electrometer amplifier (e.g., World Precision Instruments, Model FD 223) is required because the ion-selective microelectrodes have very high resistances; the amplifier must have an input impedance at least 1000 times higher than the ion-selective electrode, e.g., $10^{15}\ \Omega$. Furthermore, the input leakage current from the electrometer must be low so that no significant offset voltage (>1 mV) is produced across the ion-selective electrode (this can usually be measured and adjusted on the electrometer). Other useful features include GΩ range resistance tester and a difference-voltage output, so that a direct output equivalent–cell ion activity can be obtained. The electrometer output can be passed to a chart recorder and also via an *A/D* converter to a microcomputer. Data handling and processing are greatly facilitated by software such as that developed by I. R. Jennings (Biology Department, University of York, UK) (Miller and Sanders, 1987). The only other items of equipment needed are an electrode puller and a heating lamp for silanizing electrodes.

Microelectrodes are made from capillary glass and suppliers of suitable glass include

1. Clark Electromedical Instruments (P.O. Box 8, Pangbourne, Reading RG8 7HU, UK)
2. Hilgenberg GmbH (Postfach 9, Malsfeld, D-3509 Germany)
3. World Precision Instruments (International Trade Center, 175 Sarasota Center Blvd. Sarasota, FL 34240-9258).

B. Chemicals

Dimethyldichlorosilane (Fluka 40136), 1% v/v silanizing agent in chloroform

Tetrahydrofuran (THF) (Sigma T5267)

Ion-selective cocktail (Fluka) with polyvinylchloride (PVC) added or your own mixed cocktail

PVC (high-molecular-weight polymer, Fluka 81392)

Nitrocellulose (Whatman 7184002)

III. Methods

The preparation of ion-selective microelectrodes can be divided into five main stages:

a. pulling of class micropipettes
b. silanization of the inside surface of the ion-selective electrode barrel
c. backfilling with ion-selective cocktail
d. backfilling with aqueous salt solution
e. calibration

A detailed method that is suitable for all of the different types of ion-selective microelectrode is described below. The background to each stage is described first. The method describes the fabrication of double-barrelled ion-selective microelectrodes with one ion-sensing barrel and one membrane potential measuring barrel. Multibarrelled electrodes are an extension of the same approach.

A. Pulling

Microelectrodes are made using an electrode puller that heats the glass and pulls it to a tip in a controlled way predetermined by the operator. Normally, electrodes are pulled to give shape and dimensions appropriate for impaling the intended cell type. Multiple-barrelled microelectrodes can be prepared by twisting together individual pieces of filamented borosilicate glass or using glass that is already fused together. The twisting is done using the electrode puller. The heating is paused while the various barrels are twisted around one another and then the heating and pulling continue. There are various different types of microelectrode pullers (Blatt, 1991). Their most important feature is reproducibility, which guarantees that, when an optimum microelectrode shape for a particular cell type has been made, it can be exactly reproduced many times.

Microelectrodes are usually made from borosilicate glass, but the harder aluminosilicate glass can also sometimes be used. Filamented glass that has a glass fiber attached to the inner wall is available; this fiber assists backfilling by providing a hydraulic duct along which the solution can flow by capillarity. Multibarrelled glass of varying dimensions is also available, and this type of glass is a popular choice for much ion-selective microelectrode work. Another type of double-barrelled glass called "theta" glass can be used; this has a thin glass wall between the two preformed barrels, so that in section it resembles the Greek letter from which it derives its name.

In all multibarrelled electrodes, adjacent barrels may mutually interfere because the thin glass walls between each barrel at the electrode tip may have an impedance similar to that of the liquid ion-exchanger. In this situation, the measured potential depends on the potential across the glass as well as the potential across the liquid ion-exchanger. This problem is more acute when theta glass is used, because the final glass partition in the tip of the pulled electrode is much thinner than that in electrodes formed from individual pieces of glass capillary. Fortunately, suppliers have become aware of this problem and now sell theta glass with a specially thickened partition or septum. Ideally, all barrels of glass should be filamented to assist with backfilling. Identification of the different barrels can be done by marking them or breaking them to different lengths. The latter method has the advantage of facilitating the electrical connections, through salt bridges and half-cells, to each barrel. Eye protection should be worn at all times when pulling and breaking glass.

Before making the ion-selective microelectrode, it is important to check that the glass microelectrodes of the chosen shape and dimensions can be used to impale cells and measure stable resting membrane potentials sensitive to metabolic inhibitors when backfilled with 0.1 *M* KCl (the size of the membrane potential will depend on the cell type and the bathing solution used). An estimate of the tip diameter of the microelectrode can be obtained by measuring its electrical resistance when filled with KCl; larger tips have lower resistances. For tips 0.1–2 μm in diameter, the electrical resistances of ion-selective microelectrodes are usually in the GΩ range, whereas microelectrodes filled with 0.1 *M* KCl and lacking the ion-sensing membrane have resistances in the MΩ range. The dimensions of the microelectrodes are commonly a compromise between obtaining a good calibration response (detection limit) and a stable membrane potential. Furthermore, the electrode response time is shortened by using larger tip diameters.

B. Silanizing

The inside of the glass micropipettes must be given a hydrophobic coating, to allow the formation of a high-resistance seal between the glass and the hydrophobic ion-selective membrane. The barrel chosen to receive the ion-selective membrane is silanized by placing a few drops of a solution of 1% (w/v) silanizing agent in chloroform on its blunt open end. Care must be taken to guard that the reagent does not enter the membrane potential-sensing barrel, because the tip of the silanized barrel cannot be backfilled with an aqueous solution. There are a range of different silanizing agents that can be employed at this concentration, but dimethyldichlorosilane or tributylchlorosilane is often used. These reagents are corrosive and toxic; protective glasses and gloves must be worn and glass must be treated in a fume hood. To complete the process, the microelectrode is placed under a heating lamp giving a temperature of 120°C at the micropipette surface. The silanizing solution quickly vaporises, giving the ion-selective barrel a hydrophobic coating. After silanization there should be no liquid deposits remaining in the microelectrode tip.

C. Backfilling with Sensor Cocktail

There are two stages to backfilling; the first employs a cocktail to form the ion-selective membrane in the microelectrode tip, and the second involves backfilling with an aqueous salt solution (see Section III, D). Both steps are greatly simplified through fabricating the electrodes from filamented glass and can be done using a glass syringe and fine needle (30-gauge).

The electrodes are backfilled with the sensor cocktail containing

1. An ion-selective sensor or exchanger
2. Membrane plasticizer or solvent
3. Additives, for example, lipophilic cation or anion, to improve response characteristics
4. A membrane matrix to solidify the ion-selective membrane.

For most types of ion-selective microelectrode, the membrane cocktail can be purchased in premixed form. Alternatively, the individual components can be bought from chemical suppliers and assembled in the laboratory; such cocktails are both simple and cheap. For commercially available liquid membrane cocktails, the membrane matrix is not always included. A matrix is essential if microelectrodes are to be used in plant cells, since turgor will displace a liquid membrane from the electrode tip, thereby changing or eliminating the sensitivity to the measuring ion (Felle and Bertl, 1986; Sanders and Miller, 1986; Reid and

Smith, 1988). The matrix is typically high-molecular-weight PVC, but can also contain nitrocellulose for additional strength.

Of all of the components in the cocktail, the ion-selective sensor is the main determinant of the electrode properties (e.g., slope, selectivity, limit of detection). However, the membrane solvent can also affect electrode lifetime, stability, and selectivity. Furthermore, membrane additives, such as lipophilic ions, can be used to improve the performance of microelectrodes. The roles played by each component are described by Ammann (1986). The optimum cocktail composition is found through trial-and-error, by testing electrode performance as a function of cocktail formulation (Zhen *et al.,* 1992). Good electrodes should have a near-ideal slope, a low detection limit, and a small selectivity coefficient for physiologically important interfering ions.

D. Backfilling with Salt Solution

The second backfilling step, usually done a minimum of 48 h later, uses an aqueous salt solution to provide electrical contact between this membrane and the Ag/AgCl metal electrode (in the base of the microelectrode holder). During the 48-h period, the membrane solvent (usually THF) evaporates, leaving a solid membrane plug in the tip of the designated ion-selective barrel. Backfilling can be achieved using a fine needle and syringe, or using a plastic disposable pipette tip that has been gently heated and pulled out into a slender capillary suitable for inserting inside the glass barrel from the blunt end. It is important to try to dislodge all the air from the interface between the ion-selective membrane and the backfilling solution; this can be done using a human hair inserted from the blunt end.

E. Calibration

Ion-selective microelectrodes can be calibrated in either concentration or activity units. The electrodes actually respond to changes in activity (see Introduction), and this is the meaningful parameter for all biochemical reactions and thermodynamic calculations. Therefore, calibrating with ion activity provides a microelectrode output that can be used directly without making assumptions concerning the intracellular activity coefficient for the ion. The calibration of microelectrodes normally uses solutions that resemble the intracellular environment, in terms of pH, interfering ions, and ionic strength. Calibration of pH-selective microelectrodes is easy because standard pH buffers can be used and directly checked with a pH meter. For other types of ion-selective microelectrodes, the calibration solutions may require inclusion of a pH buffer and a background salt solution, to give an ionic strength approximately equivalent to that within the cell. Care must be taken in the choice of the salts added to control ionic strength; they must not give significant interference with measurement of the ion of interest over its likely activity range in the cell. In other words, the microelectrodes must have very small selectivity coefficients for these background ions. The calibration solutions are usually chosen to be approximately 0.14 *M* ionic strength based on the ionic strength of animal cell cytoplasm (Tsien and Rink, 1981). There are few examples of whole sap analysis to provide hints about what an appropriate figure might be for plant cells, but from measurements of giant algal cells this value would seem plausible (Okihara and Kiyosawa, 1988). Computer software can be used to calculate ion activity and the availability of a wide range of ion-selective macroelectrodes makes it easier to prepare calibration solutions for all types of ion-selective microelectrodes. Calibration solution recipes for some ion-selective microelectrodes have been published (Ca^{2+}: Tsien and Rink, 1981; Mg^{2+}: Blatter and McGuigan, 1988; NO_3^-: Miller and Zhen, 1991). However, some calibration solutions use *concentration* not *activity,* and also the term "free" ion usually means concentration of unbound ion and not activity, particularly for Ca^{2+} and Mg^{2+}. The calibration of calcium-selective microelectrodes for intracellular measurements requires the use of calcium buffering agents such as EGTA, because of the very low concentrations being measured (Tsien and Rink, 1981).

Calibration of the ion-selective microelectrode can be performed in the microscope chamber within which the intracellular measurements will be done, or in a U-shaped glass funnel near the microscope. It should be noted, finally, that the slope of the calibration curve is temperature-sensitive, and both calibrations and intracellular measurements should be done at the same temperature [see Eq. (1)]. For example, if the temperature of the calibration solutions is 4°C and the cell is at 20°C, the gradient of the electrode calibration for a monovalent ion will be 55 mV per decade change in activity, not the 58 mV expected at 20°C. As a result, intracellular ion activities will be miscalculated.

F. General Methodology for the Preparation of Ion-Selective Microelectrodes

1. An electrode puller is used to pull and twist multibarrelled glass microelectrodes suitable for measuring stable membrane potentials in the preferred type of cell. These will usually be double-barrelled if a single compartment is to be measured. Triple-barrelled electrodes incorporating a pH-sensitive electrode may be needed if cytoplasm and vacuole are to be distinguished, particularly when it is suspected that these two compartments may have similar ion activities. The following steps describe procedures for double-barrelled microelectrodes.

2. One barrel should be broken back to give a short barrel, which will be the membrane potential recording barrel. The barrel can be broken back using square-ended pliers or a razor blade on the edge of a metal plate (wear safety glasses). A razor blade is best used with double-barrelled glass that has one barrel of a smaller diameter. Pressure should be applied at the joint between the two barrels causing the smaller barrel to snap.

3. Dry the microelectrodes by placing them on the edge of an aluminium block under a heating lamp for at least 30 min before silanizing (temperature under lamp 120°C).

4. A disposable syringe and 25-gauge needle is used to introduce the silanizing agent into the blunt end of the longer barrel, which will become the ion-selective barrel. *Warning:* work in a fume hood, because the silanizing vapor is corrosive and noxious. The double-barrelled micropipette is placed under the lamp for a further 30 min.

5. If the ion-selective cocktail has been bought ready-mixed and does not contain PVC or nitrocellulose, one or both should be added by first dissolving these matrix components in 4 vol of THF, and then mixing them with the commercial cocktail. The quantity of PVC can range from 10 to 30% (w/w) and nitrocellulose 5% (w/w) of the final cocktail composition, when the THF has evaporated.

6. Backfill the ion-selective barrel of the microelectrode with the cocktail dissolved in THF/PVC mixture. Use a glass syringe (1 ml) and an all-metal 30-gauge needle (Scientific Laboratory Supplies Ltd.).

7. The microelectrodes must then be stored, tip down, in a silica-gel-dried environment for at least 48 h. During this time most of the THF evaporates leaving a solvent-cast membrane plug in the tip of the designated ion-selective barrel.

8. When the THF solvent has evaporated, the ion-selective barrel can be backfilled with an aqueous salt solution containing the ion to be measured. The second barrel, to measure the membrane potential, is usually backfilled with 0.1 *M* KCl using an all-metal 30-gauge needle and plastic syringe.

9. Most types of ion-selective microelectrode require "conditioning" for a minimum of 30 min by immersing the tip in a solution containing a high concentration (e.g., 100 m*M*) of the ion to be measured.

10. The blunt ends of double-barrelled electrodes are connected to the amplifier headstage using Ag/AgCl half-cells. The ion-selective barrel can be directly inserted into a half-cell, whereas the second barrel can be connected via a plastic tubing 0.1 *M* KCl-filled salt bridge.

11. Microelectrode calibration can be done in the chamber built to take the plant tissue, or using a U-shaped funnel.

Special points for the manufacture of triple-barrelled electrodes:

1. When using more than one type of cocktail, be sure to use a different syringe for each. It is best to devote a syringe for use with one particular cocktail only, and thus avoid any contamination by other ion sensors.

2. Backfill one ion-selective barrel, then wait at least 48 h before backfilling the second one; this avoids the mixing of the two ion-selective cocktails at the barrel tip.

G. General Practical Tips

1. Handle microelectrodes using forceps.

2. When dispensing THF, pour a few milliliters from the stock bottle into a clean glass beaker previously rinsed with THF. Cover the beaker with parafilm,

then dispense more THF using an all-metal needle and glass syringe by piercing the film with the needle; this helps to reduce solvent vapor and prevents contamination of THF.

3. When calibrating, start with the highest concentration and calibrate only in the range in which you expect to be working. There is little point in unnecessarily exposing electrodes to low ion concentrations, since most types of ion-selective membrane respond badly to long exposures to very low concentrations.

IV. Results

A. Intracellular Measurements

Several rules for acceptable measurements can be defined. After impalement, the ion-selective microelectrode should be recalibrated and should give a response very similar to that obtained before the cell impalement, particularly at activities similar to those measured *in vivo*. Sometimes the recalibration shows a displacement up or down the *Y* axis (mV output). More usually, the detection limit of the ion-selective microelectrode changes but, provided the measurement was within the linear response range of the electrode calibration curve, this is not a reason to disregard the result. Sometimes the performance of the ion-selective microelectrode can even improve with the detection limit actually becoming lower. For this reason, it can be an advantage to impale swiftly a cell with a new tip before calibrating and prior to measuring ion activity in another cell. A comparison between the electrical resistance of the ion-selective microelectrode before and after an impalement gives a good indication whether the tip will recalibrate. If the resistance declines below 1 GΩ, the ion-selective membrane has probably been dislodged during impalement and the electrode will not recalibrate. Throughout the recording, the state of the cell can be evaluated by monitoring the membrane potential (which should remain steady unless intentionally altered) or intracellular processes like cytoplasmic streaming, if visible.

When measuring changes in intracellular ion concentrations, artifacts can be caused by the differential response times of the two barrels; the ion-selective barrel normally has a slower response time than the membrane potential-sensing barrel. Compensation can be made for these differences if the response time of the electrode is known (Sanders and Slayman, 1982). The electrode response time can limit detection of rapid changes in ion activity, such as the changes in cytosolic [Ca^{2+}] occurring during signaling events.

Identifying the intracellular compartment (cytoplasm or vacuole) in which the microelectrode tip is located can be a problem for some ions, particularly if they are at similar concentrations in both compartments. In such cases, it may be possible to grow the plant under conditions in which two populations of measurements can be identified. Alternatively, a triple-barrelled microelectrode can be used where one barrel is pH- or Ca^{2+}-selective (see methods for triple-barrelled electrode manufacture). Large gradients of these two ions are known to exist across the tonoplast, with the cytoplasm maintained at relatively constant values (pH 7.2, Ca^{2+} 100 n*M*), whereas the vacuole has higher ion concentrations (pH 5–5.5, Ca^{2+} m*M*). These differences thus make compartment identfication possible. Another approach is to use tissues where the two major cell compartments can be identified under the microscope, e.g., root hairs or cell cultures that have no large vacuole. However, identifying which compartment the electrode is in can still be troublesome, particularly if the electrode deforms the tonoplast but does not penetrate it.

Leakage of salts from the tip of the membrane potential-sensing barrel has been reported (Blatt and Slayman, 1983), and this may cause significant concentration changes in small cells. Diffusion of ions from the membrane potential-recording barrel could give high local gradients of ions at the tip of a double-barrelled microelectrode. In these cases, it may be necessary to make measurements with different backfilling solutions in the membrane-potential-sensing barrel (e.g., NaCl backfilling the reference barrel of a double-barrelled K^+-selective microelectrode). Large leaks from the tip should affect cell membrane potential, and so monitoring this will quickly indicate any problems.

A further possible difficulty can arise when using ion-selective microelectrodes with inhibitors. Some inhibitor chemicals are highly lipophilic and will readily dissolve in the ion-selective membrane. These chemicals can poison the membrane, but this will be detected during the recalibration of the ion-selective microelectrode.

When statistically analyzing ion-selective electrode data, care should be taken in the calculation of means. These should be calculated using the data that are distributed normally, that is, using the log activity or output voltages not the actual ion activities (see Blatter and McGuigan, 1988). When mean activity value is used it can only be determined with 95% confidence limits, whereas -log [activity] can be given standard errors or standard deviations.

B. Fault Finding and Some Possible Problems

Faults can usually be identified by process of elimination. Begin by establishing whether a problem occurs in the wiring, or whether it is specific to the ion-selective microelectrodes. The circuitry can be tested by replacing the ion-selective microelectrode with a KCl-filled broken-tipped microelectrode. This latter electrode should give a stable zero output. If not, it may be necessary to recoat the AgCl–silver contact in the half-cell, or there may be a wiring problem. Noisy recordings can be caused by poor contact to ground, or by the presence of air bubbles in backfilling solutions. If the circuitry has no problems, this implies that the faults must be associated with the ion-selective microelectrode. If the ion-selective microelectrode does not respond to the calibration solutions, then the membrane can be checked by deliberately breaking the tip to expose a larger area of ion-selective membrane. Breaking the tip can displace the ion-selective membrane from the tip, so it is important to measure the resistance to check whether it is still in the GΩ range. If the broken tip gives a good response to changes in ion activity, then the problem is independent of the composition of the membrane. An ion-selective electrode will no longer respond to changes in ion activity when the microelectrode tip diameter becomes too fine. When a broken tip shows no voltage change in response to different calibration solutions, then a new sensor cocktail should be used. Some types of sensor cocktail have a limited lifetime, only giving responsive ion-selective electrodes for 2 to 3 months.

C. Storage of Ion-Selective Microelectrodes

Ion-selective microelectrodes should be stored without backfilling, in a silica-gel dried sealed container in the dark. Electrodes can be conveniently stored in a screw-cap glass jar containing dry silica gel, with the microelectrodes attached to the inner wall using plasticine. Ion-selective microelectrodes stored for several years in this way can still give a reasonable performance when backfilled.

V. Conclusions and Perspectives

Some variations on the above method have been reported by other authors; for example, Felle and Bertl (1986) coat the electrode tip with PVC and then backfill with ion-selective cocktail. More recently, Maathuis and Sanders (1993) reported making K^+-selective microelectrodes by backfilling the entire length of the glass pipette with ion-selective cocktail. Future developments are likely to include other types of ion-selective microelectrode for intracellular measurements, such as heavy metals. Also, triple-barrelled electrode measurements are likely to become a standard technique for determining which compartment is being measured in plant cells. Other types of electrode that are likely to be miniaturized to a size suitable for intracellular measurements include redox electrodes and enzyme electrodes, e.g., glucose electrodes.

In conclusion, ion-selective microelectrodes are a powerful tool in plant cell biology, providing direct measurements of electrochemical ion gradients inside cells.

References

Ammann, D. (1986). Ion-selective microelectrodes, principles, design and application. Berlin/Heidelberg: Springer-Verlag.

Blatt, M. R. (1991). A primer in plant electrophysiological methods. *Methods Plant Biochem.* **6,** 281–319.

Blatt, M. R., and Slayman, C. L. (1983). KCl leakage from microelectrodes and its impact on the membrane parameters of a non-excitable cell. *J. Membr. Biol.* **72,** 223–234.

Blatter, L. A., and McGuigan, J. A. S. (1988). Estimation of the upper limit of the free magnesium concentration measured with Mg-sensitive microelectrodes in ferret ventricular muscle: (1) Use of the Nicolsky-Eisenman equation and (2) in calibrating solutions of the appropriate concentration. *Magnesium* **7,** 154–165.

Bush, D. S., and Jones, R. L. (1990). Measuring intracellular Ca^{2+} levels in plant cells using the fluorescent probes, indo-1 and fura-2. *Plant Physiol.* **93,** 841–845.

Coles, J. A., and Orkland, R. K. (1985). Changes in sodium activity during light stimulation in photoreceptors, glia and extracellular space in drone retina. *J. Physiol.* **362,** 415–435.

Coster, H. G. L. (1966). Chloride in cells of *Chara australis. Aust. J. Biol. Sci.* **19,** 545–554.

Felle, H., and Bertl, A. (1986). The fabrication of H^+-selective liquid-membrane microelectrodes for use in plant cells. *J. Exp. Bot.* **37,** 1416–1428.

Fry, C. H., Hall, S. K., Blatter, L. A., and McGuigan, J. A. S. (1990). Analysis and presentation of intracellular measurements obtained with ion-selective microelectrodes. *Exp. Physiol.* **75,** 187–198.

Hajibagheri, M. A., Flowers, T. J., Collins, J. C., and Yeo, A. R. (1988). A comparison of the methods of x-ray microanalysis, compartmental analysis and longitudinal ion profiles to estimate cytoplasmic ion concentrations in two maize varieties. *J. Exp. Bot.* **39,** 279–290.

Henriksen, G. H., Bloom, A. J., and Spanswick, R. M. (1990). Measurement of net fluxes of ammonium and nitrate at the surface of barley roots using ion-selective microelectrodes. *Plant Physiol.* **93,** 271–280.

Jeschke, W. D., and Stelter, W. (1976). Measurement of the longitudinal ion profiles in single roots of *Hordeum* and *Atriplex* by use of flameless atomic absorbtion spectroscopy. *Planta* **128,** 107–112.

Lee, R., and Ratcliffe, R. G. (1991). Observations on the subcellular distribution of the ammonium ion in maize root tissue using in-vivo ^{14}N-nuclear magnetic resonance spectroscopy. *Planta* **183,** 359–367.

Kondo, Y., Bührer, T., Seiler, K., Frömter E., and Simon, W. (1989). A new double-barrelled, ionophore-based microelectrode for chloride ions. *Pflügers Arch.* **414,** 663–668.

Kühtreiber, W. M., and Jaffe, L. F. (1990). Detection of extracellular calcium gradients with a calcium-specific vibrating electrode. *J. Cell Biol.* **110,** 1563–1573.

Malone, M., Leigh R. A., and Tomos, A. D. (1989). Extraction and analysis of sap from individual wheat leaf cells: The effect of sampling speed on the osmotic pressure of extracted sap. *Plant Cell Environ.* **12,** 919–926.

Maathuis, F. J. M., and Sanders, D. (1993). Energization of potassium uptake in *Arabidopsis thaliana. Planta* **191,** 302–307.

Miller, A. J., and Sanders, D. (1987). Depletion of cytosolic free calcium induced by photosynthesis. *Nature* **326,** 397–400.

Miller, A. J., and Zhen, R.-G. (1991). Measurement of intracellular nitrate concentrations in *Chara* using nitrate-selective microelectrodes. *Planta* **184,** 47–52.

Okihara, K., and Kiyosawa, K. (1988). Ion comparison of the *Chara* internode. *Plant Cell Physiol.* **29,** 21–25.

Oparka, K. J. (1991). Uptake and compartmentation of fluorescent probes by plant cells. *J. Exp. Bot.* **42,** 565–579.

Pierce, W. S., and Higinbotham, N. (1970) Compartments and fluxes of K^+, Na^+ and Cl^- in *Avena* coleoptile cells. *Plant Physiol.* **46,** 666–673.

Reid, R. J., and Smith, F. A. (1988). Measurements of the cytoplasmic pH of *Chara corallina* using double-barrelled pH microelectrodes. *J. Exp. Bot.* **39,** 1421–1432.

Sanders, D., and Slayman, C. L. (1982). Control of intracellular pH. Predominant role of oxidative metabolism, not proton transport, in the eukaryotic microorganism *Neurospora. J. Gen. Physiol.* **80,** 377–402.

Sanders, D., and Miller, A. J. (1986). *In* "Molecular and Cellular Aspects of Calcium in Plant Development" (A. J. Trewavas, ed.), pp. 149–156. New York/London: Plenum Press.

Tsien, R. Y., and Rink, T. J. (1981). Ca^{2+}-selective electrodes: A novel PVC-gelled neutral carrier mixture compared with other currently available sensors. *J. Neurosci. Method* **4,** 73–86.

Zhen, R. G., Smith, S. J., and Miller, A. J. (1992). A comparison of nitrate-selective microelectrodes made with different nitrate sensors and the measurement of intracellular nitrate activities in cells of excised barley roots. *J. Exp. Bot.* **43,** 131–138.

CHAPTER 20

Patch-Clamping Plant Cells

Frans J. M. Maathuis and Dale Sanders
Department of Biology
University of York
York YO1 5DD, United Kingdom

I. Introduction

Biological membranes form the boundary between different cellular compartments and the external world. Transport systems within membranes facilitate the controlled passage of ions into and out of cellular compartments, thereby contributing to homeostasis. Ionic gradients are generated across membranes by pumps that utilize light, redox, or chemical potential as energy source. These gradients can be used to drive carrier-mediated movement of other ions and solutes, or be dissipated through ion channels. In the latter case some rapid signaling function, either electrical or through a change in ion activity, is usually served.

The practical analysis of ion transport systems has been dramatically boosted by the development of the patch-clamp technique by Sakmann and Neher (1983) in the late 1970s. Patch-clamping evolved from voltage clamping techniques that were applied as early as the late 1940s by Cole, Hodgkin, and others. In voltage-clamp experiments the membrane electrical potential (V_m) is clamped at a specific value by a feedback amplifier, while current passing through the membrane (I_m) is monitored with a second electrode. In patch-clamp, both V_m clamping and I_m recording are performed by one electrode. For this purpose a glass pipette is tightly sealed to the membrane with resistances in the GΩ (10^9 ohm) range. This high seal resistance enables two general experimental manipulations that have, between them, revolutionized the detail with which membrane transport systems can be studied.

First, the resultant improved signal/noise ratio allows resolution of the currents flowing through single-channel molecules residing within the patch of membrane at the tip of the pipette. Ions in such channels can turn over at rates approaching 10^8 ions s^{-1}, and therefore deliver currents in pA range. The physical stability of the membrane patch permits its detachment from the rest of the membrane (Fig. 1; see also below), thereby allowing the presence of experimentally defined solutions on both sides of the channel.

The second dramatic technical advance is achieved if the patch of membrane is destroyed (Fig. 1, see also below) and electrical access is gained to the inside of the cell. The relatively large diameter of the pipette tip (1–5 μm) enables effective control of the internal solution and hence study of potentially all electrogenic transport systems under defined conditions. These include not only populations of ion channels but also pumps and carriers which, because they turn over only at rates in the region of 10^2–10^3 s^{-1}, are not susceptible to analysis at the level of a single molecule.

Both the patch and the whole-cell recording modes can in principle be extended to organelles, providing their diameter exceeds that of the pipette tip. In practice most organelles fail to meet this criterion, although with extra manipulation patch-clamping is sometimes possible (Schönknecht *et al.,* 1988). However, the

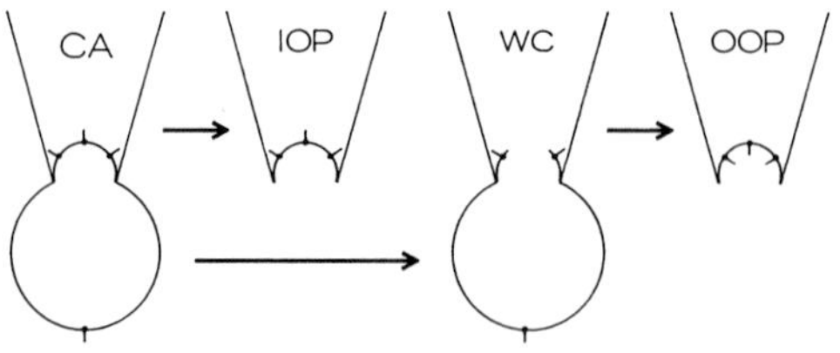

Fig. 1 Different configurations in patch-clamping. Experiments start with the cell-attached mode (CA) after which either an excised, inside-out patch (IOP) can be formed by pulling the pipette off the cell, or the whole cell (WC) is accessed by applying extra suction or voltage pulses. If the pipette is pulled off after a WC an excised outside-out patch (OOP) is formed.

large vacuoles of mature, higher plant cells are ideally suited for patch-clamping and such studies have yielded unprecedented insights into the transport properties of the vacuolar membrane (Hedrich and Schroeder, 1989, Maathuis and Sanders, 1992).

As outlined above, a high-resistance seal between pipette and membrane is crucial for successful patch-clamping and seals will only emerge if "clean" membranes are presented to the pipette glass. With respect to plant membranes, a naked vacuolar membrane is easily available in the form of isolated vacuoles. However, the plasma membrane poses difficulties since it is surrounded by the cell wall. Although introduction of laser techniques (Taylor and Brownlee, 1993) now provides an alternative way to access the membrane, most existing protocols use enzymatic degradation of cell walls and/or mechanical isolation of protoplasts. The latter methods mainly aim at optimization of protoplast yield, whereas in patch-clamp applications high yields are subordinate to optimized sealing properties and minimized damage to transport systems by protease/glycosylase activity. In this chapter we therefore include the description of both protoplast and vacuole isolation methods, specifically optimized for patch-clamping.

II. Materials and Methods

A. Vacuole Isolation

Storage tissue such as *Beta vulgaris* is particularly popular in tonoplast transport studies since vacuoles can easily be obtained by slicing or scraping a piece of tissue (e.g., Hedrich *et al.,* 1988; Davies *et al.,* 1992). This method ensures a high yield of vacuoles and a very short time span between isolation and experiments. In many cases the same strategy can be used to isolate vacuoles from root (Maathuis and Prins, 1990) and stem tissue (Maathuis and Prins, 1991). Some authors (e.g., Alexandre and Lassalles, 1991) preincubate their beet tissue in a hypertonic, EDTA-containing solution to ensure a maximum number of intact, large vacuoles that are subsequently selected individually. In cells (e.g., guard cells) or tissues (e.g., leaves) for which these simple, mechanical methods are not applicable, vacuoles must be isolated from protoplasts by osmotic or mechanical shock (Maathuis *et al.,* 1992; Raschke and Hedrich, 1992).

B. Protoplast Isolation

The isolation procedure we use is rapid and combines the use of cell wall degrading enzymes, an osmotic shock, and mechanical treatment of the tissue (Vogelzang and Prins, 1992). Roots of one *Arabidopsis thaliana* plant (grown as described in Maathuis and Sanders, 1993) with a fresh weight of about 500 mg are rinsed under tap water for approx. 30 s to remove any loosely bound debris

(Fig. 2). Next, roots are cut with a fresh razor blade into approx. 1-mm pieces while immersed in 5 ml of solution A. These steps are performed in plastic 55-mm petri dishes. After addition of enzymes (1.5% cellulysin, 10,400 units/g, CalBiochem, 0.1% pectolyase, 3600 units/g, Sigma) the petri dish is incubated at 35°C for 12–15 min. Root tissue is collected on nylon mesh (100-μm-pore size) at the bottom of a plastic funnel and washed with 5 ml of solution A followed by 10 ml of solution B. Subsequently the funnel with tissue is placed on the bottom of a clean petri dish, some solution B is added, and the tissue is squeezed with a spatula. Protoplasts, freed from the tissue, will flush through the nylon mesh after the tissue is washed with 0.5 to 1 ml solution B. The squeezing–washing routine, which causes extraction of protoplasts from the tissue, can be repeated two or three times, depending on the amount of tissue. Part of the protoplast suspension is transferred to the patch-clamp chamber while the remainder is stored at 4°C for later use.

C. Solutions

Solution A contains 600 mM mannitol (sorbitol can equally well substitute for mannitol), 10 mM KCl, 2 mM $CaCl_2$, 2 mM $MgCl_2$, 0.1% BSA, 2 mM Mes/Tris, pH 5.5. Solution B contains 300 mM mannitol, 10 mM KCl, 2 mM $CaCl_2$, 2 mM $MgCl_2$, 2 mM Mes/Tris, pH 5.5. In patch-clamp experiments, the normal

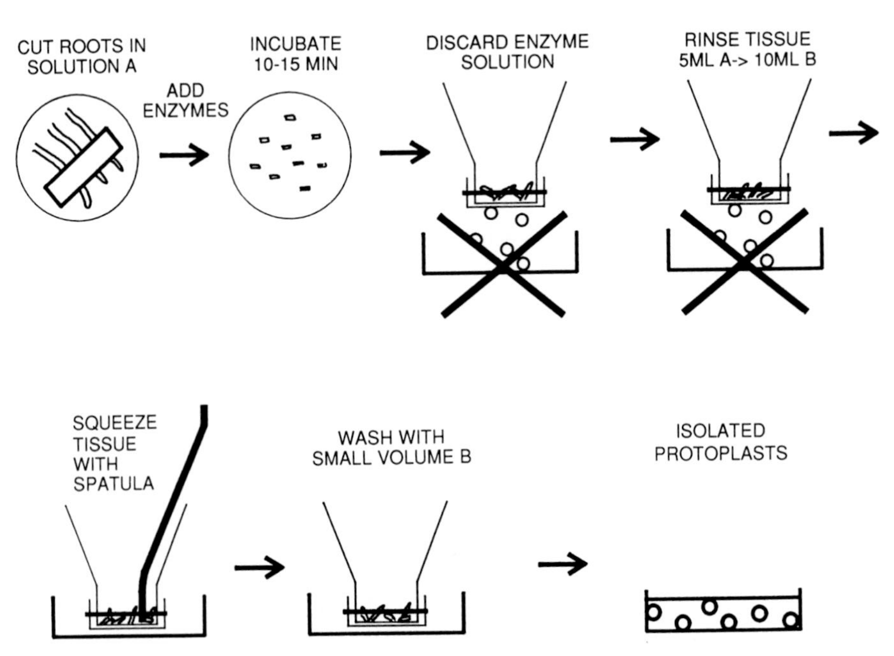

Fig. 2 Schematic representation of the protoplast isolation protocol described in the text.

bath solution comprises solution B with the mannitol concentration raised to 450 m*M*. The standard pipette solution contains 10 m*M* KCl or K-citrate, 400 m*M* mannitol, 0.5 m*M* $CaCl_2$ buffered with EGTA to a free Ca^{2+} of 200–800 n*M*, 2 m*M* $MgCl_2$, and 2 m*M* Mes/Tris, pH 7.5.

All solutions are kept for no longer than 2–4 weeks at 4°C and filtered through a 0.2-μm filter prior to usage.

D. Pipette Fabrication

Pipettes are prepared from borosilicate glass capillaries (Kimax 51, art. 34500, size 1.5 × 1.8 × 100 mm, Kimble, Ohio) and pulled on a two-stage puller (List, Darmstadt, Germany). A two-stage pull is used to ensure a relatively blunt tapered tip. The first pull is mainly to thin the glass wall and not very critical, whereas the second pull is paramount in determining the tip diameter. Larger pipette tips require less heat and may be advantageous for keeping cells in the whole cell (WC) configuration while smaller tips will reduce the amount of membrane sealed to the pipette and are therefore more desirable in cell attached (CA) and excised patch (IOP/OOP) experiments.

Since the thin glass wall of the pipette near the tip forms a considerable stray capacitance to ground, it will induce a major source of high-frequency noise. Coating with an inert, hydrophobic polymer (e.g., Sylgard 184, Dow Corning, Seneffe, Belgium) greatly reduces this capacitance, as will minimizing the bathing solution level. A thick layer of coating is applied on the last 5 mm of the pipette as close to the tip as possible while viewing at 100–150× magnification on a List coating/polishing unit. The coating is hardened by exposing the pipette to a hot air stream for a few seconds. Fire polishing in order to smooth the glass rim is normally omitted (but see below). Electrode resistance varied between 20 and 100 MΩ, depending on pipette geometry and the solution used. For pipettes with an average tip diameter and filled with 10 m*M* KCl, the electrode resistance is 30 to 50 MΩ when bathed in 10 m*M* KCl.

E. The Patch-Clamp Set-up

Basically the patch-clamp apparatus comprises a sensitive current-measuring device, a microscope plus micromanipulator, and a data storage facility. An outline of a typical set-up is shown in Fig. 3. Briefly, pipette currents are amplified by a List (Darmstadt, Germany) EPC7 or EPC9 amplifier with its output fed into a low-pass 8-pole Bessel filter (Frequency Devices, 902, Haverhill) and digitized (CED 1401 A/D converter, Cambridge, UK, or Labmaster DMA, Scientific Solutions, Solon) before storage on hard disk. Data acquisition and command voltages are under the control of "Patch 5.5" (for the CED 1401 interface, CED, Cambridge, UK) or "Pclamp" (for the Labmaster interface, Axon Instruments, Foster City) software. Inverted microscopes (Nikon Diaphot, or TMS, Tokyo, Japan) are used for easy access to the bath with the pipette and the preparation

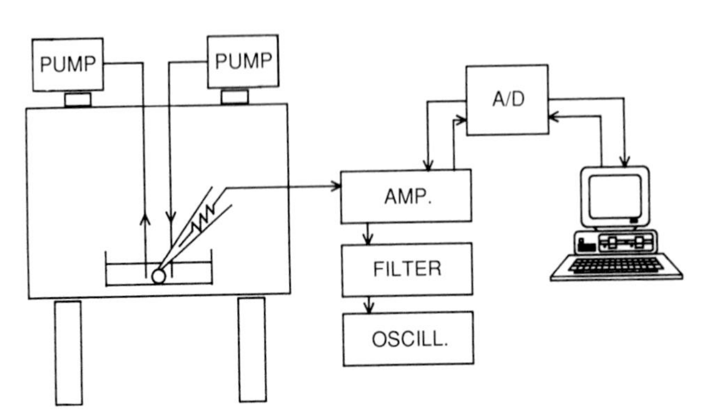

Fig. 3 Schematic diagram and connections of the patch-clamp apparatus. The graph shows a minimal set-up with micromanipulator and preparation-viewing details omitted.

is normally viewed at 40× with bright-field objectives. Microscope, micromanipulator, bath stage, and other equipment have to be thoroughly grounded and screened from electromagnetic interference by a Faraday cage. To minimize mechanical resonation, the complete set-up is mounted on a vibration isolation table.

F. Experimental Preparations

The patch-clamp chamber consists of a Teflon ring (25 mm in diameter) with a microscope coverslip glued to its bottom. Prior to use, chambers are rinsed with ethanol and water, which ensures that settled protoplasts stick to the glass. After transfer of the isolated protoplasts to the patch-clamp chamber, protoplasts are allowed to settle for 5 to 10 min.

Since isolation involves an osmotic shock, protoplasts are still in solution B, which is of low osmotic pressure (ca. 325 mOsM). In order to restore original cell volume the bath has to be perfused with fresh solution at an osmotic pressure of approx. 500 mOsM and containing the desired ionic composition for the experiment. Additionally bath perfusion has the advantage of flushing out debris not attached to the glass bottom. Bath perfusion can be an intricate procedure and a good system should allow the experimenter great control over influx and efflux of solutions while not disturbing the cell or introducing extra noise. The use of two matching peristaltic pumps (Gilson, M312, Villiers, France) with both influx and efflux tubing grounded satisfies the requirements listed above. Both pumps are placed on top of the Faraday cage and perfusion rates are kept below 400–500 μl/min.

G. Getting a Seal

Patch-clamp experiments can only be performed if a GΩ seal establishes between pipette glass and membrane. The better the seal the better the resolution of the measured currents and the better the mechanical stability will be. As stated in the Introduction, formation of seals with plasma membranes is not always straightforward and since no accurate physical explanation of the sealing process exists, it is impossible to give a general reason for this problem.

In our case the electrode is lowered in the bath and approaches the protoplast until a slight physical contact is made. With a 10-mV test pulse running, the actual resistance can be followed on an oscilloscope screen. Now gentle suction is applied to result in two- to fourfold increased resistance. In this phase, while retaining some suction, the amplifier is switched to the voltage clamp mode and the pipette is clamped at −40 to −70 mV, which usually significantly improves the sealing process. If needed, suction can be increased to obtain a higher resistance but the final stage in sealing, from approx. 0.5 to >5GΩ, normally demands no suction at all. Too much suction will result in breakage of the membrane, which is preceded by rapid invagination of a large area of membrane. To avoid this it is crucial to observe closely the test trace, since this will display profound increases in the capacitive spikes just prior to membrane rupture. The process of obtaining a seal can take anything from 10 s to 10 min but with "agreeable" cells is complete in less than 1 min.

H. Other Configurations

The large flexibility in patch-clamp configurations allows access to both membrane sides. The IOP configuration forms after the pipette is pulled back from the cell. This may sometimes involve lifting the whole cell and tapping the micromanipulator until the cell falls off. Occasionally, IOP formation results in a vesicle forming in the pipette, which can be inferred from a doubling seal resistance and distorted single-channel signals. The recommended remedy is to lift the pipette briefly out of the bath, thereby rupturing the membrane on one vesicle side. The whole cell configuration is made by applying extra suction in case protoplasts are used. Clamping the membrane to a large (± 100 mV) potential sometimes facilitates this procedure and breaking the membrane is easier when protoplasts are in a high osmolarity medium. Vacuolar membranes are ruptured by electric pulses of 500–900 mV for 10–50 ms, but these numbers can vary from tissue to tissue or even day-to-day and sometimes additional suction—while pulsing—speeds up the process.

Retraction of the pipette after formation of the whole cell/vacuole recording mode produces the OOP configuration.

III. Results and Discussion

A. Critical Aspects of the Procedure

In our view the most critical step in the procedure for patch-clamping plasma membrane is exposure of the tissue to the enzyme-containing solution. Exposure should be as short as possible to avoid detrimental side effects (e.g., proteolysis) and to improve seal frequencies, but long enough to ensure isolation of cell wall free protoplasts. This means that researchers using other types of plant material may have to optimize this step; this may also be necessary for researchers using the same plant material but grown in a different way. For instance, when *A. thaliana* is grown under K^+ starvation conditions, we frequently need to prolong the enzyme incubation to 20–25 min in order to secure proper seals. Other enzyme cocktails can be of relevance (e.g., Elzenga *et al.,* 1991) for different tissues and even a change of enzyme manufacturer may influence the outcome.

A second point worth raising is the influence of wash steps, first those to remove enzymes after incubation (residual enzyme may affect the membrane and reduces the seal frequency) and second the bath perfusion once protoplasts are settled at the bottom of the patch-clamp chamber (to remove any floating debris that may stick to the pipette). Both steps are essential for high seal frequencies.

In our experience the shape and glass type of the pipette is relatively unimportant for acquiring a seal (but see pipette fabrication) and we tend to get better results if we omit the fire polishing step. Another determining factor is the Ca^{++} concentration used in the pipette (concentrations <10–100 μM worsen seal formation).

B. General Considerations

The protocol described for patch-clamping protoplasts is to a large extent based on those published by Vogelzang and Prins (1992) and Elzenga *et al.,* (1991). It has proven successful with root and leaf tissues of at least seven different plant species and—slightly modified—with fungal hyphae (P. Whiting, personal communication). Viable protoplasts are obtained (as judged by cytoplasmic streaming) and Fig. 4 depicts single channel records from a typical *A.*

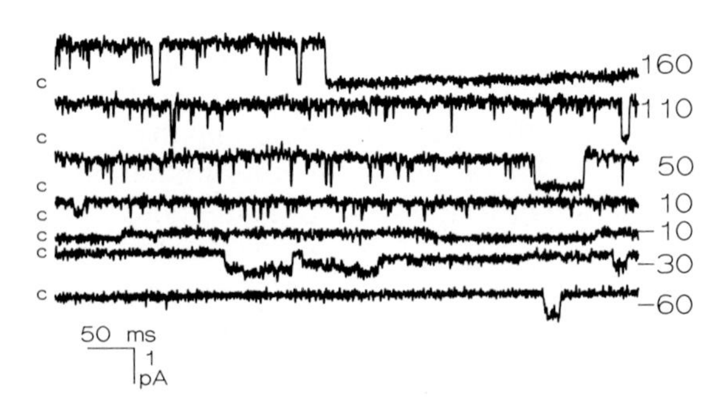

Fig. 4 Example of single channel traces from a *A. thaliana* root protoplast in the CA configuration. Clamped potentials are denoted on the right of the traces (in mV) and the closed level is denoted by "c" on the left. Both inward and outward rectifying channel activity are present.

thaliana protoplast (diameter 22 μm) in the CA mode. A high resistance seal (45 GΩ) formed within a minute using a 39 MΩ electrode with 700 n*M* Ca^{2+} in the pipette solution. The noise level is 280 fA (3 kHz bandwidth) and seals are routinely made with a success rate in the region 50%. Many factors contributing to a high seal frequency remain to be clarified and day-to-day variation is, for no seeming reason, inevitable. There is now an abundance of good literature dealing with the technical aspects of patch-clamping and electrophysiology in general (e.g., Sakmann and Neher, 1983; Standen *et al.,* 1987; Sherman-Gold, 1993). However, literature dealing with practical aspects of specific preparations is still relatively scarce.

We have described a step-by-step protocol that has proven its value and should serve as a useful basis for other researchers.

References

Alexandre, J., and Lassalles, J. P. (1991). Hydrostatic and osmotic pressure activated channel in plant vacuole. *Biophys. J.* **60,** 1326–1336.

Davies, J. M., Poole, R. J., Rea, P., and Sanders, D. (1992). Potassium transport into plant vacuoles energized directly by a proton-pumping inorganic pyrophosphatase. *Proc. Natl. Acad. Sci. U.S.A.* **89,** 11701–11705.

Elzenga, J. T. M., Keller, C. P., and Van Volkenburgh, E. (1991). Patch clamping protoplasts from vascular plants. *Plant Physiol.* **97,** 1573–1575.

Hedrich, R., Barbier-Brygoo, H., Felle, H., Fluegge, U. I., Luettge, U., Maathuis, F. J. M., Marx, S., Prins, H. B. A., Raschke, K., Schnabl, H., Schroeder, J. I., Struve, I., Taiz, L., and Ziegler, P. (1988). General mechanisms for solute transport across the tonoplast of plant vacuoles: A patch clamp survey of ion channels and protons. *Botanica Acta* **101,** 7–13.

Hedrich, R., and Schroeder, J. I. (1989). The physiology of ion channels and electrogenic pumps in higher plants. *Annu. Rev. Plant Physiol.* **40,** 539–569.

Maathuis, F. J. M., and Prins, H. B. A. (1990). Patch clamp studies on root cell vacuoles of a salt tolerant and a salt sensitive *Plantago* species. *Plant Physiol.* **92,** 23–28.

Maathuis, F. J. M., and Prins, H. B. A. (1991). Outward current conducting ion channels in tonoplasts of *Vigna unguiculata. J. Plant Physiol.* **139,** 63–69.

Maathuis, F. J. M., Flowers, T. J., and Yeo, A. R. (1992). Sodium chloride compartmentation in leaf vacuoles of the halophyte *Suaeda maritima* (L.) Dum. and its relation to tonoplast permeability. *J. Exp. Bot.* **43,** 1219–1223.

Maathuis, F. J. M., and Sanders, D. (1992). Plant membrane transport. *Curr. Opin. Cell Biol.* **4,** 661–669.

Maathuis, F. J. M., and Sanders, D. (1993). Energization of potassium uptake in *Arabidopsis thaliana. Planta* **191,** 302–307.

Raschke, K., and Hedrich, R. (1992). Patch clamp measurements on isolated guard cell protoplasts and vacuoles. *In* "Methods in Enzymology" (S. Fleischer and B. Fleischer, eds.), Vol. 174, pp. 312–330, New York: Academic Press.

Sakmann, B., and Neher, E. (1983). "Single-Channel Recording." New York/London: Plenum Press.

Schönknecht, G., Hedrich, R., Junge, W., and Raschke, K. (1988). A voltage-dependent chloride channel in the photosynthetic membrane of a higher plant. *Nature* **336,** 589–592.

Sherman-Gold, R. (1993). The Axon guide for electrophysiology and biophysics laboratory techniques. Axon Instruments, Inc. Foster City.

Standen, N. B., Gray, P. T. A., and Whitaker, M. J. (1987). Microelectrode techniques. "The Plymouth Workshop Handbook." Cambridge: The Company of Biologists Ltd.

Taylor, A., and Brownlee, C. (1993). Calcium and potassium currents in the Fucus egg. *Planta* **189,** 109–119.

Vogelzang, S. A., and Prins, H. B. A. (1992). Plasmalemma patch clamp experiments in plant root cells: Procedure for fast isolation of protoplasts with minimal exposure to cell wall degrading enzymes. *Protoplasma* **171,** 104–109.

PART II

Techniques for Manipulation and Analysis of Different Cell Types

CHAPTER 21

Methods for Mesophyll and Bundle Sheath Cell Separation

Jen Sheen

Department of Genetics
Harvard Medical School and
Department of Molecular Biology
Massachusetts General Hospital
Boston, Massachusetts 02114

I. Introduction

Mesophyll and bundle sheath cells are the dimorphic photosynthetic cell types in C4 plants that partition CO_2 fixation in two consecutive, spatially separated steps, thus eliminating photorespiration and increasing photosynthetic rates under arid, hot, and light-intensive environments (Hatch, 1992; Nelson and Lang-

METHODS IN CELL BIOLOGY, VOL. 49

dale, 1992). In order to dissect and locate precisely the photosynthetic activities and metabolic pathways in the two leaf cell types, various methods have been developed to separate mesophyll and bundle sheath cells. These methods are generally based on the differences of the two cell types in their physical positions in the C4 leaf structure (Kranz anatomy), cell wall thickness, and cell density (Kanai and Edwards, 1973; Walbot and Hoisington, 1982; Sheen and Bogorad, 1985, 1987a; Moore *et al.,* 1984, 1988; Valle *et al.,* 1989). Depending on the C4 plant species, cell separation can be achieved through either physical destruction or differential enzymatic digestion of the loosely connected and thin-walled mesophyll cells. In some dicot C4 plants where bundle sheath cells are also surrounded by thin cell walls, dextran density gradients have been used to separate mesophyll and bundle sheath protoplasts (Moore *et al.,* 1984, 1988; Boinski *et al.,* 1993).

Separated mesophyll and bundle sheath cells were initially employed in physiological and biochemical studies, including analyses of the activities of enzymes within the C4 and Calvin cycle pathways, as well as measurements of chlorophyll levels, PSII function, oxygen evolution, starch biosynthesis, nitrogen assimilation, catalase activity, photosynthetic rate, CO_2 compensation point, and protein profile (Woo *et al.,* 1970; Kanai and Edwards, 1973; Potter and Black, 1982; Tsaftaris *et al.,* 1983; Spilatro and Preiss, 1987; Valle *et al.,* 1989; Becker *et al.,* 1993). Improvement to the cell separation process, in terms both of the purity of the cell types and the quantities of cells produced, has made possible the isolation of intact protein, RNA, and DNA, and has led to studies of broad aspects of gene expression using *in vitro* translation, cDNA cloning, protein/RNA/DNA blot hybridization, methylation analysis, *in vitro* transcription, and DNA–protein/protein–protein interactions (Broglie *et al.,* 1984; Sheen and Bogorad, 1985, 1987a, 1987b; Ngernprasirtsir *et al.,* 1989; Langdale *et al.,* 1991; Schäffner and Sheen, 1991, 1992; Nelson and Langdale, 1992; Boinski *et al.,* 1993; Meierhoff and Westhoff, 1993; Sheen, unpublished; To and Sheen, unpublished).

Recently, mesophyll and bundle sheath protoplasts isolated from maize seedlings have been used successfully as a convenient and reproducible single-cell transient expression system (Sheen, 1990, and unpublished work). In contrast to the prevailing concept that isolated mesophyll protoplasts are stressed and unresponsive, we found controlled gene expression in response to a broad spectrum of physiological signals, such as metabolites, plant hormones, elicitors, light, and heat shock, and in response to the agents that induce photobleaching, and redox changes (Sheen, 1990, 1991, 1993; Schäffner and Sheen, 1991, 1992; Jang and Sheen, unpublished; Sheen, unpublished; Sheen and Jang, unpublished). In addition, this single-cell system shows fidelity in protein translocation and processing, viral RNA replication, developmental regulation, and tissue- and monocot-specific control (Sheen, 1991; Schäffner and Sheen, 1991, 1992; Sheen, unpublished). Thus, purified mesophyll and bundle sheath protoplasts (Sheen, unpublished) provide a novel and versatile tool for studies of gene regulation and signal transduction in higher plants.

In this chapter, I will describe the methods for the separation of mesophyll and bundle sheath cells from maize seedlings. The resultant cells, which can be easily manipulated, are physiologically very active. The overall purity and viability are usually greater than 95%.

II. Materials

A. Maize Seed Source and Growth Conditions

Although the methods described in this chapter are applicable to all maize seedlings and perhaps other monocot C4 plants (Meierhoff and Westhoff, 1993), the hybrid line FR992 × FR 697 from Illinois Foundation Seeds, Inc. (Champaign, IL), gives the best results if transient expression is the desired application. This maize line grows very well in the dark and gives healthy and morphologically normal etiolated leaves that respond to illumination rapidly and uniformly. Green maize leaves grown under constant light are excellent sources for protein and enzyme isolation, but generally contain less mRNA of photosynthetic genes and show lower activity for transient gene expression unless cells at the most active (spatial and temporal) developmental stage for photosynthetic gene expression are used (Jang and Sheen, unpublished).

Soak maize seeds overnight in water before planting as a monolayer in a 4 inch pot (50 to 60 seeds) filled with soaked and drained vermiculite. Cover the seed monolayer with 1 cm of wet vermiculite. Add an equal volume of peatlite mix if the vermiculite does not hold sufficient water. Grow maize seedlings under constant light (30–100 $\mu Em^{-2} s^{-1}$) or place them in a dark room after the shoots emerge from the vermiculite. Keep a constant temperature of 25°C and water only when necessary. Grow plants to the two-leaf stage (about 11 days). Only the middle portion (3 cm from the tip and 7–10 cm long) of the second leaf is used.

B. Reagents

1. Grinding buffer (0–4°C, 60 leaves/30 ml)
   - 0.4 *M* mannitol or sorbitol
   - 20 m*M* MES, pH 5.7
   - 10 m*M* β-mercaptoethanol
2. Enzyme solution (23°C, 10–20 leaves/10 ml, 0.08 g fw/leaf)
   - 1–1.5% cellulase "Onozuka" R10 or RS
   - 0.2% macerozyme R10
   - 0.6 *M* mannitol or sorbito
   - 20 m*M* MES, pH 5.7

   Dissolve the enzyme powder by stirring with a plastic loop and heat the solution at 55°C for 10 min. Cool the solution to room temperature before addition of the following:

1 mM $CaCl_2$
1 mM $MgCl_2$
5 mM β-mercaptoethanol
0.1% BSA

All chemicals can be purchased from Sigma and stored at room temperature except β-mercaptoethanol (4°C). Cellulase "Onozuka" R10 or RS and maceroxyme R10 can be obtained from Yakult Pharmaceutical, Ind. Co., Ltd. (Tokyo, Japan, fax 81-3-3575-1636) or Karlan Chemical Corp. (Torrance, CA, 800-231-9186). The enzymes are stable and can be stored at −20°C for at least 5 years. Cellulase R10 is used for green leaves, whereas cellulase RS is used for etiolated and greening leaves.

C. Tools and Equipment

Fresh razor blades (VWR)
Sidearm vacuum flask and rubber stopper
Plastic petri dish (10 cm) and beaker (50 and 500 ml)
37-μm nylon filter (Carolina Biological Supply Co., Burlington, NC, 800-334-5551)
Polytron homogenizer PT 10/35, generator PTA 10 and PTA 35 (Brinkman Instruments Co., Westbury, NY, 800-645-3050)
Microscope
Hemocytometer

III. Methods

A. Physical Destruction Method for Bundle Sheath Cell Isolation

This method is used to purify intact bundle sheath strands from which bundle sheath protoplasts, nuclei, and chloroplasts can be isolated if desired. Mesophyll cells are broken during the grinding process. Although the suspension of the first grinding is enriched for mesophyll chloroplasts and nuclei, it is heavily contaminated with bundle sheath chloroplasts and nuclei. The grinding is usually performed with a Polytron homogenizer for its efficiency and flexibility. For a large batch isolation, a Cuisinart food processor can be used instead of manual cutting to first chop the leaves into small pieces.
Isolation of bundle sheath strands is achieved as follows:

1. Harvest 60-s maize leaves (use the middle portion of the leaves, about 5 g fresh weight, 0.08 g/leaf).
2. Remove midrib with a sharp razor blade and keep de-midribbed leaves on ice.

3. Stack the 60 leaves, and cut them into 1- to 2-mm strips, without bruising leaves. Resuspend the leaf strips in 30 ml of cold grinding solution.

4. Grind the leaf strips with a Polytron using generator PTA 35 to remove mesophyll cells. Perform gentle grinding at speed 3 for 5 s to first mix the floating leaf strips and the grinding solution, which is kept in an ice-water bath. Then start vigorous grinding for 30–60 s at speed 6–8.

5. Remove the foam with Kimwipes and filter through a 37-μm nylon filter to eliminate broken mesophyll cells.

6. Repeat grinding twice or until pure bundle sheath strands are obtained. Examine the purity of bundle sheath strands under microscope. DNA, RNA, and proteins can be isolated from these bundle sheath strands for analysis (Sheen and Bogorad, 1987a). For the isolation of bundle sheath nuclei and chloroplasts, digest bundle sheath strands in 20 ml of enzyme solution (1% cellulase RS, 0.1% macerozyme R10, 0.4 *M* mannitol, 10 m*M* MES, pH 5.7, 0.1% BSA, 10 m*M* KCl, 10 m*M* β-mercaptoethanol) at room temperature for 1 h. Remove enzyme solution by filtering through a 37-μm nylon filter; wash the partially digested bundle sheath strands retained on the filter by flushing with digestion solution lacking enzymes.

7. Carry out gentle grinding either with a Polytron at speed 3 for 1 min, or with mortar and pestle in chilled grinding solution, until the solution turns green indicating the release of intact chloroplasts and nuclei. When examined under the microscope, the bundle sheath strands become transparent after grinding. Intact chloroplasts and nuclei generally are transcriptionally active. However, *in vitro* transcription and hybridization are required to determine level of transcriptional activity. Bundle sheath protoplasts can be released if the digestion (0.6 *M* mannitol) is prolonged for 2–3 h.

B. Enzymatic Digestion Method

This method allows the simultaneous isolation of mesophyll protoplasts and bundle sheath strands:

1. Excise the middle part of the second leaves. Stack 40 leaves (press gently) and cut 0.5- 1-mm strips without bruising the leaves.

2. Using a flask (250-ml flask for 20 ml of enzyme solution) with a sidearm for leaf digestion, rinse leaf strips in 40 ml of 0.6 *M* mannitol to remove the broken cells before the addition of 20 ml of enzyme solution.

3. Apply vacuum for 30 min to infiltrate the leaves with enzyme solution.

4. Continue the digestion for another 90 to 120 min with gentle shaking (40 rpm on a platform shaker). The enzyme solution should now turn green for green and greening leaves and yellow for etiolated leaves grown in the dark, indicating the release of protoplasts (check that the protoplasts are spherical under the microscope; the size of maize mesophyll protoplasts is around 25 to 35 μm).

5. Release the mesophyll protoplasts by shaking at 80 rpm for 5 min. Release is typically above 50%, based on the recovery of cell-type-specific mRNAs.

6. Pour the protoplast suspension through a 37-μm nylon filter to separate the mesophyll protoplasts and bundle sheath strands. Spin at 150 × *g* to pellet the mesophyll protoplasts in a round-bottomed tube for 2 min (speed 4 with an IEC clinical centrifuge). A higher speed may be used if the protoplast recovery is poor.

7. The pelleted mesophyll protoplasts are resuspended by gentle shaking using 10 ml of cold washing solution (0.6 *M* mannitol, 10 m*M* MES, pH 5.7, and 20 m*M* KCl).

8. Resuspend the bundle sheath strands held on the nylon filter in 10 ml washing solution in a plastic petri dish. Gently press the bundle sheath strands with a spatula to release the residual mesophyll cells. These appear as dark green spots between the bundle sheath strands. Examine the purity of bundle sheath strands under microscope. Rinse and filter to remove released mesophyll cells. Repeat the procedure until the bundle sheath strands are at least 95% pure, as judged by the absence of green mesophyll cells between the bundle sheath strands (Fig. 2).

IV. Critical Aspects of the Procedure

A. Plant Material

Provide only water and not nutrients to the maize seedlings; excess salts can make the manipulation of mesophyll protoplasts and electroporation more difficult. It is not necessary to grow plants under sterile conditions or to employ surface sterilization. Use only the middle portion of the second leaves that contain active and well-differentiated leaf cells.

B. Grinding Procedure

To obtain pure bundle sheath strands by grinding, it is important to remove the thick midvein and cut leaves to 1- to 3-mm strips for efficient grinding to eliminate the contamination of mesophyll cells.

C. Enzyme Digestion

Cutting leaf strips specifically into 0.5- to 1-mm strips is essential for both high yield and high purity; wider leaf strips limit enzyme penetration and finer strips cause more contamination of bundle sheath cells. This is perhaps the most difficult part of most people.

Although it is supposed to stabilize protoplasts, the presence of a high concentration of $MgCl_2$ (10 m*M*) during tissue digestion results in poor quality mesophyll protoplasts. The usual prolonged incubation of leaves for 16–18 h in the dark for protoplast isolation is stressful and might eliminate physiological responses of leaf cells. Unlike tobacco and *Arabidopsis* mesophyll protoplasts, maize mesophyll protoplasts are sensitive to salts during electroporation.

D. Storage

For measurement of enzymatic and photosynthetic activities, the isolation of nuclei and chloroplasts, and transient gene expression, use freshly isolated mesophyll protoplasts and bundle sheath strands. Isolated nuclei and chloroplasts can be stored at −80°C for at least a year without losing transcriptional activity. Before the isolation of proteins, RNAs, and DNAs, concentrated mesophyll protoplasts ($2–5 \times 10^7$/ml) are frozen in liquid nitrogen as small drops (50 μl), whereas bundle sheath strands are blotted dry with paper towels and frozen in liquid nitrogen. Both can be stored at −80°C for at least a year.

V. Results and Discussion

Figure 1 shows the cross section of a maize leaf with two photosynthetic cell types. Separated bundle sheath strands are displayed in Fig. 2 and purified mesophyll protoplasts are exhibited in Fig. 3. It is necessary to scan through each preparation under microscope to estimate the contamination level. With practice and patience, it is possible to separate the two cell types with high (95–99%) purity and viability. Pure bundle sheath strands should be separated by two cell layers which, in the intact leaf, comprise mesophyll cells. Contamina-

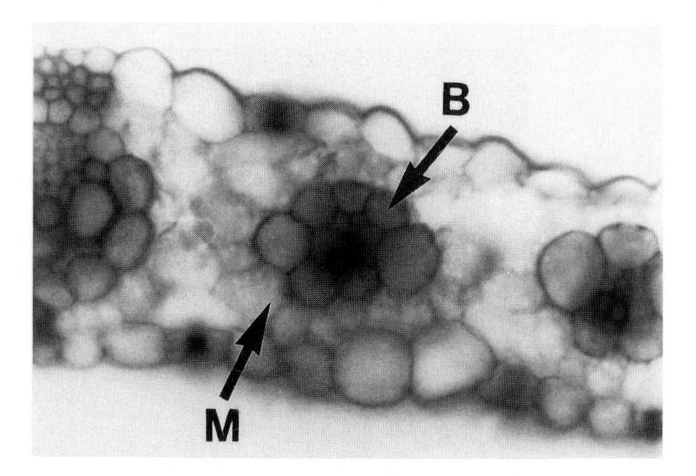

Fig. 1 Dimorphic photosynthetic cell types in a maize leaf. The mesophyll (M) and bundle sheath (B) cells are shown in the cross section of a maize leaf.

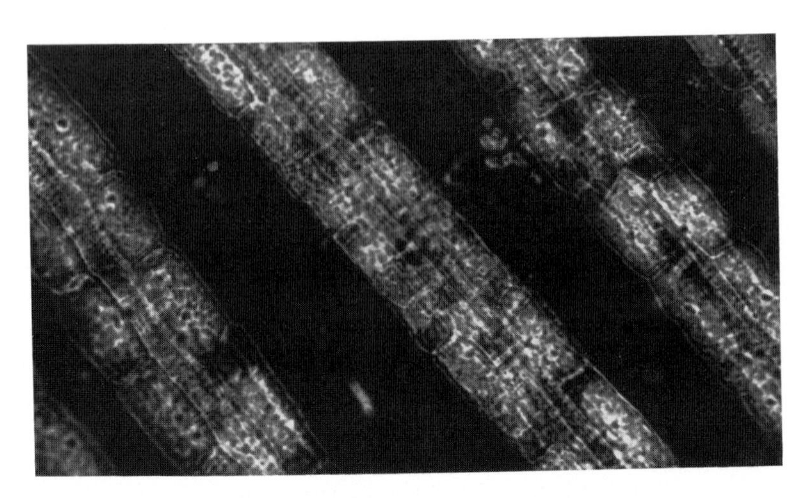

Fig. 2 Separated bundle sheath strands.

tion of mesophyll protoplasts by bundle sheath cells is indicated by the presence of rectangular cells (with cell walls) among the round mesophyll protoplasts. Cell-type-specific protein and RNA blot analysis with marker protein antibodies and marker gene probes can give more quantitative information about cross-contamination (Sheen and Bogorad, 1987a; Boinski *et al.,* 1993). Cell-type-specific RT-PCR offers the advantage of both higher sensitivity and speed (Sheen, 1991).

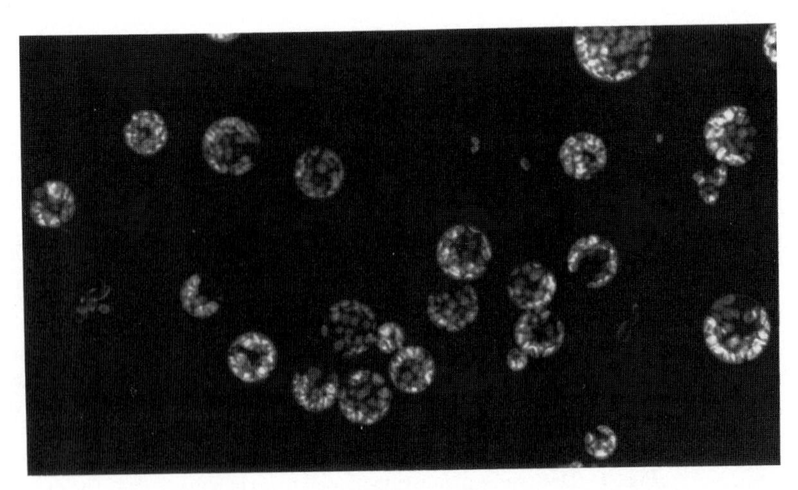

Fig. 3 Purified mesophyll protoplasts.

VI. Conclusion and Perspectives

Although immunolocalization and *in situ* hybridization methods provide information about the precise localization of the C4 enzymes and mRNAs (Nelson and Langdale, 1992), the purified cell types offer additional experimental versatility and applications, such as the measurement of enzyme activities and photosynthetic functions, and the studies of gene regulation and signal transduction using a combination of biochemical, cellular, genetic, and molecular approaches (Sheen, 1990, 1991, 1993; Schäffner and Sheen, 1991, 1992; Jang and Sheen, unpublished; Sheen and Jang, unpublished).

Unlike protoplasts isolated from undifferentiated cultured cells, maize mesophyll protoplasts show a wide range of physiological responses found in leaf cells *in planta.* This monocot system is superior to the dicot system, whose mesophyll protoplasts are easily triggered to dedifferentiate and lose photosynthetic gene regulation. Currently, mesophyll protoplasts isolated from maize seedlings provide the best cellular and molecular genetic system with active and homogeneous cell populations. Because maize leaf development is uncoupled from light, the methods can also be used to analyze photosynthetic mutants (even lethal ones) defective in light responses. With the use of marker gene promoters and assayable reporter genes, it might be possible to extend the power of this single-cell system for expression cloning and mutant complementation. Although the yield for bundle sheath protoplasts is low, these cells are potentially useful in studying the mechanisms of cell-type-specific gene regulation and nuclear–chloroplast interactions at the transcriptional and post-transcriptional levels.

References

Becker, T. W., Perrot-Rechenmann, C., Suzuki, A., and Hirel, B. (1993). Subcellular and immunocytochemical localization of the enzymes involved in ammonia assimilation in mesophyll and bundle-sheath cells of maize leaves. *Planta* **191,** 129–136.

Boinski, J. J., Wang, J.-L., Xu, P., Hotchkiss, T., and Berry, J. O. (1993). Post-transcriptional control of cell type-specific gene expression in bundle sheath and mesophyll chloroplasts of *Amaranthus hypochondriacus. Plant Mol. Biol.* **22,** 397–410.

Broglie, R., Coruzzi, G., Keith, B., and Chua, N.-H. (1984). Molecular biology of C_4 photosynthesis in *Zea mays:* Differential localization of proteins and mRNAs in the two leaf cell types. *Plant Mol. Biol.* **3,** 431–444.

Hatch, M. D. (1992). C_4 photosynthesis: An unlikely process full of surprises. *Plant Cell Physiol.* **33,** 333–342.

Kanai, R., and Edwards, G. E. (1973). Separation of mesophyll protoplasts and bundle sheath cells from maize leaves for photosynthetic studies. *Plant Physiol.* **51,** 1133–1137.

Langdale, J. A., Taylor, W. C., and Nelson, T. (1991). Cell-specific accumulation of maize phosphoenolpyruvate carboxylase is correlated with demethylation at a specific site >3 kb upstream of the gene. *Mol. Gen. Genet.* **225,** 49–55.

Meierhoff, K., and Westhoff, P. (1993). Differential biogenesis of photosystem II in mesophyll and bundle-sheath cells of monocotyledonous NADP-malic enzyme-type C_4 plant: The non-stoichiometric abundance of the subunits of photosystem II in the bundle-sheath chloroplasts and the translational activity of the plastome-encoded genes. *Planta* **191,** 23–33.

Moore, B. D., Ku, M. S. B., and Edwards, G. E. (1984). Isolation of leaf bundle sheath protoplasts from C_4 dicot species and intracellular localization of selected enzymes. *Plant Sci. Lett.* **35,** 127–138.

Moore, B. D., Monson, R. K., Ku, M. S. B., and Edwards, G. E. (1988). Activities of principal photosynthetic and photorespiratory enzymes in leaf mesophyll and bundle sheath protoplasts from the C_3-C_4 intermediate *Flaveria ramosissima. Plant Cell Physiol.* **29,** 999–1006.

Ngernprasirtsir, J., Chollet, R., Kobayashi, H., Sugiyama, T., and Akazawa, T. (1989). DNA methylation and the differential expression of C_4 photosynthesis genes in mesophyll and bundle sheath cells of greening maize leaves. *J. Biol. Chem.* **264,** 8241–8248.

Nelson, T., and Langdale, J. A. (1992). Developmental genetics of C_4 photosynthesis. *Annu. Rev. Plant Physiol. Plant Mol. Biol.* **43,** 25–47.

Potter, J. W., and Black, C. C. (1982). Differential protein composition and gene expression in leaf mesophyll cells and bundle sheath cells of the C_4 plant *Digitaria sanguinalis. Plant Physiol.* **70,** 590–597.

Schäffner, A. R., and Sheen, J. (1991). Maize rbcS promoter activity depends on sequence elements not found in dicot rbcS promoters. *Plant Cell* **3,** 997–1012.

Schäffner, A. R., and Sheen, J. (1992). Maize C4 photosynthesis involves differential regulation of maize PEPC genes. *Plant J.* **2,** 221–232.

Sheen, J. (1990). Metabolic repression of transcription in higher plants. *Plant Cell* **2,** 1027–1038.

Sheen, J. (1991). Molecular mechanisms underlying the differential expression of maize pyruvate, orthophosphate dikinase genes. *Plant Cell* **3,** 225–245.

Sheen, J. (1993). Protein phosphatase activity is required for light-inducible gene expression in maize. *EMBO J.* **12,** 3497–3505.

Sheen, J.-Y., and Bogorad, L. (1985). Differential expression of the ribulose bisphosphate carboxylase large subunit gene in bundle sheath and mesophyll cells of developing maize leaves is influenced by light. *Plant Physiol.* **79,** 1072–1076.

Sheen, J.-Y., and Bogorad, L. (1987a). Regulation of levels of nuclear transcripts for C_4 photosynthesis in bundle sheath and mesophyll cells of maize leaves. *Plant Mol. Biol.* **8,** 227–238.

Sheen, J.-Y., and Bogorad, L. (1987b). Differential expression of C4 pathway genes in mesophyll and bundle sheath cells of greening maize leaves. *J. Biol. Chem.* **262,** 11726–11730.

Spilatro, S. R., and Preiss, J. (1987). Regulation of starch synthesis in the bundle sheath and mesophyll of *Zea mays. Plant Physiol.* **83,** 621–627.

Tsaftaris, A. S., Bosabalidis, A. M., and Scandalios, J. G. (1983). Cell-type-specific gene expression and acatalasemic peroxisomes in a null *Cat2* catalase mutant of maize. *Proc. Natl. Acad. Sci. U. S. A.* **80,** 4455–4459.

Valle, E. M., Craig, S., Hatch, M. D., and Heldt, H. W. (1989). Permeability and ultrastructure of bundle sheath cells isolated from C_4 plants: Structure-function studies and the role of plasmodesmata. *Botanica Acta* **102,** 276–282.

Walbot, V., and Hoisington, D. A. (1982). Isolation of mesophyll and bundle sheath chloroplasts from maize. *In* "Methods in Chloroplast Molecular Biology" (M. Edelman, R. B. Hallick, and N.-H. Chua, eds.), pp. 211–219. New York: Elsevier Biomedical.

Woo, K. C., Anderson, J. M., Boardman, N. K., Downton, W. J. S., Osmond, C. B., and Thorne, S. W. (1970). Deficient photosystem II in agranal bundle sheath chloroplasts of C4 plants. *Proc. Natl. Acad. Sci. U. S. A.* **67,** 18–25.

CHAPTER 22

Synchronization of Cell Cultures of Higher Plants

Hiroaki Kodama[*] and Atsushi Komamine[†]

[*]Department of Biology
Faculty of Science
Kyushu University 33
Fukuoka 812, Japan

[†]Department of Chemical and Biological Sciences
Japan Women's University
2-8-1 Mejirodai, Bunkyo-ku
Tokyo 112, Japan

I. Introduction

A synchronous culture is a culture in which all cells pass through the same point in the cell cycle simultaneously. Thus, the initiation of DNA synthesis or

METHODS IN CELL BIOLOGY, VOL. 49

mitosis is observed to occur in all cells at the same time. Synchronous cultures are very useful and effective tools for investigations of particular biochemical and molecular biological events at specific phases of the cell cycle. Synchronous cultures can be established by three different methods, known as natural synchrony, selection synchrony, and induction synchrony.

Natural synchrony, in which almost all cells are observed to be at the same stage of the cell cycle without any synchronization treatment, has been noted in higher plants, for example, during male gametogenesis in lily and rape (Scott *et al.*, 1991), in primary cultures that include cultures of tuber slices of *Helianthus tuberosus* (Yeoman and Mitchell, 1970), and in tobacco mesophyll protoplasts (Cooke and Mayer, 1981).

Selection synchrony is achieved by the physical isolation of cells at a specific stage of the cell cycle from an asynchronous culture. This method is frequently utilized to obtain synchronous cultures of mammalian cells (by a mitotic detachment method) and yeasts (by a method based on density gradient centrifugation). However, no analogous appropriate selection method is available for cells of higher plants.

Induction synchrony is achieved by the arrest of almost all cells at a specific point during the cell cycle, with subsequent release of cells from growth arrest, and it is a widely used method for synchronization of cells from higher plants. The manipulations used to bring about growth arrest of cells include physical means, methods involving removal and readdition of certain components of the growth medium, and methods that involve exposure to inhibitors that reversibly block cell-cycle events. Table I shows a list of typical methods for the generation of synchronous cell-division systems that have been applied to suspension cultures of cells from higher plants.

Recent progress in the understanding of the molecular mechanisms of the cell cycle has been significant in mammalian and yeast cells and has also promoted investigations of molecular aspects of the cell cycle in plants (reviewed by Ito and Komamine, 1993). In recent studies, however, synchronous cell-division systems that allow effective molecular analysis of the plant cell cycle have been restricted to only a few systems: two systems involving nutrient-starvation methods (a method of phosphate starvation and refeeding, established by Amino *et al.*, 1983, and a method of auxin starvation and refeeding, established by Nishida *et al.*, 1992) and a system involving treatment with aphidicolin (Nagata *et al.*, 1982). These frequently used synchronous culture systems have several useful characteristics as practical experimental tools, namely, they allow high reproducibility of the degree of synchrony and the procedures for synchronization are simple. The useful characteristics also include reproducibility in terms of the proportion of cells that divide during one round of the cell cycle and the time course of the progression of the cell cycle.

Starvation of phosphate or of auxin causes the arrest of cells at the G1 phase of the cell cycle in suspension cultures of *Catharanthus roseus* cells. Thus, it is suitable for investigations of cell-cycle events during the G1 phase or the transi-

Table I
Synchronization of Cell Division Induced in Suspension Cultures of Cells from Higher Plants

Species	Method	Reference
Haplopappus	Hydroxyurea treatment	Eriksson, 1966
Acer	Cytokinin starvation and refeeding	Roberts and Northcote, 1970
Nicotiana	Cytokinin starvation and refeeding	Jouanneau, 1971
Daucus	Starvation[a] + low temperature	Okamura *et al.*, 1973
Glycine	Anaerobic treatment	Constabel *et al.*, 1974
Acer	Starvation[a]	King *et al.*, 1974
Nicotiana	Starvation[a] + light/dark cycle	Nishinari and Yamaki, 1976
Daucus	Auxin starvation and refeeding	Nishi *et al.*, 1977
Glycine	Ethylene treatment	Constabel *et al.*, 1977
Glycine	5-Fluorodeoxyuridine treatment	Chu and Lark, 1976
Nicotiana	Aphidicolin treatment	Nagata *et al.*, 1982
Daucus	Aphidicolin treatment	Sala *et al.*, 1983
Catharanthus	Phosphate starvation and refeeding	Amino *et al.*, 1983
Nicotiana	Aphidicolin treatment	Nishinari and Syono, 1986
Catharanthus	Auxin starvation and refeeding	Nishida *et al.*, 1992
Medicago	Phosphate starvation and refeeding	Kapros *et al.*, 1992
Oryza	Aphidicolin treatment	Nakasone *et al.*, 1993

[a] Including "dilution" with fresh medium or "transfer" to fresh medium of cells at stationary phase.

tion from the G1 phase to the S phase. Aphidicolin is a toxin produced by the fungus *Cephalosporium aphidicola* and it is a specific and reversible inhibitor of DNA polymerase α. Cells from a wide range of higher plants can be synchronized by the addition to the growth medium of aphidicolin at a final concentration of 5 to ~25 μg/ml. Since high mitotic indices can be obtained (about 70% in the case of tobacco cells), synchronous cultures induced by use of aphidicolin are appropriate for biochemical and morphological analyses of the events that occur from the G2 to the M phase.

In the synchronous cultures mentioned above, progression of the cell cycle is rapidly reinitiated, without any delay, after the removal of the drug or the addition of phosphate or auxin. Thus, treatment with aphidicolin and starvation of phosphate or auxin are considered to do limited damage to cells. However, the manipulations required for synchronization unavoidably disturb normal metabolic activities to some extent. Results obtained from synchronous cultures must be carefully distinguished from the effects of the factor that induces the synchrony and, if possible, results should be confirmed in another system that includes flow cytometry (Galbraith, 1990) or synchronous cultures in which synchrony has been achieved by a different method. In this chapter, we shall discuss the main methods used for synchronization of cells from higher plants. Reviews by King (1980) and Gould (1984) are valuable resources for those interested in the basic aspects of cell proliferation and growth of higher plants, as well as the introduction of synchronous cultures.

II. Application

This section provides an outline of procedures for synchronization by starvation and refeeding of phosphate or auxin in *Catharanthus roseus* cells. Synchronization by the phosphate starvation method had been considered to be restricted to suspension cultures of *C. roseus* cells (Amino *et al.,* 1983). However, recent work indicates that synchrony can be achieved by the phosphate starvation method in suspension cultures of *Medicago varia* (Kapros *et al.,* 1992) and of *Populus alba* (Maki, personal communication). The formulation of the basal culture medium may be a key factor for achieving synchrony by the phosphate starvation method. All suspension cultures amenable to synchronization by this method are maintained in Murashige-Skoog (MS) medium (Murashige and Skoog, 1962). The standard formulation of MS medium includes a relatively low concentration of phosphate, in contrast to elevated levels of nitrogen sources. Thus, these cells are maintained under conditions whereby phosphate in the MS medium limits the division of cells.

Synchronization by auxin starvation has been reported in suspension cultures of carrot cells (Nishi *et al.,* 1977) and of *C. roseus* cells (Nishida *et al.,* 1992), but strains suitable for synchronization by this means are apparently limited. In fact, among three suspension cultures of *C. roseus* maintained in our laboratory, cells of only one strain (TN21) can be well synchronized by the auxin starvation method. In cells cultured for long periods of time, this method may be unsuitable for synchronization because of habituation of cells to exogenous auxin. However, the phenomenon of auxin-induced rapid restoration of cell division is very attractive for studies of the role of auxin in the control of cell proliferation.

Synchronization by aphidicolin treatment has been reported in suspension cultures of carrot (Sala *et al.,* 1983), tobacco (Nagata *et al.,* 1982; Nishinari and Syono, 1986), and rice (Nakasone *et al.,* 1993) cells. In fact, suspension cultures of most plant cells are amenable to synchronization treatment with aphidicolin. Aphidicolin often causes inactivation of cells to some extent, depending on its concentration and the duration of treatment. Thus, experimental conditions must be determined carefully in each suspension culture. Details of procedures for synchronization treatment with aphidicolin can be found elsewhere (Sala *et al.,* 1986).

III. Plant Materials

For synchronization by the phosphate starvation method, suspension cultures of strain A (or B) of *Catharanthus roseus* L. G Don are used. These strains were initiated from a culture of stems in 1969. Cells are maintained at 27°C, in the dark, in MS medium that contains 3% (w/v) sucrose and 2.2 μM 2,4-dichlorophenoxyacetic acid (2,4-D). Cells are subcultured every 7 days by the transfer of 7 ml of the suspension of cells into 43 ml of fresh medium in a 300-ml Erlenmeyer flask, and flasks are shaken at 80 to ~90 strokes/minute on a shaker.

Strain TN21 was initiated from a culture of anthers of *Catharanthus roseus* L. cv. Little Pinky in 1988. Almost all cells in cultures of this strain are diploid. Cells of strain TN21 are maintained under the same culture conditions as described above, with the exception of the concentration of 2,4-D (4.4 μM), and they can be synchronized by the auxin starvation method.

IV. Procedures

A. Determination of Cell Number

Cell number is estimated by counting protoplasts with a hemocytometer after enzymatic maceration. The mixture for maceration of *C. roseus* A (or B) contains 0.5 ml of enzyme solution [10% (w/v) Cellulase "Onozuka" R-10 plus 5% (w/v) Macerozyme R-10; Yakult Honsha, Osaka, Japan] and 2 ml of a solution of 0.6 M mannitol and 1% (w/v) $CaCl_2$ in which cells are suspended at a concentration of 1×10^5 to $\sim 5 \times 10^5$ cells/ml. The mixture is incubated for 60 min at 27°C on a shaker operated at 60 strokes/minute.

Protoplasts of strain TN21 are prepared by enzymatic maceration of cells for 60 min with a slightly different enzyme solution, with final concentrations of 2% (w/v) Cellulase Onozuka R-10, 1% (w/v) Macerozyme R-10 and 1% (w/v) Pectolyase Y-23 (Seishin Seiyaku, Tokyo, Japan). Other conditions for preparing protoplasts of strain TN21 are the same as those for strain A (or B).

B. Determination of Percentages of Living Cells in Cultures

Cell viability is determined by staining the living cells with 0.12 mM fluorescein diacetate (Aldrich Chemical Co., WI) for 5 min by the method of Widholm (1972) and examining at least 500 cells.

C. Determination of Mitotic Indices

Cells are fixed in 2% (w/v) glutaraldehyde in 30 mM potassium phosphate buffer (pH 7). Fixed cells are stained with a solution of 0.5 μg/ml 4-6-diamidino-2-phenylindole (DAPI; Sigma, St. Louis, MO) by the method described by Kuroiwa *et al.*, (1981), or they are stained by the Feulgen method, as follows: cells are hydrolyzed in 1 M HCl for 10 min at 60°C, stained in Schiff's reagent for 3 h, and washed with sodium bisulfite solution. The mitotic index is determined by counting the number of DAPI-stained or Feulgen-stained nuclei (more than 1000) that are clearly recognized to be at metaphase or anaphase in a given population of cells.

D. Incorporation of [^{3}H]Thymidine

The rate of DNA synthesis is measured by labeling cells with [^{3}H]thymidine (111 kBq/ml suspension, 1.67 TBq/mmol; Amersham Japan, Tokyo, Japan) for 60 min at 27°C. After incubation, 1.6 ml of ice-cold ethanol is added to 0.4 ml of the suspension of labeled cells. The cells are centrifuged at $2000 \times g$ for 10 min. The pellet is washed twice with 80% ice-cold ethanol and then with 0.2 *M* ice-cold perchloric acid (PCA). Nucleic acids are solubilized by heating in 0.5 *M* PCA at 80°C for 15 min. The extract is centrifuged and radioactivity of an aliquot of the supernatant is measured in a liquid scintillation counter.

E. Flow Cytometric Analysis

Protoplasts of *C. roseus* strain A were isolated by enzymatic maceration as described above (see Section IV,A). They were then fixed in 70% (v/v) ethanol. Protoplasts stained with acridine orange were analyzed by flow cytometry using an EPICS V flow cytometer (Coulter Electronics, FL) operating at a laser wavelength of 480 nm, as described in Ando *et al.* (1987). Histograms of green fluorescence, using Peak parameters, were obtained from a total protoplast count of 20,000.

V. Critical Aspects for Synchronization

The properties of cell clusters that are necessary for successful synchronization are (*a*) a homogeneous and finely dispersed population of cells suitable for synchronization and for observations of the nucleus and chromosomes in each cell; (*b*) a high percentage of actively dividing cells (see also Section VII); and (*c*) cell clusters that can easily be macerated by cell-wall-degrading enzymes to yield protoplasts at an efficiency of almost 100%. Almost all cultures in which good synchrony has been achieved have had the properties mentioned. In the case of rice cells in suspension culture, the formulation of the basal medium was modified in order to provide finely dispersed cells, with resultant successful synchronization by aphidicolin treatment (Nakasone *et al.*, 1993).

VI. Results

A. Synchronous Cultures of *C. roseus* Cells Induced by the Phosphate Starvation Method

1. Effect of the Concentration of Phosphate on Proliferation of Cells

The growth cycle of suspension-cultured *C. roseus* cells of strain A (or B) consists of a lag phase of about 1 day, a logarithmic phase of 4 days, and a stationary phase that is reached about 6 days after subculture (Fig. 1).

Cells at stationary phase were cultured for 3 days in phosphate-free MS medium at an initial cell density of about 3×10^5 cells/ml. Then phosphate was added as KH_2PO_4 to cultures to give final concentrations of 0, 0.1, 0.15, 0.2, 0.625, and 1.25 m*M*. Cells were cultured for 9 days (except in the case of the culture with 0 m*M* phosphate) and the number of cells was counted. The number of cells in the culture in which the concentration of phosphate was 0 m*M* was determined 3 days after the addition of phosphate (Fig. 2). A linear relationship between the concentration of phosphate in the medium (0 to ~1.25 m*M*; standard MS medium contains 1.25 m*M* phosphate) and the number of cells at stationary phase was observed. Therefore, the phosphate in the MS medium was the factor that limited division of *C. roseus* cells.

2. Synchronization by the Phosphate Starvation Method

In all subsequent cultures, cells were cultured at 27°C in the dark and shaken at 80 to ~90 strokes/minute on a shaker. Cells at stationary phase were cultured

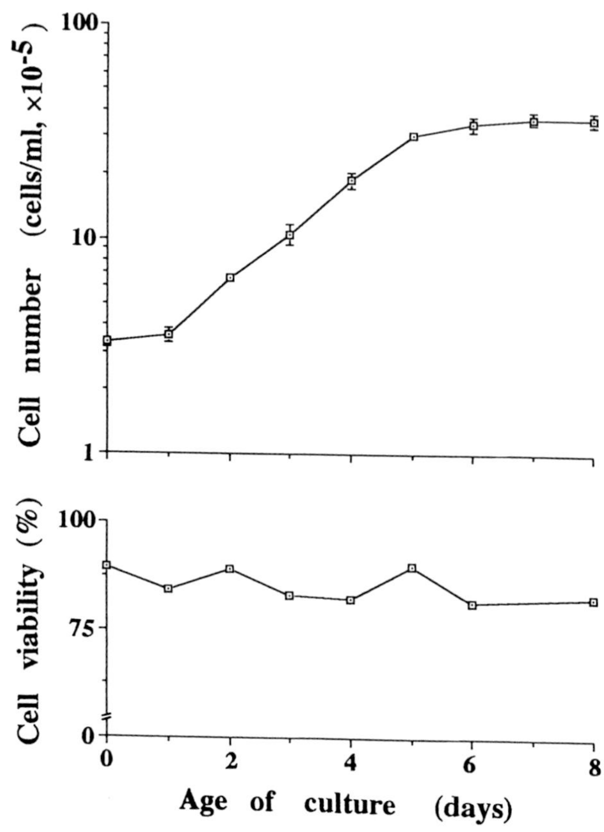

Fig. 1 Growth of cells of strain A of *C. roseus*. Changes in cell number and cell viability over the course of 8 days are shown. Vertical lines indicate standard deviations.

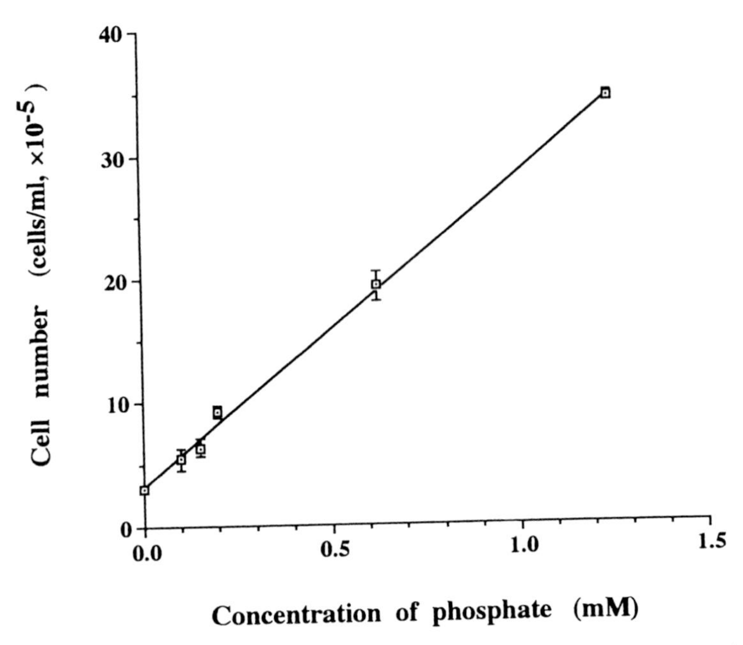

Fig. 2 Effect of the concentration of phosphate on the proliferation of *C. roseus* cells (strain A). Nine-day-cultured cells were transferred to phosphate-free medium. After culture for 3 days, phosphate was added to the medium at various concentrations, as indicated. After proliferation had ceased, cell numbers were determined. Vertical lines indicate standard deviations.

for 3 days in 100 to ~150 ml of phosphate-free medium at an initial cell density of about 3×10^5 cells/ml in 500-ml Erlenmeyer flasks. No apparent proliferation of cells was observed in the first phosphate-starved culture. Phosphate was then added directly to the medium at a final concentration of 0.14 m*M*, which allowed cells to divide once. The concentration of phosphate was estimated from the results shown in Fig. 2. Eighteen hours later the cells were collected by centrifugation at $800 \times g$ for 2 min, washed twice with phosphate-free medium, and resuspended in phosphate-free medium at a cell density of about 2×10^5 cells/ml. This suspension of cells was gently mixed by stirring with a magnetic stirrer for homogeneous dispersion of cells and divided into 10-ml aliquots in 50-ml Erlenmeyer flasks. Cell number increased two-fold during a 3-day culture under the new phosphate-starved conditions. Most cells were arrested preferentially at the early G1 phase (Ando *et al.*, 1987). In our experiments, we usually confirm the arrest of cell proliferation by counting cells at 8-h intervals. Then phosphate is added to a final concentration of 0.625 m*M* and synchronized division of cells can be observed. A diagram of the procedure of the phosphate starvation method is shown in Fig. 3.

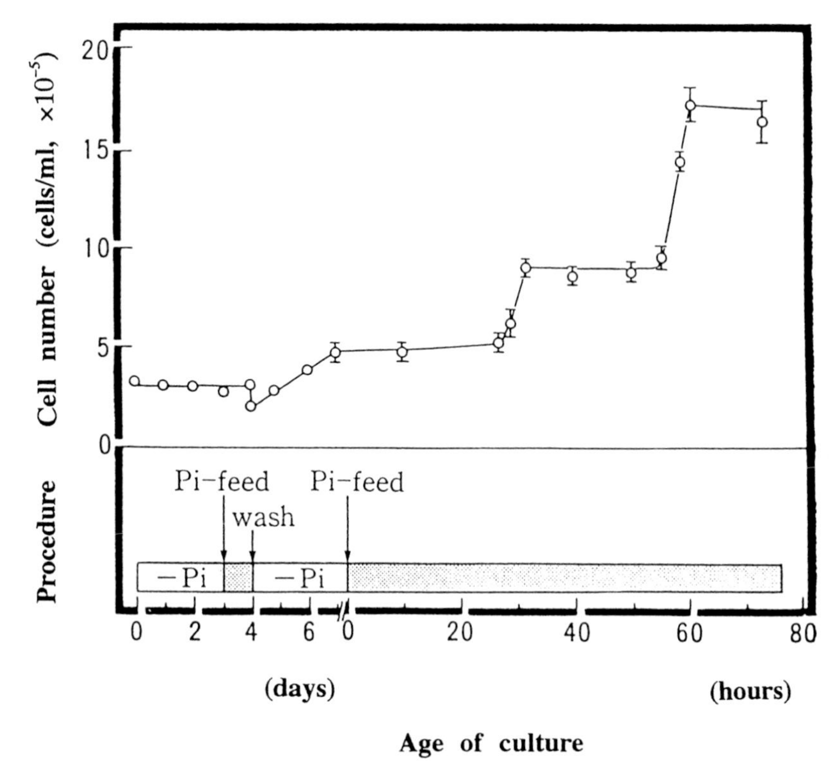

Fig. 3 Diagram of the procedure of synchronization by the phosphate starvation method. Pi indicates phosphate. Vertical lines indicate standard deviations.

3. Synchronization of DNA Synthesis and Mitosis

Synchronous division of cells occurred 27 to ~31 h after the second addition of phosphate. Cell numbers usually increased by 70 to ~80%. DNA synthesis was examined by monitoring incorporation of [^{3}H]thymidine into the DNA fraction. The S phase was 6 to ~17 h in length after the second addition of phosphate. A sharp increase in mitotic index was observed 26 to ~30 h after the second addition of phosphate (Fig. 4).

4. Distribution of the DNA Content in Population of Cells through the Cell Cycle

An analysis of the DNA contents for protoplasts obtained from a synchronous culture by flow cytometry is shown in Fig. 5. The DNA histogram of protoplasts prepared from the cells in the G1 phase showed only one peak (peak A) corresponding to a 2C level of the DNA content. Since the nuclear DNA content increased two-fold during the S phase, almost all protoplasts prepared from the

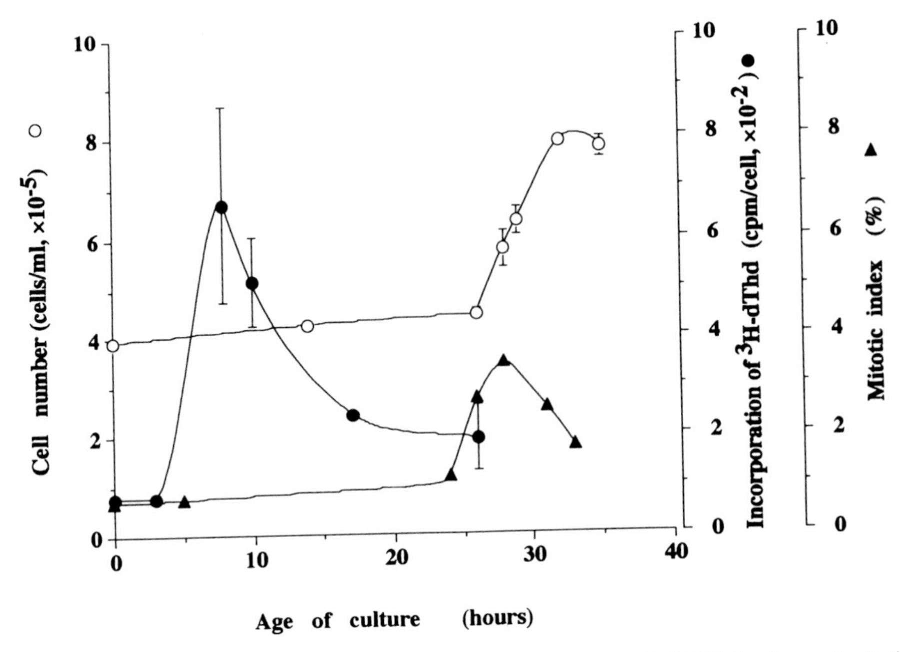

Fig. 4 Changes in cell number, incorporation of [^{3}H]thymidine into the DNA fraction, and mitotic indices in a synchronous culture of *C. roseus* cells (strain A), induced by the phosphate starvation method. Age of culture indicates the time after the second addition of phosphate. Vertical lines indicate standard deviations.

cells in the G2 phase had a 4C level of DNA content (peak B). In the histogram of protoplasts from the cells in cytokinesis, two peaks were observed and they corresponded to 2C (peak C) and 4C (peak D) DNA levels, respectively. The former seems to correspond to cells after cytokinesis and the latter to cells before cytokinesis. These flow cytometric data and the results obtained by measuring the number of cells and incorporation of [^{3}H]thymidine into the DNA fraction during the cell cycle showed a good correlation.

B. Synchronous Cultures of *C. roseus* Cells Induced by the Auxin Starvation Method

1. Effects of Auxin on the Proliferation of Cells of the TN21 Strain

The growth cycle of TN21 cells consists of a lag phase of about 1 day and a logarithmic phase of 5 to ~6 days. A stationary phase is reached after about 8 days of subculture. High cell viability (about 80%) is evident for 8 days after subculture (data not shown). Cells at stationary phase were transferred to medium free of 2,4-D (auxin-free medium) after four washes with auxin-free medium. The unique property of TN21 cells is that no increase in cell number is observed in auxin-free medium for at least for 8 days (Fig. 6). 2,4-D was added to the

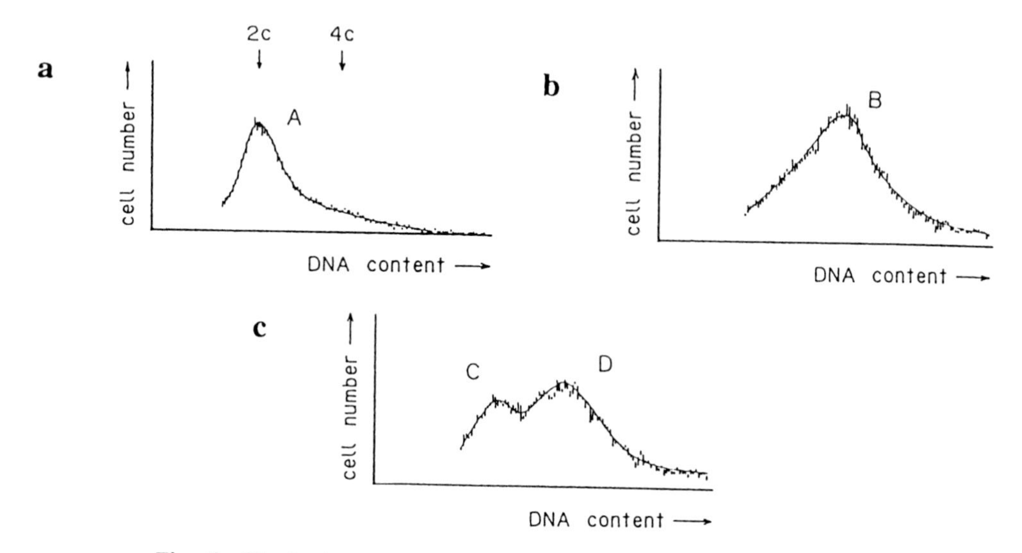

Fig. 5 Distribution of DNA contents in a synchronous culture of *C. roseus* cells induced by the phosphate starvation method. Flow cytometric analysis of acridine orange-stained protoplasts: protoplasts from cells (a) in G1 phase, (b) in G2 phase, and (c) in cytokinesis.

medium at a final concentration of 2.2 μM zero, 2, and 4 days after 2,4-D had been eliminated. Cell proliferation was reinitiated within 2 days after the addition of 2,4-D (Fig. 6). Because rapid restoration of cell growth was observed even after 4 days upon the readdition of 2,4-D, high cell viability was clearly maintained in clusters incubated without 2,4-D for at least 4 days. These results indicate that cells of the TN21 strain at stationary phase can be arrested in fresh, auxin-free MS medium and that refeeding of auxin allows cells to proliferate immediately. Therefore, proliferation of the TN21 cells can be controlled by the level of 2,4-D in the medium.

2. Synchronization by Starvation and Refeeding of Auxin

Eight-day cultured cells of the TN21 strain were washed four times by centrifugation at $800 \times g$ for 2 min with auxin-free MS medium, and then they were resuspended in auxin-free MS medium at a cell density of about 7×10^5 cells/ml. This suspension of cells was divided into 10-ml aliquots in 50-ml Erlenmeyer flasks as described above (see Section VI,A,2). After cells had been cultured for 2 days, 2,4-D was added at a final concentration of 4.4 μM. The synchronized synthesis of DNA and cell division was observed. A diagram of the procedure of the auxin starvation method is shown in Fig. 7.

3. Synchronization of DNA Synthesis and Mitosis

Synchronous division of cells occurred 12 to 15 h after the readdition of 2,4-D to cultures of TN21 cells and the cell number increased by 75%. A single

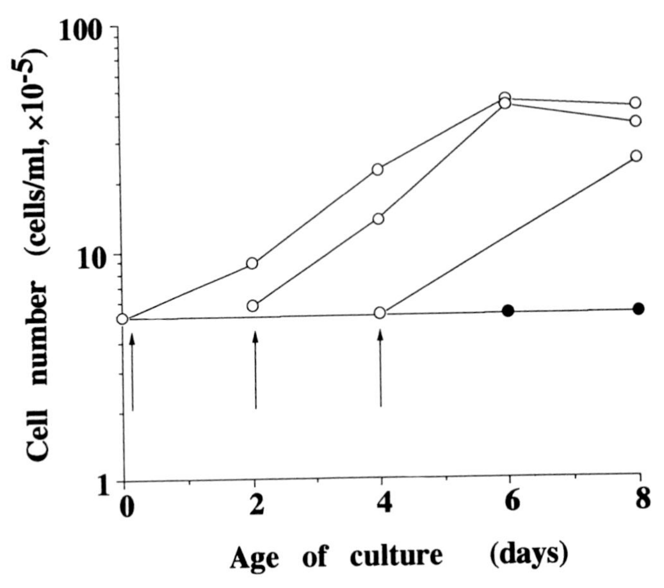

Fig. 6 Effects of 2,4-D on the proliferation of *C. roseus* cells (strain TN21) after auxin starvation. Changes are shown in cell number in auxin-free medium (●), and in medium supplemented with auxin zero, 2, and 4 days (○) after the transfer of cells at stationary phase to auxin-free medium. Arrows indicate the time at which 2,4-D was added.

and clear peak of incorporation of [^{3}H] thymidine was observed 9 h after the addition of 2,4-D. The mitotic index remained below 1% during the period when cell number hardly changed (0 to ~12 h after the addition of auxin). The mitotic index reached a maximum value 14 h after the addition of auxin, and it also showed a clear peak (Fig. 8).

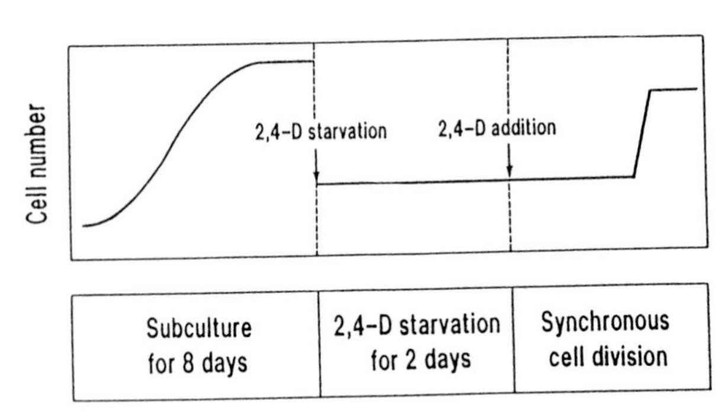

Fig. 7 Diagram of the procedure of synchronization by the auxin starvation method.

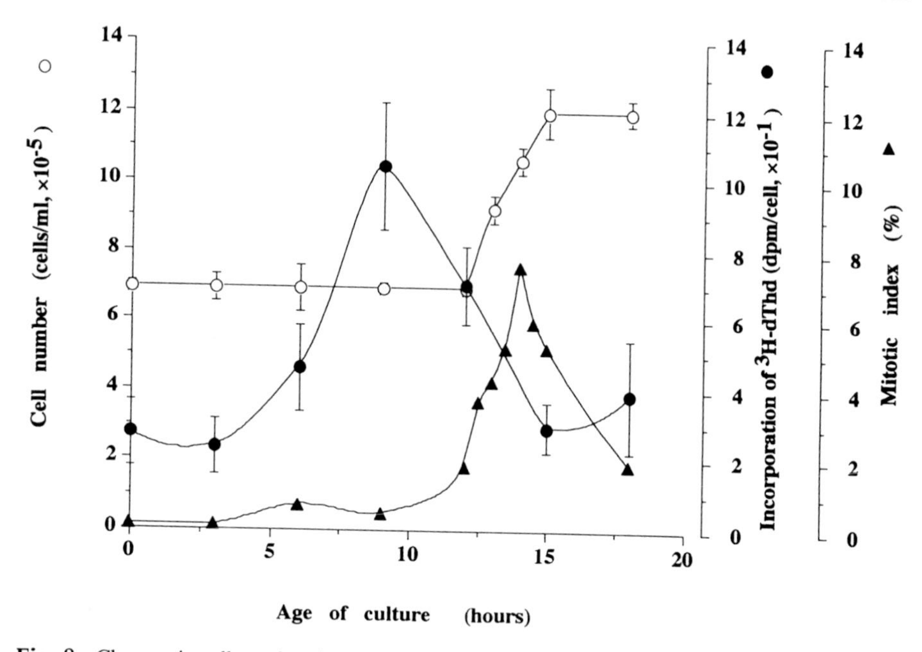

Fig. 8 Changes in cell number, incorporation of [^{3}H]thymidine into the DNA fraction, and mitotic indices in a synchronous culture of *C. roseus* cells (strain TN21) induced by the auxin starvation method. Age of culture indicates the time after the addition of auxin. Vertical lines indicate standard deviations.

VII. Discussion

The manipulations required for synchronization of cell cultures often disturb the proliferation of cells and cause a stepwise increase in cell numbers. Everett *et al.* (1981) designated this disturbed growth as "periodic growth." During periodic growth, broad peaks of maximal mitotic indices can be observed, and the rates of increases in cell numbers are nearly the same as those in rapidly growing, asynchronous cultures. True synchrony must be distinguished from periodic growth by careful interpretation of the indices that are used to assess synchrony. The indices used to assess synchrony include cell number, mitotic index, the percentage of labeled nuclei, and the distribution of the DNA content by using flow cytometry. The Scherbaum synchrony index (SI) is also appropriate for the evaluation of synchrony, and it is calculated from the following equation:

$$\mathrm{SI} = (n_2/n_1 - 1) \times (1 - t/g),$$

where n_2 is the number of cells after a synchronous division, n_1 is the number of cells before the division, t is the time during which cells divide, and g is the doubling time (Scherbaum, 1964). Scherbaum synchrony indices range from 0.6 to

0.8 in synchronous cultures of *C. roseus* cells induced by the phosphate starvation method and by the auxin starvation method, and in synchronous cultures of *Acer pseudoplatanus* cells induced by the transfer of cells at stationary phase to fresh medium (King *et al.*, 1974), whereas these indices in synchronous cultures induced by aphidicolin treatment reach about 0.9. The ratio of n_2/n_1 is strongly influenced by the percentage of nondividing cells in each culture, which can be estimated by measurement of the growth fraction or can be estimated roughly from cell viability in homogeneous, rapidly growing cultures. The growth fraction is the proportion of cells that is cycling in culture, and it is determined from maximum [^{3}H]thymidine-labeling indices (Sala *et al.*, 1986). The increase in cell number in one cell cycle is 70 to ~80% in the two kinds of synchronous culture of *C. roseus* cells. This value corresponds closely to the percentage of living cells. Therefore, the maintenance of a high growth fraction is important for obtaining good synchrony.

The timing of release of cells from the growth-arrested state during the cell cycle is also considered to be a factor that determines the degree of synchrony. The duration of the G1 phase is very variable, in contrast to that of the S, the G2, and the M phase. The high synchrony indices in synchronous cultures induced by aphidicolin treatment can be explained, at least in part, by the fact that the G1 phase is hardly detectable during the first round of the cell cycle in such cultures.

References

Amino, S., Fujimura, T., and Komamine, A. (1983). Synchrony induced by double phosphate starvation in a suspension culture of *Catharanthus roseus*. *Physiol. Plant.* **59,** 393–396.

Ando, S., Schimizu, T., Kodama, H., Amino, S., and Komamine, A. (1987). Flow cytometric analysis of the cell cycle in synchronous culture of *Catharanthus roseus*. *Agric. Biol. Chem.* **51,** 1443–1445.

Chu, Y., and Lark, K. G. (1976). Cell-cycle parameters of soybean (*Glycine max* L.) Cells growing in suspension culture: suitability of system for genetic studies. *Planta* **132,** 259–268.

Constabel, F., Kurz, W. G. W., Chatson, B., and Gamborg, O. L. (1974). Induction of partial synchrony in soybean cell cultures. *Exp. Cell Res.* **85,** 105–110.

Constabel, F., Kurz, W. G. W., Chatson, K. B., and Kirkpatrick, J. W. (1977). Partial synchrony in soybean cell suspension cultures induced by ethylene. *Exp. Cell Res.* **105,** 263–268.

Cooke, R., and Mayer, Y. (1981). Hormonal control of tobacco protoplast nucleic acid metabolism during in vitro culture. *Planta* **152,** 1–7.

Eriksson, T. (1966). Partial synchronization of cell division in suspension cultures of *Haplopappus gracilis*. *Physiol. Plant.* **19,** 900–910.

Everett, N. P., Wang, T. L., Gould, A. R., and Street, H. E. (1981). Studies on the control of the cell cycle in cultured plant cells. II. Effects of 2,4-dichlorophenoxyacetic acid (2,4-D). *Protoplasma* **106,** 15–22.

Galbraith, D. W. (1990). Isolation and flow cytometric characterization of plant protoplasts. *Methods Cell Biol.* **33,** 527–547.

Gould, A. R. (1984). Control of the cell cycle in cultured plant cells. *CRC Crit. Rev. Plant Sci.* **1,** 315–344.

Ito, M., and Komamine, A. (1993). Molecular mechanisms of the cell cycle in synchronous cultures of plant cells. *J. Plant Res. Special Issue* **3,** 17–28.

Jouanneau, J. P. (1971). Controle par les cytokinines de la synchronisation des mitoses dans les cellules de tabac. *Exp. Cell Res.* **67,** 329–337.

Kapros T., Bogre, L., Nemeth, K., Bako, L., Gyorgyey, J., Wu, S. C., and Dudits, D. (1992). Differential expression of histone H3 gene variants during cell cycle and somatic embryogenesis in alfalfa. *Plant Physiol.* **98,** 621–625.

King, P. J. (1980). Cell proliferation and growth in suspension cultures. *Int. Rev. Cytol. Suppl.* **11A,** 25–53.

King, P. J., Cox, B. J., Fowler, M. W., and Street, H. E. (1974). Metabolic events in synchronized cell cultures of *Acer pseudoplatanus L. Planta* **117,** 109–122.

Kuroiwa, T., Suzuki, T., Ogawa, K., and Kawano, S. (1981). The chloroplast nucleus: Distribution, number, size and shape and a model for the multiplication of the chloroplast genome during chloroplast development. *Plant Cell Physiol.* **22,** 381–396.

Murashige, T., and Skoog, F. (1962). A revised medium for rapid growth and bioassays with tobacco tissue cultures. *Physiol. Plant.* **15,** 473–497.

Nagata, T., Okada, K., and Takebe, I. (1982). Mitotic protoplasts and their infection with tobacco mosaic virus RNA encapsulated in liposomes. *Plant Cell Rep.* **1,** 250–252.

Nakasone, S., Minami, E., Imai, T., Akiyama, F., and Ohashi, Y. (1993). Synchronous cell division in rice suspension cultures and cell cycle specific expression of histone H3 and PCNA genes. *Bull. Natl. Inst. Agrobiol. Resour.* (*Japan*) **8,** 1–10.

Nishi, A., Kato, K., Takahashi, M., and Yoshida, R. (1977). Partial synchronization of carrot cell culture by auxin deprivation. *Physiol. Plant.* **39,** 9–12.

Nishida, T., Ohnishi, N., Kodama, H., and Komamine, A. (1992). Establishment of synchrony by elimination and readdition of auxin in suspension cultures of *Catharanthus roseus* cells. *Plant Cell Tissue Organ Culture* **28,** 37–43.

Nishinari, N., and Yamaki, T. (1976). Relationship between cell division and endogenous auxin in synchronously-cultured tobacco cells. *Bot. Mag. Tokyo* **89,** 73–81.

Nishinari, N., and Syono, K. (1986). Induction of cell division synchrony and variation of cytokinin contents through the cell cycle in tobacco cultured cells. *Plant Cell Physiol.* **27,** 147–153.

Okamura, S., Miyasaka, K., and Nishi, A. (1973). Synchonization of carrot cell culture by starvation and cold treatment. *Exp. Cell Res.* **78,** 467–470.

Roberts, K., and Northcote, D. H. (1970). The structure of sycamore callus cells during division in a partially synchronized suspension culture. *J. Cell Sci.* **6,** 299–321.

Sala, F., Galli, M. G., Nielsen, E., Magnien, E., Devreux, M., Pedrali-Noy, G., and Spadari, S. (1983). Synchronization of nuclear DNA synthesis in cultured *Daucus carota* L. cells by aphidicolin. *FEBS Lett.* **153,** 204–208.

Sala, F., Galli, M. G., Pedrali-Noy, G., and Spadari, S. (1986). Synchronization of plant cells in culture and in meristems by aphidicolin. *Methods Enzymol.* **118,** 87–96.

Scherbaum, O. H. (1964). Comparison of synchronous and synchronized cell division. *Exp. Cell Res.* **33,** 89–98.

Scott, R., Dagless, E., Hodge, R., Paul, W., Soufleri, I., and Draper, J. (1991). Patterns of gene expression in developing anthers of *Brassica napus. Plant Mol. Biol.* **17,** 195–207.

Widholm. J. M. (1972). The use of fluorescein diacetate and phenosafranine for determining viability of cultured plant cells. *Stain Technol.* **47,** 189–194.

Yeoman, M. M., and Mitchell, J. P. (1970). Changes accompanying the addition of 2,4-D to excised Jerusalem artichoke tuber tissue. *Ann. Bot.* (*London*) **34,** 799–810.

CHAPTER 23

Genetic Tagging of Cells and Cell Layers for Studies of Plant Development

Angelo Spena and Francesco Salamini
MPI für Züchtungsforschung (Erwin-Baur-Institute)
Carl-von-Linné Weg 10
D-50829 Köln, Germany

I. Introduction

Cell lineage analysis assists understanding the cellular dynamics of morphogenetic processes. In plants, patterns of cell lineage have been investigated by using chimeras, spontaneous sectors, and sectors induced at specific stages of development and by sector boundary analysis (Dawe and Freeling, 1991). In this short methodological review, approaches to the study of pattern formation are also discussed.

Although an organism can be a genetic mosaic without a visible phenotypical manifestation, in clonal analysis a cell or its clonal progeny are conveniently tagged by visible cell-autonomous traits differentiating them from the surrounding background. Mutations affecting either chorophyll or flavonoid pigments have been most often used to mark genetic mosaics (Baur, 1909; Dulieu and Bugnon, 1966; Coe and Neuffer, 1978; Christianson, 1986; Poethig *et al.,* 1986; Dellaporta *et al.,* 1991; Dawe and Freeling, 1992). Other markers are size of cells due to ploidy level (Satina *et al.,* 1940), shape of epidermal hairs (Baur, 1909), amylose content (McClintock, 1978), and morphology of epicuticular waxes (Bossinger *et al.,* 1992a).

II. Chimeras

A. Methodology

Plant chimeras can originate: (*a*) as a consequence of spontaneous or induced nuclear mutations, (*b*) as variegated phenotypes generated by sorting out of cells with mutant plastids, (*c*) by grafting, and (*d*) from callus cultures composed of mixed populations of cells (for details, see Tilney-Basset, 1986).

Plant chimeras, either periclinal or sectorial (Figs. 1A and 1B, see Color Plates), are the visible manifestation of the existence of genetic differences within layered apical meristems. Thus, they are intra-apical genetic mosaics (Bergann, 1967). When the clonal progeny of a mutated cell occupies all layers of a sector of the apical meristem, the chimera is sectorial (Fig. $1B_2$). When the mutated sector does not span all the layers, the sectorial chimera is mericlinal (Fig. $1B_1$). In periclinal chimeras, the mutated cell population completely occupies one or more, but not all, layers. Periclinal chimeras usually arise from sectorial and mericlinal chimeras. Chimeras are propagated from stem cuttings possessing axillary meristems, but are lost during sexual reproduction because plant gametes originate from the LII layer, which usually delivers only its own genotype to the progeny.

In most gymnosperms, chimeras are absent because their meristems are not layered. Exceptions include some *Chamaecyparis* and *Juniperus* species, which have apical meristems with two layers (Pohlheim, 1971). Stable chimeras do not exist in ferns, which instead of an apical layered structure have a single apical cell (Bierhorst, 1977).

For a long time, chimeras have been created by intentional grafting (Columella, 1545; Della Porta, 1589, 1592). Successful grafts cut at the stock–scion junction allow the growth of the callus layers of one plant over the tissue of the second one, and the formation of meristemoids composed of cells from both scion and stock. Intra- and interspecific chimeras have been generated by grafting plants (Krenke, 1933) or hypocotyls *in vitro* (Noguchi *et al.,* 1992), from mixed callus cultures (Marcotrigiano and Gouin, 1984), and by cocultivation of isolated protoplasts (Binding *et al.,* 1987). Chimeras can be produced by colchicine (Blakeslee *et al.,* 1939), which can induce one or more layers to become polyploid after treatment of the seeds for 2 to 5 days with alkaloid concentrations between 0.01 and 1%. Chimeric apical meristems consisting of layers from two different species, or even genera, have been efficiently produced by treatment of the freshly decapitated stock–scion junction with 0.01% *p*-chlorophenoxyacetic acid (Kaddoura and Mantell, 1991).

In periclinal chimeras, the genotype of the layers can be determined by several methods. The state of LII can be inferred from the phenotype of the selfed progeny. Shape of epidermal hairs or of wax particles, or stomatal size, or presence of chloroplasts in the guard cells of the stomata are convenient markers for LI. Leaf shape has been used to infer LII and LIII composition (for details, see Tilney-Basset, 1986). Since adventitious buds can develop from either superficial or internal tissues (Broertjes and Keen, 1980; Norris *et al.,* 1983), their phenotypes can describe the genetic state of the layers concerned. In *Pelargonium, Bouvardia,* and other species Bateson (1921) identified the genotype of LIII by analyzing adventitious buds arising from roots. Genetic mosaics can be analyzed at the histological level when visible differences exist between layers.

In transgenic plants, a cellular layer can be tagged with dominant marker genes (Christou and McCabe, 1992). In these cases, the chimeric structure arises during genetic transformation. A transgenic tobacco chimera where the *rolC* gene is used as phenotypical marker (Spena *et al.,* 1989) and the *uidA* gene as histochemical marker (Jefferson, 1987) is shown in Fig. 1D.

B. Concepts and Principles

1. Cell Fate by Position

The concept that plant chimeras are a consequence of the layered state of the apex is recent (Baur, 1909). However, the curiosity elicited by the observation of these bizarre forms of biological organization is long-standing (e.g., Pontano, 1505; Della Porta, 1589). Indeed, the *Aurantium Virgatum* (Fig. 2A, see Color Plates) and the *Aurantium Striatum* (Ferrari, 1646), having the epidermis of the orange and the internal layers of the lemon, were among the first descriptions of periclinal chimeras. In the periclinal chimera "limone aranciato" (Savastano and Parrozzani, 1912; Fig. 2B), the epidermal streaks are due to periclinal divisions of the subepidermal orange tissue, which invades the layer above. The observation of these phenomena allows the following conclusions: (*a*) a plant organ can be composed of cells from two species; (*b*) cellular invasion and substitution do not modify the developmental plan of an organ; and (*c*) layer invasion changes both cellular location and fate. This is considered to be evidence that, at least in later stages of organ formation, the development of higher plants depends largely on cell position.

2. The Layered Vision of the Plant Body

Baur (1909), studying the variety "albomarginata hort." of *Pelargonium zonale,* first suggested that leaf variegation reflected the layered structure of the apex.

The existence of layers was visualized by Satina *et al.* (1940) using polyploid periclinal chimeras of *Datura.* These authors introduced the modern terminology for the cellular layers LI, LII, and LIII. The number of layers varies from two to four in different angiosperms. In a three-layered apical meristem, LI is the external layer (protoderm), LII the subprotodermal layer, and LIII the internal tissue. In the apical meristem, LI and LII are almost exclusively characterized by anticlinal divisions, whereas LIII grows by anticlinal and periclinal divisions (Satina, 1959). The cellular thickness of the layers in the apical meristem does not reflect the state of the mature organs (Krenke, 1933). This has been elegantly visualized in cytochimeras of peach (Dermen, 1953): the LII layer is monocellular at the center of the apical dome, but in the flanks of the dome it is already pluricellular.

3. Development of Leaf Primordia

Plant organ development is either caulinar (e.g., buds) or foliar (e.g., leaves, petals). Cells starting a caulinar type of development are called initials, whereas founder cells are the cells giving rise to a foliar type of development. In a bud primordium, meristematic activity starts deep in the layers of the corpus: LII in two-layered and LIII in three-layered plants. The meristematic process is restricted to a region from which it proceeds in an outward direction. The outer layer(s) divides exclusively anticlinally. Thus the outer layer(s) of the novel bud is derived directly from the same layer(s) of the shoot apical meristem. As soon as an apical meristem is organized, the growth of the organ becomes apical.

Foliar ontogenesis starts from a group of cells distributed transversally around the stem. In some plants (i.e., grasses) their distribution forms a ring surrounding the stem. The first divisions are periclinal and they involve the most internal tunica layer (i.e., LI in monolayered, LII in two-layered apical meristems). Apical growth of the leaf primordium has a marginal role, and it ends rather early in development. Intercalary growth represents the bulk of meristematic activity and it is of primary relevance for a foliar type of development.

Leaf sectors in leaves originated from mericlinal tobacco chimeras (Dulieu and Bugnon, 1966) and from irradiated axillary tobacco buds (Poethig and Sussex, 1985) were instrumental in demonstrating the prominent role of intercalary divisions in leaf development. Type and pattern of leaf sectors, in fact, while demonstrating the existence of leaf founder cells, rule out the hypothesis of an apical mode of development sustained by apical leaf initials. The existence of sectors that start at the base of the leaf and then fan out from the midrib toward the margin but do not extend to the margin of the blade has proven the prominent role of intercalary divisions in the foliar type of development and provided a unifying vision of leaf development in monocots and dicots.

4. Ontogenetic Variation of the Components of the Plant Body

Periclinal chimeras allow analysis of the relative contributions of each meristem layer to mature organs (Satina and Blakeslee, 1941; Dermen, 1951; Dulieu, 1970;

Stewart and Burk, 1970; Stewart *et al.*, 1974). The contribution differs not only among species but also within individual plants (Dermen, 1953; Stewart and Dermen, 1979). Within organs, a defective or excessive proliferation of one layer is compensated by the adjacent layer. For example, in the leaves of three-layered plants, LI forms the epidermis, LII forms the mesophyll of the leaf margins and a thin layer above and below the leaf core, and LIII forms the core tissue. However, the part played by any one layer in mesophyll development is highly variable (Fig. 3A, see Color Plates). In peach ploidy chimeras, LIII forms most of the stem, but roots produced at different points along its circumference differ in ploidy, indicating that the primary phloem, where adventitious roots are formed, might be formed from tissue derived by either LII or LIII (Dermen and May, 1966).

The contribution of each layer to mature organs is even more variable among different species. LI, with the notable exception of root formation, usually gives rise only to the epidermis. However, periclinal chimeras of plants with an LI thicker than four cells show that this layer alone can be responsible for the formation of all tissues present in lateral organs (Neilson-Jones, 1969). In several monocots, LI also contributes to the subepidermal layers of the leaf margin. The foliar primordium may even originate from a monocellular tunica alone, as in oat, rye, and wheat (Rösler, 1928).

5. Cellular Interactions

In floral organs, periclinal chimeras have been used to clarify the existence of correlative and/or positional influence among layers. If LI and LII differ genetically, in some instances it can be shown that a phenotype in one layer is determined by the genotype of the other layer, indicating a non-cell-autonomous action of some genes of the latter.

Darwin (1878) noted that *Laburnocytisus adamii,* an interspecific chimera, had malformations of the pistil. Later Bateson (1916) reported that in *Pelargonium zonale* "Double new life," the petaloid stamens were caused by the interaction between the cell layers forming the chimeric structure. A direct influence of LI on LII and LIII was demonstrated by Stewart *et al.* (1972) working with a graft-chimera that had an LI of *Camellia sasanqua* and an LII and LIII of *C. japonica. C. sasanqua* has perfect flowers, whereas *C. japonica* produces flowers without androecium and gynoecium. Unexpectedly, the periclinal chimera had flowers with male and female organs, while its sexual progeny was composed only of *C. japonica* seedlings. It was concluded that LI *C. sasanqua* cells influenced the developmental plan of the cells of the two layers underneath.

Interspecific and intraspecific periclinal chimeras of tomato have revealed the influence of LIII on the number of floral organs and on floral meristem size (Szymkowiak and Sussex, 1992).

Periclinal chimeras expressing the homeotic gene *Floricaula* in each of the three layers have been used to show that its action is not cell-autonomous, regardless of the layer expressing the transcriptional factor (Hantke, 1994). Since the FLORICAULA protein does not appear to diffuse from one layer to another, the data suggest that *Floricaula* activates a signal that is transmittable from one layer to the others.

The analysis of cellular interactions between layers is not limited to systems where floral organs are considered. For example, Becraft and Freeling (1991) have studied cell interactions during leaf differentiation in maize and revealed cellular interactions between the LI and the LII layers in the formation of the ligule, a tissue fringe separating leaf blade and sheath.

6. Apical Initials: Number and Permanence

Initials are cells of the meristem from which all other ones derive (Esau, 1977). When one initial divides, one of the daughter cells generates clones participating in the building of the differentiated plant body. The second cell remains in its position, ensuring the persistence of the meristem. The number of apical initials has been deduced from the size of somatic sectors. In several species the largest sectors encompass either one-half or one-third of the stem (Mason, 1930, Stewart and Dermen, 1970). Thus the number of initials in each layer (apparent cell number ACN; Table I) cannot be higher than the reciprocal of the cited fractions, and corresponds to two to three cells. In sectorial chimeras, the width of stem sectors might change suddenly due to substitution of one initial cell. The magnitude of these sudden changes is consistent with the given estimates of number of initials (Stewart and Dermen, 1970; for a detailed discussion, see Tilney-Basset, 1986).

Permanence or impermanence of apical initial cells is still a controversial issue. After division, one of the two daughters of an initial cell can remain initial (permanence), or after some cell divisions, one of the derivative cells is recruited as initial (impermanence; Klekowsky, 1988) Persistence of stem sectors along many internodes has been interpreted as evidence for the relative permanence of the initials (Stewart, 1978; Stewart and Dermen, 1970). This has been questioned on mathematical grounds by Klekowsky and Kazarinova-Fukshansky (1984a,b). Experiments carried out in *Juniperus, Nicotiana,* and *Arabidopsis* support the existence of impermanent initials (Ruth *et al.,* 1985; Dulieu, 1970; Furner and Pumfrey, 1992). Bossinger *et al.* (1992a) have shown that clonal populations of meristem cells can modify their relative contribution to the vegetative apex of maize, an observation interpreted in favor of the existence of impermanent initials.

7. Atypical Divisions and Rearrangement of Cell Layers

In 1863, Hofmeister observed that the plane of division is usually perpendicular to the long axis of the cell. Later, Errera (1886) developed this observation into a rule, according to which cell divisions occur parallel to the wall of minimal area.

In plant chimeras, division planes parallel to the longer axis of the cell (periclinal divisions) provide the basis for the appearance of "variant" variegations.

Table I
Apparent Cell Number (ACN) Calculated in Experiments Based on Sectorial Chimeras, Sector Boundary Analysis or Induced Sectors

Initials or founder cells of	Species	Mosaic organ considered	ACN	Reference
Apical meristems	Palm[a]	Stem	3	Mason (1930)
	Cranberry[a]	Leaves	3	Bain and Dermen (1944)
	Cotton[a]	Leaves	3	Christianson (1986)
	Juniper[a]	Leaves	2–3	Stewart and Dermen (1970)
	Poinsettia[a]	Leaves	3	Stewart and Dermen (1970)
	Privet[a]	Leaves	2–3	Stewart and Dermen (1970)
	Spirea[a]	Leaves	2–3	Stewart and Dermen (1970)
	Poinsettia[a]	Stem	2	Robinson (1931)
	Maize[b]	Leaves	2	Steffensen (1968)
	Potato[b]	Tuber	2	Howard (1969)
	Potato	Tuber	3	Klopfer, 1965
	Barley[b]	Anthers	3	Lindgren *et al.* (1970)
	Epilobium[a]	Leaves/Stem	4	Michaelis (1957)
Floral meristems	Fig[a]	Fruit	3	Condit (1928)
	Carnation[a]	Flower	3	Stewart and Dermen (1970)
	Apple[a]	Fruit	2	Clayberg (1963)
	Tomato[a]	Fruit	2	Walkof (1964)
	Gerbera[a]	Flower	3	Unpublished observation
	Orange[a]	Fruit	3	Robinson (1927)
Cotyledon	Cotton[c]		8	Christianson (1986)
Leaf	Tobacco[b]		100	Poethig and Sussex (1985)
	Maize[b]		250	Poethig (1984)
Ear	Maize[b]		2–4	Coe and Neuffer (1978)
Tassel	Maize[b]		2–4	Coe and Neuffer (1978)
Root	Broadbean[b]		3[d]	Brumfeld (1943)
	Crepis capillaris[b]		3	Brumfeld (1943)
	Carrot[a]		2	Lahmprecht and Svenson, 1949

[a] ACN in sectorial chimeras is the reciprocal of the fraction of the largest sector observed. In some of the cited experiments the ACN has been calculated after a shift was observed in the size of sectorial chimeras. In such cases the ACN is the reciprocal of the fractional increase.
[b] ACN in induced sectors is the reciprocal of the fraction of the area covered by the average sector.
[c] ACN in gynandromorph analysis is the reciprocal of the fraction of the area covered by the smallest sector observed.
[d] Apical intials of the only one root layer.

These rare events (Fig. 1C) are indicated by displacement (perforation and loss of the outer layer) and replacement (duplication of one layer with loss of the more internal one) and are easily detectable as sudden changes in the chimeral phenotype (Dermen, 1960; Bergann and Bergann, 1962). In tobacco leaves, the frequency of periclinal divisions of LI cells (Fig. 3B) is betwen 1.7 and 3×10^{-3} of that of anticlinal divisions (Stewart and Burk, 1970). A higher frequency (1×10^3 of that of anticlinal divisions) has been recorded for the androecium and gynoecium by analyzing the progeny of chimeras with either LI or LIII genetically tagged (Stewart and Burk, 1970). In the apical meristem, histological examinations have recorded 1 periclinal division for every 680 anticlinal divisions in the LI of *Ligustrum ovalifolium* (Stewart and Dermen, 1970), and 1 for every 333 in *Hedera helix* (Rogers and Bonnet, 1989). In the maize anther, the frequency of cellular replacement (LI invading LII) is 1 for every 634 cells (Dawe and Freeling, 1990). X-ray irradiation increases the frequency of layer rearrangements and hence represents a method to obtain chimera derivatives with modified apical meristems (Bergann, 1967).

For a discussion concerning the morphogenetic role of atypical periclinal cell divisions, see Bossinger *et al.* (1992b).

III. Spontaneous Sectors

A. Methodology

In 1931, Barbara McClintock examined L. J. Stadler's collection of maize plants derived from homozygous recessive mutant lines crossed with irradiated pollen carrying corresponding wild-type alleles (McClintock, 1984). Some of the variegated plants had a ring chromosome with fused broken ends. Ring chromosomes are unstable, and their loss results in variegation if a dominant marker is only present on the ring chromosome (McClintock, 1932). Such chromosomal abnormalities can be used in clonal analysis. This method is similar to the one proposed for *Drosophila,* where chromosomal non-disjunction was already known and used in 1929 (Sturtevant, 1929; Stern, 1936).

In plants, spontaneous sectors are frequently induced by the excision of transposable elements. These are mobile fragments of DNA, which, when inserted into a gene, switch off gene expression (McClintock, 1965). Transposon excision can reactivate the gene and generate somatic mosaics (Fig. 4, see Color Plates). The existence of mosaics with sharp borders is, *per se,* proof of cell autonomy (e.g., Hake and Freeling, 1986; Bennetzen *et al.,* 1988; Poethig, 1988; Spena *et al.,* 1989).

A drawback in cell lineage analysis based on spontaneous sectors is that transposon excision could be tissue-dependent. To avoid this problem, the analysis should be restricted to sectors appearing before the inception of the primordia of the organ under study, when tissues are still not differentiated. This prerequisite is fullfilled when the excision takes place in cells not yet committed to a specific structure. In cell lineage analysis of the leaf, sectors occupying a corresponding position in more than one leaf are assumed to result from a genetic event taking place in the meristem before primordium inception (discussed in Cerioli *et al.,* 1994).

Using switches based on transposon excision, spontaneous sectors have been generated in transgenic plants to study the effects of mosaicism on hormonal metabolism (Spena, 1990).

B. Concepts and Principles

1. Endosperm Development

Maize endosperm development has been followed by studying transposon excision at the loci *Waxy* (*Wx;* amylose syntesis) and *Anthocyaninless* (*A;* anthocyanin synthesis; McClintock, 1978). After the first three to six divisions that follow the double fertilization, cell lineages proliferate in the endosperm as radially expanding cones with the last divisions leading to the formation of the aleurone layer (Coe and Neuffer, 1978).

2. Cell Identity

In *Anthirrinum majus,* reactivation of the *deficiens* gene results in petaloid sectors appearing in a background of sepal tissue (Fig. 4; Sommer *et al.,* 1991). This shows that determination of petal specific cells is cell autonomous. A similar conclusion has been drawn from experiments carried out in *Impatiens balsamina,* where changes in photoperiod causes the formation of sepals with patches of petaloid tissue (Battey and Lyndon, 1984).

Mosaics due to the somatic activation of a cytokinin synthesizing gene have shown that an increase of cytokinins causes *in planta* formation of adventitious buds on leaves. Thus, cytokinins can override the final phase of leaf development by inducing differentiated cells to resume division (Estruch *et al.,* 1991).

3. The Ontogenetic Contribution of LI and LII to the Maize Gynoecium

In maize, carpel primordia develop according to a foliar mode of development, to which several founder cells located on the flanks of the apical meristem contribute. Visible markers are not available for the early stages of gynoecium development. Therefore, to evaluate the contribution of meristematic layers to the gynoecium, Dellaporta *et al.* (1991) have studied the teguments of the seed, which are derived from the gynoecium. In these tissues, flavonoid pigments can be used as markers. The *Ac* transposable element was used to generate somatic sectors by excision from the locus *P* (*Pericarp color*). By following two phenotypically different types of transposition of *Ac* (the first characterized by dark red sectors that do not enter the silk attachment region, and the second with light red sectors originating at the silk attachment region), Della Porta *et al.* (1991) concluded that the pericarp of the maize seed derives from both LI and LII. In particular, the finding of subepidermal transpositions transmitted to the offspring shows unequivocally that LII participates in gynoecium formation. The epidermis of the gynoecium is single-layered, but at the more apical region of the abgerminal side it is multilayered. From this multilayered region derives the silk, a tissue of LI origin.

4. The Role of Early Cell Divisions in Leaf Development

In unstable *glossy* mutants of maize, sectors marked by wild-type juvenile waxes have a strong tendency to start and end at positions that correlate with the location of the long cells of the ribs (Fig. 5A). Based on this observation, Cerioli *et al.* (1994) arrived at the following conclusions: (*a*) a clonal tye of development exists during the early phases of the formation of leaf epidermis and (*b*) in the protoderm only a few cells have a role in the generation of a leaf module (epidermal stripe of cells delimited by two lateral ribs). These results confirm the observation of Bugnon *et al.* (1969), who, using sectorial chimeras of

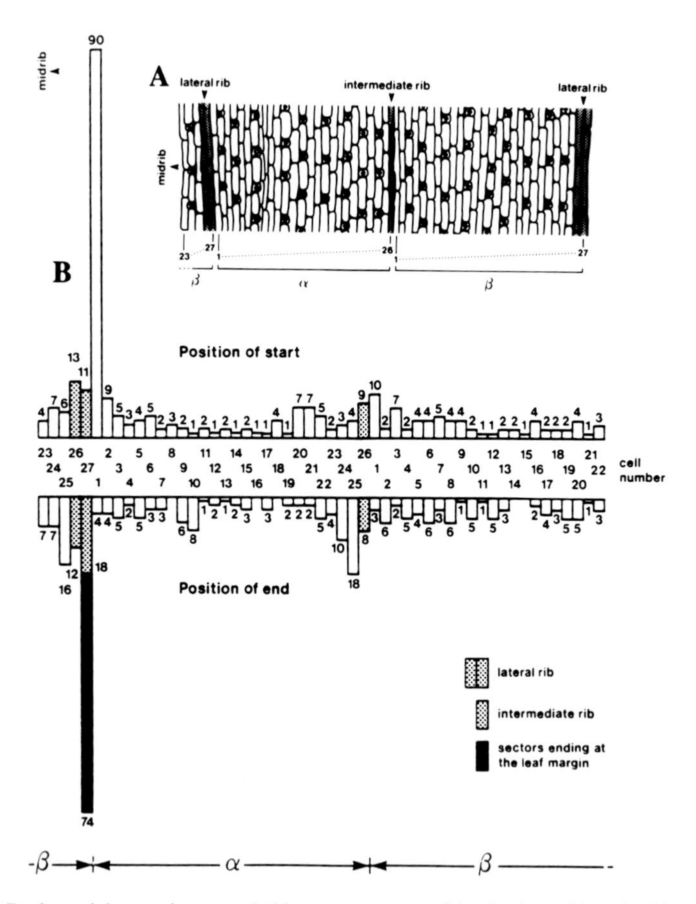

Fig. 5A Preferential sectoring revealed by transposon excision in the epidermis of juvenile leaves of maize. (A) A leaf developmental module of the maize epidermis consisting of the submodules alpha and beta. The module is delimited by two lateral ribs; the submodules are divided by an intermediate rib. Position of cells in the submodule is also indicated. (B) Position of starts and ends of sectors marked by the presence of epicuticular waxes (from Cerioli *et al.*, 1994).

several species (Fig. 5B), noticed that during the early stages of leaf primordium development, the direction of growth of the main and major veins coincides with the shape and decurrence of sectors (Fig. 5B). However, although this correlation is strict in early stages of leaf development, it can be relaxed either during later developmental stages (Fig. 5B,10) or when the major veins are *de facto* secondary veins (Figure 5B,8).

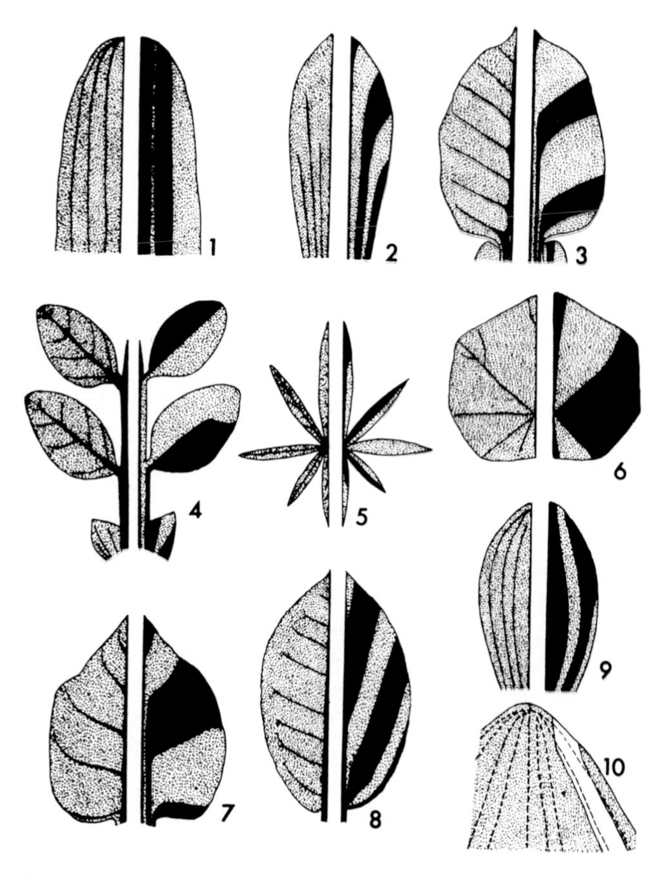

Fig. 5B Distribution on leaves of chlorophyll-deficient sectors (right half-leaves) and their relation to the decurrence of main and major veins (left half-leaves), observed in sectorial chimeras of the following species: 1: *Triticum monococcum* L. 2: *Linum grandiflorum*. Desf. 3: *Nicotiana tabacum* L. 4: *Vicia faba* L. var. *minor.* 5: *Lupinus polyphyllus* Lindl. 6: *Tropaelum majus* L. 7: *Scindapsus* sp. 8: *Elaeagnus pungens* Thunb. 9: *Polygonatum multiflorum* L. In all leaf sectorings, with the exception of 8, an almost prefectly overlapping of the pattern of distributions of the cellular clones and the direction of the main midvein is observed. 10: Details of a leaf of *Polygonatum multiflorum* L. with a sector deficient in chlorophyll, which follows the direction of the veins at the base of the leaf, but that in its distal portion deviates before terminating on the leaf margin; the veins remain parallel to the margin (from Bugnon *et al.,* 1969).

IV. Sectors Induced at Specific Stages of Development

A. Methodology

Stadler (1930) noticed that the size of sectors induced in maize by X-rays decreased if the irradiation after fertilization was delayed. These sectors represent the lineage of one mutated cell. Thus, the induction of a clone of mutated tissue can follow an experimental schedule that incorporates a temporal measure. Provided that the X-ray treatment does not cause extensive cell death, and that the marker gene does not alter cell growth, this method can be used to obtain fate maps of cells of the embryo, or of other meristematic tissues, and to estimate their apparent cell number (ACN; Table I).

A fate map relates cells present in a meristem at the time of irradiation to the contribution of their progenies to the plant body. Fate maps of the shoot apical meristem have been proposed in maize, sunflower, and *Arabidopsis.* The data on which these fate maps are based were obtained by irradiating dry seeds (Steffensen, 1968; Jegla and Sussex, 1989; Furner and Pumfrey, 1992; Irish and Sussex, 1992), germinating seeds (McDaniel *et al.*, 1988), or developing embryos (Poethig *et al.*, 1986). The number of plants considered varied between 10^3 (McDaniel and Poethig, 1988; Jegla and Sussex, 1989) and 8×10^4 (Furner and Pumfrey, 1992). After irradiation, the appearance and size of the somatic sectors, together with their position in the plant, are recorded. Sectors appear with frequencies from 0.4% (Furner and Pumfrey, 1992) to 10% (Jegla and Sussex, 1989) to 16% (McDaniel and Poethig, 1988). Although wild-type plants can be used (Jegla and Sussex, 1989; Irish and Sussex, 1992), marker gene affecting anthocyanin (Poethig *et al.*, 1986) or chlorophyll pigmentation (Steffensen, 1968) are usually preferred. Presentations of the data obtained report the position of the start and end of sectors along the shoot in relation to node number.

In these studies, the ACN is the reciprocal of the fraction of an organ occupied by the average somatic sector. Stem ACN is calculated by dividing the circumference of the stem by the width of the sector (Mason, 1930). When the sectors are not visible on the stem, the ACN of a node at the time of irradiation is obtained by multiplying the fraction of the leaf lamina that is sectored by the fraction of the stem circumference covered by the leaf petiole (Jegla and Sussex, 1989). The ACN is based on the assumption that all cells present at the time of irradiation contribute equally to organ development. Its inaccuracy has an inherent approximation factor of two because the mutation can take place at the four (G2) or at the two strand stage (G1) of DNA duplication (discussed in: Poethig, 1987).

B. Concepts and Principles

1. The Formation of the Apical Meristem in the Maize Embryo

Irradiation of maize proembryos between 28 and 45 h after pollination predominantly generates solid mutant plants (Steffensen, 1962). Irradiation of 52–68 h induces sectors with the border passing through the midvein of successive leaves, indicating that at this stage of development two cells have been recruited to form the shoot apical meristem. At this stage the shoot apical meristem starts to acquire its identity. Histological analysis has shown that the maize embryo has a layered structure at approximately 8–10 days after pollination (DAP) (transition stage) (Randolph, 1936).

In the experiment of Steffensen (1962), the finding that most plants are either solid or 50% variegated suggests either that one cell of the proembryo divides to generate the two founder cells of the shoot apical meristem or that two cells of the proembryo are recruited as founder cells. Sectors covering half-lamina of successive leaves must have taken place before layer formation and organ inception (Bossinger *et al.,* 1992b). Consistent with this interpretation, sectors induced at the midembryo stage are not restricted to one layer, whereas at the late embryo stage, Poethig *et al.* (1986) have found sectors limited to one layer.

2. Contribution of Embryonic Cells to Adult Structures

The fate of the cells present in the shoot apical meristem of the dormant seed can be deduced by sector analysis. Anatomical studies have shown that in most plants the shoot apex has the form of a conical dome (Fig. 6). The initials of the meristem are assumed to be positioned at the most distal point of the structure (for maize, see Poethig *et al.,* 1986). In contrast, inception of the first leaf primordium takes place starting from the most basal cells of the shoot meristem, whereas successive primordia originate from cells—or from progenies of cells—positioned progressively closer to the initials (Fig. 6). This representation of the shoot apex is consistent with the finding that, in fate map studies, sectors intercepting the basal nodes of the adult plant are narrower than those found on higher nodes. This result is expected since the number of cells present at the basal circumference of the dome is higher than the one measured in other positions of the meristematic dome. A logical corollary of this mode of organization of the apical meristem is that in sector studies, the ACN calculated for lower nodes is higher than that in more apical nodes (Fig. 6). Fate maps of plant meristems are usually drawn as concentric rings of cells representing *in fieri* plant parts with the most external ring responsible for the organization of the basal part of the plant (Fig. 6).

A remarkable finding of fate map studies in plants is that sectors starting at the same position may end at very different nodes. Even more evident is the observation that a sector originating from a specific cell of the meristem can contribute cellular clones to both vegetative and reproductive organs (Fig. 6; Poethig *et al.,* 1986; McDaniel and Poethig, 1988; Jegla and Sussex, 1989; Irish and Sussex, 1992; Furner and Pumfrey, 1992). Consequently, it has been concluded that a precise fate map cannot be assigned to the cells present in the apical meristem at a given developmental stage. Due to the large variability in sector ending, it has been proposed that, in plants, fate maps should be more correctly called probability maps (Irish and Sussex, 1992).

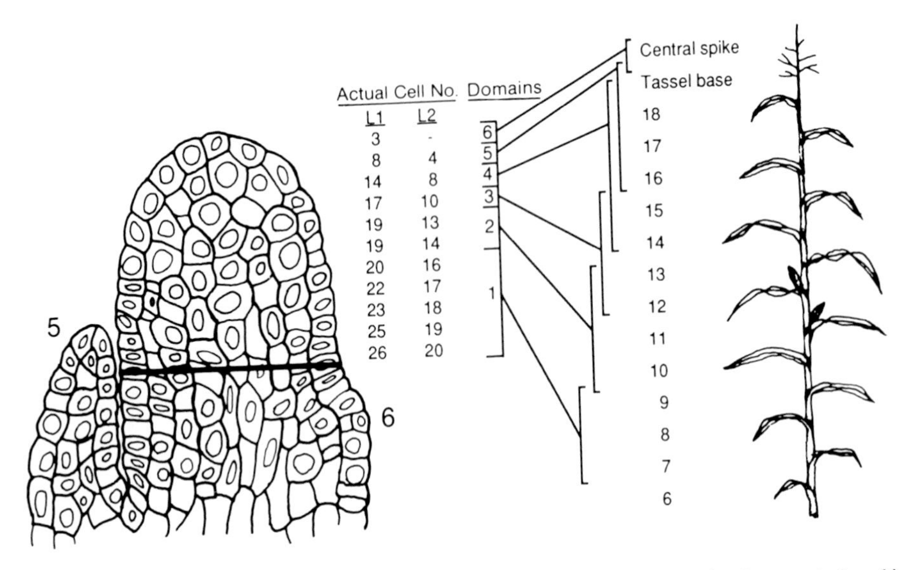

Fig. 6 Fate map of the shoot apical meristem of maize deduced from the study of sectors induced in germinating embryos by γ-rays. The drawing on the left reproduces the longitudinal section of the apical meristem of the germinating embryo. The horizontal line delimits the meristem proper from the region with incoming leaf primordia (the numbers 5 and 6 indicate the primordia of leaves 5 and 6). The parts of the plant produced by the meristem cells are shown on the right. Fates for domains of cells in the meristem were assigned, based on sector size and extension, to parts and organs of the adult plant. The actual cell number of LI and LII present in the meristem at the time of irradiation is also shown, as calculated from sector size (from McDaniel and Poethig, 1988. Copyright Springer-Verlag).

V. Sector Boundary Analysis

A. Methodology

Sector boundary analysis was first proposed by Sturtevant (1929) in *Drosophila,* where it is based on gynandromorph mosaics generated by the loss of one X-chromosome during early divisions. The mosaic border can run across areas undergoing morphogenesis. Structures originating at the border that arise from a single cell will always appear solid (i.e., phenotypically either of male or female type). When the structure originates from two cells and if the boundary passes between them, the structure will be 50% variegated. The number of founder cells (ACN; Table I) of the structure under analysis is estimated as the reciprocal of the smallest area of the two contrasting phenotypes forming the structure.

This type of analysis was adapted to plants by Christianson (1986) using semigamic cotton. Semigamy is a type of fertilization where a male nucleus enters an egg cell without fusing with the female nucleus (Battaglia, 1946). The two nuclei divide independently and generate cells producing mosaic embryos with the phenotypes of both parents: a plant equivalent of gynandromorphs. Pollination of a phenotypically virescent strain of *Gossipium barbadense* with the phenotypically green *Gossipium hirsutum* generates an F1 with 1–10% variegated plants, either haploid/haploid or haploid/diploid (Turcotte and Feaster, 1967). This type of genetic mosaic allowed Christianson (1986) to describe a critical stage of embryo development: the transition from a structure without a layered meristem (the proembryo), to one with a layered meristem (the embryo at the globular stage).

B. Concepts and Principles

1. The Concept of Compartment

The concept of compartment refers to the observation that, in an insect body, the border between two distinct domains is not trespassed by cellular clones. The existence of compartments has been demonstrated in *Drosophila* (Garcia-Bellido *et al.,* 1973), where they represent polyclonal groups of cells recruited in the early phases of embryo development to generate precise territories in the developing and/or adult body (Lawrence and Morata, 1993). The boundaries of a compartment frequently correspond to a structural feature. In plant embryo development, Christianson (1986) defined the proembryo compartments as cells from which specific tissues or organs are generated.

In the development of *Drosophila,* each group of cells sequestered in the larva as an imaginal disc has a precise fate, and its cellular clones will only form specific domains of the insect body. In plants, the making of a complex organ like a leaf also admits a role for a clonal type of development, particularly in early phases of primordia formation (Cerioli *et al.,* 1994). However, the existence of the shoot apical meristem generates an open developmental system where a clone of cells contributes to successive leaves. Thus, the concept of compartment, if it can be adapted to plants at all, has to be restricted to the fate of cells recruited from an apical meristem to form an organ (or parts of it), without implying that clones of identical lineage cannot be found elsewhere in the plant. It is nevertheless interesting that both in the work of Christianson (1986) and Cerioli *et al.* (1994), the border limiting the clonal propagation of cells on the leaf lamina is frequently represented by veins, units with a distinct morphology that divide the leaf lamina into recurrent developmental modules (Fig. 5).

Also, Poethig and Sussex (1985) have noted discontinuities in sectors at the boundaries of lateral veins in tobacco leaves. These authors have interpreted the observation as reflecting the fact that, in young tobacco leaves, vascular tissue occupies half of the leaf primordium, but significantly less in the mature leaf. On the basis of this observation the cited authors concluded that sectors tend to have a higher probability to start in positions corresponding to vascular tissues (Poethig and Sussex, 1985; for a similar interpretation in *Arabidopsis,* see Irish and Sussex, 1992).

2. Distinct Compartments in the Cotton Embryo

The cotyledons, the first and second leaves and the shoot apical meristem of cotton are not generated by the same cell lineage (Christianson, 1986). This conclusion is based on the finding that 30 of 44 chimeric seedlings of semigamic origin had tissues restricted to the cotyledons that were derived either from *G. barbadense* (virescent) or from *G. hirsutum* (green). The fraction of the cotyledon occupied by a sector was never smaller than one-eighth. Consequently, Christianson (1986) proposed that each cotyledon has eight founder cells (ACN).

Four chimeric seedlings were sectored in the first leaf (half green–half virescent) without concomitant sectoring of the shoot apex. This finding indicated that there were two initials of the first leaf, which were different from the initials of the cotyledons and shoot apex. Also, the second leaf (derived from one initial) had a cell ancestry distinct from that of the other organs. Similarly, the formation of the shoot apical meristem either *in vitro* from leaf tissue (Christianson, 1985) or *in planta* (Tian and Marcotrigiano, 1993) appears to take place by recruiting cells different from those forming the first leaves and lower part of the stem. The topographical relationships between the five compartments defined by Christianson are shown in Fig. 7 (see Color Plates). The figure represents an hypothetical anatomy of the cotton proembryo as deduced from the analysis of chimeric plants.

In this formulation, Christianson identifies compartments as progenitors of organs. However, a second and somewhat different interpretation has been provided by the same author (Christianson, 1986). On the basis of the observation that sector borders coincide with primary or secondary veins in cotyledons, and with midveins in leaves, Christianson postulates the existence of "16 cotyledonary compartments." This second formulation emphasizes the clonal restriction on the development of the vegetative tissues caused by veins (see also Section IV,B,1).

In cotton, anatomical studies have implied that the aerial part of the plant originates from a quartet of cells. Late in proembryo development only three cells are recruited as apical initials. This is deduced from the existence of sectorial chimeras with sectors covering one-third of the mature plant (see Section II,B,5). Moreover, the observation that the six plants showing chimerism of the apex were such in all layers strongly favors the interpretation that three initial cells may even be recruited at the proembryo stage as a three-celled compartment, already fated to form the apical initials and hence to generate all the plant parts derived from them (Christianson, 1986).

VI. Pattern Determination

A. Methodology

Walbot (1985) and Sussex (1989) have described the relevant developmental differences between plants and animals. The lack of a sequestered germ-line, the continuous embryogenic state of meristems, and the late commitment of cells to a specific fate are typical of plants. However, the cellular feature with the most profound implications on plant cell growth and differentiation is the presence of cell walls. This condition prevents cell rotation and migration, and increases the morphogenetic relevance of early cell divisions that already define the adult cell arrangements.

In commenting on the existence of maize plants half white–half green with the border corresponding to the plane that sets the bilateral symmetry of the plant, Steffensen (1968) suggested that the maize shoot originates from two precisely oriented cells. Christianson (1986) interpreted such phenotypes as being derived from an event creating something which functions like cartesian coordinates" in the orientation of the future symmetry of the plant. In this review, this "something" is called and treated as pattern determination (see Dawe and Freeling, 1991, where the same phenomenon is discussed as pattern imprinting). The methods used to clarify this phenomenon are some of those previously discussed.

B. Concepts and Principles

1. Pattern Determination in Cotton Embryos

In cotton, histological studies have implied that the formation of a quartet of cells in the proembryo is the first stage in the organization of the apical meristem (Gore, 1932). Christianson (1986) reasoned that sectors observed in cotyledons of chimeric seedlings might be cellular projections of the quartet organization of the proembryo. In fact, when the two cotyledons are divided in 16 hypothetical clonal units (Figs. 7A and 7B), 22 of the 44 observed sectors appeared to span either 4, or 8 or 12 clonal units. This finding is interpreted as support for the role of the proembryonic quartet of cells in the origin of the aerial part of the seedling.

In Christianson's experiment, pattern determination is seen as an answer to the question whether the orientation of the four cells of the quartet determines the left/right and back/front symmetry of the seedling. As shown in Fig. 8A (see Color Plates), it is conceivable that the two planes of symmetry in seedlings coincide with the two orientations of the cell walls dividing the quartet. We wish, however, to underline the relevance of an additional interpretation of Christianson's data: a 45° deviation of the planes of symmetry from the planes of the quartet can be interpreted as a delay in the mechanism of pattern determination, which, therefore, becomes operative at a putative eight-celled stage of the proembryo where the two planes of symmetry are aligned along the planes of the more recent cell divisions (Fig. 8C).

2. Pattern Determination in Maize

a. Shoot

Chimeric seedlings of maize with the mutated sector covering 50% of the five juvenile leaves have been analyzed by Bossinger *et al.* (1992a). Such sectors were generated in *glossy-1* mutable plants by transposon excision using the presence of epicuticular waxes as a marker for LI-derived tissues. Two hundred thirty-five plants, with reversions due to a single excision taking place early in the organization of the shoot apical meristem, were analyzed. One-third of the plants had sector borders located precisely on the plane of symmetry, which passes through the leaf midribs, while another 9.1% were a variant characterized by an increase or a decrease in the width of the reverted sector during development. Thus, almost half of the sectored plants were characterized, at least in their first leaves, by coincidence of sector boundary and midrib. As proposed by Steffensen (1968), these observations could indicate that the plane separating the cells founding the apical meristem in the proembryo determines the future plane of symmetry of the seedling. However, Bossinger *et al.* (1992a) found "half-alternate" plants, where the border between wild-type and mutant tissue was positioned in a plane normal to the one coincident with the midrib; this occurred in 7.9% of the cases analyzed. This experiment supports the conclusion that in the early phase of vegetative meristem organization in maize, a mechanism of pattern determination based on the spatial arrangement of founder cells determines the left–right and back–front orientation of the seedling. However, the existence of "half-alternate" mosaics strongly supports the possibility that the left–right plane either coincides with the plane along which the founder cells divide, or it is perpendicular to it.

b. *Anther*

Sectors were induced by irradiating germinating seedlings that were heterozygous for a number of dominant genes affecting anthocyanin pigmentation. Nine large sectored tassels were selected where both LI and LII had originated from the same mutated cell. At the borders of these large sectors, 101 chimeric anthers were considered for sector boundary analysis (Dawe and Freeling, 1992).

Based on sector areas, the anther was deduced to originate from four cells, surrounded by a ring of eight cells. The presence of the ring of eight cells was felt necessary to explain the observation that 40% of the sectors cut the anther in half, whereas 6% spanned one-eighth of the anther. As in cotton, a nonrandom distribution of sector boundaries was observed: in 77% of cases the sector borders passed between microsporangia, whereas the rest usually deviated by 45° (Fig. 9, see Color Plates). The authors conclude that the orientation of the four founder cells predicts the orientation of the four microsporangia, i.e., the symmetry of the mature anther. This conclusion is remarkably similar to the one proposed for the cotton embryo. Sector borders deviating by 45° with respect to the planes of symmetry of the anther can be explained as similar to the deviations observed for the cotton seedlings (see Fig. 8C).

c. *Leaf Vein*

Each maize leaf primordium originates from at least 250 cells present all around the flanks of the shoot apex (Poethig, 1984). Spontaneous sectors have been used to show that intermediate and small veins—developing in the internal layer of the leaf mesophyll with a basipetal direction—represent the transverse fusion of two cell lineages (Langdale *et al.*, 1989). When the future leaf consists of only two subepidermal layers, the adaxial subepidermis periclinally initiates a third layer. Cells generated by this layer have distinct fates: one daughter cell of each division gives rise to bundle sheath and vascular cells of half a vein, whereas the second cell gives rise to differentiated cells of a mesophyll photosynthetic unit. This type of development takes place transversally and results in the formation of a developmental unit that can be considered the building block of the vein. The elongation of the vein in the direction leaf tip to base proceeds by the addition of new building blocks to the incipient vein, and may incorporate different longitudinal cell lineages. Thus the development of the maize vein consists of a transversal stem-cell type (Dawe and Freeling, 1991) of process, locally adjusted by positional information from the existing differentiated vein (Fig. 10).

VII. Perspectives

The genetic approach to plant development based on cell lineage studies is almost one century old (Baur, 1909). In the future, the technology of plant transformation might allow the expansion of the number of systems amenable to cell lineage studies (Spena, 1990; Christou and McCabe, 1992; Fig. 1D). At the same time, genes with radical effects on plant morphology and/or body organization have been either cloned or are in the process of being isolated. The consequent availability of riboprobes and antibodies specific for these genes will allow the study of their expression and interactions during development. It is

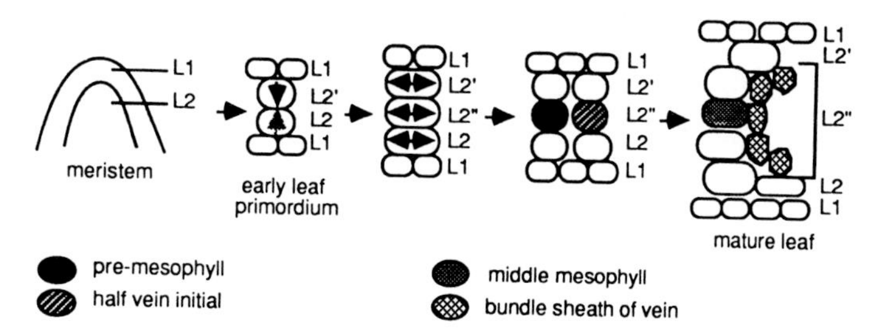

Fig. 10 Model based on spontaneous sector analysis proposed by Langdale *et al.* (1989) to describe the pattern of vein formation in maize leaves. In the leaf blade, the type of veins considered in the study differentiate first at the tip, and proceed basipetally. The programmed divisions of the central (L2") primordial mesophyll cell generate middle mesophyll and half vein initial cells. If the mesophyll daughter cell divides again and repeats the process, an alternating "two mesophyll cells-vein" veination pattern is produced. The model has been based on the observation that middle mesophyll-bundle sheath sectors end most frequently in the middle of a vein (from Dawe and Freeling, 1991. Copyright Blackwell Scientific Publications).

our opinion that cell lineage studies are beginning to attract novel interest. Their inherent power to clarify developmental issues will be greatly magnified by incorporating in proper experiments the use of molecular probes specific for cells or tissues or compartments.

Acknowledgments

We thank Jane Langdale, Peter Starlinger, and Riccardo Velasco for critical reading of the manuscript. We thank Suzanne Schwartz-Sommer for providing Fig. 4 and Elke Kemper for assistance in preparing Fig. 1D.

References

Bain, H. F., and Dermen, H. (1944). Sectorial polyploidy and phyllotaxy in the cranberry (*Vaccinium macrocarpon* Ait). *Am. J. Bot.* **31,** 581–587.

Bateson, W. (1916). Root-cuttings, chimaeras and "sports." *J. Genet.* **6,** 75–80.

Bateson, W. (1921). Root cuttings and chimaeras II. *J. Genet.* **11,** 91–97.

Bateson, W. (1926). Segregation. *J. Genet.* **16,** 201–236.

Battaglia, E. (1946). Richerce cariologiche e embriologiche sul genere *Rudbeckia* (Asteraceae). *Nuovo Giorn. Bot. Italiano* **53,** 483–511.

Battey, N. H., and Lindon, R. F. (1984). Changes in apical growth and phyllotaxis on flowering and reversion in *Impatiens balsamina* L. *Ann. Bot.* **54,** 553–567.

Baur, E. (1909). Das Wesen und die Erblichkeitsverhältnisse der "Varietates albomarginatae hort." von *Pelargonium zonale. Zietschrift für induktive Abstammungs- un Vererbungslehre.* **1,** 330–351.

Becraft, P. W., and Freeling, M. (1991). Sectors of *liguleless-1* tissue interrupt an inductive signal during maize leaf development. *Plant Cell* **3,** 801–807.

Bennetzen, J. L., Blevins, W. E., and Ellingboe, A. H. (1988). Cell-autonomous recognition of the rust pathogen determines *Rp1*-specified resistance in maize. *Science* **241,** 208–210.

Bergann, F. (1967). The relative instability of chimerical clones—the basis for further breeding. *Abhandl. Deut. Akad. Wiss. Berlin.* **2,** 287–300.

Bergann, F., and Bergann, L. (1962). Über Umschichtungen (Translokationen) an den Sproßscheiteln periklinaler Chimären. *Der Züchter.* **32,** 110–119.

Bierhorst, D. W. (1977). On the stem apex, leaf initiation and early leaf ontogeny in filicalean ferns. *Am. J. Bot.* **64,** 125–152.

Binding, H., Witt, D., Monzer, J., Mordhorst, G., and Kollmann, R. (1987). Plant cell graft obtained by co-culture of isolated protoplasts. *Protoplasma* **141,** 64–73.

Blakeslee, A., Bergner, D., Satina, S., and Sinnot, E. W. (1939). Induction of periclinal chimeras in *Datura stramonium* by colchicine treatment. *Science* **89,** 402.

Bossinger, G., Maddaloni, M., Motto, M., and Salamini, F. (1992a). Formation and cell lineage patterns of the shoot apex of maize. *The Plant J.* **2,** 311–320.

Bossinger, G., Lundquist, U., Rohde, W., and Salamini, F. (1992b). Genetics of plant development in barley. *In* "Barley Genetics VI" (L. Munck, ed.), pp. 989–1022. Copenhagen, Denmark: Munksgaard International Publishers Ltd.

Broertjes, C., and Keen, A. (1980). Adventitious shoots: Do they develop from one cell? *Euphytica* **29,** 73–87.

Brumfield, R. T. (1943). Cell-lineage studies in root meristems by means of chromosome rearrangements induced by X-rays. *Am. J. Bot.* **30,** 101–110.

Bugnon, F., Dulieu, H., and Turlier, M.-F. (1969). Rapports entre les directions fondamentales de croissance dand l'ébauche et la nervation foliaires. *C.R. Acad. Sci. Paris* **268,** 48–50.

Cerioli, S., Marocco, A., Maddaloni, M., Motto, M., and Salamini, F. (1994). Early event in maize leaf epidermis formation as revealed by cell lineage studies. *Development* **120,** 2113–2120.

Christianson, M. L. (1985). Competence, determination, and clonal analysis in plant development. *In* "Somatic embryogenesis—Proceedings of a San Miniato Workshop" (M. Terzi, L. Pitto, and Z. R. Sung, eds.), pp. 146–151. Rome: IPRA.

Christianson, M. L. (1986). Fate map of the organizing shoot apex in Gossypium. *Am. J. Bot* **73,** 947–958.

Christou, P., and McCabe, D. E. (1992). Prediction of germ-line transformation events in chimeric R_o transgenic soybean plantlets using tissue-specific expression patterns. *The Plant J.* **2,** 283–290.

Clayberg, C. D. (1963). Delicious apple chimera (half-red, half-yellow). *Fruit Varieties Hort. Dig.* **17,** 58.

Coe, E. H., and Neuffer, M. G. (1978). Embryo cells and their destinies in the corn plant. *In* "The Clonal Basis of Development" (S. Subtelny and I. M. Sussex, eds.), pp. 113–129. Academic Press: New York.

Columella, L. I. M. (1545). De re Rustica. Ch. IX in Lib. de Arborebus, p. 476, Lyon.

Condit, I. J. (1928). Other fig chimeras. *J. Hered.* **19,** 49–52.

Darwin, C. (1878). "Das Variiren der Thiere und Pflanzen im Zustande der Domestication." Vol. 1, p. 433. Stuttgart: E. Schweizerbart'sche Verlagshandlung.

Dawe, R. K., and Freeling, M. (1990). Clonal analysis of the cell lineages in the male flower of maize. *Dev. Biol.* **142,** 233–245.

Dawe, R. K., and Freeling, M. (1991). Cell lineage and its consequences in higher plants. *The Plant J.* **1,** 3–8.

Dawe, R. K., and Freeling, M. (1992). The role of initial cells in maize anther morphogenesis. *Development* **116,** 1077–1085.

Dellaporta, J. B. (1589). "Magia Naturalis." Liber 2, Ch. 2 Napoli.

Della Porta, J. B. (1592). "Villae," p. 169, Frankfurt.

Dellaporta, S. L., Moreno, M. A., and Delong, A. (1991). Cell lineage analysis of the gynoecium of maize using the transposable element Ac. *Development suppl.* **1,** 141–147.

Dermen, H. (1951). Ontogeny of tissues in stem and leaf of cytochemical apples. *Am. J. Bot.* **38,** 753–760.

Dermen, H. (1953). Periclinal cytochimeras and origin of tissues in stem and leaf of peach. *Am. J. Bot.* **40,** 154–168.

Dermen, H. (1960). Nature of plant sports. *Am. Hort. Mag.* **39,** 123–173.

Dermen, H., and May, C. (1966). Colchiploidy of *Ulmus pumila* and its possible use in hybridization with *U. americana. Forest Sci.* **12,** 140–146.

Dulieu, H. (1970). Les mutations somatiques induites et l'ontogénie de la pousse feuillée. *Ann. Melior. Plantes.* **20,** 27–44.

Dulieu, H., and Bugnon, F. (1966). Chimères mériclines et ontogénie foliaire chez le Tabac (*Nicotiana tabacum* L.) *C. R. Acad. Sci.* (*Paris*) **263,** 1714–1717.

Errera, L. (1886). Sur une condition fondamentale d'équilibre des cellules vivantes. *C. R. Acad. Sci.* (*Paris*) **103,** 822–824.

Esau, K. (1977). "Anatomy of Seed Plants." New York: Wiley.

Estruch, J. J., Prinsen, E., Van Onckelen, H., Schell, J., and Spena, A. (1991). Viviparous leaves produced by somatic activation of an inactive cytokinin-synthesizing gene. *Science* **254,** 1364–1367.

Ferrari, J. B. (1646). Hesperides sive de malorum aureorum cultura et usu. p. 397. Roma.

Furner, I. J., and Pumfrey, J. E. (1992). Cell fate in the shoot apical meristem of *Arabidopsis thaliana. Development* **115,** 755–764.

Garcia-Bellido, A., Ripoll, P., and Morata, G. (1973). Developmental compartmentalization of the wing disc of *Drosophila. Nature New Biol.* **245,** 251–253.

Gore, U. R. (1932). Development of the female gametophyte and embryo in cotton. *Am. J. Bot.* **19,** 795–807.

Hantke, S. S. (1994). Molecular analysis of *floricaula,* a homeotic gene in *Antirrhinum majus.* Ph.D.-Thesis, Universität Köln.

Hofmeister, W. (1863). Zusätze und Berichtigungen zu den 1851 veröffentlichen Untersuchungen der Entwicklung höherer Krytogamen. *Jahr. Wiss. Bot.* **3,** 259–293.

Irish, V. F., and Sussex, I. M. (1992). A fate map of the *Arabidopsis* embryonic shoot apical meristem. *Development* **115,** 745–753.
Jefferson, R. A. (1987). Assaying chimeric genes in plants: The GUS gene fusion system. *Plant Mol. Biol. Rep.* **5,** 387–405.
Jegla, D. E., and Sussex, I. M. (1989). Cell lineage patterns in the shoot meristem of the sunflower embryo in the dry seed. *Dev. Biol.* **131,** 215–225.
Kaddoura, R. L., and Mantell, S. H. (1991). Synthesis and characterization of *Nicotiana-Solanum* graft chimeras. *Ann. Bot.* **68,** 547–556.
Klekowsky, E. J. (1988). "Mutation, Developmental Selection, and Plant Evolution." New York: Columbia Univ. Press.
Klekowsky, E. J., and Kazarinova-Fukshansky, N. (1984a). Shoot apical meristems and mutation: Fixation of selectively neutral cell genotypes. *Am. J. Bot.* **71,** 22–27.
Klekowsky, E. J., and Kazarinova-Fukshaansky, N. (1984b). Shoot apical meristems and mutation: Selective loss of disadvantageous cell genotypes. *Am. J. Bot.* **71,** 28–34.
Klopfer, K. (1965). Erfolgreiche experimentelle Entmischungen und Umlagerungen periclinalchimärischer Kartoffelklone. *Züchter* **35,** 201–214.
Krenke, N. P. (1933). "Wundkompensation, Transplantation und Chimären bei Pflanzen," pp. 601–666. Berlin: Springer-Verlag.
Lambrecht, H., and Svenson, V. (1949). Zwei Chimären von *Daucus carota* L. sowie allgemeines über Art und Entstehung von Chimären. *Agric. Hort. Genet.* **7,** 96–111.
Langdale, J. A., Lane, B., Freeling, M., and Nelson, T. (1989). Cell lineage analysis of maize bundle sheath and mesophyll cells. *Dev. Biol.* **133,** 128–129.
Lawrence, P. A., and Morata, G. (1993). A no-wing situation. *Nature* **366,** 305–306.
Lindgren, D., Erikson, G., and Sulovska, K. (1970). The size and appearance of the mutated sector in barley spikes. *Hereditas* **65,** 107–132.
McClintock, B. (1965). The control of gene action in maize. *In* "Genetic Control of Differentiation." Brookhaven Symposia in Biology, **18,** 162–184.
McClintock, B. (1932). A correlation of ring-shaped chromosomes with variegation in *Zea mays. Proc. Natl. Acad. Sci. U.S.A.* **18,** 677–681.
McClintock, B. (1978). Development of the maize endosperm as revealed by clones. *In* "The Clonal Basis of Development" (S. Subtelny and I. M. Sussex, eds.), p. 217. New York: Academic Press.
McDaniel, C. N., and Poethig, S. R. (1988). Cell-lineage patterns in the shoot apical meristem of the germinating maize embryo. *Planta* **175,** 13–22.
Marcotrigiano, M., and Gouin, F. R. (1984). Experimentally synthesized plant chimeras I. *In vitro* recovery of *Nicotiana tabacum* L. chimeras from mixed callus cultures. *Ann. Bot.* **54,** 503–511.
Mason, S. C. (1930). A sectorial mutation of a Deglet Noor date palm. *J. Hered.* **21,** 157–163.
Michaelis, P. (1957). Genetische, entwicklungsgeschichtliche und cytologische Untersuchungen zur Plasmavererbung. *Planta* **50,** 60–106.
Neilson-Jones, W. (1969). "Plant Chimeras." London: Methuen.
Noguchi, T., Hirata, Y., and Yagishita, N. (1992). Intervarietal and interspecific chimera formation by *in vitro* graft-culture method in *Brassica. Theor. Appl. Gen.* **83,** 727–732.
Norris, R., Smith, R. H., and Vaughn, K. C. (1983). Plant chimeras used to establish *de novo* origin of shoots. *Science* **220,** 75–76.
Poethig, R. S. (1984). Cellular parameters of leaf morphogenesis in maize and tobacco. *In* "Contemporary Problems of Plant Anatomy" (R. A. White and W. C. Dickinson, eds.), pp. 235–259. New York: Academic Press.
Poethig, R. S. (1987). Clonal analysis of cell lineage patterns in plant development. *Am. J. Bot.* **74,** 581–594.
Poethig, R. S. (1988). A non-cell-autonomous mutation regulating juvenility in maize. *Nature* **336,** 82–83.
Poethig, R. S., Coe, E. H., and Johri, M. M. (1986). Cell lineage patterns in maize embryogenesis: A clonal analysis. *Dev. Biol.* **117,** 392–404.

Poethig, R. S., and Sussex, I. M. (1985). The cellular parameters of leaf development in tobacco: A clonal analysis. *Planta* **165,** 170–184.

Pohlheim, F. (1971). Untersuchungen zur Sproßvariation der *Cupressaceae.* 1. Nachweis immerspaltender Periklinalchimären. *Flora* **160,** 264–293.

Pontano, J. J. (1505). De hortis Esperidum sive de cultu citriorum. Liber 2, Venezia.

Randolph, L. F. (1936). Developmental morphology of the caryopsis in maize. *J. Agric. Res.* **53,** 881–916.

Robinson, T. R. (1927). An orange chimera. *J. Hered.* **18,** 48.

Robinson, T. R. (1931). A chimera in the Poinsettia. *J. Hered.* **22,** 359.

Rogers, S. O., and Bonnet, H. T. (1989). Evidence for apical initial cells in the vegetative shoot apex of *Hedera helix* cv. Goldheart. *Am. J. Bot.* **76,** 539–545.

Rösler, P. (1928). Histologische Studien am Vegetationspunkt von *Triticum vulgare. Planta* **5,** 28–69.

Ruth, J., Klekowsky, E. J., and Stein, O. L. (1985). Impermanent initials of the shoot apex and diplontic selection in a juniper chimera. *Am. J. Bot.* **72,** 1127–1135.

Satina, S., Blakeslee, A. F., and Avery, A. G. (1940). Demonstration of the three germ layers in the shoot apex of *Datura* by means of induced polyploidy in periclinal chimeras. *Am. J. Bot.* **27,** 895–905.

Satina, S., and Blakeslee, A. F. (1941). Periclinal chimeras in *Datura stramonium* in relation to development of leaf and flower. *Am. J. Bot.* **28,** 862–871.

Satina, S. (1959). Chimeras. *In* "Blakeslee: The Genus Datura." pp. 132–151. New York: Ronald Press.

Savastano, L., and Parrozzani, A. (1912). Di taluni ibridi naturali degli agrumi. *Ann. R. Staz. Sper. Agrumi Frutt. Acireale* **1,** 37–63.

Sommer, H., Nacken, W., Beltran, P., Huijser, P., Pape, H., Hansen, R., Flor, P., Saedler, H., and Schwarz-Sommer, Z. (1991). Properties of *deficiens,* a momeotic gene involved in the control of flower morphogenesis in *Antirrhinum majus. Development Suppl.* **1,** 169–175.

Spena, A., Aalen, R., and Schulze, S. C. (1989). Cell-autonomous behaviour of the *rolC* of *agrobacterium rhizogenes* during leaf development: A visual assay for transposon excision in transgenic plants. *The Plant Cell* **1,** 1157–1164.

Spena, A. (1990). Unstable liasions: The use of transposons in plant genetic engineering. *Trends Gen.* **6,** 76–77.

Stadler, L. J. (1930). Some genetic effects of X-rays in plants. *J. Heredity* **21,** 3–19.

Steffensen. D. M. (1962). Patterns of sectoring in seedling with reference to early embryonic development. *Maize Genet Coop. Newsletter* **36,** 24.

Steffensen, D. M. (1968). A reconstruction of cell development in the shoot apex of maize. *Am. J. Bot.* **55,** 354–369.

Stern, C. (1936). Somatic crossing over and segregation in *Drosophila melanogaster. Genetics* **21,** 625–730.

Stewart, R. N. (1978). Ontogeny of the primary body in chimeral forms of higher plants. *In* "The Clonal Basis of Development" (S. Subtelny and I. M. Sussex, eds.), pp. 131–160. New York: Academic Press.

Stewart, R. N., and Burk, L. G. (1970). Independence of tissues derived from apical layers in ontogeny of the tobacco leaf and ovary. *Am. J. Bot.* **57,** 1010–1016.

Stewart, R. N., and Dermen, H. (1970). Determination of number and mitotic activity of shoot apical initial cells by analysis of mericlinal chimeras. *Am. J. Bot.* **57,** 816–826.

Stewart, R. N., and Dermen, H. (1979). Ontogeny in monocotyledons as revealed by studies of the developmental anatomy of periclinal chloroplast chimeras. *Am. J. Bot.* **66,** 47–58.

Stewart, R. N., Meyer, F. G., and Dermen, H. (1972). *Camellia* + "Daisy Eagleson", a graft chimera of *Camellia sasanqua* and *C. japonica. Am. J. Bot.* **59,** 515–524.

Stewart, R. N., Semeniuk, P., and Dermen, H. (1974). Competition and accomodation between apical layers and their derivatives in the ontogeny of chimeral shoots of *Pelargonium* x *Hortorum. Am. J. Bot.* **61,** 54–67.

Sturtevant, A. H. (1929). The claret mutant type of *Drosophila simulans.* A study of chromosome elimination and cell lineage. *Z. Wiss. Zool.* **135,** 323–356.

Sussex, I. M. (1989). Developmental programming of the shoot meristem. *Cell* **56,** 225–229.
Szymoniak, E. J., and Sussex, I. (1992). The internal meristem layer (L3) determines floral meristem size and carpel number in tomato periclinal chimeras. *Plant Cell* **4,** 1089–1100.
Tian, H., and Marcotrigiano, M. (1993). Origin and development of adventitious shoot meristems initiated on plant chimeras. *Dev. Biol.* **155,** 259–269.
Tilney-Basset, R. A. E. (1986). "Plant Chimeras." London: Arnold.
Turcotte, E. L., and Feaster, C. V. (1967). Semigamy in Pima cotton. *J. Hered.* **58,** 55–57.
Walbot, V. (1985). On the life strategies of plants and animals. *Trends Genet.* **1,** 165–169.
Walkof, C. (1964). A pericarp chimera in the tomato. *Can. J. Genet. Cytol.* **6,** 46–51.

CHAPTER 24

Chemically Induced Mitotic Synchrony in Root Apical Meristems

Betty Prewett and Thomas Jacobs
Department of Plant Biology
University of Illinois
Urbana, Illinois 61801

I. Introduction

In the biochemical and molecular analysis of any developmental pathway, it is essential to have a ready source of bulk tissue, uniformly enriched in selected stages of the pathway. The mitotic cell division cycle is a circular pathway, and cell populations naturally enriched for a single stage of the cycle are rare. Therefore, one must artificially impose synchrony in mitotic populations in order to obtain material enriched in any particular cell cycle stage, G1, S, G2, or M.

Systems in which mitotic synchrony have been most frequently imposed are *in vitro* grown cell cultures. The high surface-to-volume ratio and the aqueous

METHODS IN CELL BIOLOGY, VOL. 49

environment of cultured cells greatly facilitates their metabolic labeling and pharmacological manipulation. However, cells in culture do not necessarily behave as they would in the intact organism, their more "natural" environment. On the other hand, cells in intact metazoans are more difficult to treat uniformly with chemicals, as only their surface tissues are directly accessible. Furthermore, *in vivo,* tissues invariably comprise diverse cellular populations, both in and out of the proliferative state.

The higher plant root represents an attractive system for *in vivo* cell cycle studies. Roots are conveniently organized with a distal subpopulation called the apical meristem that is highly enriched in proliferating cells. More proximal domains of this linear organ system represent a gradient of increasing maturation, a useful resource for developmental studies. In addition, roots have evolved efficient systems to take up water and dissolved solutes. The apoplastic space of the angiosperm root rapidly equilibrates with its external aqueous environment. This feature makes roots exceptionally amenable to chemical manipulation. One further advantage of roots for biochemical analyses is that they lack many of the proteins constituting the photosynthetic machinery found elsewhere in the plant which can, by their great abundance, obscure or distort quantitative measurements of other less abundant cellular components, such as those that regulate the cell division cycle.

II. Materials and Recipes

Large plastic or porcelain-coated metal trays
Aluminum foil
Bleached paper toweling
Whatman 3MM filter paper or equivalent
Stiff plastic mesh (5-mm pore size, Small Parts, Inc., Miami, FL)
Aquarium air bubblers with tubing and aeration stones
Rubbermaid Style 3690 plastic tubs [32 cm(l) × 28 cm(w) × 13 cm(d)]
Mini-BeadBeater with tubes and baked 0.5-mm zirconium beads (BioSpec Products, Bartlesville, OK)
Clinical centrifuge (IEC)
Benchtop ultracentrifuge (Beckman TL-100)
Polypropylene pestles (Kontes No. 749520) and 1.5-ml microcentrifuge tubes
1-ml disposable syringes and 18-gauge needles
Nylon mesh (20-μm-pore size, Small Parts, Inc., Miami, FL)
Snap-cap plastic tubes (Falcon No. 2063)
Ultracentrifuge tubes (Beckman No. 349622)

Hoagland's Solution (10 liters)	
Hoagland's A (100×)	100 ml
Hoagland's B (100×)	100 ml
Hoagland's Nitrate (100×)	100 ml
H_2O	700 ml

Hoagland's A (100×) (1 liter)	
$CaCl_2 \cdot 2H_2O$	36.8 g
Iron chelate (Sprint 330, CIBA-Geigy)	7.6 g
H_2O to 1 liter	

Autoclave 20 min, liquid cycle

Hoagland's B (100×) (1 liter)	
KH_2PO_4	6.8 g
KCl	18.8 g
$MgSO_4 \cdot 7H_2O$	25.2 g
Hoagland's micronutrients (10,000×)	10 ml
H_2O to 1 liter	
Autoclave 20 min, liquid cycle	

Hoagland's Nitrate (100×) (1 liter)	
KNO_3	25.28 g
H_2O to 1 liter	
Autoclave 20 min, liquid cycle	

Hoagland's Micronutrients (10,000×) (100 ml)	
$ZnSO_4 \cdot 7H_2O$	0.10 g
$MnSO_4 \cdot H_2O$	0.78 g
$CuSO_4 \cdot 5H_2O$	0.04 g
H_3BO_3	1.45 g
$MoO_3 \cdot 2H_2O$	0.01 g
H_2O to 100 ml	
Filter sterilize	

MB (50 ml)	*Final*	*50 ml*
Tris, pH 8 (1 *M* stock)	70 m*M*	3.5 ml
EGTA (0.4 *M* stock)	20 m*M*	2.5 ml
$MgCl_2$ (1 *M* stock)	15 m*M*	750 μl
sucrose (1 *M* stock)	250 m*M*	12.5 ml
Dithiothreitol (1 *M* stock)	5 m*M*	250 μl
Leupeptin (50 mg/ml stock)	3 μg/ml	3 μl
ß-Glycerophosphate (0.9 *M* stock)	60 m*M*	3.33 ml
H_2O	21.67 ml	
PMSF (10 mg/ml stock)[1]	100 μg/ml	(500 μl)
Make fresh from sterile stocks		

[1] Phenylmethylsulfonylfluoride, dissolved in isopropanol. Add just prior to initiating homogenization.

Wash Buffer (2×) (500 ml)	*Final*	*500 ml*
Tris, pH 7.4 (1 *M* stock)	10 m*M*	10 ml
EDTA (0.5 *M* stock)	10 m*M*	20 ml
NaCl (5 *M* stock)	100 m*M*	20 ml
H_2O	450 ml	
Make from sterile stocks		
Dilute a small amount of 2× stock 1:1 with water before use		

Fixative (10 ml)	*Final*	*10 ml*
Formaldehyde (37% w/v stock)	4% w/v	1.1 ml
Wash Buffer (2× stock, above)	5 ml	
H_2O	3.9 ml	
Make fresh from sterile stocks		

NIB (Nuclear Isolation Buffer, 5 ml)	*Final*	*5 ml*
Wash buffer (2 ti stock, above)	2.5 ml	
Triton-X 100 (10% stock)	0.1%	50 μl
H_2O	2.45 ml	
Make from sterile stocks		

Nuclear Stain (7 ml)	*Final*	*7 ml*
PEG 6000–8000 (Sigma No. 5413)	3% w/v	0.21 g
Propidium iodide (2 mg/ml stock)	50 μg/ml	175 μl
RNase A (500 U/ml, BRL)	9 U/ml	126 μl
Triton-X 100 (10% w/v stock)	0.1% v/v	70 μl
Na-citrate, pH 7.2 (1 *M* stock)	3.56 m*M*	25 μl
H_2O	to 7 ml	
Make fresh from sterile stocks		

Nuclear Salt Solution (7 ml)	*Final*	*7 ml*
PEG 6000–8000 (Sigma No. 5413)	3% w/v	0.21 g
Propidium iodide (2 mg/ml stock)	50 μg/ml	175 μl
Triton-X 100 (10% w/v stock)	0.1% v/v	70 μl
NaCl (5 *M* stock)	376 m*M*	526 μl
H_2O	to 7 ml	
Make fresh from sterile stocks		

Propidium Iodide Stock (2 mg/ml)	*1 ml*
Propidium iodide	2 mg
H_2O	1 ml
Store in dark at 4°C for up to 2 weeks	

III. Aspects of the Procedure

A. Mitotic Synchrony

Synchronization of the mitotic cell cycle is achieved by selectively but reversibly blocking the process at a defined step for a period of time equal to or greater than the time required to complete one cycle. Individual cells arrive at the arrest point at different times during the treatment period, depending upon the stage of the cycle in which they happened to be when the blocking agent was administered. The agent is then removed, freeing cells to proceed through the cycle in synchrony. Samples are collected and analyzed at appropriate time points following removal of the blocking agent. These harvests will be enriched for cells passing through the stage of the cycle that occurs at that particular interval following the arrest point.

Two caveats should be acknowledged. First, the initial cell population is essentially never uniformly sensitive to the blocking agent. For example, the target population, whether a cell culture or part of an intact organism, invariably contains noncycling cells that are impervious to the mitotic inhibitor. These cells will represent a nonmitotic and therefore nonsynchronizable background, ultimately limiting the percentage synchrony, and consequently the developmental uniformity, of the harvested population that one can expect in any experiment.

Second, it is frequently overlooked that, at the time the mitotic blocker is removed, subsets within the arrested cell population will have spent differing amounts of time in the mitotically blocked state, depending upon the stage of the cycle they happened to occupy at the time the blocker was added. This diversity within the arrested and subsequently released population can contribute to unanticipated behaviors within the presumably synchronous population. There is no reason to assume that arrested cells will not respond differentially to short vs long treatments with a given chemical blocking agent. For example, the kinetics with which cells resume progress through the cycle following removal of the agent might depend upon the length of time spent under its influence. For this reason, it is probably best to employ different blockers in parallel experiments, in order to validate results obtained with any one agent. For a discussion of chemical blocking agents applicable to plant cell synchrony experiments, the reader is referred to the thoughtful review by Gould (Gould, 1984).

A variety of mitotic blockade strategies is available, both chemical and physical. For the pea root apical meristems under investigation in our laboratory, 5-aminouracil (5-AU) has proven to be an economical, convenient, and reliable blocking agent (Clowes, 1965; Van't Hof, 1966; Van't Hof and Lamm, 1991). 5-AU causes mitotic arrest early in G1 and is fully reversible by removal of the drug. Whether 5-AU treatment starves cells for thymidine through a false-feedback mechanism or directly inhibits an enzyme of DNA synthesis is not known (Prensky and Smith, 1965; Díez *et al.*, 1976).

B. Plant Growth

The garden pea, *Pisum sativum* cv. Alaska, has been the primary subject of our plant cell division studies. Peas are genetically uniform, easily grown for bulk harvest, and consistently offer high and clean yields of both protein and nucleic acids. Pea roots are also infectible by Rhizobium bacteria, a focus of some of our cell division control studies.

We grow peas hydroponically. Seeds are first germinated for three days on 30 cm(l) × 46 cm(w) × 2-cm(d) porcelain-coated metal trays, lined with 16 single layers of bleached white paper toweling, topped with a single sheet of Whatman 3MM filter paper or equivalent. Prior to sewing the seeds, trays are assembled, covered with foil, and autoclaved, after which the filter paper is soaked with 350 ml of sterile water. Consistent moisture and sowing density are important to ensure reproducible and uniform growth of seedlings. Use of sterile technique throughout germination helps to avoid interference from contaminating microorganisms.

Three-day-old seedlings are transferred to hydroponics. Such a system ensures that the root apices are continuously bathed in nutrient solution, affording greatest control over chemical treatments. Our hydroponics system consists simply of 32 cm(l) × 28 cm(w) × 13-cm(d) Rubbermaid plastic tubs (style 3690) filled to within 2 cm of the top with 10 liters of Hoagland's solution (Hoagland and Arnon, 1950), continuously aerated by an aquarium bubbler. A stiff plastic mesh with 5 × 5-mm openings rests atop of the tub. Roots of germinated seedlings are threaded through the mesh, through which their imbibed cotyledons cannot pass. Each tub accommodates 850–900 seedlings. Seedlings are germinated and grown hydroponically in complete darkness at 20°C.

C. Flow Cytometry

As cells pass through S phase into G2 following release from the 5-AU blockade, nuclear DNA content doubles from 2C to 4C. At M phase, chromosomes are equally distributed between daughter cells and their G1 nuclear DNA content returns to 2C. Thus, nuclear DNA content provides a convenient marker for cells in G1, S, and G2, and measurement of this parameter is an essential indicator of the effectiveness of any mitotic synchronization protocol.

We assay nuclear DNA content in pea meristem cells by flow cytometry. Nuclei are fixed, isolated, stained with propidium iodide, and analyzed by published procedures (Sgorbati *et al.*, 1986). The flow cytometer passes a single-file stream of nuclei past a laser beam, exciting propidium iodide fluorescence directly proportional to the amount of DNA present. The fluorescence of each nucleus is detected by a photomultiplier tube and recorded as a histogram (see discussions of flow cytometry elsewhere in this volume). In our system, S phase is completed by 6 h after release from the 5-AU blockade and mitosis begins approximately 2 h thereafter. We estimate that 60–80% of the sampled cells are dividing synchronously. The remainder of the cells in this distal 3 mm of the root are no longer in the proliferative state, but are in a noncycling 2C or 4C "G0" state (Van't Hof, 1973).

D. Protein Extraction

A variety of analyses can be performed on mitotically synchronous plant cells. In various studies, we have extracted whole cell proteins and RNAs and have analyzed these by direct blotting and enzymatic methods. We will confine our more generic discussion here to protein extraction. As in any such procedure, tissue is disrupted in an appropriate buffer and the resulting slurry is clarified by centrifugation. The particular challenge in root tip analyses is the small sample size. Both an efficient extraction procedure and highly sensitive assays are required. Although a discussion of the specific enzyme assays we employ in our studies would be inappropriate in the present context, a word about our extraction strategy is in order.

We use a Mini-BeadBeater (Biospec Products, Bartlesville, OK) and Beckman Model TL-100 tabletop ultracentrifuge for protein extraction from harvests of approximately 100 root tips of 2–3 mm each. The Mini-BeadBeater is designed to agitate vigorously a tube containing tissue, buffer, and small glass or zirconium beads. The beads collide with the tissue, breaking cells and releasing their contents into the surrounding buffer. One hundred pea root tips is about the minimum practical sample size for our assays, and yields about 1 mg of protein. Larger samples provide disproportionately greater yields of protein, but require more hands for efficient and timely processing.

IV. Methods

A. Cell Cycle Synchronization and Sample Collection (Fig. 1)

1. Surface sterilize pea seeds by shaking gently in 95% ethanol for 30 min.
2. Further sterilize seeds by shaking gently in full-strength commercial bleach for 10 min. Do not allow seeds to soak in bleach longer than 10 min or germination will be impaired.
3. Rinse seeds four times in sterile distilled water.
4. Soak seeds overnight in sterile distilled water with aeration (e.g., in a large flask containing a pipet attached to a house air line).
5. Spread seeds onto soaked germination trays, cover with foil, and place trays in a 20°C dark incubator for 3 days.
6. Thread seedling roots through plastic mesh over hydroponics tanks containing aerated Hoagland's solution. Place in 20°C dark incubator for 12 h.
7. Start now to dissolve 2 g 5-AU (Sigma No. A4005) in 4 liters of water for each tub of Hoagland's/5-AU to be used. 5-AU takes a while to dissolve (final concentration of 5-AU in tank will be 0.2 mg/ml).
8. Position the plastic mesh holding germinated seedlings over a tank of Hoaglands/5-AU. Leave tank, with aeration, in 20°C dark incubator for 12 h.

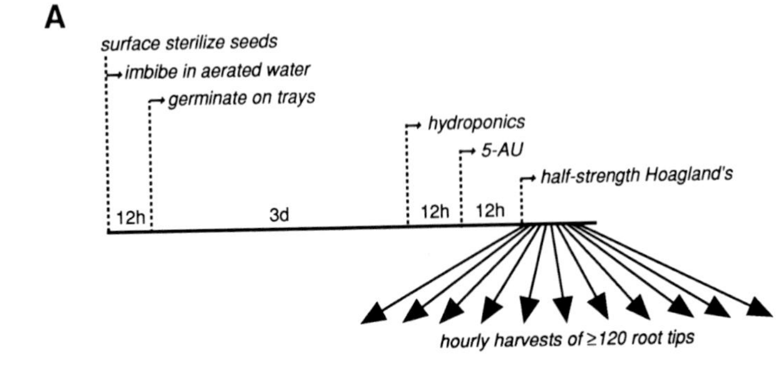

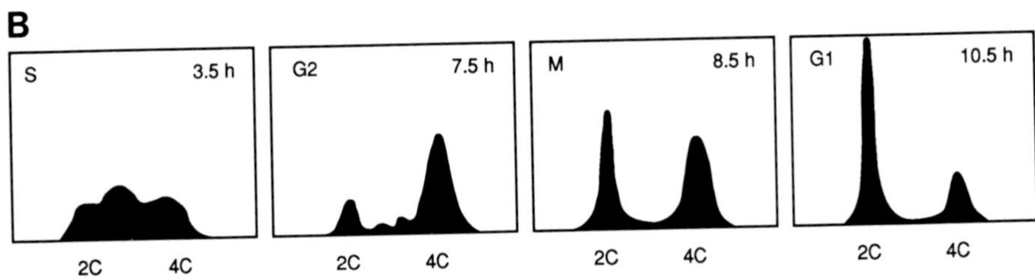

Fig. 1 Time course of pea root tip mitotic synchronization protocol. (a) Steps in procedure are shown above and intervals between them are indicated between vertical dotted lines. Root tip harvests at 1-h intervals are indicated by downward arrows. (b) Flow cytometer histograms representative of S, G2, M, and G1 time points with 2C and 4C peaks labeled.

9. Release roots from 5-AU block by rinsing in water and transferring to tank of fresh, aerated Hoagland's. Return to 20°C, dark incubator.

10. Harvest root tips for flow cytometry and protein extraction at desired intervals as follows.

   a. Flow cytometry

      i. Prepare a 1.5-ml microcentrifuge tube with 100 μl fixative on ice for each harvest of 20 root tips.

      ii. Remove roots from tank, singly or in small groups, and rinse in sterile distilled water.

      iii. With razor blade or scalpel, excise distal 3 mm from 20 root tips for each time point and collect into prepared tube.

      iv. Incubate 10 min in fixative.

      v. Rinse tips with wash buffer three times for 3 min each.

      vi. Fixed root tips may be stored in wash buffer overnight at 4°C.

   b. Protein extraction

      i. Excise distal 3 mm from ≥100 root tips for each time point.

ii. Harvest root tips into 500 μl MB in a Mini-BeadBeater tube on ice.

iii. Process root tips as described below before next time point.

11. Continue to harvest hourly samples as needed.

B. Soluble Protein Extraction (as soon as sample is collected for each time point; all steps at 4°C; reagents on ice)

1. Add 5 μl PMSF to chilled tips in 500 μl MB.

2. Add enough sterile 0.5-mm zirconium beads (we bake them overnight at 140°C) to bring total volume to 1 ml.

3. Agitate each tube in Mini-BeadBeater for 30 s, six to eight times, cooling briefly on ice between agitations.

4. Heat a 23-gauge needle and poke a hole in the bottom of the bead beater tube. Slide pierced tube into the bottom of a 5-ml snap-cap tube (Falcon No. 2063).

5. Spin the liquid out of the Mini-BeadBeater tube into the surrounding snap-cap tube in a clinical centrifuge at top speed for 5 s.

6. Rinse the beads with 500 μl MB/PMSF (as above); spin as in previous step and pool with primary extract.

7. Transfer pooled extracts to a 0.5 × 2-in. thick-walled polycarbonate ultracentrifuge tube (Beckman No. 349622).

8. Centrifuge 30 min at 4°C, 150,000 × *g* (60,000 rpm in 100.3 rotor of Beckman TL-100 table-top ultracentrifuge).

9. Transfer supernatant to a clean microfuge tube and store at −80°C.

C. Nuclear Isolation and Staining for Flow Cytometry (the following day; all reagents on ice)

1. Replace wash buffer with 100 μl NIB.

2. Crush fixed tissue with four to six manual strokes of a polypropylene pestle in the 1.5-ml microcentrifuge tube. Rinse pestle into same tube with additional 50 μl NIB.

3. Place a square of nylon mesh (pore size 20 μm) between a 1-ml syringe and an 18-gauge needle (mesh should protrude from the Luer-lock). Pipette suspension of nuclei into the syringe, insert plunger, and push suspension gently through the mesh into a clean 1.5-ml microcentrifuge tube on ice.

4. Pellet nuclei at 300 × *g* for 5 min at 4°C.

5. Gently resuspend nuclei in 50 μl NIB.

6. Add 500 μl nuclear stain and incubate at 37°C for 30 min.

7. Add 500 μl nuclear salt solution and incubate on ice for 1 h.

8. Analyze nuclei by flow cytometry.

V. Perspectives

The principal constraint in this synchronization protocol is one of personnel. Careful and timely root tip excision is, of necessity, a labor-intensive process requiring at least two to three people and, for some, a dissecting microscope. Harvesting more than a few hundred root tips in 1 h requires additional hands dedicated to processing the tissue. If the time required for harvesting a given time point's batch of root tips exceeds the interval between the time points, then the definition of a time point itself obviously becomes problematic. Alternative approaches would be required for studies aimed at the purification of a low-abundance protein from a particular stage of the cell cycle, as true "bucket biochemistry" cannot be practiced with merely hundreds of root tips, despite their being enriched in macromolecules compared to mature plant tissues. These limitations notwithstanding, efficient affinity matrices and sensitive assays for specific cellular components render the yields from harvests of as few as 100 root tips fully adequate for many analytical objectives.

The procedure outlined above has not been applied by our group to any plant species besides pea. However, there is no reason to believe that it, or a slight variation on it, would not be applicable to other species, especially those with large seeds. More creative adaptations would obviously be required for smaller seeded and rooted species.

Key control points of the eukaryotic cell cycle occur at the G1/S and G2/M transitions. The 5-AU procedure provides an unperturbed G2/M passage. However, 5-AU-treated root tip meristems do not maintain synchrony long enough to pass through the G1/S transition in sufficient synchrony for biochemical analyses of this control point to be of value. In order to observe the G1/S/G2 passages, unperturbed by the synchronizing agent itself, a protocol employing a G2-M blocker, such as a reversible anti-microtubule drug, is preferred. Several possibilities in this area have been reported (Morejohn and Fosket, 1991).

References

Clowes, F. (1965). Synchronization in a meristem by 5-aminouracil. *J. Exp. Bot.* **16,** 581–586.

Díez, J., González-Fernández, A., and López-Sáez, J. (1976). Mechanism of mitotic synchronization induced by 5-aminouracil. *Exp. Cell Res.* **98,** 79–89.

Gould, A. R. (1984). Control of the cell cycle in cultured plant cells. *CRC Crit. Rev. Plant Sci.* **1,** 315–344.

Hoagland, D., and Arnon, D. (1950). "The Water-Culture Method for Growing Plants without Soil," Calif. Agric. Expt. Sta. Cir. 347.

Morejohn, L., and Fosket, D. (1991). The biochemistry of compounds with anti-microtubule activity in plant cells. *Pharmacol. Ther.* **51,** 217–230.

Prensky, W., and Smith, H. (1965). The mechanism of 5-aminouracil-induced synchrony of cell division in *Vicia faba* root meristems. *J. Cell Biol.* **24,** 401–414.

Sgorbati, S., Levi, M., Sparvoli, E., Trezzi, F., and Lucchini, G. (1986). Cytometry and flow cytometry of 4′,6-diamidino-2-phenylindole (DAPI)-stained suspensions of nuclei released from fresh and fixed tissues of plants. *Physiol. Plant.* **68,** 471–476.

Van't Hof, J. (1966). Experimental control of DNA synthesizing and dividing cells in excised root tips of *Pisum. Am. J. Bot.* **53,** 970–976.

Van't Hof, J. (1973). The regulation of cell division in higher plants. *In* "Basic Mechanisms in Plant Morphogenesis" (P. Carlson, H. Smith, A. Sparrow, and J. Van't Hof, eds.), Vol. 25, pp. 152–165. Brookhaven, NY: Brookhaven National Laboratory.

Van't Hof, J., and Lamm, S. S. (1991). Single-stranded replication intermediates of ribosomal DNA replicons of pea. *EMBO J.* **10,** 1949–1953.

CHAPTER 25

Manipulation of Pollen Grains for Gametophytic and Sporophytic Types of Growth

V. Raghavan
Department of Plant Biology
The Ohio State University
1735 Neil Avenue
Columbus, Ohio 43210

I. Introduction

A single-celled pollen grain born out of a reduction division of the pollen mother cell represents the beginning of a short-lived male gametophytic phase in angiosperms. This cell not only has the capacity to undergo terminal differentiation into committed sperm cells, but can also enter into a pathway of continued growth and differentiation, thus attaining immortality. Moreover, pollen grains constitute the only haploid cell type in the reproductive life of angiosperms that are available at defined stages of development in quantities large enough to allow application of biochemical procedures. These attributes have made pollen grains appealing models for a steadily growing number of investigations on the

METHODS IN CELL BIOLOGY, VOL. 49

physiology, cytology, and molecular biology of cell differentiation and dedifferentiation.

The methods described in this chapter relate to three experimental designs using pollen grains as the starting material. These are (*a*) the culture of pollen grains to study the requirements for their germination and growth of pollen tubes; (*b*) isolation of viable sperm cells from pollen grains; and (*c*) induction of sporophytic type of growth in pollen grains.

Pollen grains of many species germinate in high numbers within minutes after sowing in a relatively simple medium; growth of pollen tubes is rapid and is sensitive to a wide variety of physiologically active substances; the short experimental duration provides immunity from microorganisms and eliminates the need for complete aseptic techniques; use of large cell populations facilitates studies that involve quantification; techniques used are relatively simple, allowing continuous records to be made of the quantitative and cytological aspects of germination and pollen tube growth. In recent years, analysis of pollen tubes by electron microscopic and immunofluorescence methods has made important contributions to our knowledge of the subcellular localization of the cytoskeletal elements of rapidly elongating plant cells. In the field of fertilization physiology, isolation of sperm from pollen grains has brought us a step closer to developing an *in vitro* fertilization system. Induction of sporophytic type of growth in pollen grains by tissue culture technology has become the method of choice for the production of haploid plants in quantity for genetic and breeding purposes. Perhaps the area of greatest promise lies in the use of pollen grains as gene vectors. For these reasons, pollen grains have not only continued to hold the sustained interest of botanists of many persuasions, but they have enjoyed a veritable renaissance of interest as experimental systems in cell and developmental biology.

As the literature pertaining to pollen germination, sperm isolation, and induction of pollen sporophytic growth is relatively vast, no attempt is made here to present a comprehensive account of the techniques used in various laboratories. Rather, the emphasis will be on a few selective methods that have been found to be reliable and of general applicability, and thus can be employed for different species with minor modifications.

II. Materials and Methods

This section presents a list of the pollen sources, as well as the methods commonly employed for experiments in the areas outlined above. It should be understood that theoretically it is possible to use pollen grains of any plant for the three types of experimental applications, although pollen grains of each species will have their own special requirements for optimum results. The choice of material is determined primarily by its availability and the long-term research objectives. For critical experiments it may be necessary to have available in the greenhouse a continuing supply of plants of a known cultivar at the desired stage of floral development for collection of pollen grains.

A. Pollen Germination

Pollen grains have found their widest use in the laboratory, to date, in studies relating to germination and pollen tube growth. A recently published laboratory manual by Shivanna and Rangaswamy (1992) is especially recommended for beginners as well as for the experienced for access to a wide variety of protocols employed in pollen germination studies.

Germination experiments begin with the collection of pollen grains. There are many ingenious ways such as tapping the flowers, allowing anthers to dehisce under low humidity, and splitting open anthers to collect pollen grains and keep them for a reasonable length of time in prime condition for germination. Since the objective in all instances is to obtain viable pollen grains, this is best achieved by determining the germination responses of collections made at different times before and after anthesis of the flower for each species under investigation. Pollen grains of *Brassica napus, Hyoscyamus niger, Nicotiana tabacum, Tradescantia paludosa,* and *Zea mays,* among others have been extensively used for germination experiments.

Pollen grains of some plants begin to germinate readily when they are sown in distilled water. Bursting of pollen grains releasing their contents is often observed when the osmolality of the growth medium is lower than that of the milieu of the pollen grain. This is, however, eliminated by increasing the osmolality of the medium by adding sucrose or mannitol. Supplementation of the medium with small quantities of boric acid and calcium nitrate has also been shown to increase the germination percentage and growth of pollen tubes. The following basal medium, prepared in distilled water according to the formulation of Brewbaker and Kwack (1963), has been found to be suitable for pollen germination studies in a wide variety of plants.

Sucrose 10%

H_3BO_3 100 mg/liter

$Ca(NO_3)_2 \cdot 4H_2O$ 300 mg/liter

$MgSO_4 \cdot 7H_2O$ 200 mg/liter

KNO_3 100 mg/liter

Essential to the continuous monitoring of pollen germination and pollen tube growth is the selection of a suitable method of culture. Microscopic observation of the pollen grains is facilitated by the hanging drop culture. In the protocol usually followed, pollen grains are suspended in a drop of the liquid medium on a coverglass and the latter is inverted over the cavity of a depression slide. To prevent desiccation of the medium, the edges of the coverglass are sealed with molten wax or petroleum jelly. Alternatively, pollen grains are sown on a drop of the medium placed on a slide and the latter is kept in a humid chamber.

For some experiments, pollen grains are germinated on the surface of a solid medium secured by the addition of agar or gelatin. Solid cultures are specially useful in experiments on pollen tube chemotropism, i.e., the directional growth of pollen tubes to a source of a chemical or substances released by the tissues of the ovary placed at a distance.

With all types of cultures, estimation of the percentage of pollen germination and the average length of the pollen tube may be obtained by microscopic examination within 24 h after sowing. There is no better criterion to assess germination than the appearance of one or more pollen tubes through the germination pores. Although pollen grains of many plants begin to germinate within a few minutes to a few hours after sowing, final count of germination should be delayed until almost all viable pollen grains have germinated. In a similar way, optimal growth in length of the pollen tube occurs within a short period of time after it emerges from the pollen grain, although growth at a reduced rate continues for a prolonged period. For cytological studies, germinated pollen grains are fixed and stained with acetocarmine.

B. Sperm Isolation

Isolation of sperm cells from pollen grains and pollen tubes has become an important objective for development of an *in vitro* fertilization system in angiosperms. Some of the successful isolation attempts have been undertaken with tricellular pollen grains, that is, pollen grains that harbor a vegetative cell and two sperm cells. A recent review (Chaboud and Perez, 1992) has surveyed from a historical perspective sperm isolation procedures. As currently used, the protocol generally involves releasing sperm by immersing pollen grains in a medium of high osmolality, followed by Percoll gradient centrifugation. For maize sperm isolation, about 0.1 to 1 g pollen grains are suspended in Brewbaker and Kwack (1963) medium containing 15% sucrose and gently agitated for 30 min. After filtration through 50- and 20-μm sieves, aliquots of the second filtrate are layered on a discontinuous 15 to 40% Percoll density gradient made up in the same medium and centrifuged at $9000 \times g$ for 40 min to free the sperm from pollen contaminants. Another round of centrifugation generally yields good quality sperm cells. Viability of sperm is routinely determined by Evans blue as an exclusion dye or by fluorochrome reaction (Dupuis *et al.*, 1987). Modifications of this protocol have been used to isolate sperm from pollen grains of *Plumbago zeylanica, Lolium perenne, Lilium longiflorum,* and *Spinacia oleracea* (Chaboud and Perez, 1992).

C. Induction of Sporophytic Growth in Pollen Grains

Sporophytic growth was originally induced in pollen grains when anthers of *Datura innoxia* were cultured at an appropriate stage of development in a nutrient medium supplemented with certain organic additives and hormones. It was found that a small number of the enclosed pollen grains produced multicellular units, which proceeded through typical stages simulating zygotic embryogenesis to form haploid embryoids and plantlets. Later work has resulted in the simplification of the nutrient medium as well as in the demonstration of the ability of isolated pollen grains to go through the embryogenic type of development. Sporophytic mode of growth of pollen grains has been documented in nearly 200 species of plants. Individual protocols used in the anther culture of several cereals, trees, vegetables, and medicinal plants are described in a volume edited by Bajaj (1990). In this section, I will present methods for the induction of embryogenic growth of pollen grains in cultured anthers of *Hyoscyamus niger,* which has been extensively used in my laboratory (Raghavan, 1990). Because of their recent use in molecular studies, methods for isolated pollen cultures in *Brassica napus* and *Nicotiana tabacum* will also be briefly described.

1. Anther Culture of *Hyoscyamus*

Hyoscyamus niger includes both annual and biennial varieties. The annual variety has a long-day flowering habit, whereas the biennial variety responds to vernalization, sometimes combined with a specific photoperiodic regime to initiate flowers. For anther culture, flower buds, ca. 6 mm long, containing uninucleate pollen grains are collected from an annual variety grown under long days at 20°C. They are sterilized in 12.5% Clorox for 5 min followed by several rinses in sterile distilled water. Anthers are excised from flower buds under aseptic conditions and transferred to French square bottles containing 10 ml of solid or liquid medium. Bourgin and Nitsch's (1967) medium containing 2% sucrose has been found most suitable for anther culture of *H. niger* (Table I); however, virtually any mineral salt medium currently employed in plant tissue culture work that gives a good balance of major salts, vitamins, and a source of iron is ideal. Addition of hormones such as IAA, 2,4-D, or kinetin induces callus formation from pollen grains. The cultures are generally maintained in a culture room illuminated with weak fluorescent and incandescent light. Progress of pollen embryogenesis is monitored by acetocarmine squashes of anthers sacrificed at intervals after culture. Multicellular pollen grains are observed in about 48 to 72 h after culture and these subsequently go through stages reminiscent of zygotic embryogenesis and evolve into plantlets. Plantlets generally emerge from anthers in about 3 weeks after culture.

2. Pollen Culture of *Brassica*

Several laboratories have developed protocols, which differ from one another only in minor details, for optimization of pollen embryogenesis from isolated pollen cultures of *Brassica napus.* The following information is summarized from Huang (1992). Donor plants are grown at 10/5°C day/night temperatures at a photoperiod of 16 h. Flower buds, 3 to 4 mm long, containing pollen developmental stages close to the first haploid mitosis are sterilized by immersing them in a commercial bleach containing ca. 6% sodium hypochlorite for 15 min fol-

Table I
Bourgin and Nitsch's Medium

$Ca(NO_3)_s \cdot 4H_2O$	500 mg/liter
KNO_3	125 mg
$MgSo_4 \cdot 7H_2O$	125 mg
KH_2PO_4	125 mg
$MnSO_4$	25 mg
H_3BO_3	10 mg
$ZnSO_4 \cdot 7H_2O$	10 mg
$Na_2MoO_4 \cdot 2H_2O$	0.25 mg
$CuSO_4 \cdot 5H_2O$	0.25 mg
$FeSO_4 \cdot 7H_2O$/ Na_2ETA	5 mg/liter of a stock solution containing 5.57 g $FeSO_4 \cdot 7H_2O$ and 7.45 g $Na_2 \cdot EDTA$ per liter of water
Myoinositol	100 mg/liter
Nicotinic acid	5 mg
Glycine	2 mg
Pyridoxine HCl	0.5 mg
Thiamine HCl	0.5 mg
Folic acid	0.5 mg
Biotin	0.05 mg
Sucrose	20 g
pH adjusted to 5.5	

lowed by rinses in sterile water. The buds are then macerated in B5 medium Gamborg *et al.,* 1968; see Chapter 29, this volume) containing 750 mg/liter $CaCl_2$ and 13% sucrose. The homogenate is filtered through a 40- to 100-μm nylon mesh. A pollen fraction is separated from the filtrate by mild centrifugation (100 × *g* for 5 min) and cleaned by suspending it in an aliquot of the fresh medium, followed by centrifugation. The procedure is repeated two or three times. The pollen grains are then suspended in Millipore-filtered Lichter medium (Lichter, 1981) without potato extract (Table II) and cultured in the dark at 33°C for 3 days and at 25°C subsequently. Changing the medium 24 h after culture to a fresh aliquot of the same medium is recommended for some genotypes to increase the yield of embryoids. Embryoids at the cotyledonary stage of development are seen in cultures in about 2 weeks; the yield is generally of the order 10% of the pollen placed in culture.

3. Pollen Culture of *Nicotiana*

Kyo and Harada (1986) have developed a method using Percoll density gradient centrifugation to obtain a homogeneous embryogenic pollen population of *Nicotiana tabacum.* If these pollen grains are first subjected to a starvation diet (by culturing in a medium lacking sucrose and glutamine) and then transferred to a regular medium, they divide in the embryogenic pathway. Flower buds containing pollen grains at the early, mid-, and late-binucleat stages are collected

Table II
Lichter Medium

	(mg/liter)
$Ca(NO_3)_2 \cdot 4H_2O$	500
KNO_3	125
$MgSo_4 \cdot 7H_2O$	125
KH_2PO_4	125
$MnSO_4 \cdot 4H_2O$	25
H_3BO_3	10
$ZnSO_4 \cdot 4H_2O$	10
$Na_2MoO_4 \cdot 2H_2O$	0.25
$CuSO_4 \cdot 5H_2O$	0.25
$CoCl_2 \cdot 6H_2O$	0.025
Sodium salt of EDTA (7.45 mg/liter) and $FeSO_4 \cdot 7H_2O$ (5.57 mg/liter), 5 ml	
Glycine	2
Myo-inositol	100 mg
Nicotinic acid	5 mg
Pyridoxine HCl	0.5 mg
Thiamine HCl	0.5 mg
Folic acid	0.5 mg
Biotin	0.05 mg
Glutathione	30
Glutamine	800
Serine	10
Sucrose	At various levels

from plants grown in the greenhouse under natural light conditions. Anthers excised from flower buds are sterilized by immersion in 8% sodium hypochlorite solution for 10 min, followed by several rinses in water. They are homogenized in medium A (lacking sucrose and containing glutamine; see Table III), and the homogenate is filtered through a 53-μm-pore-size nylon mesh. The pollen pellet

Table III
Kyo and Harada Medium[a]

	(mM)
KCl	20
$MgSO_4$	1
$CaCl_2$	1
KH_2PO_4	1
Glutamine	3
Mannitol	300

[a] Medium B as above, but lacks glutamine; medium C as above, but contains 1 mM sucrose.

is washed by suspending it in medium A followed by centrifugation (150 × g for 1 min). The pellet suspended in a freash aliquot of medium A is used for density gradient centrifugation. The pollen pellet is layered over a discontinuous Percoll gradient (50, 60, 70%) prepared by mixing with 3.3× concentrated A medium. Following centrifugation at 450 × g for 5 min, the pollen band is collected, diluted with an equal volume of medium A, and subjected to Percoll gradient centrifugation again. The pollen grains from the second centrifugation are suspended in medium B (lacks both sucrose and glutamine) and cultured in the dark for 2 days. Subsequently, the pollen grains are collected by centrifugation and cultured in medium C (contains both sucrose and glutamine). Multicellular pollen grains are observed in about 10 days after culture.

III. Critical Aspects of the Procedures

Pollen quality is a prerequisite to germination experiments and sperm isolation. Pollen grains of the vast majority of plants are highly dehydrated cells at the time they are dispersed from the anther and the quality of pollen grains is dependent on their degree of hydration at the time of collection. Optimum germination occurs at a certain percentage of water content for pollen of each species. It is therefore useful to standardize conditions for growth of donor plants and for time of collection of pollen grains relative to the time of anthesis. Since pollen grains of many species show a population effect, the amount of pollen loaded into each culture may also affect their germination.

In anther/pollen culture studies for inducing sporophytic development of pollen grains, special consideration should be given to the stage of pollen development in the anthers at the time of culture. In most cases anthers containing uninucleate pollen grains are most responsive to culture. The critical stage is established for each species in a preliminary experiment in relation to the length of flower bud; this eliminates the necessity of determining the stage of pollen development in anthers of each flower bud at the time of culture. However, it is recommended that one anther from each flower bud is fixed in acetocarmine at the time of culture for determination of the pollen developmental stage later.

Although it is not stated explicitly, familiarity with procedures used in a tissue culture laboratory is essential for success in some of the procedures described above. This applies to long-term pollen germination experiments and for anther and pollen culture experiments for inducing sporophytic growth. Besides surface sterilization of flower buds or anthers, medium and glassware should also be sterilized. All operations are done in a sterile transfer room or in a laminar flow hood.

IV. Conclusions and Perspectives

Some the methods described above for the study of developmental potential of angiosperm pollen grains are similar to those currently used for culture of spores of lower plants and for the culture of other plant organs such as embryos. Although methods for pollen germination and anther and pollen culture have been successfully applied for a broad spectrum of plants, methods for the isolation of sperm from pollen grains are still in their initial stages and isolation of sperm from pollen tubes has hardly been attempted. If experience is any indication, one can hope that when the potential use of sperm from pollen tubes is fully recognized, their isolation will become a minor problem. On the whole, the protocols described here with pollen grains will provide a level of information about growth of single cells and totipotency of male germ cells that is impossible to obtain with any other system in the angiosperm plant body.

References

Bajaj, Y. P. S., ed. (1990). "Biotechnology in Agriculture and Forestry, Vol. 12. Haploids in Crop Improvement I." Berlin: Springer-Verlag.

Bourgin, J. P., and Nitsch, J. P. (1967). Obtention de *Nicotiana* haploïdes á partir d'étamines cultivées *in vitro*. *Ann. Physiol. Vég.* **9,** 377–382.

Brewbaker, J. L., and Kwack, B. H. (1963). The essential role of calcium ion in pollen germination and pollen tube growth. *Am. J. Bot.* **50,** 859–865.

Chaboud, A., and Perez, R. (1992). Generative cells and male gametes: Isolation, physiology, and biochemistry. *Int. Rev. Cytol.* **140,** 205–232.

Dupuis, I., Roeckel, P., Matthys-Rochon, E., and Dumas, C. (1987). Procedure to isolate viable sperm cells from corn (*Zea mays* L.). *Plant Physiol.* **85,** 876–878.

Gamborg, O. L., Miller, R. A., and Ojima, K. (1968). Nutrient requirements of suspension cultures of soybean root cells. *Exp. Cell Res.* **50,** 151–158.

Huang, B. (1992). Genetic manipulation of microspores and microspore-derived embryos. *In Vitro Cell Dev. Biol.* **28P,** 53–58.

Kyo, M., and Harada, H. (1986). Control of the developmental pathway of tobacco pollen *in vitro*. *Planta* **168,** 427–432.

Lichter, R. (1981). Anther culture of *Brassica napus* in a liquid culture medium. *Z. Pflanzenphysiol.* **103,** 229–237.

Raghavan, V. (1990). *In* "Biotechnology in Agriculture and Forestry, Vol. 12. Haploids in Crop Improvement I" (Y. P. S. Bajaj, ed.), pp. 290–305. Berlin: Springer-Verlag.

Shivanna, K. R., and Rangaswamy, N. S. (1992). "Pollen Biology. A Laboratory Manual." Berlin: Springer-Verlag.

CHAPTER 26

Root Border Cells as Tools in Plant Cell Studies

Lindy A. Brigham, Ho-Hyung Woo, and Martha C. Hawes

Departments of Plant Pathology and Molecular and Cellular Biology
University of Arizona
Tucson, Arizona 85721

I. Introduction

Root border cells lend themselves to a wide range of studies by virtue of their unique morphology. Border cells are populations of single cells that separate from the outer cells of the root cap and can be collected by gentle agitation in water (reviewed in Hawes and Brigham, 1992). The cells of the root cap originate in the root cap meristem (Feldman, 1984). As the cells progress through the root cap, they undergo cytological and morphological changes associated with specialized functions including gravity sensing and mucilage secretion (Rougier, 1981). Upon reaching the outer edge of the root cap, the middle lamellae of the cells are degraded, and the cells separate from each other and from the root cap. Cell separation is the determinative developmental event that defines border cells (Hawes and Brigham, 1992), which remain transcriptionally active after separation (Brigham *et al.,* in press). The cells stay loosely adhered to each other and to the root cap within a water soluble mucilage, until removed by gentle agitation in water or mechanical abrasion (Fig. 1).

Substantial evidence is consistent with the hypothesis that border cells constitute a uniquely differentiated part of the root system that functions to modulate

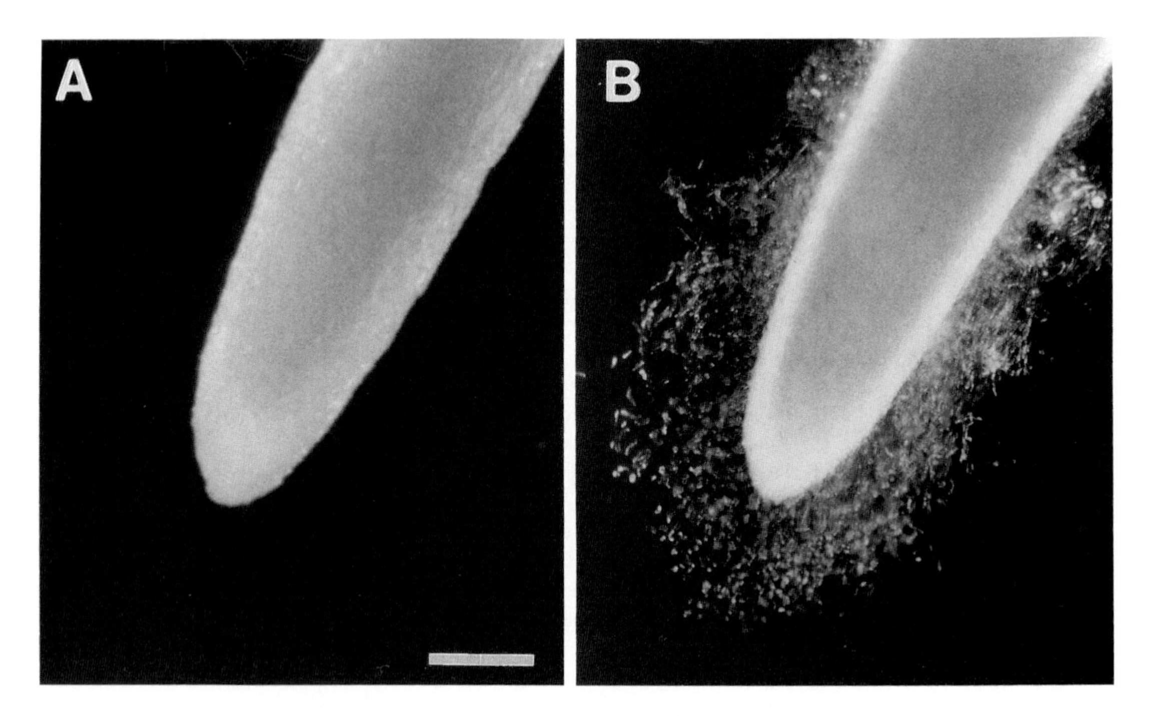

Fig. 1 Border cells from a single pea root. In the absence of water, border cells remain appressed to the tip, forming a smooth, slightly irregular surface (A). After immersion of the tip for 20 s in a 20-μl droplet of water, without agitation, masses of separated cells become dispersed in the medium surrounding the root tip (B) (Hawes and Pueppke, 1986). Bar, 0.5 mm.

microbial populations in the rhizosphere, and most work on border cells has been focused on such interactions (reviewed in Hawes, 1990; Hawes and Brigham, 1992). However, as populations of single, metabolically active cells with intact cell walls, they provide tools to study a wide range of biological questions. Few other plant "tissues" can be so easily distinguished and dissected without sophisticated equipment. Unlike protoplasts, border cells survive in a wide range of osmotic conditions, including distilled water, without lysis or observable cellular damage. In this paper, specific conditions for manipulation of pea root border cells are provided. In addition, diverse applications of root border cells in assays for research and teaching are summarized.

II. Materials

Seeds, bleach, absorbent paper, petri dishes, agar, forceps, and water are used.

III. Methods

A. Plant Material

We present information on the garden pea (*Pisum sativum* L.) because it provides a good source of root border cells. The seeds, which are available from numerous commercial sources, germinate and grow rapidly. The large roots, each of which yields up to 4000 border cells, can be manipulated without magnification. The methods described can be adapted to many other species (Hawes and Pueppke, 1986).

B. Preparation of the Seeds

Dry seeds are first immersed in 95% ethanol for 15 min, drained, and then immersed in full-strength commercial bleach (5.25% sodium hypochlorite) for 30 min; these steps are repeated. Peas are rinsed five times in sterile distilled water, with 5 min in each rinse to allow contaminated seeds to be detected by swelling, by floating, or by the presence of softened or nonuniform surfaces; only those seeds that appear as they did before processing are retained. Lack of contamination is verified after collection of border cells (below) by plating 50 μl of border cell suspension on a rich medium such as Luria Broth, and incubating overnight at 30°C.

Contamination varies among seed lots and genotypes. Wrinkled seeded varieties like Little Marvel generally harbor more contaminants than smooth seeded varieties like Alaska; with Little Marvel, it is not uncommon to discard 30 to 50% of the original batch of seeds. Seeds are not allowed to imbibe in water since this can contribute to the spread of any contaminants left after sterilization.

Imbibition in water containing antibiotics has proven unsuccessful with pea, because antibiotic concentrations sufficient to kill contaminants are deleterious to seedling development.

C. Germination and Growth

The sterilized seeds are placed on sterile germination paper, filter paper, or white paper towels (brown towels can contain chemicals that inhibit germination) overlaid on water solidified with 1.2% agar in petri plates or other dishes. Agar is optional, but if paper alone is used it is important to ensure throughout germination that the paper remains damp, but free of standing water. The seeds are incubated at 18 to 22°C in the dark. Under these conditions, the radicle will emerge in 3 to 4 days.

D. Border Cell Collection

Border cells are removed from the root tip by gentle agitation in liquid. Mass collection, by immersion of whole seedlings in a large volume of water, is not recommended since contamination by seedborne contaminants is almost impossible to avoid. Using destructive methods like agitation of excised root tips to release border cells results in substantial cell and tissue debris which can confound interpretation of assays. To exploit the unique potential for nondestructive cell isolation in this system, each seedling is lifted individually, and the *tip* (3 to 5 mm) of the intact root is immersed in a drop of water to initiate release of the border cells (Fig. 1). After 30 to 60 s, a pasteur pipette is used to dislodge the cells by taking up and releasing the liquid several times. For many experiments, the cells are now ready to use in assays.

E. Border Cell Number

In pea, a few border cells can be collected by the time the radicle has emerged to 5 to 6 mm in length; cell number increases until 3400 ± 600 cells are present when the root is 2.5 cm long. Border cells from a single pea root collected into a volume of 100 μl will yield a final cell concentration of approximately 3.4×10^4/ml. After border cells are removed, the synthesis of a new set of cells is initiated (Hawes and Lin, 1990).

The best method to determine cell number is to mix the suspension gently before counting the number in a small fraction of the sample, and then extrapolating to the entire volume. Approximate yields that can be expected from species in several families are provided in Table I.

In addition to single cells, border cell populations from some species include small, monolayer clusters of two or more cells. Clustering is genotype dependent. For instance, among 10 maize cultivars, 3 released border cells that were 100% separate from each other (unpublished results). In contrast, among border cell

Table I
Range of Border Cells per Root

Plant family	Cell number
Agavaceae	600–1500
Amaranthaceae	80–200
Brassicaceae[a]	0
Chenopodiaceae[a]	0
Cucurbitaceae	1000–3800
Gramineae	1800–2500
Leguminosae	2000–4000
Malvaceae	2900–3100
Pinaceae	3000–5500
Solanaceae	10–100
Umbelliferae	850–1000

[a] Border cells were not detected in seedlings of Arabidopsis, cabbage, bail, or in *Chenopodium amaranticolor* under conditions developed in our laboratory. We have not ruled out the possibility that border cell separation in these species occurs later in development or under different environmental conditions.

populations from each of 30 pea cultivars tested, up to 30% of the cells were in clusters of two or more cells. For many purposes this is not a problem because the cells are as easily visualized whether in clusters or not. However, if uniform single cells are required, the suspension can be filtered through a 20-μm mesh screen to remove clusters. Alternatively, genotypes without clumps can be selected by microscopic screening.

F. Washing Border Cells

If the cells need to be concentrated into a smaller volume, the suspension is transferred into a conical centrifuge tube and spun at 500–600 $\times$ *g* for 1 to 3 min to pellet the cells. If it is crucial that cells be free of extracellular exudates from the root, the procedure is repeated.

G. Viability of Border Cells

Viability can be detected by standard methods. In most cases, microscopic examination (100$\times$ magnification) of 30 or more cells to detect those with collapsed cytoplasm can give a good approximation of the viability of the population.

Cytoplasmic streaming can be detected at 400× magnification; visualization of the process is made easier if cells are stimulated by vortexing for a few seconds prior to observation. Alternatively, uptake of vital stains can be used to measure viability. Fluorescein diacetate is the most accurate and rapid (Hawes and Wheeler, 1982). A 2- to 3-μl droplet of 0.5% fluorescein diacetate in acetone is added to a clean glass slide and air-dried before a 20-μl droplet of border cells is added. Within 5 min, living cells can be distinguished from dead cells by staining which is detectable at 100× magnification with a microscope outfitted with an ultraviolet radiation source.

The viability of pooled border cell populations from most species we have tested is higher than 90% (Hawes and Pueppke, 1986). However, viability of border cells from a few species appears to be naturally low. For instance, border cells from tobacco may be only 60% viable when collected under the conditions described (Hawes and Pueppke, 1986), and the viability of sunflower border cells is less than 50% (unpublished). If cell viability is significantly lower than expected, border cells from individual seedlings should be compared to determine whether damage occurred to some seedlings during germination. Border cells may have been allowed to dry out by exposing the root to air, or there may be contaminating microorganisms that escaped sterilization. If contamination problems cannot be alleviated easily, procuring an alternative seed source is recommended if at all feasible.

H. Assay Conditions

The basic protocol for using border cells to study cellular interactions is to mix border cells with the agent of interest for defined periods, and then measure the response. Examples of the ways border cells have been exploited are outlined below, but the system can be adapted readily for other uses. Border cells require no osmoticum and can survive for nearly 24 h in distilled water, so assay media can be complex or simple. Long-term survival and growth can be obtained using tissue culture medium (Hawes and Pueppke, 1986), but the cells dedifferentiate in response to growth regulators, and developmental uniformity is sacrificed (Fig. 2).

IV. Special Considerations

A. Microbial Contamination

Sterilization protocols that result in aseptic populations of living border cells must be determined empirically for different species, genotypes, and seed lots. Many commercial seed lots, while guaranteed against certain pathogens and for a maximum germination ratio, contain bacterial and fungal contaminants that can spread to roots and cause problems in certain experiments. Different seed

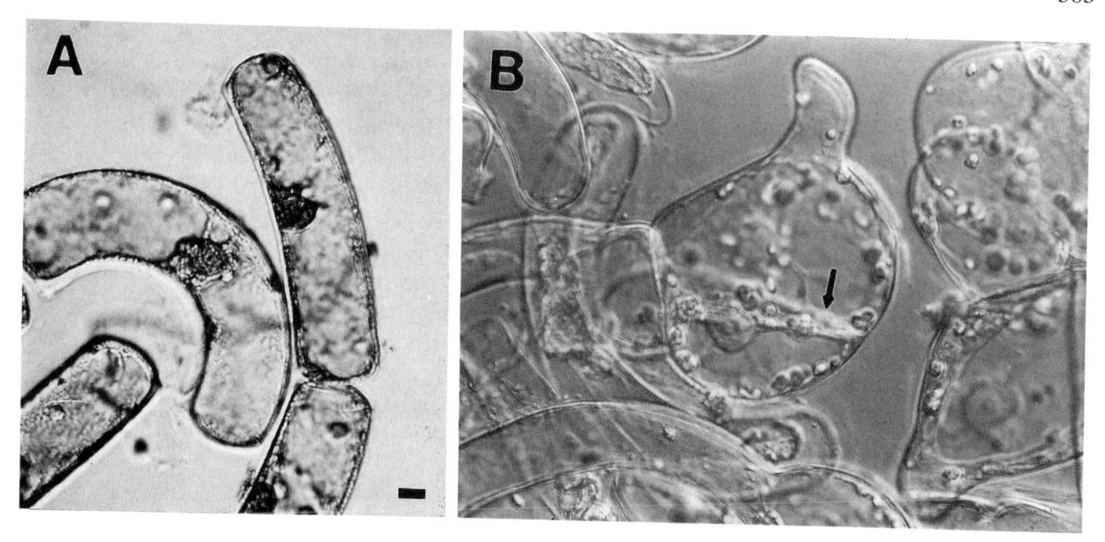

Fig. 2 Root border cell suspensions from pea (A) and alfalfa (B). In distilled water or other medium without plant hormones, border cells retain their characteristic elongated shape (A); the nucleus and other cell structures are distinguished easily. Within 3 days in tissue culture medium containing auxin and cytokinin (B), border cells dedifferentiate, undergo changes in morphology, and begin to divide (arrow) (Hawes and Pueppke, 1986; Hawes *et al.*, 1991). Bar, 4 μm.

lots from the same company may vary in the amount of seed contamination. In some cases, it can be very difficult to eliminate these microorganisms. Using the same protocol described for pea, for instance, up to 90% of common bean seeds (obtained from commercial sources) must be discarded to eliminate contamination, and even then microorganisms may be detected after germination.

B. Premature Loss of Border Cells

We emphasize that border cells naturally separate from the root by exposure to abrasion or water. It is therefore critical that the root tips not penetrate the agar when the seeds are germinated. Growth of the tip through agar dislodges border cells. Any contact with water, however brief, also releases the border cells from the root tip.

C. Availability of Border Cells

Some important experimental systems like *Arabidopsis thaliana* do not release border cells under the conditions developed for pea and other species, and others like tobacco release such small numbers that obtaining sufficient populations is too labor intensive to be practical for most purposes (Table I).

D. Specialization of Border Cells

It is important to remember that, unlike cell suspension cultures, border cells are not undifferentiated populations domesticated for growth in culture. Instead, they are uniquely differentiated to carry out functions whose specialized nature is reflected in patterns of protein synthesis and gene expression markedly distinct from those of other cell types (Brigham *et al.,* in press). Expression of transferred genes in border cells also can be distinct from that which occurs in other tissues. For instance, chimeric reporter genes expressed under the control of promoters of "stress" genes like chalcone synthase and phenylalanine ammonia lyase are expressed constitutively in the root tip, but not in border cells (Nicoll *et al.,* submitted). Although this does not preclude their utility in many types of experiments, their specialized nature needs to be considered in evaluating their suitability for addressing particular biological questions.

V. Applications of Border Cells in Teaching and Research

Border cells have been used primarily to study cellular interactions with plant-associated bacteria and fungi, but the system can be adapted to a wide range of physiological, biochemical, and molecular biological assays. They can be especially useful for classroom teaching because of the low cost and simplicity of obtaining required materials (Hawes, 1988). Examples of experiments using border cells are outlined below; detailed protocols are provided in the referenced publications. Most of the assays can be performed using border cells from a single plant. For instance, one pea or corn root provides enough cells for 40 replicate assays to detect binding or toxin sensitivity, and 10 replicate assays to detect chemotaxis.

A. Cell Structure

Border cells can be used to demonstrate principles of cell structure and biology. Cells are collected into liquid medium and examined microscopically. Even without staining, cytoplasmic streaming, plasmolysis, and the appearance of the nucleus and other cell structures can be observed using a simple teaching microscope (Fig. 2) (Hawes, 1983; Hawes and Wheeler, 1982). Border cells from some species can be distinguished from each other by their appearance, and these differences can be exploited in assays (unpublished results). For instance, cells from legumes generally are larger and more elongated than maize cells, whereas carrot border cells are smaller and more uniform in shape than those of either cereals or legumes. Cytoplasmic inclusions like starch granules are more obvious in pine and wheat border cells than in those of other species. In many genotypes of sorghum and sugarcane, pigmentation is expressed, resulting in pink or purple border cells.

B. Cell Wall Effects

Border cells provide a convenient method for detecting impact of the cell wall on cellular responses to microorganisms or their metabolites, because single cells with intact walls can be compared directly with isolated protoplasts from the same cell type (Hawes, 1983). Ease of border cell wall removal can vary with species. For instance, oat border cells yielded protoplasts only after a 2-h incubation in 5% commercial cell wall degrading enzymes (5% Cellulysin, w/v, Calbiochem-Behring) (Hawes, 1983). In contrast, cotton border cells released uniform populations of protoplasts after incubation for 30 to 60 min in 1% Cellulysin (unpublished results).

C. Chemotaxis, Attachment, and Agglutination

Border cells have been used to measure genotype- and cell-specific chemotaxis and binding of bacteria and fungi to host cells (Hawes *et al.*, 1988; Goldberg *et al.*, 1989), and to evaluate their relationship with susceptibility to infection (Hawes and Smith, 1989; reviewed in Hawes, 1990, Hawes and Brigham, 1992). A defined number of border cells is mixed with a suspension of the microorganism and incubated for minutes to hours before examining microscopically to detect chemotaxis, binding, and agglutination.

Border cells can be used as a substitute for red blood cells in lectin assays. Using standard procedures for hemagglutination assays, hapten-specific binding to border cell-specific surface molecules can be detected (Hawes and Palevitz, unpublished). For instance, wheat germ agglutinin (WGA) specifically reacts with *N*-acetylglucosamine. When WGA (0.5 mg/ml w/v) was mixed with a dispersed suspension of wheat border cells (600 cells) in wells of a microtiter plate, the cells agglutinated within minutes into a mass that could be detected without magnification. Among six tested hapten sugars, only the addition of *N*-acetylglucosamine reversed the agglutination and caused immediate dispersal of the cell clump.

D. A Source of Biologically Active Chemicals

Border cells provide a quantifiable source of biologically active chemicals that specifically support growth of certain microorganisms but not others (Goldberg *et al.*, 1989; Hawes and Pueppke, 1987). Border cell exudates also can induce sporulation of bacteria (Gochnauer *et al.*, 1990), and activate the expression of reporter genes under the regulatory control of nodulation and virulence promoters (Zhu *et al.*, submitted).

E. Toxin Assays

Plant resistance or susceptibility to fungal toxins determined by single genes can be detected using border cell assays (Hawes and Wheeler, 1982, 1984; Hawes,

1983). Toxins are added to border cell suspensions, and viability is measured using cytoplasmic streaming or vital stains. Border cells from plants that are susceptible to infection by the pathogens are killed within minutes of exposure to toxin, whereas border cells from resistant plants are insensitive (Hawes, 1983; Hawes and Wheeler, 1984).

F. Fungal Infection

Genotype-specific variation in ability of fungi to infect plant cells can be measured using populations of border cells (Goldberg *et al.,* 1989; Sherwood, 1987). In the absence of exogenous nutrients, border cells can synthesize putative defense structures called papilla in response to fungi (Sherwood, 1987). The ability to detect differences in responses among individual cells made it possible to demonstrate that border cells from resistant plants produced more papillae, and had fewer successful penetrations, than did cells from susceptible plants.

VI. Summary and Perspectives

Perhaps the most important feature of using border cells to study cellular interactions is that, unlike other plant cells, they can be collected nondestructively. No tissue is torn, excised, digested, or homogenized to procure these cell populations. Although the same can be said for cell suspension cultures, border cells provide several important advantages over cultured cells:

1. Unlike suspension cultures, which consist primarily of large, nonuniform cell clumps, border cells compose populations of separated cells and/or small monolayer clusters of cells. This allows uniform exposure of cells to assay conditions, and greatly facilitates light or scanning microscopic observation of cellular responses (Hawes and Wheeler, 1982; Sherwood, 1987).
2. Border cells are taken directly from the plant in their normal developmental state, and are not exposed to the drastic physiological and genetic disturbances inherent with cell suspensions grown in liquid culture for weeks, months, or years.
3. Within families that produce border cells, experiments are not confined to those species or genotypes that happen to grow well in culture or are available in cell suspension. Border cells to be used in assays can be collected from seedlings of any genotype of interest, including mutants or individual transgenic roots (Nicoll *et al.,* submitted).
4. No special equipment or facilities are required to obtain populations of border cells for assays, so protocols are accessible to anyone with a microscope and a supply of seeds.

References

Brigham, L. A., Woo, H-H., Nicoll, S. M., and Hawes, M. C. (1995). Differential expression of proteins and mRNA from border cells and root tips of *Pisum sativum* L., *Plant Physiol.* in press.

Feldman, L. J. (1984). The development and dynamics of the root cap meristem. *Am. J. Bot.* **71,** 1308–1314.

Gochnauer, M. B., Sealey, L. J., and McCully, M. E. (1990). Do detached root-cap cells influence bacteria associated with maize roots? *Plant Cell Envir.* **13,** 793–801.

Goldberg, N. P., Hawes, M. C., and Stanghellini, M. E. (1989). Specific attraction to and infection of cotton root cap cells by zoospores of *Pythium dissotocum. Can. J. Bot.* **67,** 1760–1767.

Hawes, M. C. (1983). Sensitivity of isolated oat root cap cells and protoplasts to victorin. *Physiol. Plant Pathol.* **22,** 65–76.

Hawes, M. C. (1988). The use of isolated root cap cells to teach cellular aspects of host-parasite recognition. *Plant Disease* **72,** 916–917.

Hawes, M. C. (1990). Living plant cells released from the root cap: A regulator of microbial populations in the rhizosphere? *Plant Soil* **129,** 19–27.

Hawes, M. C., and Brigham, L. A. (1992). Impact of root border cells on microbial populations in the rhizosphere. *Adv. Plant Pathol.* **8,** 119–148.

Hawes, M. C., and Lin, H. J. (1990). Correlation of pectolytic enzyme activity with the programmed release of cells from the root cap of *Pisum sativum. Plant Physiol.* **94,** 1855–1859.

Hawes, M. C., and Pueppke, S. G. (1986). Isolated peripheral root cap cells: Yield from different plants, and callus formation from single cells. *Am. J. Bot.* **73,** 1466–1473.

Hawes, M. C., and Pueppke, S. G. (1987). Correlation between binding of *Agrobacterium tumefaciens* by root cap cells and susceptibility of plants to crown gall. *Plant Cell Rep.* **6,** 287–290.

Hawes, M. C., and Smith, L. Y. (1989). Requirement for chemotaxis in pathogenicity of *Agrobacterium tumefaciens* on roots of soil-grown pea plants. *J. Bacteriol.* **171,** 5668–5671.

Hawes, M. C., Smith, L. Y., and Howarth, A. J. (1988). Selection and characterization of *Agrobacterium tumefaciens* mutants deficient in chemotaxis to root exudates. *Mol. Plant Microbe Interact.* **1,** 182–186.

Hawes, M. C., Smith, L. Y., and Stephenson, M. B. (1991). Root organogenesis from single cells released from the root cap of Medicago sp. *Plant Cell Tissue Organ Culture* **27,** 303–308.

Hawes, M. C., and Wheeler, H. (1982). Factors affecting victorin-induced root cap cell death: Temperature and plasmolysis. *Physiol. Plant Pathol.* **20,** 137–144.

Hawes, M. C., and Wheeler, H. (1984). Detection of effects of nuclear genes on susceptibility to *Helminthosposium maydis* race T by a root cap cell bioassay for HMT-toxin. *Physiol. Plant Pathol.* **24,** 163–168.

Nicoll, S. M., Brigham, L. A., Wen, F., and Hawes, M. C. (1995). Expression of transferred genes in transgenic hairy roots of *Pisum sativum.* Submitted for publication.

Rougier, M. (1981). Secretory activity of the root cap. *In* "Encyclopedia of Plant Physiology: Plant Carbohydrates" (W. Tanner and F. A. Loewus, eds.), Vol. II, pp. 542–574. Berlin: Springer-Verlag.

Sherwood, R. T. (1987). Papilla formation in corn root-cap cells and leaves inoculated with *Colletotrichum graminicola. Phytopathology* **77,** 930–934.

Zhu, Y., Pierson, L. S., and Hawes, M. C. (1995). Induction of microbial genes for pathogenesis and symbiosis by chemicals from root border cells, submitted for publication.

PART III

Signal Transduction and Information Transfer

CHAPTER 27

In Vivo Footprinting of Protein–DNA Interactions

Anna-Lisa Paul and Robert J. Ferl
Department of Horticultural Sciences
University of Florida
Gainesville, Florida 32611

I. Introduction

Gene regulation is a complex processing of the environmental and developmental signals that serve to initiate transcription. *In vivo,* there are a variety of components that influence gene regulation: the organization of the gene within the genome, the degree of packaging associated with the gene, the direct interactions of proteins with the gene (especially trans-acting factors), and finally, secondary structures of the DNA itself (e.g., Z-DNA, H-DNA). All of these components are interconnected to constitute the eukaryotic structure we define as chromatin. In experimental practice, the process of isolating intact chromatin

METHODS IN CELL BIOLOGY, VOL. 49

invariably compromises much of its structure, and few of these influences of gene expression can be effectively mimicked through *in vitro* analyses with linear, cloned segments of genes. Thus, a means of creating a "window" into a living cell to examine the relationship between chromatin structure and gene activation as it occurs *in vivo* is vital to a comprehensive understanding of transcriptional regulation.

In vivo footprinting with the chemical reagent dimethyl sulfate (DMS) creates such a window. DMS freely passes through the cell wall and membranes of living cells. It interacts with chromatin primarily by methylating DNA at the N-7 of guanines in the major groove (Maxam and Gilbert, 1980). The ability of DMS to access a particular nucleotide will be altered if there is a protein in close association with the DNA near that position. The modification (and subsequent cleavage) of the DNA will be either enhanced or repressed depending upon the microenvironment which that particular protein exerts on the DNA.

When compared to DMS reactions conducted with protein-free ("naked") genomic DNA *in vitro,* the sequencing patterns resulting from the variable DMS interactions *in vivo* are referred to as "footprints," as they indicate where a protein was directly associated with the DNA. The footprints are visualized with the process of genomic sequencing. Genomic sequencing, a technique developed by Church and Gilbert (1984) to characterize individual nucleotides within eukaryotic chromosomes, is essentially a means of producing a genomic DNA blot from a sequencing gel. Genomic sequencing is a powerful tool that facilitates the characterization of genomic DNA at nucleotide resolution *in vivo,* thus changes in chromatin structure, methylation, and protein interactions can be observed in their native state. The use of indirect end-labeling and strand specific probes allows each nucleotide within the region of interest to be examined without the limitation imposed by restriction enzymes and other endonucleases, and the positions of the reactive nucleotides can be identified precisely.

Genomic sequencing was first applied to plants for the investigation of cytosine methylation in maize (Nick *et al.,* 1986). To date, however, the primary use for genomic sequencing in plant research has been in footprinting the *in vivo* interactions of DNA binding factors in maize (Ferl and Nick, 1987; Paul and Ferl, 1991), *Arabidopsis* (Ferl and Laughner, 1989), parsley (Schulze-Lefert *et al.,* 1989), and wheat (Hammond-Kosack *et al.,* 1993).

II. Materials

A. General Considerations

Although the set-up for *in vivo* footprinting and conventional genomic sequencing involves some specialized equipment and reagents, the major considerations are more biological in nature.

The first biological consideration pertains to the DNA sequence of the gene or section of DNA to be analyzed. The sequence must be known for two reasons.

First, it is obviously necessary to know the sequence of the region of analysis to identify individual bases involved in a footprint. Second, the sequence can be used to choose a potential restriction site for indirect end-labeling and additional sites that can be used to design subclones that will facilitate the production of single-stranded probes for hybridization (see below). The restriction site to be used for indirect end-labeling (predicted from the plasmid sequence) should be confirmed as actually available in genomic DNA with a simple Southern. For example, if the clone used for the sequence analysis was derived from a library with a different allele than the system to be studied, it is possible that a polymorphism might exist at the site you have chosen. The second biological tool that is required is the set of subclones mentioned above. The subclones must be made in vectors capable of producing single-stranded probes homologous to the region of genomic DNA that abuts the restriction site chosen for indirect end-labeling. The scheme for indirect end-labeling and subclone design should be contrived such that the probes are sufficiently long for good hybridization signals, but short enough so that the restriction site used for indirect end-labeling is within 200 bases of the region of interest. Finally, a homogenous population of cells where the gene is uniformly expressed (such as cultured cell suspensions) will yield more easily interpreted results than a mixed population of cells (as in a plant organ such as roots or leaves).

B. Specific Materials, Equipment, and Recipes

The following list describes the system used in our lab. In most cases, a variety of adaptations can be applied to the same purpose, and are indicated where we are aware of them ourselves.

1. *Dimethyl sulfate (DMS):* The 99+% liquid from Aldrich Chemicals. DMS is stored at 4°C under argon. DMS is considered to be a potent carcinogen. The reactions involving the direct use of DMS should be carried out in a chemical fume hood while wearing gloves and protective clothing. Waste DMS can be broken down into harmless components with exposure to NaOH (see Methods).

2. *Piperidine:* The 99.5% liquid from Fisher Scientific. Piperidine is also stored at 4°C under argon.

3. *Sequencing apparatus:* Any standard apparatus will suffice (we have used set-ups from both IBI and BRL), as long as the gel can be cast 0.75 mm thick and is 30–40 cm long. The thickness is necessary to facilitate loading large amounts of genomic DNA (up to 20 μg) and to give the gel strength to hold up to the rigors of electroblotting.

4. *Electroblotting apparatus:* We use a 20-liter horizontal electrotransfer tank built by Polytech Products (95 Properzi Way, Somerville, MA 02143). It consists of a submersible sandwich that holds the gel and nylon membrane in close contact throughout the transfer. The sandwich is made from two 50 × 40-cm plastic grids that hold two pieces of Scotch-Brite cut to the same size. The membrane/gel

piece is supported between the Scotch-Brite, and the whole sandwich is held tightly together with large rubber bands. If necessary, a smaller electrotransfer apparatus can be employed by cutting the membrane/gel into manageable pieces, then reassembling the membrane pieces after hybridization. There are two problems with this approach; first, it takes a few times to empirically determine where your footprints will lie in respect to the pieces you have made (you do not want to piece it such that they fall near a cut) and second, the edges of genomic blots tend to accumulate more unwanted background hybridization than toward the center of the blot.

5. *Hybridization apparatus:* We use a water bath that contains rotating Lucite tubes (2-cm inner diameter), made by Polytech Products (see above). The membrane is wrapped around a plexiglass rod (1.2-cm diameter) that is about the same length as the width of the membrane and placed inside a Lucite tube with 5–10 ml of hybridization buffer. The incubator ovens set up to accommodate roller bottles also work well for genomic sequencing size blots.

6. *Vectors suitable for generating single stranded probes:* We have had success with DNA probes produced by synthesis from M13 clone templates, and RNA probes produced by *in vitro* transcription systems.

7. *Recipes for solutions:*

TESE:	50 m*M* Tris, pH 8, 50 m*M* NaCl, 400 μg/ml ethidium bromide, 2% *N*-lauroyl sarcosine
1 × TE:	10 m*M* Tris, pH 8, 1 m*M* EDTA
10 × TBE:	0.89 *M* Tris, pH 8, 0.89 *M* boric acid, 26 m*M* EDTA
Hybridization solution:	0.5 *M* Na phosphate, pH 7.2 (adjust pH with H_3PO_4), 7% SDS (ultra pure, BRL), 1% bovine serum albumin (Sigma A-4378), 1 m*M* EDTA
Wash solution:	40 m*M* Na phosphate, 1 m*M* EDTA, 33 m*M* NaCl, 0.1% SDS

III. Methods

A. DMS Treatments

The steps outlined below are geared for using a 50-ml cell suspension culture containing about 5 g of cell mass after filtration.

1. Add 100 μl of DMS to the culture flask and swirl the continuously for 1–2 min. This is usually sufficient to produce DMS modifications in a 1-kb section of DNA in intact cells, but this step should be optimized for each new system. For example, if none of the parent band from the restriction digest is left unreacted, reduce the incubation time or concentration of DMS in the reactions.

2. Recover the cells promptly after treatment by vacuum filtration, then wash by slowly pouring a liter of deionized water over the cells as they are being filtered. The media and wash containing residual DMS should be collected into

vacuum flask containing enough NaOH to keep the solution at a minimum of 0.3 *M* to inactivate the remnant DMS.

3. Freeze the filtered cells in liquid N_2 and store at −80°C.

B. Isolation and Genomic DNA

Although a variety of methods of DNA isolation can be applied to the cells recovered from the DMS treatments, we have been most successful recovering genomic DNA from CsCl gradients. Whatever method is chosen, it is important that the same method be used to isolate both the control DNA and the DNA from the *in vivo* DMS treatments. The following protocol is a compilation of several procedures (e.g. Shure *et al.*, 1983) and yields high-quality, genomic DNA.

1. Freeze the cells (ca. 5 g) in liquid N_2, then grind to a fine powder in a small electric coffee grinder that has been prechilled with a little liquid N_2 or dry ice.
2. Drop the powdered cells into a 50-ml screw-top centrifuge tube containing 5 ml of TESE buffer, then mix well with a glass rod to wet the powder evenly. Stir occasionally while the mixture comes to room temperature.
3. Centrifuge 10 min at 17,000 × *g* at 5°C. Transfer the supernatant to a clean, 50-ml screw-top centrifuge tube and add 1 g of CsCl per milliliter of supernatant.
4. Dissolve the CsCl by gently rocking the tube back and forth, then centrifuge as above, but at 20°C.
5. Transfer the supernatant to ultracentrifuge tubes (note: it is sometimes necessary to add extra ethidium bromide at this point when excessive amounts are lost to the pellet and pellicle; this is almost always necessary when isolating DNA from leaf tissue by this method). Recovering the genomic DNA after ultracentrifugation (we typically spin 5 ml samples in a Beckman VTi65 rotor for 4 h) at concentrations of at least 0.1 mg/ml will enable the remaining steps to be handled in one microfuge tube per sample.

C. Preparing the DNA for Genomic Sequencing

The subsequent steps apply to both the naked genomic DNA (protein free control) and the genomic DNA isolated from the DMS-treated cells. The control samples require a few extra steps to provide a reference pattern of *in vitro* DMS cleavages that occurs when no proteins are associated with the DNA.

1. Dilute 20 μg of both the *in vivo*-treated and the control DNA samples to a volume of 200 μl and digest with the restriction enzyme to facilitate indirect end-labeling.
2. After restriction, set the tubes containing the DNA from the *in vivo* DMS treatments aside. To the control DNA only, add 1 μl of DMS, vortex to dissolve the DMS, then incubate at room temperature for 1 min. Extract immediately with 200 μl of phenol:chloroform:isoamyl alcohol (25:24:1).

3. Once the *in vitro* DMS reactions have been stopped by the organic extraction, they can be set aside and the restricted DNAs from the *in vivo* DMS treatments can be extracted with phenol : chloroform : isoamyl alcohol. Then extract all samples with chloroform : isoamyl alcohol (24 : 1). Precipitate the DNA from the aqueous phase with 80 μl of 7.5 *M* ammonium acetate and 500 μl of 95% ethanol for at least 15 min on ice.

4. Resuspend the air-dried pellet in 50 μl of 10% piperidine (note: the piperidine should be diluted in water just prior to use). Place the samples in a rack designed to keep the lids of the microfuge tubes closed and incubate at 90°C for 20 min.

5. Place the tubes on ice for a minute while still in the rack, then open the tubes and carefully add 250 μl of water. Freeze the samples in liquid N_2 and drive off the liquid by lyophilizing (can use a speed-vac without heat). Resuspend the dry pellets in 50 μl of distilled water, and repeat the lyophilization.

6. Bring the samples up in 5 μl of sequencing dye made with deionized formamide, boil for 3 min, and load on a standard sequencing gel. We typically use 6% acrylamide, but this can be varied. As mentioned under Materials, the gel must be 0.75 mm thick.

7. After electrophoresis, dismantle the gel plates from the sequencing apparatus and separate the gel plates so that the gel remains on the bottom plate.

8. Cover the gel with a piece of plastic wrap and mark the outline of the area of the gel to be transferred on the plastic. Cut through the plastic wrap and the gel along the outline with a scalpel, carefully remove the plastic from the gel, and overlay the exposed gel surface with a dry piece of Whatman 3MM paper. Smooth the paper over the gel surface to ensure that the gel has adhered to the paper then lift the gel/paper piece off the plate. Lay the gel/paper piece with gel side facing up on one surface of the electrotransfer sandwich support.

9. Mark one side of a piece of nylon membrane slightly larger than the size of the gel piece to be transferred with an indelible pen, then prewet in 1 × TBE.

10. Wet the exposed surface of the gel with TBE; we find that having a squirt bottle filled with TBE is helpful. Carefully lay the wet nylon membrane on the gel with a rolling motion. Have the marked surface of the membrane be in contact with the sequencing gel. If any air bubbles are trapped between the gel and the membrane, they can be removed by repeating the rolling process.

11. Assemble the rest of the electrotransfer sandwich and electrotransfer the DNA from the gel to the membrane for 1.5–2 h at 1.8 A.

12. After transfer, peel the membrane away from the gel, and crosslink the DNA to the membrane by UV irradiation if required for the type of nylon membrane used. The marked surface of the membrane indicates the side of the membrane to be irradiated. Irradiation is done according to the manufacturer's specifications. We have used a 6-min exposure at 35-cm distance from a bank of four 15 W GE germicidal bulbs (No. GT15T8) in our own work.

D. Probes and Hybridization

It is critical that the probe be single-stranded and of a very high specific activity (10^9–10^{10} cpm/μg), since the individual bands to be visualized will be present in minute amounts in a typical reaction from a single copy gene. We generate probes by priming an M13 clone containing sequence homology just outside of the region of the gene to be examined that abuts the restriction site chosen for indirect end labeling.

1. The M13 clones are designed by cloning a restriction fragment of 100–200 bp that has one end in common with the restriction site chosen for the genomic digests into both M13mp18 and M13mp19. This strategy produces orientations of the probe that will be specific for either the top or the bottom strand.

2. The single-stranded M13 clone is first annealed to the standard 17mer sequencing primer, then a radiolabeled single strand is synthesized in a reaction mixture containing 4.5 μg of the annealed phage/primer (in a volume of 10 μl), 1 μl each dGAT, dATP, and dTTP (at 2 m*M*), 4 μl 10× Taq polymerase buffer, 1 μl Taq polymerase and 25 μl (250 μCi)[^{32}P]CTP. Incubate the reaction mixture at 65°C for 30 min.

3. The labeled single-stranded DNA is separated from the vector on a short, preparative sequencing gel, then the DNA is eluted from the acrylamide by cutting the gel slice containing the labeled DNA into small pieces (ca. 2 mm^2) and eluting in hybridization buffer for at least 1 h at 65°C. We typically pre-hybe the genomic blots for an hour at 65°C in the hybridization buffer. After prehybridization, discard the pre-hybe solution and add the eluted probe (gel pieces included).

E. Other Methods of Genomic Sequencing

There is an alternative to genomic sequencing through indirect end-labeling with a strand-specific probe. DMS modifications introduced *in vivo* can be analyzed through ligation-mediated PCR (LMPCR) (e.g., Mueller and Wold, 1989). Although it is possible that PCR reactions can introduce sequence artifacts, the utilization of polymerase enzymes with a higher degree of fidelity than Taq polymerase has reduced this possibility (Garrity and Wold, 1992). LMPCR has been applied to plant systems, and detailed protocols can be found in Sorenson (1992) and Hammond-Kosack *et al.* (1993).

IV. Typical Results and Discussion

The reactivity of DMS with a guanine residue of DNA can be influenced by the presence of a DNA binding protein. The degree of modification can be either enhanced or suppressed, depending upon the nature of the amino acid residue in contact with the particular guanine. A pattern of DMS reactivity introduced in genomic DNA *in vivo* that differs from the *in vitro* pattern in naked DNA indicates where proteins interact with the gene in the living cell. Thus, the *in vivo* interactions of regulatory proteins, such as *trans*-acting factors, and other aspects of chromatin structure can be evaluated as they occur in response to environmental and developmental changes in plant cells. An example of an *in vivo* footprint is shown in Fig. 1.

Our analyses of the *Adh* genes of maize and *Arabidopsis* provide good examples of the type of experiments that can be designed to identify *cis* elements and the accompanying *trans*-acting factors within the regulatory portion of a gene. The maize *Adh1* gene shows four points of DNA–protein interactions *in vivo*. Two of the footprints are present only when the gene is transcriptionally active, and contain sequence elements similar to known regulatory elements in other plants. The other two footprints are constitutively present, and coincide with the two *cis* anaerobic response elements known for maize *Adh1* (the ARE: Walker *et al.*, 1987). We monitored the footprints over an 8-h induction period and could correlate footprint acquisition with increasing mRNA levels, suggesting that the factors responsible for the inducible footprints played a role in the induction of the gene. *In vivo* experiments performed using leaves, which do not express

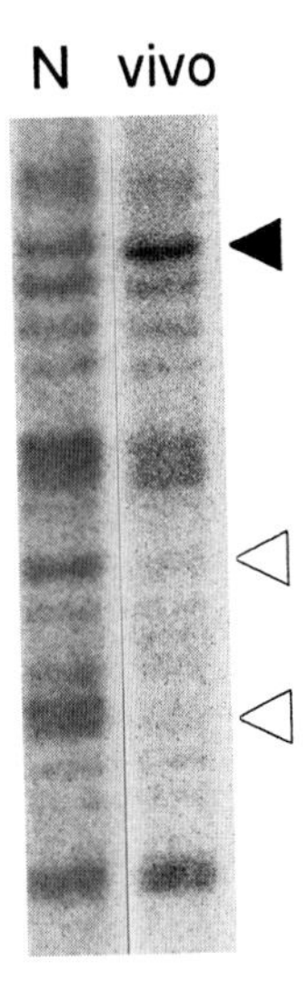

Fig. 1 An example of an *in vivo* footprint. A lane of naked (protein free) genomic DNA (N) treated with DMS *in vitro* is compared to a lane from an *in vivo* (vivo) DMS treatment of a maize cell suspension. The bands indicated by triangles show guanine residues where the reactivity with DMS has been either enhanced (solid triangle) or inhibited (open triangles) through the action of a protein associated with the DNA at that position *in vivo*.

Adh, showed no footprints. The value of using a combination of *in vivo* footprinting with *in vitro* DNA–protein analyses was demonstrated in a study of the G-box factors associated with the *Arabidopsis Adh* promoter. *In vivo* footprinting had identified a G-box at −210. A specific DNA binding protein was characterized, and footprinted *in vitro* and site-directed mutagenesis demonstrated that this G-box has a dramatic contribution to transient expression of *Adh.* However, the G-box in *Adh* is homologous to the G-Box in *RbcS* genes of *Arabidopsis* and other plants. Leaves contain an abundance of the G-box binding factor. Since the G-box factor is present in leaves, but *Adh* is not expressed, we were in a unique position to tell whether the presence of a DNA binding protein in a cell is necessarily correlated with its actual binding to a target sequence. *In vivo* footprinting of the *Adh* G-box site in leaves revealed that the site was not occupied, even though the factor was clearly present (McKendree *et al.,* 1990). In this case, influences other than the match between target site and binding protein dictate whether this factor is bound to its *Adh* site.

V. Conclusions and Perspectives

There are many potential methods for defining *cis*-elements and characterizing their respective *trans*-acting factors. Deletion/site-directed mutagenesis, followed by transgenic analysis is the favored method for functionally defining *cis*-elements, whereas *in vitro* DNA binding studies by DNase I footprinting or band-shift is the most popular method for searching for protein–DNA interactions. These are meritorious methods and have been used to great advantage in many systems. The value of *in vivo* DMS footprinting is based on the ability of DMS to interact with the genome in its natural state to reveal points of protein–DNA interactions of the native chromatin within living cells. These interactions precisely define *cis* elements as areas of protein contacts and provide a characteristic set of nucleotide interactions that serve as a unique signature of any given protein–DNA interaction. Thus DMS footprinting offers the ability to define *cis* elements, the ability to determine whether the elements are occupied by *trans*-acting factors during any given stress response, and the ability to distinguish even subtle differences in the binding signature that might indicate the occupancy of an element by a different factor.

References

Church, G. M., and Gilbert, W. (1984). Genomic sequencing. *Proc. Natl. Acad. Sci. U.S.A.* **81,** 1991–1995.

Ferl, R. J., and Laughner, B. (1989). *In vivo* detection of regulatory factor binding sites of *Arabidopsis thaliana Adh. Plant Mol. Biol.* **12,** 357–366.

Ferl, R. J., and Nick, H. N. (1987). *In vivo* detection of regulatory factor binding sites in the 5′ flanking region of maize *Adhl. J. Biol. Chem.* **262,** 7947–7950.

Garrity, P. A., and Wold, B. (1992). Effects of different polymerases in ligation-mediated PCR, enhanced genomic sequencing and *in vivo* footprinting. *Proc. Natl. Acad. Sci. U.S.A.* **89,** 1021–1025.

Hammond-Kosack, M. C. U., Holdsworth, M. J., and Bevan, M. W. (1993). *In vivo* footprinting of a low molecular weight glutenin gene (LMWG-1D1) in wheat endosperm. *EMBO J.* **12,** 545–554.

Maxam, A. M., and Gilbert, W. (1980). Sequencing end-labelled DNA with base-specific chemical cleavages. *Methods Enzymol.* **65,** 499–560.

McKendree, W. L., Paul, A.-L., DeLisle, A. J., and Ferl, R. J. (1990). *In vivo* and *in vitro* characterization of protein interactions with the dyad G-box of the *Arabidopsis Adh* gene. *Plant Cell.* **2,** 207–214.

Mueller, P. R., and Wold, B. (1989). *In vivo* footprinting of a muscle specific enhancer by ligation mediated PCR. *Science* **246,** 780–786.

Nick, H., Bowen, B., Ferl, R. J., and Gilbert, W. (1986). Detection of cytosine methylation in the maize alcohol dehydrogenase gene by genomic sequencing. *Nature* **319,** 243–246.

Paul, A.-L., and Ferl, R. J. (1991). *In vivo* footprinting reveals unique *cis* elements and different modes of hypoxic induction in maize *Adh1* and *Adh2*. *Plant Cell.* **3,** 159–168.

Schulze-Lefert, P., Dangl, J. L., Becker-André, M., Hahlbrock, K., and Schulz, W. (1989). Inducible *in vivo* DNA footprints define sequences necessary for UV light activation of the parsley chalcone synthase gene. *EMBO J.* **8,** 651–656.

Shure, M., Wessler, S., and Fedoroff, N. (1983). Molecular identification and isolation of the waxy locus in maize. *Cell* **35,** 225–233.

Sorenson, M. B. (1992). Methylation of B-hordein genes in the barley endosperm is inversely correlated with gene activity and affected by the regulatory gene Lys3. *Proc. Natl. Acad. Sci. U.S.A.* **89,** 4119–4123.

Walker, J. C., Howard, E. A., Dennis, E. S., and Peacock, W. J . (1987). DNA sequences required for anaerobic expression of the maize *alcohol dehydrogenase 1* gene. *Proc. Natl. Acad. Sci. U.S.A.* **84,** 6624–6628.

CHAPTER 28

The Interaction Trap: *In Vivo* Analysis of Protein–Protein Associations

Brenda W. Shirley[*] and Inhwan Hwang[†]

[*] Department of Biology
Virginia Polytechnic Institute and State University
Blacksburg, Virginia 24061-0406

[†] Plant Molecular Biology and Biotechnology Research Center
Gyeongsang National University
Chinju
Kyeong Nam 660-701, South Korea

I. Introduction

Protein–protein interactions contribute to the function and regulation of virtually every cellular process, from the level of transcription factor dimerization to the assembly of enzyme complexes and the cytoskeleton. A number of approaches to gene cloning on the basis of protein–protein interactions have been developed

METHODS IN CELL BIOLOGY, VOL. 49

in recent years. These include methods for screening phage expression libraries with labeled target proteins and the oligonucleotide-based cloning of genes encoding proteins identified by coimmunoprecipitation with proteins for which antibodies are available, by copurification with histidine-tagged target proteins, or by immunoblotting techniques such as Farwesterns. However, these methods are not applicable to all situations, particularly when the interactions between the proteins of interest are weak or short-lived.

At least some of these limitations have been overcome by an elegant and powerful new genetic method named the two-hybrid system, which was developed by Stan Fields and colleagues at SUNY-Stony Brook (Fields and Song, 1989; Chien *et al.*, 1991) and a variation of this method, named the interaction trap, developed in Roger Brent's laboratory at Harvard Medical School (Gyuris *et al.*, 1993; Zervos *et al.*, 1993). Both methods take advantage of the modular properties of transcription factors, which allow DNA-binding and transcriptional activating functions to be carried on separate peptides. As illustrated in Fig. 1, the assays are based on the requirement that two fusion proteins interact to activate the transcription of reporter genes in yeast. The fusion proteins are constructed on separate plasmid vectors; in one vector, DNA sequences encoding a known protein are inserted adjacent to sequences encoding DNA-binding and dimerization domains (from the yeast transcriptional activator protein, GAL4, or the bacterial repressor protein, LexA). A second vector contains sequences encoding another known protein or a cDNA library fused to sequences encoding a transcriptional activation domain (the GAL4 activation domain or a bacterial acid patch that activates transcription in yeast). Interaction between the fusion proteins creates a transcription factor which activates reporters that can be screened (β-galactosidase) or selected for (HIS3 or LEU2) in yeast.

One application of the two-hybrid system and interaction trap has been to identify interactions between the products of previously cloned genes, such as helix–loop–helix-containing transcription factors (Staudinger *et al.*, 1993) and RNA polymerase subunits (Lalo *et al.*, 1993). It has also proved possible to analyze deletion constructs in these assays; in at least some cases peptide fragments retain much of the interactive function of the parent protein. For example, deletion analyses were used to identify specific interaction domains required for dimerization of HIV Tat proteins and the yeast DNA recombination and repair

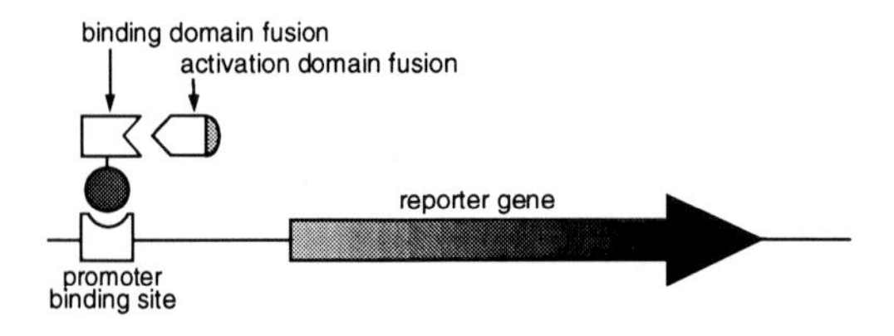

Fig. 1 Components of the two-hybrid system or interaction trap.

proteins RAD1 and RAD10 (Bardwell *et al.*, 1993; Bogerd *et al.*, 1993). The two-hybrid system and interaction trap can also be used to quantify these protein–protein interactions by using liquid culture β-galactosidase assays. In addition, it appears that these assays are not limited to the analysis of proteins that associate with each other in the nucleus; for example, the two-hybrid system has been used to characterize the multimerization of retroviral gag polyproteins that are normally found only outside the nucleus (Luban *et al.*, 1992), and we have preliminary results indicating that two cytosolic enzymes of the Arabidopsis flavonoid biosynthetic pathway specifically interact with each other in the interaction trap (M. K. Pelletier and B. W. Shirley, unpublished data).

The two-hybrid system and interaction trap have also been used successfully to screen expression libraries for clones whose products interact with a target protein, or "bait." Several novel proteins have been identified using this approach, including SAP1, part of a ternary complex that binds to the serum response element in c-*fos* (Dalton and Triesman, 1992), Mxi1, a protein that interacts with the mammalian transcription factor Max (Zervos *et al.*, 1993), and Cdi1, a protein that interacts with Cdc2 protein kinases (Gyuris *et al.*, 1993). These experiments also demonstrate the remarkable sensitivity of the method as the fleeting interactions of kinases and phosphatases with their substrates have been sufficient to identify specific target proteins in library screens (Yang *et al.*, 1992; Durfee *et al.*, 1993). An added feature of this approach is that partial cDNAs isolated in library screens can localize C-terminal DNA-binding domains, providing immediate information about specific regions involved in protein–protein interactions (Gyuris *et al.*, 1993).

The two-hybrid system and the interaction trap both rely on the ability of fusion proteins to activate transcription of reporter genes in yeast. Although different elements were used to construct these two systems, the underlying theory and experimental approach are the same. The interaction trap provides additional controls for confirming the targeting of fusion proteins to the yeast nucleus. This article describes several methods we have used in characterizing interactions between the products of previously cloned genes and to construct and screen an Arabidopsis library using the interaction trap.

II. Materials

Bacterial and yeast strains and cloning vectors: The following special materials are required to set up the interaction trap: yeast strains EGY40 (*MATα ura3- trp1- his3- leu2-*) and EGY48 (*MATα ura3- trp1- his3- LEU2::pLexAop6-LEU2*), *Escherichia coli* strain KC8 (*purF::Tn5 hsdR leuB600 trpC9830 lacD74 strA galK hisB436*), a "bait" vector, pL202pl or pEG202, the "prey" or library vector, pJG4-5, reporter plasmids, pJK101 (for repression assays) and pJK103 or pSH18-34 (for activation assays and library screening), and control plasmids, pSH17-4 (carrying a transcriptionally active LexA-GAL4 fusion) and pRFHM1 (carrying a transcriptionally inert LexA–Bicoid fusion). All of these strains and vectors can be obtained by contacting Roger Brent's laboratory (Department of Molecular Biology, Massachusetts General Hospital, Boston, MA 02114). Additional information on submitting requests for these materials is available through the MGH Department of Molecular Biology Gopher Server (currently under the Arabidopsis Research Companion).

III. Methods

This section describes in detail several of the methods that we have used to generate bait and prey fusions with previously cloned Arabidopsis sequences and for the construction of an Arabidopsis expression library in the prey vector. In addition, methods for testing baits in repression and activation assays, for high-efficiency transformation of plasmids into yeast, and for characterizing the positive clones isolated in library screens are described. Additional details for many of these methods can be found in the primary references cited in this section. The Brent laboratory has also posted valuable information on the MGH Department of Molecular Biology Gopher Server, including details of the construction of the yeast strains and plasmid vectors, sequences of fusion cloning sites in pEG202 and pJG4-5, a list of libraries that have been constructed by various groups, and technical information that is periodically updated.

A. Construction of Bait and Prey Fusions Using Cloned Genes

The first step in the use of the interaction trap for the analysis of interactions between two known proteins or for screening an expression library with a single known protein is to construct a bait fusion. To do this, sequences encoding a protein of interest are cloned in-frame behind (C-terminal to) sequences for LexA, which provide DNA binding and dimerization functions. Two bait vectors are available for the interaction trap: pL202pl, which contains unique *Eco*RI and *Sal*I cloning sites, and pEG202, which contains a multilinker that adds unique sites for *Nco*I, *Not*I, and *Xho*I between the *Eco*RI and *Sal*I sites in pL202pl. In the likely event that the protein of interest lacks convenient sites for in-frame cloning into these vectors, a straightforward approach is the use of oligonucleotides to prime PCR reactions from a cDNA clone or cDNA library. If a cDNA clone or appropriate library is not available, we routinely use reverse transcription-linked PCR (RT-PCR) to synthesize DNA fragments from mRNA of tissues that express the gene of interest at high levels. The products of these reactions span all or part of the coding region, are free of introns, provide a stop codon, and are flanked by appropriate restriction sites for in-frame fusion to LexA.

1. Oligonucleotide Primers

As an example, the oligonucleotide primers used to generate a full-length Arabidopsis chalcone synthase bait in pL202pl had the following sequences (lower case letters indicate the linkers, bold letters the start and stop codons):

sense primer: 5′ cgggaattc**ATG**GTGATGGCTGGTG 3′
antisense primer: 5′ ccggtcgac**TTA**GAGAGGAACGCTGT 3′

These primers introduced an *Eco*RI site upstream of the start codon and as *al*I site downstream of the stop codon. For analysis of interactions between two specific gene products, the same approach can be used to generate coding-region inserts for in-frame cloning into the *Eco*RI and *Xho*I sites in pJG4-5, which fuses the protein to the C-terminus of the B42 transcriptional activator (Ruden *et al.*, 1991). Furthermore, *Eco*RI–*Sal*I fragments from bait fusions and *Eco*RI–*Xho*I fragments from prey constructs can be cloned into the reciprocal vectors since *Sal*I and *Xho*I have complementary ends. These types of swapping experiments can provide useful controls for characterizing the interactions between specific proteins, for example, as described by Lalo *et al.* (1993).

2. RT–PCR Reactions (Belyavsky *et al.*, 1989)

a. To anneal the antisense primer to the RNA, mix 2 μM primer with 10 μg Arabidopsis total RNA in a final volume of 11 μl. Float the tube in a beaker containing 100 ml of water that has been heated to 80°C. Allow to cool slowly to room temperature.

b. To the tube add 1 μl RNaseIn (United States Biochemical Corp.), 1 μl dNTP mix (10 mM each of dATP, dCTP, dGTP, dTTP; prepared from 100 mM solutions, Pharmacia), 4 μl 5× reverse transcriptase buffer (supplied with the enzyme), 2 μl 100 mM EDTA (supplied with the enzyme) and 1 μl (200 units) MMLV reverse transcriptase (SuperScript reverse transcriptase, Gibco BRL). Incubate at 37°C for 30 min.

c. Electrophorese a 2-μl (1 μg RNA) aliquot on a 1% agarose/TBE minigel to confirm that the RNA was not degraded during this procedure.

d. Amplify 5 μl of the reverse transcription reaction in a 100-μl PCR solution containing 0.1 mg/ml RNase A, 1 μM sense primer, 1 μM antisense primer, 5 U Taq DNA polymerase (Cetus, Norwalk, CT) and 1× buffer [10 mM Tris–HCl, pH 8.3, 50 mM KCl, 1.5 mM $MgCl_2$, 0.001% (w/v) gelatin]. Cycle the reaction for 1 min at 94°C, 1 min at the estimated T_m of the primers (Suggs *et al.*, 1981), and 3 min at 72°C, 30 times.

e. Examine a 10-μl aliquot of the PCR reaction on a minigel.

Note: It may be advisable to sequence the RT-PCR products prior to construction of bait or prey fusion, as nucleotide changes have on occasion been introduced during the RT-PCR procedure (B. W. Shirley, unpublished observations). If this is to be done, the RT-PCR products are first cloned into an appropriate bacterial vector, such as pBluescript KS+, and then sequenced using standard methods. Alternatively, the RT-PCR products can be cloned directly into pL202pl or-pEG202 (and/or pJG4-5, if the interaction of two known gene products is to be analyzed), as described below, and several clones used as bait or prey in parallel experiments.

3. Cloning into Shuttle Vectors

Precipitate the remainder of the PCR reaction, wash with 80% ethanol and then digest with the appropriate restriction enzyme(s). At the same time digest vector DNA with the corresponding restriction enzyme(s) and treat with calf intestinal phosphatase. Electrophorese both reactions on a low-melting-point agarose/TAE gel. Excise the bands containing vector and insert DNA and ligate using T4 DNA ligase as described by Shea and Williamson (1991). In some cases the efficiency of these cloning experiments can be improved significantly by isolating the PCR products using the Magic PCR Preps DNA Purification System (Promega) prior to restriction endonuclease digestion.

B. Transformation of Bacterial and Yeast Strains

All of the plasmids used in the interaction trap are shuttle vectors that confer ampicillin resistance in *E. coli* and URA, TRP, or HIS prototrophy in the yeast strains EGY40 and EGY48. Ligations for the construction of the bait and prey fusions are initially screened in *E. coli;* we routinely use JM109 and standard transformation and miniprep methods for these experiments. The miniprep DNA can then transformed into yeast using a variety of methods. Electroporation methods, such as the method of Becker and Guarente (1991), are the least labor-intensive and provide sufficiently high-transformation efficiencies for the routine introduction of plasmid constructs into yeast. The reproducibly high-transformation efficiencies that are needed for library screening can be obtained using the method described in Section III,E. Transformed yeast colonies are selected on CM dropout glucose medium lacking the appropriate amino acid(s) (Ausubel *et al.,* 1989).

C. Testing the Bait

A basic requirement of the interaction assay is that the LexA fusion protein, the bait, cause little or no transcriptional activation of reporter genes in the absence of the activation fusion, the prey. In addition, the introduced sequences must not affect the ability of the LexA domain to bind the Co1E1 domains in the promoters of the reporter genes. The interaction trap provides two assays for testing the feasibility of using a particular fusion as a bait.

1. Activation Assay (to Demonstrate that the Product of the Fusion Construct Does Not, by Itself, Activate Transcription of the Reporter Genes)

a. Introduce the clone of interest into the cloning site of pL202pl or pEG202 so that it is in-frame with the LexA binding and dimerization domain as described in III,A.

b. Transform the construct into EGY48 cells containing the reporter plasmid JK103 (or the new, more sensitive pSH18-34), as described in III,B. Test for lack of β-galactosidase activity on Ura^-His^- CM dropout Gal/Raf/X–Gal plates (Ausubel *et al.*, 1989). Also, confirm that the yeast cells remain auxotrophic for leucine by comparing growth on $Ura^-His^-Leu^+$ and $Ura^-His^-Leu^-$ CM dropout Glu plates. Two control plasmids are available for comparison. The first plasmid, pSH17-4, encodes a LexA-GAL4 fusion protein that activates transcription in the absence of an activation domain fusion (via the GAL4 activation domain) and provides a good positive control for activation of the β-galactosidase and LEU2 reporter genes. The products of the pL202pl and pEG202 plasmids (LexA fused to the amino acids encoded by the polylinkers) do cause some transcriptional activation. Therefore a second control plasmid, pRFHM1, which carries a LexA–Bicoid fusion construct that does not by itself activate transcription of the reporter genes, is available as a negative control for the activation assay.

c. In experiments where the interaction of two known proteins is to be tested it is also critical to show that the prey fusion in pJG4-5 also does not activate transcription by itself, i.e., that the introduced sequences do not encode a fortuitous Co1E1 binding domain. To do this, transform the bait fusion into yeast cells containing JK103 and pRFHM1 and confirm that the *lac*Z and LEU2 genes are not expressed as described in part b, but using Ura^-Trp^- CM dropout Gal/Raf/X–Gal plates.

2. Repression Assay

The interaction trap provides a second assay to confirm that lack of transcriptional activation by the "bait" is not simply because the fusion protein is excluded from the nucleus or interferes with LexA binding to ColEI sites. This repression assay tests the ability of the fusion protein to block transcription of a β-galactosidase gene construct containing most of the GAL1 upstream activating sequence (UAS) and two LexA binding sites between the UAS and the transcription start site. Yeast cells carrying JK101 will produce high levels of β-galactosidase activity when grown on galactose medium. To test for the ability of the bait to bind to the LexA binding sites, transform the bait construct into EGY40 yeast cells containing the reporter plasmid JK101. Test for the loss of β-galactosidase activity compared to the parent strain on Ura^-His^- CM dropout Gal/Raf/X–Gal medium. Even a small reduction in β-galactosidase activity is indicative of a good candidate for a bait fusion, since a twofold decrease in β-galactosidase activity should correspond to 50% occupancy of operator sites; successful baits typically exhibit a 2- to 20-fold repression of *lac*Z gene transcription in this assay (Finley and Brent, MGH Gopher Server). The control plasmid pRFHM1 serves as a good positive control in the repression assay, reducing the activity of the β-galactosidase reporter construct on pJK101 by 2- to 5-fold. In the rare situation that the repression assay indicates that the bait may not be entering the nucleus, a derivative of pEG202 is available in which sequences encoding the SV40 T-antigen nuclear localization signal have been inserted between LexA and the polylinker.

D. Constructing an Interaction Library in the Prey Vector

Interaction libraries are constructed in pJG4-5, which contains the *E. coli* ampicillin resistance gene and a TRP1 marker for selection in yeast. We have constructed a library using total RNA extracted from 3-week-old Arabidopsis plants (Ausubel *et al.*, 1989), from which poly(A^+) RNA was purified using commercially available oligo(dT)–cellulose columns. A cDNA construction kit (Stratagene) was used to prepare double-stranded cDNA according to the manufacturer's protocol; this procedure introduces a *Xho*I site at one end of the resulting cDNA, providing for directional cloning into the library vector. Special adaptors were then attached to the cDNA products and to pJG4-5 to ensure high-efficiency ligation while preventing insert multimerization. The details of this method are provided below. Other methods for constructing libraries in pJG4-5 are described by Gyuris *et al.* (1993) and by Gyuris and Brent (MGH Gopher Server).

1. Preparation of Adaptors

Two slightly different adaptors are used to modify the cDNA products and pJG4-5 prior to ligation, as illustrated in Fig. 2. The blunt ends of the cDNA adaptors are attached to the products of second-strand synthesis, leaving *Eco*RI-compatible overhangs. The vector adaptors are ligated in the opposite orientation to pJG4-5 linearized with *Eco*RI, leaving single G overhangs. Because the adaptors lack 5′-phosphates, only one strand of the remaining adaptor is covalently attached during the ligation reaction. Adaptors are removed from one end of the cDNAs and pJG4-5 by digestion with *Xho*I. When heated at 65°C and purified by electrophoresis, both the cDNAs and the pJG4-5 are left with a *Xho*I overhang at one end and a long (12 nucleotide) compatible overhang at the other end, ensuring high-efficiency ligation of single inserts into the plasmid vector.

Oligonucleotides for adaptors:

Top-1 strand:	5′ AATTCGGATCCC 3′
Top-2 strand:	5′AATTCGGATCC 3′
Bottom strand:	5′ GGGATCCG 3′

The oligonucleotides should not be phosphorylated; 5′ hydroxyl groups are used to generate the long overhangs needed for efficient library construction as described above. For the cDNA adaptor, mix 2.5 μg each of the top-1 strand and bottom strand oligonucleotides in a total volume of 7 μl. For the plasmid vector adaptor, mix 10 μg each of the top-2 strand and bottom strand oligonucleotides in a total volume of 6 μl. Heat at 65°C for 10 min, then incubate at room temperature for 30 min.

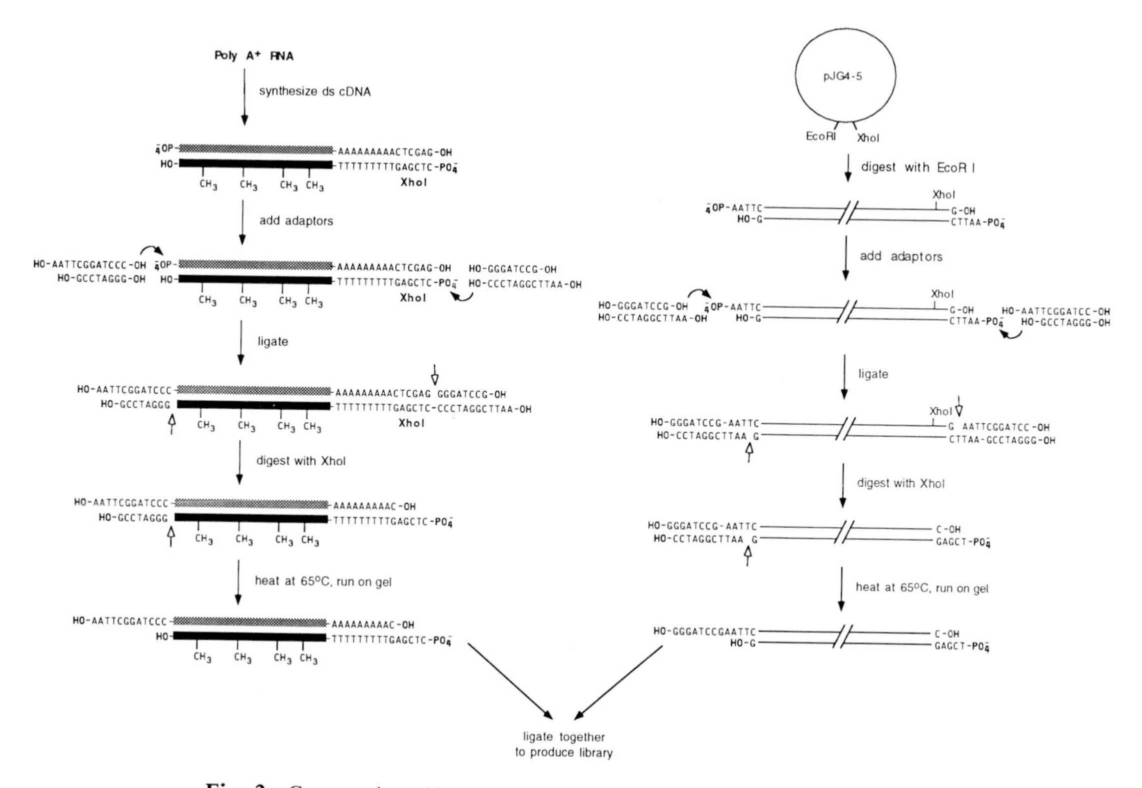

Fig. 2 Construction of interaction libraries using specialized adaptors. Open arrows indicate gaps remaining after ligation due to 5′-hydroxyl groups on the adapters. Details of the procedures are given in the text.

2. Preparation of cDNA for Ligation to Vector

a. Addition of Adaptor to cDNA

Add the adaptors prepared in step 1 (in 7 μl) to the cDNA (in 10μl). Set up the ligation reaction by adding 1 μl 10× T4 DNA ligase buffer, 1 μl 10 m*M* ATP, and 1 μl (7 weiss units) T4 DNA ligase. Incubate at 14°C overnight. Add 20 μl TE, then phenol/chloroform and chloroform extract. Precipitate the DNA with 2 vol 100% ethanol at −20°C overnight. Spin in a microcentrifuge at 4°C for 30 min. Remove supernatant, carefully add 100 μl cold 80% ethanol to the pellet, and spin at 4°C for 10 min. Remove the supernatant and dry the pellet in a SpeedVac. Dissolve the pellet in 20 μl dH_2O.

b. Digestion of Adaptor-cDNA

Digest the adaptor-cDNA with 50 units *Xho*I in a 50-μl reaction volume at 37°C for 5 h. Extract with an equal volume of phenol/chloroform, and then with chloroform. Ethanol precipitate and wash as in step 2. Dissolve the dried pellet in 20 μl dH_2O.

c. Size Selection and Purification

Prepare a 1% low-melting-point agarose/TAE minigel containing 20 ng/ml ethidium bromide. Heat the cDNA at 65°C for 10 min and load immediately on one side of the gel. Electrophorese at 80 V for 1 h. Excise the area of the gel containing the desired size range of cDNA (generally 0.5 to 3 kb) based on the size of marker bands. Remove an identical area from the adjacent part of the gel. Turn the agarose block containing the cDNA around and insert into this space so that the smallest cDNA fragments are at the top of the gel, facing the negative electrode. Seal the block into position with molten low-melting-point agarose. Electrophorese the gel exactly as before (80 V for 1 h). Cut the concentrated cDNA band from the gel and melt at 67°C for 10 min. Add 2 vol of dH_2O, mix well, and immediately add an equal volume of phenol. Vortex vigorously for 1 min, then spin in a microcentrifuge for 1 min to separate the two phases. Extract the aqueous phase once more with phenol. Reduce the volume of the aqueous phase to 50 μl by extraction with sec-butanol (Maniatis *et al.*, 1982). Reextract the aqueous phase (be careful to take the correct phase) with 200 μl of phenol and then with 100 μl chloroform. Ethanol precipitate the DNA as in step 2a. Dissolve the pellet in 10 μl dH_2O and estimate the concentration of cDNA by a spot test (Maniatis *et al.*, 1982).

3. Preparation of Vector DNA

a. Ligation of adaptor: Digest 10 μg of the plasmid vector pJG4-5 with 50 units *Eco*RI in a 100-μl reaction volume at 37°C for 5 h. Extract with phenol/chloroform and then with chloroform. Ethanol precipitate the cDNA and dissolve the pellet in 10 μl dH_2O. Ligate the vector adaptor from step 1 (in 6 μl) to the 10 μg of *Eco*RI-digested vector (in 10 μl) in a total volume of 20 μl as described in step 2, but using 2 μl (14 weiss units) T4 ligase. Incubate at 15°C overnight. Extract with an equal volume of phenol/chloroform, then with chloroform. Ethanol-precipitate the DNA overnight and wash as in step 2a. Dissolve the dried pellet in 20 μl dH_2O.

b. Digest the vector-adaptor with 50 units *Xho*I in a 100-μl reaction volume at 37°C for 5 h. Extract with an equal volume of phenol/chloroform and then with chloroform. Ethanol-precipitate and wash as in step 2a. Dissolve the pellet in 20 μl dH_2O. Heat the DNA at 65°C for 10 min, then immediately load on a 0.8% low-melting-point agarose/TAE minigel containing 20 ng/ml ethidium bromide. Electrophorese at 100 V for 1 h and cut out the linearized vector DNA. Phenol extract, reduce the volume with sec-butanol, reextract with phenol, ethanol-precipitate, and wash as in step 2c. Dissolve the pellet in 20 μl dH_2O.

4. Ligation of the Vector and cDNA

Mix 600 ng vector DNA and 100 ng cDNA in a 10-μl total volume. Heat at 67°C for 5 min, then incubate at room temperature for 30 min. Add 1.5 μl 10×

ligation buffer, 1.5 μl 10 m*M* ATP, 1.0 μl (7 weiss units) T4 DNA ligase. Incubate at 14°C overnight. Extract with an equal volume of phenol/chloroform, then with chloroform. Ethanol-precipitate and wash as in step 2a. Dissolve the pellet in 5 μl dH_2O.

5. Amplification of Library in *E. coli*

a. Determination of library titer: Electroporate bacterial cells with 0.1 ml of the ligated DNA from step 4. Plate various amounts to determine the number of colony forming units (cfu) per microliter of ligation product. We have found that *E. coli* strain MC1061 gives very good results in this procedure.

b. Amplification: Scale up the electroporation and spread 5×10^5 cfu per large bioassay plate (24.5 × 4.5 cm) containing LB and ampicillin at a concentration of 50 μg/ml. Incubate at 37°C overnight. Add 20 ml LB to each plate, swirl gently, then collect the cells. Add glycerol to a final concentration of 15% (v/v) for long-term storage and mix well. Snap-freeze and store at −80°C.

c. DNA extraction: Add 5 ml of the frozen culture to 2 liters LB medium containing 50 μg/ml ampicillin and incubate for 8 h. Prepare DNA using a standard alkaline–SDS lysis method, including purification through a CsCl gradient.

E. High-Efficiency Transformation into Yeast Cells

The plasmid cDNA library is transformed into yeast cells according to a modification of the methods of Gietz *et al.* (1992) and Hill *et al.* (1991) as follows:

1. Prepare yeast cells (EGY48/pJK103 or pSH18-34/pL202pl-bait) for transformation using lithium acetate as described in Gietz *et al.* (1992). Note: We have found that some bait proteins have a significant effect on the growth rate and the relationship between OD and cell density of liquid cultures. It is therefore essential to determine empirically the optimum cell density for transformation of EGY48 cells containing pL202pl constructs prior to transformation with pJG4-5 containing a cDNA library, as efficiencies of at least 10^5 cfu/μg DNA are required to obtain an adequate mRNA representation.
2. Add 0.3 ml of 40% PEG3300 in 1× LiAc/TE, pH 7.5, to 0.1-ml aliquots of cells. Mix well and incubate for 1 h at 30°C.
3. Add DMSO to approximately 10% (v/v) final concentration and mix well. Heat-shock at 42°C for 5 min.
4. Pellet the cells by spinning at 2000 rpm for 5 min at room temperature. Remove the supernatant and resuspend the cells in 1 ml of sterile dH_2O. Pellet the cells again by spinning at 2000 rpm for 5 min at room temperature.
5. Remove the supernatant and add 1 ml YPD. Incubate for 1 h at 30°C.
6. Spin down the cells at 2000 rpm for 5 min at room temperature and wash twice with sterile dH_2O. Resuspend the cells in 1 ml TE, pH 7.5.

7. Plate 0.1 ml cells onto $Ura^-His^-Trp^-$ CM dropout glucose plates.

8. Incubate at 30°C for 2 to 3 days.

9. For transformation of yeast cells with library DNA, scale-up the transformation 10-fold and plate the transformed cells on large bioassay plates (24.5 × 24.5 cm) containing $Ura^-His^-Trp^-$ CM dropout glucose medium. After 2 to 3 days of incubation at 30°C, add 20 ml sterile dH2O and collect the transformant in a sterile tube. Plate immediately on selective media as described in III,F. An alternative method that allows storage of aliquots of transformed yeast cells is described by Gyuris *et al.* (1993) and Finley and Brent (MGH Gopher Server).

F. Identifying Positive Clones in the Interaction Trap

In the interaction trap, the LEU2 reporter provides a selection system that allows large numbers of cDNA clones to be assayed simultaneously. The *lac*Z reporter provides a secondary screen to eliminate false positives by confirming that leucine prototrophy is conferred by an interaction between two fusion proteins and not by activation of the LEU2 promoter via cis- or trans-acting yeast mutations (Gyuris *et al.,* 1993; Hanes and Brent, MGH Gopher Server). The transformed yeast cells are screened as described by Zervos *et al.* (1993) and Gyuris *et al.* (1993):

1. Plate approximately 10^7 transformants on a single 24 × 24-cm $Ura^-His^-Trp^-Leu^-$ CM dropout Gal/Raf plate. Incubate at 30°C for 2 to 3 days (do not incubate too long).

2. Pick colonies and streak onto $Ura^-His^-Trp^-Leu^-$ CM dropout Gal/Raf/X–Gal medium and then onto $Ura^-His^-Trp^-Leu^-$ CM dropout Glu/X-Gal medium. Incubate at 30°C.

3. Select colonies that are blue on the galactose medium but not on glucose.

4. Repeat the color screen once more to confirm the galactose-dependent *lac*Z^+ phenotype of the colonies.

G. Recovering Library Plasmids from Yeast Cells

The library-derived plasmids that are positive in rescreening (III,F) can be separated from the other plasmids in the yeast cells by selecting for TRP1 gene expression in bacteria. Plasmid DNAs are first isolated from galactose-dependent *lac*Z^+ yeast colonies by the miniprep method of Hoffman and Winston (1987). The Trp^+ library-derived plasmids are separated from the other shuttle plasmids by electroporation into *E. coli* strain KC8 (carrying a TrpC mutation) and selecting transformants on Trp- ampicillin plates as described by Zervos *et al.* (1993) and Gyuris *et al.* (1993). Colonies from these plates are grown in LB broth containing 50 μg/ml ampicillin and plasmid DNAs are isolated using a standard bacterial miniprep procedure.

Finley and Brent (MGH Gopher Server) describe a useful method for identifying identical library plasmids if a large number of positive clones are isolated in the initial screen. After isolating yeast plasmids by the miniprep method, a PCR reaction is performed with primers complementary to the sequences adjacent to the cloning site in pJG4-5. The resulting products are digested with *Hae*III and/or *Alu*I and compared on a minigel.

H. Further Characterization of Putative Positive Clones

The putative positive clones are further tested by reintroduction into control yeast cells that contain a reporter construct and either pL202pl or the pL202pl-bait construct. The transformed cells are tested again for galactose-dependent expression of the LEU2 and ß-galactosidase genes.

1. Transform DNA from positive clones into yeast cells containing pL202pl and JK103. Also transform the DNA into control cells containing pL202pl-bait and JK103. Perform the color screen as described in III,3 using Ura$^-$His$^-$Trp$^-$Leu$^-$ CM dropout Gal/Raf/X–Gal medium and Ura$^-$His$^-$Trp$^-$Leu$^-$ CM dropout Glu/X-Gal medium to confirm the galactose-dependent *lac*Z$^+$ phenotype of the transformants.

2. Introduce the positive clones into yeast cells containing a more sensitive reporter construct such as pSH18-34. Repeat the color screen as in step 1.

IV. Critical Aspects of the Procedure

Several aspects of the interaction trap should be emphasized at this point. First, it is crucial that appropriate controls be performed at all steps of the procedure, beginning with characterization of bait fusions in the activation and repression assays and ending with experiments to confirm that activation of both the LEU2 and the *lacZ* reporter genes is absolutely dependent on the presence and expression of both the bait and the prey fusion proteins. Detailed discussions of the identification and elimination of potential false positives are available for the two-hybrid system (Bartel *et al.,* 1993) and the interaction trap (Gyuris *et al.,* 1993; Brent *et al.,* MGH Gopher Server). Perhaps the most critical aspect of the successful use of the interaction trap is that there be a strategy for confirming the significance of the interactions detected in these experiments, for example, using functional assays to characterize novel gene products (Hardy *et al.,* 1992; Gyuris *et al.,* 1993) or by illustrating specific and/or coordinate patterns of gene expression (Zervos *et al.,* 1993; Gyuris *et al.,* 1993). This issue should be carefully considered before initiating experiments involving the use of the interaction trap, particularly in efforts to isolate novel genes. Third, in at least some cases, the assays have been used to identify specific domains required for the interaction between two proteins. However, it is likely that at least some types of interactions will not be amenable to simple deletion analysis, for example, if the interactions are mediated by surface domains comprised of two or more domains in the linear protein sequence or if other parts of the protein are necessary for the correct conformational arrangement of the interaction domain. These possibilities must be taken into account in the design of experiments to characterize the interactions of specific proteins.

A number of reports of the use of the two-hybrid system or interaction trap to screen expression libraries have been published. The outcome of these experiments has ranged from the identification of a single true positive when the yeast repressor/activator protein 1 (RAP1) was used to screen a yeast library (Hardy *et al.*, 1992) to 412 LEU2+ colonies detected using Cdc2 to screen a HeLa library. Clearly, the sensitivity of the reporter genes, the characteristics of the bait (including its stability and affinity for promoter binding sites), the stability of the interactions between the bait and prey, the number of cDNAs screened, and the representation of potential target proteins in the library will all impact the final results obtained in individual experiments. Numerous options for altering these characteristics are becoming available, such as reporters of varying sensitivities, which may permit fine-tuning of experiments as the need arises. Furthermore, recent experiments using the human thyroid-hormone receptor to screen a HeLa library have led to the remarkable observation that the spectrum of positive clones obtained differs with the absence and presence of thyroid hormone (Lee *et al.*, 1995). Thus it also appears that, even in yeast cells, it may sometimes be possible and even necessary to manipulate the intracellular environment in which the interactions occur in order to identify specific target proteins. Finally, it should be noted that libraries constructed for the two-hybrid system and the interaction trap are not interchangeable. However, numerous libraries have already been generated for both systems, many of which are available for screening by other laboratories; an Arabidopsis two-hybrid library has recently been deposited with the Ohio State Arabidopsis Biological Resource Center.

V. Conclusions and Perspectives

The two-hybrid system has provided a powerful new approach to addressing innumerable questions of fundamental biological importance. This method has filled the long-standing need for a general and sensitive technique for detecting and characterizing interactions among the products of cDNAs and/or previously cloned genes. As with any important new technology, the method continues to be modified, adapted, and improved. The interaction trap introduced several improvements over the original two-hybrid system, including the selectable LEU2 reporter and the activation and repression assays for characterizing bait fusions. In addition, the relatively weak activation domain and the LexA DNA-binding domain provided technical advantages that increased the spectrum of fusion proteins that could be detected and minimized the number of false positives (Gyuris *et al.,* 1993). More sensitive reporter genes have now been developed for the interaction trap as well as a vector that allows fusion of the bait to the amino terminus of LexA (Brent *et al.,* MGH Gopher Server). The two-hybrid system has also recently been adapted to include a histidine selection scheme (Durfee *et al.,* 1993) and has inspired the development of vectors and reporter genes that can be used to analyze the interactions of fusion proteins in mammalian cells, thus taking into account the effects of endogenous regulatory proteins and specific physiological changes (Vasavada *et al.,* 1991; Chakraborty *et al.,* 1992). These innovations, together with novel applications of the original assays, such as screening libraries in the presence or absence of accessory molecules (Lee *et al.,* 1995), promise that the utility of these assays will continue to increase and that we will see its use expand to address questions in all areas of molecular cell biology.

Acknowledgments

We are sincerely thankful to the many members of the Brent laboratory, particularly Russ Finley, Erica Golemis, Jenö Gyuris, and Steve Hanes, for their generosity in providing technical advice and sharing materials and strains prior to publication. We also thank Jenö Gyuris, Erica Golemis, Helen Chertkov, and Roger Brent as well as Jae Lee and David Moore for sharing their unpublished results. Finally, we thank Howard Goodman for the productive and enjoyable years we spend as postdoctoral fellows in his laboratory at Massachusetts General Hospital.

References

Ausubel, F. M., Brent, R., Kingston, R. E., Moore, D. D., Seidman, J. G., Smith, J. A., and Struhl, K. (1989). "Current Protocols in Molecular Biology," New York: Green Publishing Associates/Wiley–Interscience.

Bardwell, A. J., Bardwell, L., Johnson, D. K., and Friedberg, E. C. (1993). Yeast DNA recombination and repair proteins Rad1 and Rad10 constitute a complex in vivo mediated by localized hydrophobic domains. *Mol. Microbiol.* **8,** 1177–1188.

Bartel, P., Chien, G., Sternglanz, R., and Fields, S. (1993). Elimination of false positives that arise in using the two-hybrid system. *BioTechniques* **14,** 920–924.

Becker, D. M., and Guarente, L. (1991). High-efficiency transformation of yeast by electroporation. *Methods Enzymol.* **194,** 182–187.

Belyavsky, A., Vinogradova, T., and Rajewsky, K. (1989). PCR-based cDNA library construction: General cDNA libraries at the level of a few cells. *Nucleic Acids Res.* **17,** 2919–2932.

Bogerd, H. P., Fridell, R. A., Blair, W. S., and Cullen, B. R. (1993). Genetic evidence that the Tat proteins of human immunodeficiency virus types 1 and 2 can multimerize in the eukaryotic cell nucleus. *J. Virol.* **67,** 5030–5034.

Chakraborty, T., Martin, J. F., and Olson, E. N. (1992). Analysis of the oligomerization of myogenin and E2A products in vivo using a two-hybrid assay system. *J. Biol. Chem.* **267,** 17498–17501.

Chien, C. T., Bartel, P. L., Sternglanz, R., and Fields, S. (1991). The two-hybrid system: A method to identify and clone genes for proteins that interact with a protein of interest. *Proc. Natl. Acad. Sci. U.S.A.* **88,** 9578–9582.

Dalton, S., and Treisman, R. (1992). Characterization of SAP1, a protein recruited by serum response factor to the c-fos serum response element. *Cell* **68,** 597–612.

Durfee, T., Becherer, K., Chen, P.-L., Yeh, S.-H., Yang, Y., Kilburen, A. E., Lee, W.-H., and Elledge, S. J. (1993). The retinoblastoma protein associates with the protein phosphatase type 1 catalytic subunit. *Genes Dev.* **7,** 555–569.

Fields, S., and Song, O. (1989). A novel genetic system to detect protein-protein interactions. *Nature* **340,** 245–246.

Gietz, D., St. Jean, A., Woods, R. A., and Schiestl, R. H. (1992). Improved method for high efficiency transformation of intact yeast. *Nucleic Acids Res.* **20,** 1425.

Gyuris, J., Golemis, E., Chertkov, H., and Brent, R. (1993). Cdil, a human G1 and S phase protein phosphatase that associates with cdk2. *Cell* **75,** 791–803.

Hardy, C. F. J., Sussel, L., and Shore, D. (1992). A RAP1-interacting protein involved in transcriptional silencing and telomere length regulation. *Genes Dev.* **6,** 801–814.

Hill, J., Donald, K. A., Griffiths, D. E., and Donald, G. (1991). DMSO-enhanced whole cell yeast transformation. *Nucleic Acids Res.* **19,** 5791.

Hoffman, C. S., and Winston, F. (1987). A ten-minute DNA preparation from yeast efficiently releases autonomous plasmids for transformation of Escherichia coli. *Gene* **57,** 267–272.

Lalo, D., Carles, C., Sentenac, A., and Thuriaux, P. (1993). Interactions between three common subunits of yeast RNA polymerases I and III. *Proc. Natl. Acad. Sci. U.S.A.* **90,** 5524–5528.

Lee, J. W., Ryan, F., Swaffield, J. C., Johnston, S. A., and Moore, D. D. (1995). Interaction of thyroid-hormone receptor with a conserved transcriptional mediator. *Nature* **374,** 91–94.

Luban, J., Alin, K. B., Bossolt, K. L., Humaran, T., and Goff, S. P. (1992). Genetic assay for multimerization of retroviral gag polyproteins. *J. Virol.* **66,** 5157–5160.

Maniatis, T., Fritsch, E. F., and Sambrook, J. (1982). "Molecular Cloning: A Laboratory Manual," Cold Spring Harbor, NY: Cold Spring Harbor Laboratory Press.

Ruden, D. M., Ma, J., Li, Y., Wood, K., and Ptashne, M. (1991). Generating yeast transcriptional activators containing no yeast protein sequences. *Nature* **350,** 250–252.

Shea, C., and Williamson, J. C. (1991). Rapid and inexpensive protocol for generating >95% recombinants in subcloning experiments. *BioTechniques* **10,** 176–177.

Staudinger, J., Perry, M., Elledge, S. J., and Olson, E. N. (1993). Interactions among vertebrate helix-loop-helix proteins in yeast using the two-hybrid system. *J. Biol. Chem.* **268,** 4608–4611.

Suggs, S. V., Hirose, T., Miyake, T., Kawashima, E. H., Johnson, M. J., Itakura, K., and Wallace, R. B. (1981). Use of synthetic oligodeoxyribonucleotides for the isolation of specific cloned DNA sequences. *ICN-UCLA Symp. Mol. Cell. Biol.* **23,** 682–693.

Vasavada, H. A., Ganguly, S., Germino, F. J., Wang, Z. X., and Weissman, S. M. (1991). A contingent replication assay for the detection of protein-protein interactions in animal cells. *Proc. Natl. Acad. Sci. U.S.A.* **88,** 10686–10690.

Yang, X., Hubbard, E. J. A., and Carlson, M. (1992). A protein kinase substrate identified by the two-hybrid system. *Science* **257,** 680–682.

Zervos, A. S., Gyuris, J., and Brent, R. (1993). Mxil, a protein that specifically interacts with Max to bind Myc-Max recognition sites. *Cell* **72,** 223–232.

CHAPTER 29

Cloning Plant Genes by Complementation of Yeast Mutants

Christophe d'Enfert,[*] Michèle Minet,[†] and François Lacroute[†]

[*] Unité de Mycologie
Institut Pasteur
28 rue du docteur Roux
75724 Paris Cédex 15, France

[†] Centre de Génétique Moléculaire
CNRS
91190 Gif sur Yvette, France

I. Introduction

A better understanding of the cell biology of plants will require the characterization of a variety of the basic functions of the cell. It is now clear that a wide array of these functions are shared by most eukaryotic cells, ranging from lower eukaryotes like yeasts to highly differentiated organisms, and involves proteins with similar activities. Although proteins with similar functions from individuals of different taxa may show a high level of amino acid sequence conservation, some show significant divergence (Botstein and Fink, 1988). This situation may preclude the identification of plant genes encoding functional homologues of

METHODS IN CELL BIOLOGY, VOL. 49

proteins from other eukaryotic origins by conventional techniques based on DNA similarity, e.g., Southern hybridization or amplification of conserved sequences by the polymerase chain reaction.

The genetic flexibility of lower eukaryotes like the yeasts *Saccharomyces cerevisiae* and *Schizosaccharomyces pombe* has allowed the identification of a collection of recessive mutations affecting different aspects of their cell biology (Mortimer *et al.*, 1989; Nasim *et al.*, 1989). Most of these mutations confer a specific phenotype to the mutant strain which differentiates it from the wild-type strain. This facilitates the cloning of the wild-type allele by direct complementation of the mutant phenotype after transformation with a genomic library. Assuming that a similar function is present in the eukaryotic organism of interest, expression of its structural gene (as a cDNA) under the control of a yeast promoter may correct the defect of the yeast mutant. The utility of this approach was demonstrated in several instances by using cloned cDNAs from various eukaryotes to complement the mutant phenotype of appropriate yeast mutants (Katakoa *et al.*, 1985; DeFeo-Jones *et al.*, 1985). These results paved the way for the identification of functional homologues of yeast proteins by direct complementation of mutations using cDNA libraries constructed in yeast expression vectors. Since the pioneering experiments of Lee and Nurse (1987), who cloned a human homologue of the $p34^{cdc2}$ kinase by complementation of a *S. pombe cdc2* mutant, this approach has been extensively used to identify mammalian (mostly human) and insect genes involved in different aspects of cell biology such as cell cycle control, transcription control, metabolic pathways, carbohydrate metabolism, and signal transduction (Lew *et al.*, 1991; Koff *et al.*, 1991; Becker *et al.*, 1991; Minet and Lacroute, 1990; Thon *et al.*, 1993; Colicelli *et al.*, 1989).

This mutant complementation strategy, although successful with other eukaryotic organisms, had not been applied for the cloning of plant genes until recently. Minet *et al.* (1992) and Ellerstrom *et al.* (1992) demonstrated that the method could be used to complement auxotrophic mutants of *S. cerevisiae* with genes from *Arabidopsis thaliana* and rape. Since then, we and others have identified *A. thaliana* genes that encode functional homologues of *S. cerevisiae* proteins involved in protein secretion, ion transport, and cell cycle control (d'Enfert *et al.*, 1992; Sentenac *et al.*, 1992; Anderson *et al.*, 1992; F. Lacroute, unpublished results). Identification of complementing activity is facilitated by the ready availability of numerous *S. cerevisiae* mutants and of *A. thaliana* cDNA expression libraries [for example, the cDNA expression library described by Minet *et al.* (1992) is available from the American Type Culture Collection (Rockville, Maryland)]. It can be completed within a month, although, as discussed below, it may present several pitfalls. Here we present the procedure used by Minet *et al.* (1992) to construct an *A. thaliana* cDNA expression library and transformation strategies that can be used to introduce the cDNA library into mutant *S. cerevisiae* strains and to recover complementing plasmids.

II. Materials and Methods

A. cDNA Library Construction

1. Overview of the Experiment

To construct the cDNA library, we use pFL61, a multicopy *S. cerevisiae* expression vector (Fig. 1) described by Minet *et al.* (1992). pFL61 allows the cloning of cDNAs at two incompatible *Bst*XI sites (Aruffo and Seed, 1987), thus avoiding its recircularization during the ligation step. cDNAs are cloned downstream of the *S. cerevisiae* phosphoglycerate kinase (*PGK1*) promoter and upstream of the *PGK1* terminator. Cloning in this locus, together with the high copy number of the vector, allows high-level constitutive expression in *S. cerevisiae* when the cDNA is cloned in the proper orientation. However, many inserts in the opposite orientation to the *PGK1* promotor can complement yeast mutants, suggesting

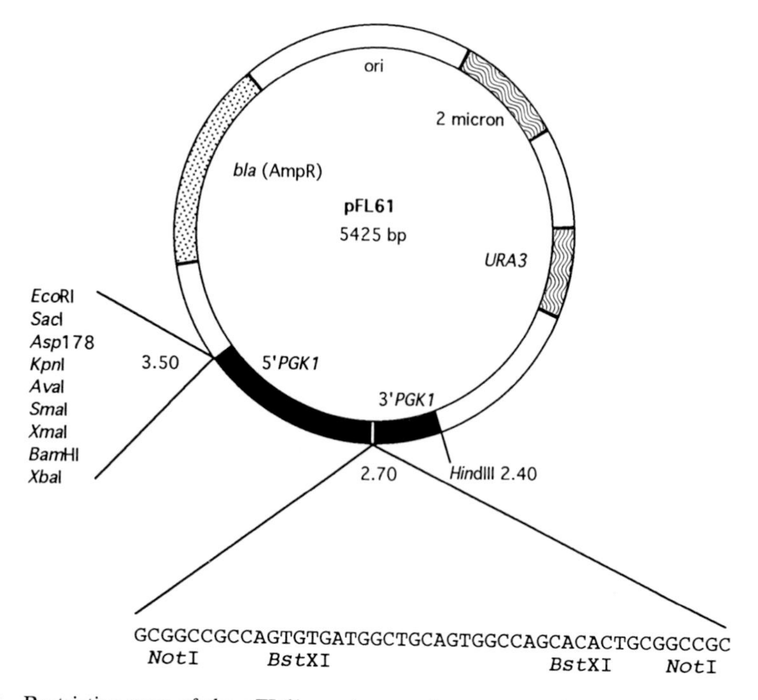

Fig. 1 Restriction map of the pFL61 yeast expression vector and sequence of the *Not*I–*Bst*XI linker (Minet *et al.*, 1992). The restriction sites indicated are one-cut sites. The promoter (5′*PGK1*) and terminator (3′*PGK1*) regions of the *S. cerevisiae PGK1* gene are indicated by black boxes. The *S. cerevisiae* 2-μ replication origin and the *URA3* gene for complementation of *S. cerevisiae ura3* mutations are indicated by gray boxes. The *bla* gene for selection of the plasmid in *E. coli* is indicated by a stippled box.

the presence of a promotor activity in the terminator region (our unpublished results). Furthermore, cloned cDNAs become flanked by *Not*I sites, facilitating their recovery for further analysis. The *URA3* gene is used as a selectable marker for transformation of *S. cerevisiae.*

The procedure that is outlined below describes the construction of a cDNA library derived from young seedlings (stage two leaves) of *A. thaliana.* After preparation of the poly(A)$^+$RNAs, cDNAs are synthesized and modified by the addition of *Bst*XI adaptors at their ends. The cDNAs are then gel-purified and ligated into *Bst*XI-restricted pFL61. The cDNA library is introduced into and propagated in *Escherichia coli.* Classical molecular biology procedures are according to Sambrook *et al.* (1989).

2. Materials

Materials are stored at room temperature unless otherwise stated. Germination medium contains the salt mixture described by Murashige and Skoog (1962), 1% sucrose, 100 mg l^{-1} inositol, 1 mg l^{-1} thiamine, 0.5 mg l^{-1} pyridoxine, 0.5 mg l^{-1} nicotinic acid, 8 g l^{-1} agar.

Liquid nitrogen

TES: Tris–HCl 10 m*M*, pH 8, EDTA 0.5 *M*, 5% SDS (sodium dodecyl sulfate); 4°C

Phenol equilibrated with Tris–HCl, pH 8; 4°C

Phenol–chloroform (1:1) made with Tris–HCl, pH 8, equilibrated phenol; 4°C

4 *M* NaCl

Ethanol; −20°C

DEPC-treated water: 0.1% diethyl pyrocarbonate (DEPC) in distilled water; allow to stand at 37°C overnight and autoclave

Oligo(dT)–cellulose type 7 (Pharmacia, 27-5543-01); 4°C

Solutions for oligo(dT) chromatography:

- 0.1 *M* NaOH
- DEPC-treated 10 *M* LiCl
- 0.5 *M* LiCl, 10 m*M* Tris–HCl, pH 7.5, 1 m*M* EDTA, 0.1% SDS
- 0.15 *M* LiCl, 10 m*M* Tris–HCl, pH 7.5, 1 m*M* EDTA, 0.1% SDS
- 2 m*M* EDTA, 0.1% SDS

cDNA Synthesis System Plus (Amersham, RPN1256); −20°C

*Bst*XI adaptors: B1: 5′-CTAAATTACTCACA-3′; −20°C
B2: 3′-GATTTAATGA-5′

1 m*M* ATP; −20°C

T4 Polynucleotide kinase (Biolabs, No. 201S) and accompanying 10× buffer; −20°C

T4 DNA Ligase, 2000 U/μl (Biolabs, No. 202CS) and accompanying 10× buffer; −20°C

pFL61 (Minet *et al.*, 1992)

*Bst*XI (Biolabs, No. 113S); −20°C

SeaPlaque GTG Agarose (FMC Bioproducts)

TBE: 89 m*M* Tris, 89 m*M* boric acid, 2 m*M* EDTA

20 m*M* Tris–HCl, pH 8, 1 m*M* EDTA

20 m*M* Tris–HCl, pH 8, 10 m*M* $MgCl_2$

LB: 1% NaCl, 1% Bacto-Tryptone (Difco), 0.5% Yeast Extract (Difco); adjust to pH 7.5 with NaOH, and autoclave for 10 min at 120°C

Electroporation device: Bio-Rad Gene Pulser Apparatus (Bio-Rad165-2076) and Pulse Controller (Bio-Rad 165-2098) equipped with Gene Pulser/*E. coli* Pulser cuvettes, 0.2-cm electrode gap (Bio-Rad 165-2088)

SOC: 2% Bacto-Tryptone (Difco), 0.5% yeast extract (Difco), 10 m*M* NaCl, 2.5 m*M* KCl, 10 m*M* $MgCl_2$, 10 m*M* $MgSO_4$, 20 m*M* glucose. Adjust at pH 7.5 with NaOH and autoclave for 10 min at 120°C

10 mg/ml ampicillin; aliquot and store at −20°C

*Not*I (Biolabs, No. 189S); −20°C

100% Glycerol

3. Procedure

a. Preparation of poly(A)$^+$ RNAs from A. thaliana Seedlings

Surface-sterilized seeds of *A. thaliana* (L) Heynh (Landsberg *erecta* ecotype) are germinated on germination medium and subjected to a 16-h light photoperiod until they reach the two-leaf stage. Young seedlings (ca. 200 plantlets) are then collected with their roots, frozen in liquid nitrogen, and ground in a mortar with 10 ml of frozen TES. Once thawed, the crude extract is extracted twice with 1 vol of phenol–chloroform. The resulting aqueous phase is brought to 0.4 *M* NaCl and extracted twice with phenol–chloroform. Nucleic acids contained in the aqueous phase are then precipitated by the addition of 2 vol of ice-cold ethanol and collected by a 10-min centrifugation at 10,000 × *g*. The nucleic acid pellet is washed with 75% ice-cold ethanol and dried under vacuum. Poly(A)$^+$ RNAs are immediately enriched by batch chromatography with 10 mg of oligo(dT) cellulose as described in Ausubel *et al.* (1987). After elution, the poly(A)$^+$ RNAs are ethanol-precipitated, resuspended in DEPC-treated water, quantified by absorbance at 260 nm (25 units A_{260} = 1 mg), and stored at −80°C.

b. cDNA Synthesis

cDNAs are synthesized from 5 μg poly(A)$^+$ RNAs using Amersham cDNA Synthesis System Plus. After denaturation of the poly(A)$^+$ RNAs by a 5-min incubation at 95°C, synthesis of the cDNA first strand is initiated with AMV reverse transcriptase in the presence of oligo(dT) and synthesis of the cDNA second strand uses RNaseH and the Klenow fragment of *E. coli* DNA polymerase. Double-stranded cDNAs are then blunt-ended using T4 DNA polymerase. All reactions are carried out according to the supplier's instructions. We find useful to include ^{32}P-labeled dCTP during the synthesis of both strands in order to quantify cDNA recovery after synthesis and during the subsequent steps of the experiment. However, addition of the radioactive nucleotide can be restricted to 1 μCi and to the second-strand synthesis. Analysis of the resulting cDNA molecule on an alkaline agarose gel, as described by the supplier, gives a good indication of the quality of the cDNA.

c. Preparation of the BstXI Adaptors

One nanomole of each of the B1 and B2 oligonucleotides is mixed and phosphorylated with 200 units of T4 polynucleotide kinase in the presence of 10 m*M* ATP in a final volume of 250 ml. After a 30-min incubation at 37°C, the mixture is incubated for 10 min at 90°C and allowed to cool slowly to room temperature to favor the annealing of the two oligonucleotides and the formation of the adaptor molecules. After the addition of 1 μl glycogen (10 mg/ml), the adaptors are ethanol-precipitated and resuspended in 20 μl H_2O.

d. Ligation of the Adaptors to the cDNAs

Phenol–chloroform-extracted cDNAs are ethanol-precipitated and resuspended in 20 μl H_2O. The cDNAs are then mixed with 4 μl of *Bst*XI adaptors and the ligation is carried out in a final volume of 40 μl with 10,000 units of T4 DNA ligase for at least 24 h at 16°C. A high amount of T4 DNA ligase and a long incubation time are crucial to the success of the experiment.

e. Gel Purification of the cDNAs and of BstXI-Cleaved pFL61

Prior to their ligation to pFL61, the cDNAs are gel-purified in order to remove excess *Bst*XI adaptors and to separate the different size classes. Size fractionation is required to prevent the overrepresentation of short cDNAs in the final cDNA library. Gel purification of the cDNAs is achieved by running the cDNAs on a 0.8% agarose–TBE gel made with low-melting agarose at 3 V/cm. Three size classes are recovered from the gel: 0.2 to 1 kb, 1 to 2.5 kb and >2.5 kb. Omission of the cDNAs shorter than 0.2 kb (even 0.5 kb) is essential since they often represent truncated cDNAs. In order to recover the cDNAs, about 2 vol of 20 m*M* Tris–HCl, pH 8, 1 m*M* EDTA is added to the gel slice, which is incubated at 65°C until melted. cDNAs are extracted once with phenol, then brought to 0.75 *M* NaCl and extracted once with phenol and once with phenol–chloroform. Direct extraction of the cDNAs with phenol–chloroform is to be avoided since it will result in the loss of material. DNA in the aqueous phase is ethanol-precipitated and resuspended in 20 μl H_2O. The amount of recovered cDNAs in each size class is estimated by counting the radioactivity of each sample and comparing these values to that obtained after cDNA synthesis.

Parallel purification of 10 μg of *Bst*XI-cleaved pFL61 is carried out in order to remove the internal *Bst*XI adaptor (Fig. 1), thereby preventing the recircularization of the vector during ligation. The gel slice containing *Bst*XI-cleaved pFL61 is processed in a manner similar to that described for the cDNAs, the DNA pellet being resuspended in 20 μl H_2O. The vector may be phenol-extracted, ethanol-precipitated, and redigested by *Bst*XI before gel purification to ensure full digestion by the enzyme.

f. Cloning of the cDNAs

The construction of the cDNA library is completed by ligating the purified cDNAs in *Bst*XI-cleaved pFL61. cDNAs of each size class are individually mixed in equimolar amounts with gel-purified vector and incubated with 2000 units T4 DNA ligase at 4°C for at least 24 h. Mixing of equimolar amounts of vector and cDNAs is optimal since the purified vector cannot recircularize and the cDNAs cannot ligate to each other. Knowledge of the amount of cDNAs recovered after gel purification will therefore help in preparing the ligation mixture. For instance, if 200 ng of the 1- to 2.5-kb size class is to be ligated, 200 × 5.4 (pFL61 size)/1.8 (average size of the cDNA class), i.e., 600 ng of *Bst*XI-cleaved pFL61, should be used for the ligation. However, discrepancies in the molar ratio of the vector and the inserts can be counterbalanced by ligating at low DNA concentrations ($j/i = 5$; Sambrook *et al.,* 1989).

g. Transformation of the cDNA Library into E. coli, Propagation, and Quality Control

The ligation mixture is the actual cDNA library and could be used to transform directly the yeast mutant of choice. However, given the low efficiency of yeast transformation and the low recovery of plasmids from yeast, it is advisable to first propagate the cDNA library in *E. coli* so that large amounts of plasmid DNA can be prepared to test the cDNA library in several recipient yeasts strains.

Several protocols have been described for high-efficiency transformation of *E. coli.* We favor transformation by electroporation, although the use of commercially available competent *E. coli* cells (Stratagene) is a very convenient alternative when an electroporation device is not available. Electrocompetent *E. coli* cells are prepared by growing a large volume (2 liters of LB) to early log phase ($A_{600} = 0.3$) and washing the cells twice with 800 ml of ice-cold distilled water, once with 400 ml ice-cold distilled water, and once with 400 ml ice-cold 15% glycerol. The cell pellet is resuspended in 2.5 ml 15% glycerol and 60-μl aliquots of electrocompetent *E. coli* are frozen on dry ice. For electroporation, an aliquot of cells is rapidly thawed, 1 μl DNA (1–100 ng of vector DNA) is added together with 3 μl 20 m*M* Tris–HCl, pH 8, 10 m*M* $MgCl_2$. The mixture is then submitted to a pulse at 2.5 kV, 25 μF, 200 W using Bio-Rad 0.2-cm cuvettes (E_o = 12.5 kV/cm) and transferred to a tube containing 1 ml SOC. After a 1-h incubation at 37°C, the cells are plated at various dilutions on LB agar plates containing 100 μg/ml ampicillin and incubated at 37°C for 16 h. Approximately 40 plates are used for each size class. Electroporation conditions must be optimized according to the *E. coli* strain and to the electroporation device and we therefore recommend that the reader refer to the manufacturer's instructions. Typical transformation efficiencies are in the range 10^8–10^9 transformants/μg. When starting the experiment with 2 μg of poly(A)$^+$ RNAs, 5.10^5 to 10^6 transformants are expected for each size class.

After transformation, the quality of the cDNA library is tested by examining the length of the cDNA inserts of eight random transformants for each size class by *Not*I restriction. The average size of these cDNA inserts should fit that of the different size class. Transformants of the 120 transformation plates are scrapped off and resuspended in a small volume of LB. An aliquot is brought to 50% glycerol and frozen at −80°C. The remainder is directly used to prepare plasmid DNA of the cDNA library. When fresh DNA is required for further experiments, frozen cells are spread on LB plates containing 100 μg/ml ampicillin, harvested after incubation, and used to prepare plasmid DNA in order to reduce the degeneracy of the cDNA library.

B. Complementation of *Saccharomyces cerevisiae* Mutants with the cDNA Library

1. Overview of the Procedure

Selection of a recombinant plasmid carrying a cDNA insert capable of complementing the mutation of choice is achieved by transforming the whole cDNA library into mutant *S. cerevisiae* and selecting transformants that display a wild-type phenotype. The selection scheme will vary according to the mutation studied and cannot be discussed in detail here. However, two main strategies can be used to obtain the desired transformant. The first strategy involves the selection of transformants on the appropriate medium immediately after transformation. The second strategy involves the initial selection of random transformants on a medium permissive for the mutation of interest, followed by the selection of the desired transformant by transferring (replica plating) the whole population of transformants onto an appropriate medium. Since pFL61 carries the *URA3* gene, the transformation event can be easily selected by using *ura3-52* mutant of *S. cerevisiae* and plating the transformation mixture on a medium lacking uracil. We therefore recommend the use of a strain with a *ura3-52* mutation in addition to the mutation to be complemented. A double mutant carrying the *ura3* mutation may be constructed as described in Guthrie and Fink (1991). Both strategies have been shown to work equally well (Minet *et al.,* 1992; d'Enfert *et al.,* 1992) and the choice is made according to the mutation studied: the first strategy is best adapted to mutations that do not affect cell viability (e.g., auxotrophic mutations), whereas the second is to be favored when dealing with a mutation that is lethal to the cell (e.g., thermosensitive mutations). Intermediate procedures can be designed by allowing the transformants to grow for a certain time under permissive conditions and then shifting the cells to nonpermissive conditions. Below, we describe a procedure that allows the recovery of uracil prototrophic transformants. High-transformation efficiency is obtained using lithium acetate-treated *S. cerevisiae* as described by Gietz *et al.* (1992), a method that we prefer to the techniques employing spheroplasts or electroporation (Becker and Guarente, 1991).

2. Materials

All solutions must be sterilized by autoclaving for 10 min at 120°C and stored at room temperature unless otherwise stated.

YPAD: 1% yeast extract (Difco), 2% Bacto-Peptone (Difco), 2% D-glucose, 0.003% adenine sulfate

Distilled water

10× TE: 0.1 *M* Tris–HCl, pH 7.5, 0.01 *M* EDTA; filter sterilize

10× LiAc: 1 *M* lithium acetate, pH 7.5, adjusted with acetic acid; filter sterilize

TE/LiAc buffer: 1× TE, 1× LiAc; make fresh every time

Carrier DNA: calf thymus DNA (Sigma) is resuspended in 10 m*M* Tris–HCl, pH 8, at 10 mg/ml and denatured by autoclaving twice for 20 min with a dry exhaust

50% polyethylene glycol (PEG) 4000; filter sterilize

PEG solution: 40% PEG 4000, 1× TE, 1× LiAc; make fresh every time

SD plates: 0.67% yeast nitrogen base without amino acids (Difco), 2% glucose, 1.5% Bacto-agar (Difco), appropriate supplements except uracil

3. Procedure (Gietz *et al.*, 1992)

Cells are inoculated into YAPD medium and grown overnight to an $A_{600} = 0.4$ (2×10^7 cells/ml). The cells are then diluted to 2×10^6 cells/ml in 100 ml fresh YAPD and grown to an $A_{600} = 0.2$. Cells are collected by centrifugation (5 min, $3000 \times g$), washed once with 20 ml distilled water, resuspended in 2 ml of distilled water, and transferred to a sterile 2-ml centrifuge tube. Cells are pelleted (3 min, 5000 rpm), washed with 2 ml TE/LiAc buffer, and finally resuspended in 0.5 ml TE/LiAc buffer (2×10^9 cells/ml). Fifty microliters of these competent yeast cells is mixed with 1 μg transforming DNA and 50 μg carrier DNA in microfuge tubes. Three hundred microliters of PEG solution is added and mixed. After a 30-min incubation at 30°C (25°C when using thermosensitive mutants) with gentle shaking, the cells are heat-shocked for 15 min at 42°C (37°C when using thermosensitive mutants). Cells are collected by centrifugation (5 s) and resuspended in 1 ml TE and appropriate dilutions are plated on SD plates lacking uracil. Typical transformation efficiencies are in the range of 10^6 transformants/μg for plasmid DNA.

C. Analysis of the Complementing Plasmids

1. Overview of the Procedure

Once transformants with the appropriate phenotype have been obtained, it is essential to determine whether the complementing activity is plasmid-linked.

This is achieved by two independent approaches. First, cosegregation of the plasmid and of the complementing activity is demonstrated by curing the transformed strains of their plasmid and studying the resulting phenotype. Second, the transforming plasmids are prepared from the transformants, propagated in *E. coli,* and reintroduced into the mutant strain to test whether they restore the wild-type phenotype.

2. Materials

YPD: 1% yeast extract (Difco), 2% Bacto-Peptone (Difco), 2% D-glucose

YPD plates: YPD + 1.5% Bacto-agar (Difco)

SD: 0.67% yeast nitrogen base without amino acids (Difco), 2% glucose, appropriate supplements except uracil

STES: 0.5 *M* NaCl, 0.2 *M* Tris–HCl, pH 7.6, 10 m*M* EDTA, 1% SDS

Acid-washed glass beads

Phenol–chloroform made with Tris–HCl, pH 8, equilibrated phenol

3. Procedures

a. Segregation Analysis

The transformant strain is grown for 24 h in a medium that allows for the loss of the plasmid (e.g., YPD), plated at a cell density of ca. 200 cells (1 $A_{600} = 5 \times 10^7$ cells) per plate on the same medium, and incubated at the appropriate temperature until the appearance of colonies. Colonies are replica-plated on SD plates lacking uracil as an indicator of the presence of the plasmid and on plates selecting for the complementation of the mutation. Cells that have lost the plasmid should be unable to grow on the selective medium, indicating a plasmid-linked complementing activity.

b. Recovery of Plasmids from Yeast Transformants

Transformants are grown for 24 h in 2 ml of SD lacking uracil at 30°C. After centrifugation (2 min, 5000 rpm), the cell pellet is resuspended in 50 μl STES and acid-washed glass beads are added up to the meniscus. The slurry is vortexed for 1 min and, after addition of 60 μl phenol–chloroform, vortexed for an additional 1 min. After centrifugation, the aqueous phase is recovered and used to transform *E. coli.* Fifty to 200 transformants are usually recovered when $CaCl_2$-treated *E. coli* (Sambrook *et al.,* 1989) are used for transformation. Plasmid is then prepared from *E. coli* transformants and reintroduced in the mutant strain by transformation as described above. Upon transformation, the mutant should regain the wild-type phenotype.

III. Critical Aspects of the Procedures

Most of the critical parameters of the procedures have been raised above. However, we would like to stress three important aspects of the overall strategy:

1. Yeast expression vectors other than pFL61 have been used to construct expression libraries and involve cloning strategies that differ from that outlined in this review. Especially, it may be advantageous to choose a vector that, in contrast to pFL61, allows controlled expression of the cloned gene. Examples of such vectors may be found in Guthrie and Fink (1991) and Elledge *et al.* (1991).

2. The identification of a complementing plasmid relies on the identification of a few interesting clones out of a large population of useless transformants. It is therefore crucial to define a selection scheme that allows the mutant and the wild-type phenotypes to be identified unambiguously. In this regard, a good knowledge of the behavior of the mutant strain in various conditions and of the strategy used to clone the *S. cerevisiae* wild-type gene is of considerable importance. It should be remembered that complementation of yeast mutations is sometimes due to a multicopy suppressor whose overexpression can bypass or counteract the effect of the mutation.

3. The construction of a good cDNA library represents a certain amount of work but can be completed within 2 weeks. However, the obtention of a complementing plasmid will probably require more time and several trials. If the cDNA library is of good quality, i.e., complementation of auxotrophic mutants of *S. cerevisiae* is easily achieved, four or five trials must be considered a maximum effort for a given selection scheme.

IV. Results and Discussion

Typical results that are to be expected during the cDNA library construction have been reported by Minet *et al.* (1992). Starting with 5 μg poly(A)$^+$ RNAs, they recovered 1.5, 1, and 0.4 μg of the cDNAs of the short (0.2–1 kb), medium (1–2.5 kb), and large (>2.5 kb) class, respectively, after gel purification, and eventually obtained 3.5×10^5, 5×10^5, and 3×10^5 *E. coli* transformants of the different classes per microgram of starting poly(A)$^+$ RNAs. This cDNA library has been used for the complementation of a variety of *S. cerevisiae* mutants, as shown in Table I. It may be difficult to use this approach to identify plant genes encoding homologues of yeast proteins that are part of a multiprotein complex. Indeed, coevolution of the various partners of the complex may preclude the reconstitution of a functional complex in yeast with a component from a quite different organism. A good illustration of this may be the inability to complement the yeast *wbp1* mutation with cDNA from *A. thaliana* since Wbp1p is one of the six different subunits of *S. cerevisiae* oligosaccharyl transferase (M. Aebi, personal communication). However, d'Enfert *et al.* (1992) have shown that in the case of the GTP-binding protein Sarlp and of the Sarlp-specific nucleotide exchange factor Secl2p (Barlowe and Schekman, 1993), divergence can be restricted to one of the interacting molecules: the *A. thaliana* homologue of Sarlp is 64% identical to the yeast protein, whereas the *A. thaliana* Sec12p homologue is only 19% identical to the yeast protein and yet high level expression of either

Table I
Complementation of *Saccharomyces cerevisiae* mutants by *Arabidopsis thaliana* cDNAs

S. cerevisiae mutant	Function/phenotype	Complementation	Reference
ura1	Uracil auxotroph	+	Minet *et al.*, 1992
ura2	Uracil auxotroph	+	Minet *et al.*, 1992
ura4	Uracil auxotroph	+	Minet *et al.*, 1992
ura5-ura10	Uracil auxotroph	+	Minet *et al.*, 1992
ade2	Adenine auxotroph	+	Minet *et al.*, 1992
his3	Histidine auxotroph	+	Minet *et al.*, 1992
leu2	Leucine auxotroph	+	Minet *et al.*, 1992
trp1	Tryptophan auxotroph	+	Minet *et al.*, 1992
sec12	Sar1p-guanine nucleotide exchange factor; thermosensitive for growth	A.t.STL2 A.t.SAR1	d'Enfert *et al.*, 1992
trk1	K^+ transport system; required for growth at low K^+ concentrations	+	Sentenac *et al.*, 1992
wbp1	Oligosaccharyl transferase subunit; thermosensitive for growth	–	[a]M. Aebi
yred	Cytochrome P450 reductase	+	[a]D. Pompon
rna14	mRNA processing; thermosensitive for growth	–	[b]F. Lacroute
rna15	mRNA processing; thermosensitive for growth	–	[b]F. Lacroute
cdc28	Cell cycle control $p34^{cdc2}$ kinase; thermosensitive for growth	+	[b]F. Lacroute

[a] Personal communication.
[b] Unpublished data.

proteins is sufficient to complement a thermosensitive *sec12* mutation. These results suggest that the approach of cloning plant genes by direct complementation of yeast mutants can also be successful even when dealing with proteins that belong to multicomponent complexes.

V. Conclusion and Perspectives

The method that we have described above is highly efficient for identifying plant genes with functional yeast homologs and is not dependent upon any sequence homology of the encoded proteins. Although it has been used to complement *S. cerevisiae* mutations, there are no technical limitations to the adaptation of this strategy to cloning genes by complementation of mutations obtained in other genetically amenable lower eukaryotes, e.g., *S. pombe, Aspergillus nidulans,* or *Neurospora crassa.* There is no doubt that the cloning of plant genes by functional complementation of yeast mutations will help in defining the basic functions of the plant cell: ironically, this may be a prerequisite to understanding what makes a plant a plant and not a yeast!

References

Anderson, A. A., Huprikar, S. S., Kochian, L. V., Lucas, W. J., and Gaber, R. F. (1992). Functional expression of a probable *Arabidopsis thaliana* potassium channel in *Saccharomyces cerevisiae*. *Proc. Natl. Acad. Sci. U.S.A.* **89,** 3736–3740.

Aruffo, A., and Seeds, B. (1987). Molecular cloning of a CDC28 cDNA by a high-efficiency COS cell expression system. *Proc. Natl. Acad. Sci. U.S.A.* **84,** 8573–8577.

Ausubel, F. M., Brent, R., Kingston, R. E., Moore, D. D., Seidman, J. G., Smith, J. A., and Struhl, K. (1987). "Current Protocols in Molecular Biology." New York: Greene Publishing Associates/Wiley–Interscience.

Barlowe, C., and Schekman, R. (1993). *SEC12* encodes a guanine-nucleotide-exchange factor essential for transport vesicle budding from the ER. *Nature* **365,** 347–349.

Becker, D. M., and Guarante, L. (1991). High-efficiency transformation of yeast by electroporation. *Methods Enzymol.* **194,** 182–187.

Becker, D. M., Fikes, J. D., and Guarente, L. (1991). A cDNA encoding a human CCAAT-binding protein cloned by functional complementation in yeast. *Proc. Natl. Acad. Sci. U.S.A.* **88,** 1968–1972.

Botstein, D., and Fink, G. R. (1988). Yeast: An experimental organism for modern biology. *Science* **240,** 1439–1443.

Colicelli, J., Birchmeier, C., Michaeli, T., O'Neill, K., Riggs, M., and Wigler, M. (1989). Isolation and characterization of a mammalian gene encoding a high-affinity cAMP phosphodiesterase. *Proc. Natl. Acad. Sci. U.S.A.* **86,** 3599–3603.

DeFeo-Jones, D., Tatchell, K., Robinson, L. C., Sigal, I. S., Vass, W. C., Lowy, D. R., and Scolnick, E. M. (1985). Mammalian and yeast *ras* gene products: Biological function in their heterologous systems. *Science* **228,** 179–184.

Elledge, S. J., Mulligan, J. T., Ramer, S. W., Spottswood, M., and Davis, R. W. (1991). Lambda YES: A multifunctional cDNA expression vector for the isolation of genes by complementation of yeast and *Escherichia coli* mutations. *Proc. Natl. Acad. Sci. U.S.A.* **88,** 1731–1735.

Ellerstrom, M., Josefsson, L. G., Rask, L., and Ronne, H. (1992). Cloning of a cDNA for rape chloroplast 3-isopropylmalate dehydrogenase by genetic complementation in yeast. *Plant Mol. Biol.* **18,** 557–566.

d'Enfert, C., Gensse, M., and Gaillardin, C. (1992). Fission yeast and a plant have functional homologues of the Sarl and Sec12 proteins involved in ER to Golgi traffic in budding yeast. *EMBO J.* **11,** 4205–4211.

Gietz, D., Jean, A. S., Woods, R. A., and Schietsl, R. H. (1992). Improved method for high efficiency transformation of intact yeast cells. *Nucleic Acids Res.* **20,** 1425.

Guthrie, C., and Fink, G. R. (1991). Guide to yeast genetics and molecular biology. "Methods in Enzymology," Vol. 194. New York: Academic Press.

Katakoa, T., Powers, S., Cameron, S., Fasano, O., Goldfarb, M., Broach, J., and Wigler, M. (1985). Functional homology of mammalian and yeast *RAS* genes. *Cell* **40,** 19–26.

Koff, A., Cross, F., Fisher, A., Schumacher, J., Leguellec, K., Philippe, M., and Roberts, J. M. (1991). Human cyclin E, a new cyclin that interacts with two members of the *CDC2* gene family. *Cell* **66,** 1217–1228.

Lee, M. G., and Nurse, P. (1987). Complementation used to clone a human homologue of the fission yeast cell cycle control gene *cdc2*. *Nature* **327,** 31–35.

Lew, D. J., Dulic, V., and Reed, S. (1991). Isolation of three novel human cyclins by rescue of G1 cyclin (Cln) function in yeast. *Cell* **66,** 1197–1206.

Minet, M., and Lacroute, F. (1990). Cloning and sequencing of a human cDNA coding for a multifunctional polypeptide of the purine pathway by complementation of the *ade2-101* mutant in *Saccharomyces cerevisiae*. *Curr. Genet.* **18,** 287–291.

Minet, M., Dufour, M. E., and Lacroute, F. (1992). Complementation of *Saccharomyces cerevisiae* auxotrophic mutants by *Arabidopsis thaliana* cDNAs. *Plant J.* **2,** 417–422.

Mortimer, R. K., Schild, D., Contopoulou, C. R., and Kans, J. A. (1989). Genetic map of *Saccharomyces cerevisiae*, edition 10. *Yeast* **5,** 321–403.

Murashige, T., and Shoog, F. (1962). A revised medium for rapid growth and bioassays with tobacco tissue cultures. *Physiol. Plant.* **15,** 479–497.

Nasim, A., Young, P., and Johnson, B. (1989). "Molecular Biology of Fission Yeast." New York: Academic Press.

Sambrook, J., Fritsch, E. F., and Maniatis, T. (1989). "Molecular cloning: A laboratory manual," 2nd ed. Cold Spring Harbor: Cold Spring Harbor Laboratory Press.

Sentenac, H., Bonneaud, N., Minet, M., Lacroute, F., Salmon, J. M., Gaymard, F., and Grignon, C. (1992). Cloning and expression in yeast of a plant potassium ion transport system. *Science* **256,** 663–665.

Thon, V. J., Khalil, M., and Cannon, J. F. (1993). Isolation of human glycogen branching enzyme cDNAs by screening complementation in yeast. *J. Biol. Chem.* **268,** 7509–7513.

CHAPTER 30

Differential mRNA Display

T. Lynne Reuber and Frederick M. Ausubel

Department of Molecular Biology
Massachusetts General Hospital
Boston, Massachusetts 02114

I. Introduction

Differential RNA display was devised by Liang and Pardee (1992) as a method to compare gene expression in two or more cell types and to clone differentially expressed genes rapidly. The principle of the technique is to amplify specific subpopulations of mRNA, using reverse transcription and PCR to produce a set of "RNA fingerprints." To do this, mRNA is reverse-transcribed in subsets using specific anchored oligo(dT) primers (see below) that recognize different fractions of the total mRNA population. The resulting cDNA is then amplified with the

METHODS IN CELL BIOLOGY, VOL. 49

same anchored oligo(dT) primer and a short arbitrary primer. Labeled dATP is included in the reactions and the labeled products are separated on a DNA sequencing gel and visualized by autoradiography. Each pair of primers produces a distinct pattern of bands. The band patterns obtained for each cell type with each primer pair are compared; differentially expressed bands are cut out of the gel, and the DNA is eluted and reamplified. The amplified products are used to probe an RNA blot to confirm that they represent differentially expressed mRNA species, and can then be used to probe a cDNA or genomic DNA library to recover a full-sized clone of the gene of interest.

The key to displaying a useful number of bands (i.e., neither too few nor too many) lies in the choice of primers. For reverse transcription of specific subpopulations of mRNA, Liang and Pardee (1992) used a set of 12 oligo(dT) primers that each contained two additional 3′ nucleotides, allowing hybridization only to the 5′ end of the poly(A) tail of mRNA (for example, $T_{12}CA$). The 12 primers represent all possible combinations of two nucleotides, excluding T as the penultimate base. Therefore, 12 sets of reactions are needed to amplify all the mRNA in the cell. A recent modification of the technique used in the RNAmap kit sold by GenHunter Corp. uses a set of four anchored oligo(dT) primers that are degenerate at the penultimate base (for example, $T_{12}VA$, where V represents a mixture of A, C, and G). Using these primers, only 4 sets of reverse transcription reactions are needed. Although we used this modification of the original technique, the protocol given below is the same for either type of anchored oligo(dT) primer.

The ideal size of the arbitrary primers used for PCR amplification was found to be 10 nucleotides. In theory, 10-mers would not hybridize frequently enough to give the 50–100 bands per primer pair that are typically observed. However, 10-mers have been shown to hybridize with mismatches at the 5′ end, requiring only about six exact matches at the 3′ end to function in the PCR amplification (Bauer *et al.*, 1993; Liang *et al.*, 1992; Liang and Pardee, 1992). The selection of appropriate arbitrary 10-mers and the number of 10-mers needed to cover the total RNA population have been discussed elsewhere (Bauer *et al.*, 1993). In general, any random 10-mer that is not self-complementary is acceptable. We have found the 10-mer kits marketed by Operon for genetic mapping useful for this purpose.

II. Methods

A. RNA Preparation

Any method of RNA preparation should be suitable for this protocol. For *Arabidopsis*, a standard protocol for preparation of plant RNA (Ausubel *et al.*, 1993) was used. It is critical that the mRNA not be degraded; care should be taken in RNA preparation and handling.

B. DNase Treatment of RNA

DNase treatment of RNA is necessary to remove contaminating DNA that might be amplified in the PCR reactions. As a precaution against possible RNase contamination of commercial DNase I, human placental RNase inhibitor is added to the reactions.

1. Materials

diethylpyrocarbonate (DEPC)
DNase I (RNase free), Bethesda Research Laboratories
RNase inhibitor (human placental, 10 U/μl), BRL
DEPC-treated water
10× PCR buffer: 100 m*M* Tris, pH 8.3
15 m*M* $MgCl_2$
500 m*M* KCl
1 mg/ml gelatin
3:1 phenol:chloroform
absolute ethanol (preferably from a bottle used only for RNA preparation)
70% ethanol (diluted with DEPC-treated water)
3 *M* sodium acetate (DEPC-treated)

2. Protocol

The RNA concentration should be adjusted to approximately 1 μg/μl before treatment. Reactions are carried out in microcentrifuge tubes as follows:

For each sample:

	(μl)
Total RNA	50 (50 μg)
10× PCR buffer	5.7
RNase inhibitor	1
DNase I	2 (diluted to 10 U/μl immediately before use in 0.1× TE)

Mix by pipetting up and down, and incubate for 30 min at 37°C. Add 40 μl of 3:1 phenol/chloroform, vortex each sample for 1 min, spin samples in a microcentrifuge for 5 min, and collect the aqueous phase of each sample. Add 5 μl of 3 *M* sodium acetate (DEPC-treated) and 150 μl of absolute ethanol to each sample to precipitate the RNA, allow the samples to stand at −20°C for at least 2 h, and spin the samples in a microcentrifuge for 10 min at 4°C. Wash the RNA pellets with 0.5 ml 70% ethanol and resuspend each in 50 μl of DEPC-treated water. Requantitate the RNA by measuring the OD_{260} and dilute the samples to 0.1 μg/μl. Accurate RNA quantitation is important because differences in initial RNA concentration can cause differences in the pattern and intensity of bands obtained in the final PCR step. It is also helpful at this step to run an aliquot of the RNA on an agarose gel to ensure that the RNA has not been degraded.

C. Reverse Transcription of RNA

1. Materials

MMLV reverse transcriptase (BRL or GenHunter)

5× reverse transcriptase buffer (generally included with reverse transcriptase):

250 m*M* Tris–HCl, pH 8.3

375 m*M* KCl

15 m*M* $MgCl_2$

0.1 *M* dithiothreotol (DTT, generally included with reverse transcriptase)

dNTP solution: 250 μ*M* each dATP, dCTP, dGTP, dTTP (Pharmacia or GenHunter)

set of four anchored oligo(dT) primers, 10 μ*M* solutions: $T_{12}VA$, $T_{12}VC$, $T_{12}VG$, $T_{12}VT$ (GenHunter)

2. Protocol (adapted from the instructions to the GenHunter RNAmap kit)

For each reaction (20 μl total volume):

	(μl)	Final concentration
Distilled H_2O	7.4	
5× reverse transcriptase buffer	4	1×
0.1 *M* DTT	2	10 m*M*
dNTPs (250 μM each)	1.6	20 μ*M*
Oligo(dT) primer (one of the four)	2	1 μ*M*
mRNA (0.1 μg/μl)	2	0.01 μg/μl

Incubate the samples at 65°C for 5 min to denature the RNA and transfer to 37°C for 10 min. Add 1 μl of MMLV reverse transcriptase (200 U/μl) to each tube. Incubate at 37°C for an additional 50 min. Stop the reactions by heating to 95°C for 5 min and place the samples on ice or store at −20°C if they will not be used immediately. Each reaction is sufficient for 10 PCR reactions.

D. PCR

1. Materials

10× PCR buffer (as above)

dNTP solution, 25 μ*M* each dATP, dCTP, dGTP, dTTP (Pharmacia or GenHunter). Note that this is a lower dNTP concentration than that used in the reverse transcription reaction and in the standard PCR reaction. The lower dNTP concentration increases the specificity of the PCR amplification and the efficiency of product labeling (Liang and Pardee, 1992).

set of oligo(dT) primers, 10 μM solutions (GenHunter)

10-mer oligonucleotide primers, 2 μM solutions (GenHunter or Operon)

[α-^{35}S]dATP (1200 Ci/mmol, 12.5 mCi/ml) (New England Nuclear)

Taq DNA polymerase, 5U/μl

mineral oil

programmable thermal cycler

2. Protocol (adapted from the instructions to the GenHunter RNAmap kit)

For each PCR reaction:

	(μl)	Final concentration
dH_2O	9.2	
10× PCR buffer	2	1×
dNTPs (25 μM)	1.6	2 μM
oligo(dT) primer (same as used for reverse transcription)	2	1 μM
[^{35}S]dATP	1	0.5 μM
Taq DNA polymerase	0.2	0.05 U/μl

Mix and aliquot these components. Then add 2.0 μl of a 10-mer primer (0.2 μM final concentration) and 2.0 μl of the reverse transcription mix and mix by pipetting up and down (good mixing is critical for reproducible PCR). Cover each reaction mixture with 2–3 drops of mineral oil. The PCR conditions are as folows: a 5-min initial denaturation at 94°C, followed by 40 three-step cycles of a 30-s denaturation at 94°C, a 2-min annealing at 40°C, and a 30-s elongation at 72°C, and then a final 5-min elongation at 72°C.

E. Separation of Products and Reamplification of Differential Bands

1. Materials

loading dye: 95% formamide
0.05% bromophenol blue
0.05% xylene cyanol

3 M sodium acetate

absolute ethanol

10 mg/ml glycogen (molecular biology grade, BRL)

2. Protocol (adapted from the instructions to the GenHunter RNAmap kit)

Add 3.5 μl of the completed PCR reaction to 2 μl of loading dye and heat to 80°C for at least 2 min. Load 2–5 μl onto a DNA sequencing gel (6% acrylamide).

Electrophorese until the xylene cyanol dye is nearly to the bottom of the gel. In a 6% gel, xylene cyanol runs with DNA fragments of approximately 100 bp (Ausubel *et al.*, 1993). Dry the gel without fixation and autoradiograph (overnight–48 h). It is helpful to spread a small amount of powder (magnesium carbonate works well) on the dried gel to prevent it from sticking to the film. The film and dried gel should be taped together during the exposure and marked with needle punches so that the developed film can be reoriented with the gel.

The simplest way to recover differentially expressed bands is to pin the film to the dried gel through the needle holes and cut the bands out through the film (include the filter paper backing). To reamplify the bands, soak each dried gel and paper slice in 100 μl of dH_2O in a microcentrifuge tube for a few minutes and boil the tube for 15 min. Spin briefly and collect the supernatant. Add 10 μl of 3 *M* sodium acetate and 5 μl of glycogen (as a carrier) and precipitate the DNA with 450 μl of absolute ethanol. Allow the solutions to stand at −80°C for at least 30 min and spin 10 min at 4°C. Wash the DNA pellet with cold 85% ethanol and resupend in 10 μl of dH_2O.

Use 4 μl of this DNA solution for PCR reamplification using the same primers that generated the band. The reaction conditions are the same as in the first PCR amplification, except that the final dNTP concentration is 20 μ*M*, the total volume is increased to 40 μl, and no label is added. After the first PCR amplification, 4 μl of the product is used as the template for a second round of PCR amplification using the same conditions, and 20 μl of each reaction is analyzed on an agarose gel. Most products can be seen after the first reamplification, and nearly all after the second reamplification. Generally, more secondary PCR products appear in the second reamplification. The size of the PCR product should be checked against the estimated size of the original band.

F. Confirmation of Differential Bands

The reamplified PCR products can be purified from the agarose gel using the MerMaid kit from Bio 101, which is useful for fragments less than 500 bp long. The products can then be labeled with a random priming kit (Boehringer Mannheim), and used directly to probe an RNA blot. If only a small amount of fragment is recovered (less than 20 ng), it can be labeled by PCR using the same PCR conditions and primers used to reamplify the fragment, with the substitution of [^{32}P]dCTP for unlabeled dCTP. Fragments that recognize differentially expressed transcripts can then be used to probe a DNA library to isolate a full-length clone of the gene of interest.

III. Critical Aspects of the Technique

Although most of the bands obtained with any pair of primers are reproducible, a number of artifacts can be obtained. Therefore, potential differential bands should be confirmed in a second, independent set of reverse transcription and PCR reactions before proceeding with reamplification and testing. We have found it most efficient to carry two independent RNA preparations for each cell type or treatment through the entire procedure, and load them on adjacent lanes on the sequencing gel. Only bands that are consistently differential in both independent samples are isolated.

IV. Potential Modifications of the Procedure

Several modifications to the technique have been made in various laboratories. We have used the protocol given above with success, but the modifications to the procedure described below may give better results.

A. Primer Choice

The use of anchored oligo(dT) primers that are degenerate at the penultimate base would seem to increase the efficiency of the technique. In this case, only 4 primers rather than 12 are needed to reverse transcribe all species of RNA in the cell. However, one comparison of the two methods in another laboratory indicated that the band patterns obtained were more reproducible with the original set of nondegenerate oligo(dT) primers (E. van der Knaap, personal communication).

B. Band Labeling

The original procedure used [^{35}S]dATP to label PCR products. However, ^{35}S-labeled compounds can break down under thermal cycling conditions, producing volatile radioactive compounds that contaminate the PCR machine. We have not found contamination to be a significant problem when reactions are done in 0.5 ml microcentrifuge tubes, but other types of tubes may create more of a problem. [^{33}P]dATP can be substituted for [^{35}S]dATP at 2 μCi (60 n*M*) per reaction (Bauer *et al.*, 1993). In general, ^{33}P labeling gives clearer bands and better resolution than ^{35}S labeling and ^{33}P is reportedly more stable under thermal cycling conditions. However, ^{33}P is more expensive than ^{35}S. Another solution is end-labeling of the anchored oligo(dT) primers with ^{32}P (E. van der Knaap, personal communication).

C. Separation of PCR Products

Bauer *et al.* (1993) have shown that the PCR products obtained from a single mRNA species can produce a cluster of two or more bands on a standard denaturing sequencing gel. These clusters of bands apparently result from slightly different mobilities of the two labeled strands of each product and from the addition of an extra A at the 3′ ends of some PCR products by Taq DNA polymerase. Therefore, the band patterns obtained by separating PCR products on a sequencing gel are misleadingly complex. Bauer *et al.* have modified the differential display technique by separating PCR products on nondenaturing gels, which give simpler band patterns.

D. Confirmation of Differential Products

Although the reamplified PCR products can be used directly to probe RNA blots, it has been found that these products are generally heterogeneous. When the PCR products were cloned and several clones were characterized by restriction analysis, several species were often present (R. A. Dietrich and J. Dangl, unpublished data). Therefore, better results will almost certainly be obtained if the PCR products are cloned and characterized to ensure that a single species is being used as a probe. The TA Cloning kit marketed by Invitrogen has been found to be useful for cloning of differential display products.

V. Results and Discussion

We have used differential RNA display to look for *Arabidopsis* genes involved in conferring resistance to bacterial pathogens. We compared RNA populations at two time points after infection in a wild-type *Arabidopsis* ecotype that is resistant to the infecting bacteria and in an *Arabidopsis* mutant that lacks resistance to these bacteria. The band pattern obtained with one primer pair is shown in Fig. 1. Most bands were present in all eight lanes. The arrow marked "a" indicates a band that was consistently present at higher levels in the mutant lanes. Arrows "b" and "c" indicate anomalous bands that were overexpressed only in one lane. In general, we obtained about 50–100 clear, useful bands per primer pair. In most cases, fragments smaller than approximately 200 bp tended to form a continuous ladder of faint bands, which rarely showed consistent differences among samples (Fig. 1). Most of the potential differential bands we have isolated are at least 300 bp in size, and none are smaller than 200 bp. The modifications discussed in the previous section may improve the band patterns obtained.

To date, we have screened 10 different 10-mers with the four anchored oligo(dT) primers. Of 26 potential differential bands that we investigated further, we were able to reamplify 23 from the sequencing gels; these were used to probe blots of total RNA from pathogen-infected plants. Only 6 of these 23 probes generated clear signals on RNA blots. Two of these hybridized to transcripts that were more highly expressed in wild-type plants than in mutant plants, whereas the other four hybridized to transcripts that did not show consistent differences in expression between wild-type and mutant plants. Genomic or cDNA clones corresponding to the two differentially expressed transcripts were

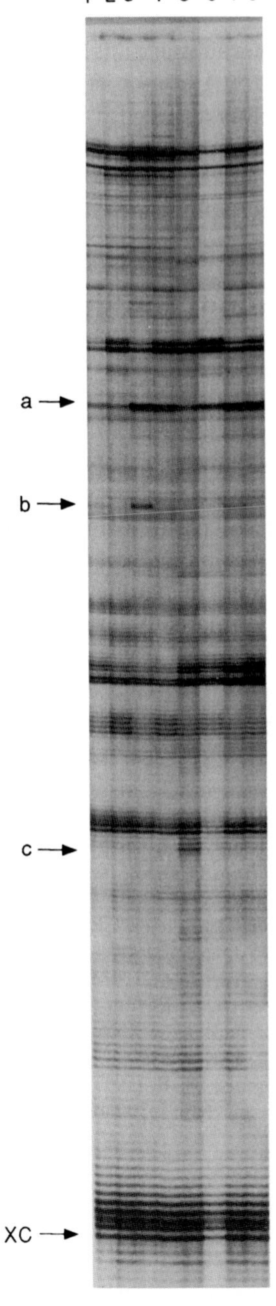

Fig. 1 Band patterns obtained from *Arabidopsis* RNA with one primer pair. Lanes 1 and 2, RNA from wild-type plants at 3 h after bacterial infection; lanes 3 and 4, RNA from mutant plants 3 h after infection; lanes 5 and 6, RNA from wild-type plants 9 h after infection; lanes 7 and 8, RNA from mutant plants 9 h after infection. (a) Band that was consistently more intense in the mutant lanes (3, 4, 7, and 8) than in the wild-type lanes (1, 2, 5, and 6). (b) and (c) Anomalous bands that were more intense only in one lane. XC, position of the xylene cyanol dye that comigrates with fragments of approximately 100 bp.

isolated, and preliminary analysis indicated that they represent novel pathogen-induced genes of *Arabidopsis*. The other bands (17 of 23) that did not hybridize to the RNA blots may represent genes that are expressed at very low levels, or they may result from PCR-generated artifacts. Using these probes on poly(A)$^+$ RNA blots to increase the sensitivity of hybridization may help distinguish between these possibilities.

VI. Conclusions and Perspectives

Differential RNA display is a promising technique for isolating differentially expressed genes. It has several major advantages over other methods such as differential hybridization and subtractive hybridization. Because it is based on PCR, it is more sensitive than these methods and has a better chance of detecting less abundant mRNAs. It requires little RNA, an advantage in systems where large amounts of tissue are hard to come by. Finally, it allows comparison of multiple samples in one experiment, so several tissues, treatments, or time points can be examined in parallel. One disadvantage of differential display in our hands is that a relatively large number of candidate bands must be checked to find a few differential transcripts. However, the technique is still being refined, and further improvements may increase its efficiency. In general, the unique advantages of this technique will make it useful in many diverse systems.

References

Ausubel, F. M., Brent, R., Kingston, R. E., Moore, D. D., Seidman, J. G., Smith, J. A., and Struhl, K. (1993). "Current Protocols in Molecular Biology." New York: Greene Publishing Associates/Wiley–Interscience.

Bauer, D., Müller, H., Reich, J., Riedel, H., Ahrenkiel, V., Warthoe, P., and Strauss, M. (1993). Identification of differentially expressed mRNA species by an improved display technique (DDRT-PCR). *Nucleic Acids Res.* **21,** 4272–4280.

Liang, P., Averboukh, L., Keyomarsi, K., Sager, R., and Pardee, A. B. (1992). Differential display and cloning of messenger RNAs from human breast cancer versus mammary epithelial cells. *Cancer Res.* **52,** 6966–6968.

Liang, P., and Pardee, A. B. (1992). Differential display of eukaryotic messenger RNA by means of the polymerase chain reaction. *Science* **257,** 967–971.

CHAPTER 31

Molecular Methods for Isolation of Signal Transduction Pathway Mutants

Joanne Chory, Hsou-min Li, and Nobuyoshi Mochizuki
Plant Biology Laboratory
The Salk Institute for Biological Studies
P.O. Box 85800
San Diego, California 92186-5800

I. Introduction

In higher eukaryotes, the use of classical genetics to approach the analysis of regulatory pathways is often met with complications, including the large gene families that can code for a particular protein, the relatively long life cycle, and the pleiotropic effects that such mutations might have. Perhaps the greatest limitation to finding regulatory mutations is to predict the phenotype of such mutants. Promoter fusions have proven to be powerful tools for the analysis of gene regulation in a variety of systems. Their utility in the selection of *trans*-acting regulatory mutations has been elegantly demonstrated, but has not been

METHODS IN CELL BIOLOGY, VOL. 49

widely applied (e.g., Guarante *et al.*, 1982; Bonner *et al.*, 1984). We have recently applied promoter fusion methodology to the study of the phototransduction pathways in *Arabidopsis thaliana* (Susek *et al.*, 1993; Li *et al.*, 1994; Li and Chory, unpublished results). This chapter will review the methodology for Arabidopsis transformation, mutagenesis, and positive and negative genetic selections based on selectable marker gene cassettes. Although we will discuss the methodology in terms of our own results using an Arabidopsis light-regulated promoter, the methods described here should be generalizable for the study of any signal transduction pathway.

Several criteria need to be met for performing these sorts of molecular genetic studies in higher plants. The plant system chosen must be easily transformable and a good genetic organism. Moreover, the signal transduction or developmental pathway under analysis must have well-defined downstream events that are manifested by tightly regulated transcriptional activation or repression. For these reasons, we chose *A. thaliana* as our genetic system and the nuclear *CAB3* gene as an indicator of light-regulated, developmental gene expression (Leutwiler *et al.*, 1986; Meyerowitz, 1989). The transcription of *CAB* genes is tightly regulated, being transcribed in the light in green plants, with little or no detectable levels in etiolated seedlings. In addition, *CAB* genes are expressed in a tissue-specific manner, transcripts being most abundant in leaves and lower or undetectable in other organs. Finally, the developmental stage of the chloroplast appears to regulate the expression of *CAB* genes. For example, in photooxidative mutants of maize and in a variety of plants where chloroplast development is arrested with an inhibitor, *CAB* genes are not transcribed (e.g., Taylor, 1989). Thus, *CAB* gene transcription is regulated by light, intrinsic developmental signals, and must also be sensitive to signals originating from the chloroplast.

The *CAB* promoter–marker gene chimeras needed for our studies were introduced into Arabidopsis at a single site in each transgenic line. The constructs (Fig. 1) contain a fully regulated *CAB3* promoter sequence fused to either of two selectable marker genes: (*a*) the *hph* (hygromycin phosphotransferase) gene, which confers hygromycin resistance allowing for positive selection strategies (Gritz and Davies, 1983), or (*b*) the Arabidopsis *ADH* (alcohol dehydrogenase) gene, which allows for negative selection using the suicide substrate, allyl alcohol. Allyl alcohol is converted to the toxic intermediate acrolein by alcohol dehydrogenase (Rando, 1974; Chang and Meyerowitz, 1986). [The *ADH* construct is transformed into an adh^- mutant of Arabidopsis (Jacobs *et al.*, 1988)]. Both constructs show low basal expression from the *CAB3* promoter and carry a screenable marker *uidA* gene (*Escherichia coli* β-glucuronidase, GUS) under control of a second *CAB3* promoter. Our strategy was to mutagenize and select for plants that aberrantly expressed the marker transgenes from the *CAB3* promoter under a variety of conditions. Following selection, we also screened for GUS activity, which is under the control of the second *CAB3* promoter. This step is important so that true signal transduction mutants can be distinguished from *cis*-acting promoter mutations.

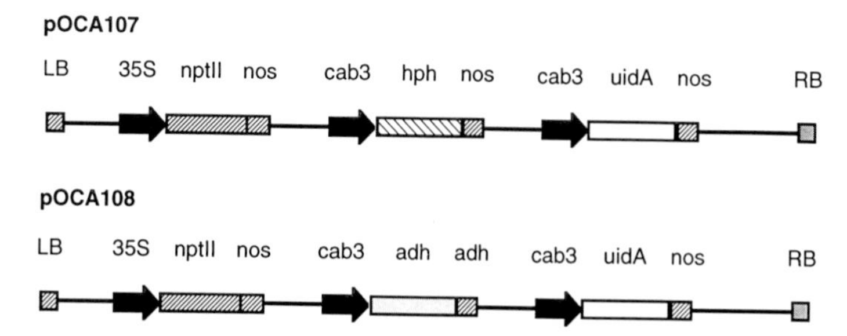

Fig. 1 Promoter fusion constructs for selecting signal transduction mutants. pOCA107 allows selection for hygromycin resistance in the dark or in the presence of norflurazon. The *uid*A gene allows for assaying of β-glucuronidase activity. In pOCA108, negative selection with allyl alcohol is performed to kill plants in which the *CAB* promoter is still active. As for pOCA107, screening for GUS activity subsequent to selection helps delineate promoter mutations from *trans*-acting mutations. In both cases, the selection for the transformation event is by selection for kanamycin resistance (*nptII*), which is expressed from a highly and constitutively expressed plant promoter from cauliflower mosaic virus (35S).

II. Method I: Transformation of *Arabidopsis thaliana*

A. Considerations

Your selectable/screenable marker gene chimeras should be constructed by standard cloning protocols in an *Agrobacterium tumefaciens* disarmed vector. Several protocols are available for transforming Arabidopsis explants using *A. tumefaciens.* The protocols are similar in that they generally use kanamycin to select for transformed cells, although hygromycin selection also works. *Agrobacterium* transformation of Arabidopsis is based on protocols described for other dicotyledonous plants. However, Arabidopsis transformation is unusual in that roots are used as the source of tissue for transformation and regeneration. The methods for transformation of Arabidopsis are constantly being updated and are usually discussed via the internet on the Arabidopsis bulletin board. A slightly modified version of the procedure of Valvekens *et al.* (1988) is used here. Other variations are described in papers referenced at the end of this chapter (Clarke *et al.*, 1992; Huang and Ma, 1992; Koncz *et al.*, 1992). Certain ecotypes of Arabidopsis are easy to transform and regenerate. These include the ecotypes *Nossen, Bensheim,* and *RLD,* although the standard ecotypes used for genetic studies (*Landsberg* and *Columbia*) are also transformable. Seeds are available from the Arabidopsis stock center at Ohio State University or commercially from Lehle Seeds (Tucson, AZ).

B. Media for Transformation

1. Germination Medium (GM)
   1× Murashige and Skoog salt mixture (GIBCO or Sigma)
   1% sucrose

B5 Vitamins (IX):
- 100 mg/liter inositol
- 1.0 mg/liter thiamine
- 0.5 mg/liter pyridoxine
- 0.5 mg/liter nicotinic acid

(adjust to pH 5.7 with 1 *N* KOH)

2. 0.5/0.05 callus-inducing medium (CIM)
   - 1× Gamborg's B5 medium (without 2,4-dichlorophenoxyacetic acid (2,4-D), kinetin, and sucrose) (Sigma)
   - 2% glucose
   - 0.5 g/liter MES
   - (adjust to pH 5.7 with 1 *N* KOH)
   - 0.8% phytagar (for solid 0.5/0.05 medium)
   - 0.5 mg/liter 2,4-D
   - 0.05 mg/liter kinetin
3. 0.5/0.05 T200
   - As 0.5/0.05, but supplemented with 200 mg/liter timentin
4. 0.15/5 shoot-inducing medium (SIM)
   - Gamborg's B5 medium (Sigma)
   - 2% glucose
   - 0.5 g/liter MES (pH 5.7)
   - 0.8% phytagar
   - 5 mg/liter N^6-(2-isopentenyl) adenine (2ip)
   - 0.15 mg/liter indole-3-acetic acid (IAA)
5. 0.15/5 T200 K50
   - As 0.15/5, but supplemented with
     - 200 mg/liter timentin
     - 50 mg/liter kanamycin
6. 12/0.1 root-inducing medium (RIM)
   - Gamborg's B5 medium (Sigma)
   - 2% glucose
   - 0.5 g/liter MES (pH 5.7)
   - 0.8% phytagar
   - 12 mg/liter indole-3-butyric acid (IBA)
   - 0.1 mg/liter kinetin
7. GM K50
   - As GM, but supplemented with 50 mg/liter kanamycin

Notes: (*a*) Hormones can be dissolved in dimethyl sulfoxide (DMSO) or follow the supplier's recommendations; remember to filter-sterilize. Antibiotics are dissolved in water and subsequently filter-sterilized. Hormones and antibiotics are added after autoclaving and cooling of the media to 65°C. (*b*) Petri dishes are sealed with pressure-sensitive tape (Scotch 3M) to minimize condensation.

C. Basic Protocol

1. Growth of Arabidopsis Plants

1. Seed sterilization: i. Wash seeds in 95% ethanol for 1 min. Remove the ethanol by aspiration. ii. Resuspend seeds in 1:3 diluted bleach (containing 3 drops of Tween 20 per 50 ml bleach) for 10 min. Shake gently. iii. Wash seeds in sterile, distilled water five times. iv. After last wash, dispense seeds in 0.5–1 ml 0.1% agar. Shake to disperse seeds evenly in the solution.
2. Growth of seedlings: Inoculate approximately 80 surface-sterilized seeds in 75 ml liquid GM in a 250-ml Erlenmeyer flask on a shaker (100 rpm) for 10–14 days (10 mg seeds/6 flasks GM).

2. Transformation of Root Explants

1. Remove the seedlings and some of the growth medium into a sterile petri dish. The seedlings will be in one intertwined mass.
2. Tear off roots with forceps, taking care that no green parts remain attached to the roots.
3. Incubate roots on solid 0.5/0.05 medium for 4 h; take care that the roots are entirely in contact with the medium.
4. Transfer callus-induced roots to a sterile petri dish containing less than 5 ml liquid 0.5/0.05 media; cut the roots into 0.5-cm explants.

Note: One root explant is composed of multiple root segments and can be considered a cutting of about 0.5 cm through an entire root system and *not* as a cutting through one branch of a root system. When performing infections or washings the explants sometimes fall apart, but then 5–10 root segments are restacked for further incubation.

5. Add 0.5–1 ml of a late log phase *Agrobacterium* culture (28°C; 200 rpm; Luria broth) that has been resuspended in 0.5 vol of liquid 0.5/0.05 media. Shake gently for about 2 min.
6. Blot root explants onto a sterile filter paper to remove most of the liquid; subsequently put them on solidified 0.5/0.05 medium.
7. Incubate up to 30 explants per 100 mm petri dish in the growth room for 2 days to allow *Agrobacterium* transformation. After 2 days of coculturing with *Agrobacterium,* the explants should be completely overgrown by the bacteria.
8. Transfer the explants to 10–20 ml of liquid 0.5/0.05 T200 medium; mix to wash off agrobacteria; blot root explants for a few seconds on sterile filter paper;

transfer explants to solified 0.15/5 T200 K50 medium, taking care that root explants are in close contact with the medium.

9. Incubate in growth room for 3 weeks. After 1–2 weeks tiny, green calli appear on the yellowish root explants. About 1 week later the green calli form shoots; these shoots are initially often vitreous (watery) but turn into "normal" structures a few days later.

10. Transfer the explants to fresh solid 0.15/5 T200 K50 medium every 3–4 weeks.

11. Transfer "normal" shoots (at least two leaves) to solid 12/0.1 for 4 days; then transfer to GM.

Shoots should be incubated on 12/0.1 at relatively high densities. To obtain seeds *in vitro* the transformants should be cultured at very low density (two to four shoots petri dish) and the lid of the petri dish should be absolutely free of condensation. Rooted transformants should be transferred to soil to set seed.

3. Germination of F1 Progeny

To test for transformations, F1 seedlings are germinated on GM K50.

1. Plate seeds (after drying for about 1 week) on GM K50; seal with pressure-sensitive tape.
2. Put petri dish in the dark at 4°C (refrigerator) overnight.
3. Incubate petri dish in growth room for 2 weeks. Sensitive seedlings do not form roots or leaves, and show white cotyledons; transformed seedlings are phenotypically normal.

III. Method II: Screen/Selection for Signal Transduction Pathway Mutants

A. General Considerations

To increase the chances of obtaining desired mutants and to minimize the number of false positives, the promoter used in the transgene construct should have certain properties. For instance, if you seek *trans*-acting regulatory mutations that result in overexpression of a certain gene, the promoter of that gene should have no or very low basal levels of expression at the developmental stage at which mutants are sought. If you are looking for mutants with reduced levels of expression, the promoter should have a high and stable level of expression. As mentioned in the Introduction, it is also advantageous to make a transgenic construct with the promoter sequences fused to two different reporter genes. After transformation of Arabidopsis, the transgenic plants should be characterized for the expression of the reporter genes. The reporter genes should have the same expression pattern as the endogenous gene from which the promoter was derived. Large numbers of seeds from the transgenic line can then be propagated for mutagenesis and screening.

Several things should be taken into consideration in designing a mutant screen. First, you should conduct a detailed kinetic study for the regulated expression of the promoter and determine the time point that best distinguishes between mutant and wild-type plants. Whenever possible, plants should be grown under conditions in which a large number of seedlings can be treated with the selection drugs easily and evenly. However, these growth conditions should not alter normal physiological processes, especially the expression of the gene of interest. In addition, a range of concentrations of the selection drug should be tested to facilitate the choice of a concentration that minimizes false positives while still allowing the recovery of mutants. Three different examples of screening conditions, including both positive and negative selection strategies, are outlined below. The conditions outlined here apply specifically to the identification of signal transduction pathway mutants that are affected in the regulated expression of the *CAB3* promoter, however, the protocols should be generally applicable to the analysis of other signal transduction pathways as well.

B. Materials

Mutagens: e.g., ethyl methanesulfonate (EMS)

γ-ray or X-ray source

1,2:3,4-diepoxybutane (DEB)

MS medium: Murashige and Skoog salt mixture (GIBCO)

Gamborg's vitamin mix (Sigma), 2% (w/v) sucrose, pH 5.8, with KOH.

Hygromycin B (Boehringer Mannheim)

Allyl alcohol (Sigma)

Norflurazon (Sandoz)

GUS fixation buffer (0.3 *M* mannitol; 10 m*M* MES, pH 5.6; 0.3% formaldehyde)

GUS wash buffer (50 m*M* sodium phosphate, pH 7)

X-Gluc solution: (Dissolve 5 mg X-gluc in 0.1 ml dimethyl formamide and then 50 m*M* sodium phosphate buffer, pH 7, to 5–10 ml total vol)

C. Basic Protocols

1. Mutagenesis

Protocols for several different mutagenesis strategies are described.

EMS: Weigh 25,000 to 50,000 transgenic seeds in an Ehrlenmeyer flask (1000 seeds weigh about 20 mg) and add 50 to 100 ml sterile water. IN A FUME

HOOD, add EMS to 0.3% (v/v). Incubate seeds in this EMS solution with gentle shaking overnight at room temperature. Rinse with sterile water three to five times. Used EMS solutions can be decontaminated by addition of an excess of 1 *M* NaOH.

γ-ray: Imbibe seeds overnight in water; then irradiate with a cobalt-60 source at a dosage of 30 krad.

DEB: Imbibe seeds overnight in water and then resuspended in a solution of 22 m*M* DEB at room temperature for 4 h with shaking. Rinse away the DEB with several water washes.

Mutagenized seeds (M_1 seeds) are sown in soil and the plants are allowed to self-fertilize to obtain homozygous recessive mutations. Seeds from these self-fertilized M_1 plants (M_2 seeds) are then used for the mutant screens.

2. Mutant Screens

a. Positive Selection for Aberrant High Expression of a Promoter

Figure 2 illustrates a generalized scheme for isolation of mutants using promoter fusions. Individual examples are detailed below.

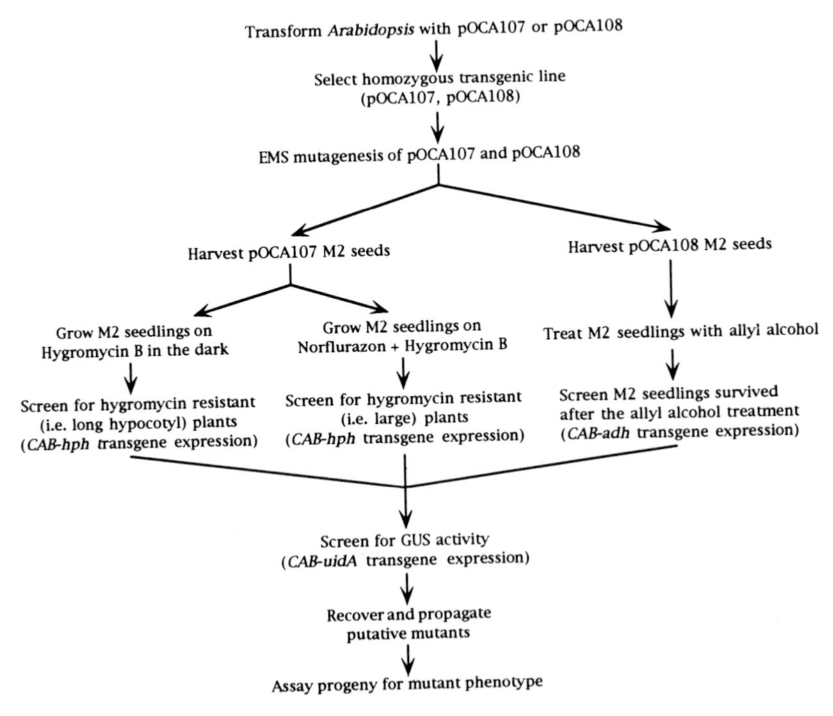

Fig. 2 Generalized scheme for mutant screens.

Example 1: Mutants That Overexpress CAB in the Dark
Note: This protocol is designed to identify mutants that aberrantly express *CAB* in the dark, a growth condition in which *CAB* expression is normally very low (about 50- to 100-fold lower than *CAB* transcription in light-grown seedlings). This protocol can be adapted to select for mutants in which a promoter is constitutively derepressed.

1. Pour MS media containing 20 to 40 μg/ml hygromycin B in petri dishes of 150-mm diameter. Let plates sit (with lids on) in the hood overnight. Because these plates are going to be wrapped in layers of aluminum foil after the sowing of seeds, excess moisture in the plates should be removed.

2. Sterilize seeds by washing 1 min with 95% ethanol, 10 to 15 min with 33% (v/v) house bleach containing 0.02% Tween 20, and then five to six times with sterile water. Do the last one or two washes in the hood. Seeds can be resuspended in sterile 0.1% agarose to facilitate dispensing. About 1000 seeds can be sown on one 150-mm petri dish. Try to disperse the seeds on the plates as evenly as possible. Controls lines should be sown on every plate. Take extra precaution in sterilizing and sowing of seeds since these plates cannot be checked for contamination once they are put into the dark.

3. Cold treat the seeds on plates for 1 to 2 days followed by 1 day of light treatment to stimulate germination.

4. Wrap plates in two layers of aluminum foil and put them into a dark growth chamber for 5 to 8 days. Hygromycin-resistant mutants (i.e., mutants that overexpress the *CAB* promoter controlling the hygromycin phosphotransferase gene) should have longer hypocotyls than the wild-type seedlings (Fig. 3).

5. Potential mutants are rescued to MS medium plates without hygromycin. Seedlings will have almost no roots at this point since the *CAB* promoter is not expressed in roots. Try to lay the rescued seedlings on plates so that the entire seedling is in contact with the medium. This will increase the seedling survival rate.

6. Potential mutants that recover and set seeds are further screened for the expression of the second reporter gene (the GUS gene) following growth in the dark for the same length of time as for the hygromycin selection in the previous generation. Etiolated seedlings are harvested and assayed for the activity of GUS by the fluorometric assay (Jefferson, 1987). About 20 etiolated seedlings will provide enough tissue for one assay.

Example 2: Mutants That Express CAB in the Absence of Chloroplast Development
Note: This protocol is specific for the identification of mutants in an interorganellar signal transduction pathway between the chloroplast and the nucleus. The selection relies on the use of a herbicide called norflurazon, which is a noncompetitive inhibitor of the carotenoid biosynthetic enzyme phytoene desaturase. The presence of norflurazon in the growth medium causes seedlings to photobleach

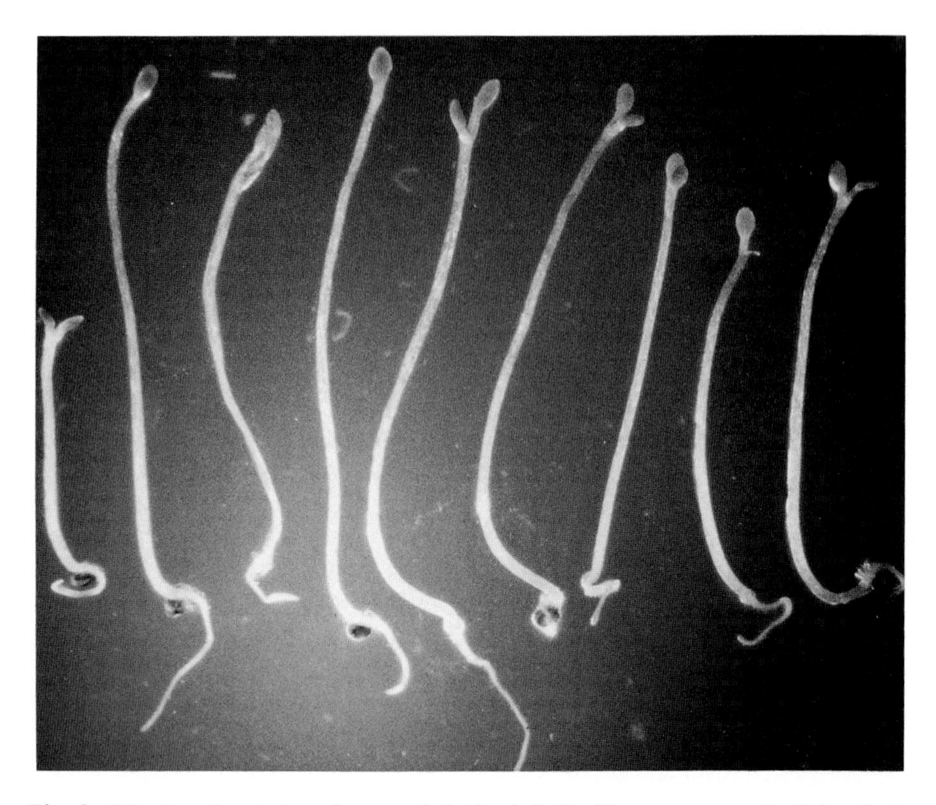

Fig. 3 Selection of mutants on hygromycin in the dark. Seedlings were grown for 7 days in the dark on media containing 20 μg/ml of hygromycin B. The seedling on the left is wild type, followed by eight hygromycin-resistant putative mutants (Li *et al.,* 1994). Reprinted with permission from Cold Spring Harbor Press, New York.

due to the generation of oxygen free radicals (normally scavenged by carotenoids present in thylakoid membranes). In the presence of norflurazon, chloroplasts do not develop and the transcription of several nuclear-encoded genes (e.g., *CAB, RBCS*) for chloroplast-localized proteins is repressed. This protocol could be generalized for other signal transduction pathway mutants if an inhibitor of a regulated response is available.

1. Pour MS medium containing 5 m*M* norflurazon and 20 mg/ml hygromycin B in 150-mm-diameter petri dishes.
2. Sterilize M2 seeds and sow on the plates as described above.
3. Incubate seeds on plates under continuous high fluence rate light (2×10^{16} quanta/s/cm^2) after the cold treatment at 4°C for 1 to 2 days.

4. After 7–10 days, *CAB3-hph* transgene expression is monitored by visual inspection for large seedlings (Fig. 4).

5. Putative hygromycin-resistant seedlings are then assayed for *CAB3-uidA* transgene expression. Snip off one of the cotyledons of each putative hygromycin-resistant seedling and submerge it in fixation solution in a microfuge tube. This fixation step is recommended to prevent recovery from photobleaching during the incubation. After incubation at room temperature for 30–45 min wash with 50 m*M* Na-PO_4, pH 7, twice, then add X-gluc solution. Incubate it at 37°C for 12–24 h. The remainder of the seedling is transferred to an MS plate (without norflurazon and hygromycin) and allowed to recover and set seeds.

6. M3 plants of putative mutants grown in the presence of norflurazon are reexamined for GUS activity by both the histochemical and the fluorimetric

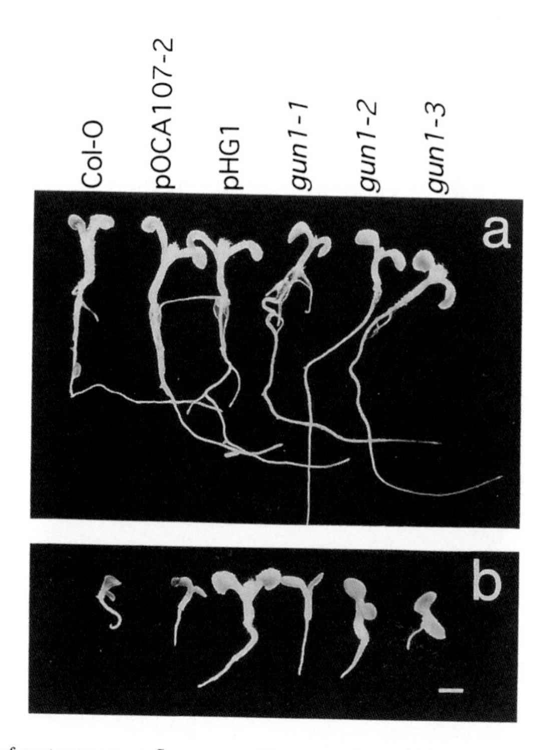

Fig. 4 Selection of mutants on norflurazon and hygromycin in bright white light. Wild-type Columbia (Col-O), transgenic wild-type (pOCA107-2), a positive control for growth on hygromycin (pHG1), and *gun* mutants were germinated and grown for 7 days in the presence of norflurazon with or without hygromycin B (Susek *et al.,* 1993). (a) In the absence of hygromycin B, all photobleached plants are the same size. (b) In the presence of hygromycin B, the *gun* mutants and PHG1 appear large owing to their hygromycin resistance. In contrast, the hygromycin-sensitive pOCA107-2 and Columbia plants are small. Scale bar, 1 mm. Reprinted with permission from *Cell* Press.

assays (Jefferson, 1987). Ten to 20 seedlings from 5-day-old photobleached seedlings are sufficient for a fluorimetric assay.

b. Negative Selection for Reduced Expression of a Promoter

Mutants with Reduced CAB Expression in the Light

Note: This protocol is designed to find *trans*-acting mutations that result in plants with a decreased response to a specific stimulus. It should be effective for the identification of mutants in any situation for which a promoter is highly transcribed.

1. Sterilize seeds as described above and sow about 300 seeds into each well of a six-well tissue culture dish (Costar). Each well should contain 9 ml of liquid MS medium.
2. Cold-treat seeds in culture dishes for 1 to 2 days then move dishes to a shaker. Let seeds germinate and grow in the liquid medium for 5 days under continuous light with shaking.
3. Replace the liquid MS medium in the wells with MS medium containing 2.5 to 3 m*M* allyl alcohol and incubate for 1 to 1.5 h. Remove the medium containing allyl alcohol and rinse the plant tissue twice with MS medium. Transfer the plant tissue onto solid MS medium in petri dishes.
4. Initially, cotyledons from almost all the plants will be killed by the allyl alcohol treatment—turning white then brown in about 2 days. Plants that survive will gradually make green leaves in the next few weeks.
5. Seeds from potential mutants that survive the allyl alcohol treatment are sown and the seedlings tested for the expression of the GUS gene by the fluorimetric assay (Jefferson, 1987).

IV. Genetic Characterization

Now that you have putative mutants, the first thing you need to do is an additional check for the expression of the endogenous mRNA using RNA gel blot analysis. If the expression of the endogenous gene is also elevated or reduced as reflected by the reporter genes, these mutants should then be back-crossed to the wild type to eliminate any mutations other than the one that causes the gene expression phenotype. From the phenotype of the F1 and F2 seedlings of the back-cross, you should be able to determine whether the mutation is dominant or recessive and whether the phenotype is caused by a defect in a single gene. Mutant plants from the F2 population can be further back-crossed and crossed to other ecotypes in preparation for mapping of the mutant loci. Linkage of the mutant loci to the transgene is determined by the segregation ratio in F2 seedlings (the number of mutants in the F2 population that contain the transgene) from crosses to lines that do not contain the transgene. Mutants should also be crossed to one another to determine the number of complementation groups defined by the new collection of mutants.

V. Results and Discussion

We have successfully implemented the three screening protocols described and some representative results are outlined below (Susek *et al.*, 1993; Li *et al.*, 1994; Li and Chory, unpublished). To isolate mutants that overexpressed *CAB* in the dark, 98,000 M2 seeds were screened. From these, 375 putative mutants were selected as hygromycin resistant (longer hypocotyls than that of the wild type). Forty of these lines also had higher GUS activities than the wild type in the dark. After rescreening for the expression of both reporter genes in the next few generations, 8 mutants consistantly showed longer hypocotyls on hygromycin-containing media and had higher GUS activity than the wild type in the dark. RNA gel blot experiments indicated that 7 of the mutants had elevated *CAB* mRNA levels in the dark compared to the wild type. Three of these mutants were characterized in detail because they had the highest levels of elevation of *CAB* mRNA. The *CAB* overexpression phenotype in all three mutants resulted from single recessive mutations independent of the transgene. The three mutants also complemented one another, indicating that they had defined three new loci controlling the expression of *CAB* in the dark.

We screened 100,000 EMS-mutagenized M2 seedlings to isolate mutants that expressed *CAB* in the presence of norflurazon in bright light. We found 227 photobleached plants that appeared hygromycin-resistant and showed GUS histochemical staining. Of these, 138 recovered and were fertile. We assayed their M3 and M4 progeny and found 12 independent mutants with heritable mutant phenotypes. The mutants accumulate endogenous *CAB* and *RBCS* mRNAs following growth on norflurazon. These 12 mutations (called *gun* for **g**enomes **un**coupled) define at least 3 new loci that are implicated in an intracellular signal transduction pathway between the chloroplast and the nucleus. In addition *gun*1 mutants are unable to green in the light following germination and growth in the dark, suggesting that *GUN*1 also modulates the coordinate changes in the nucleus and chloroplast genomes during early stages of photosynthetic growth.

To isolate mutants with reduced *CAB* transcription in the light, 56,000 M2 seeds were screened by treatment with allyl alcohol. One hundred seventy-two plants survived and set seeds. Although experiments are still in progress, at least two mutants with reduced endogenous *CAB* mRNA levels have been identified. The two mutations are both recessive and complement each other, thus identifying two new loci that positively regulate *CAB* gene expression in the light.

VI. Conclusions

The experiments described here have identified at least seven new regulatory genes that control *CAB* gene expression under a variety of conditions. The methodology should be generally applicable to the study of any regulated plant promoter and should prove useful in describing the important controlling elements involved in signal transduction in plants.

References

Bonner, J. J., Parks, C., Parker-Thornburg, J. Mortin, M. A., and Pelham, H. R. B. (1984). The use of promoter fusions in Drosophila genetics: Isolation of mutations affecting the heat shock response. *Cell* **37,** 979–991.

Chang, C., and Meyerowitz, E. M. (1986). Molecular cloning and DNA sequence of the *Arabidopsis thaliana* alcohol dehydrogenase gene. *Proc. Natl. Acad. Sci. U.S.A.* **83,** 1408–1412.

Clarke, M. C., Wei, W., and Lindsey, K. (1992). High-frequency transformation of *Arabidopsis thaliana* by *Agrobacterium tumefaciens. Plant. Mol. Biol. Rep.* **10,** 178–189.

Gritz, L., and Davies, J. (1983). Plasmid-encoded hygromycin B resistance: The sequence of hygromycin B phosphotransferase gene and its expression in *Escherichia coli* and *Saccharomyces cerevisiae. Gene* **25,** 179–188.

Guarante, L., Yocum, R. R., and Gifford, P. (1982). A *GAL*10-*CYC*1 hybrid yeast promoter identifies the *GAL*4 regulatory region as an upstream site. *Proc. Natl. Acad. Sci. U.S.A.* **79,** 7410–7414.

Huang, H., and Ma, H. (1992). An improved procedure for transforming *Arabidopsis thaliana* (*Landsberg erecta*) root explant. *Plant Mol. Biol. Rep.* **10,** 372–383.

Jacobs, M., Dolferus, R., and van den Bossche, D. (1988). Isolation and biochemical analysis of ethyl methanesulfonate-induced alcohol dehydrogenase null mutants of *Arabidopsis thaliana* (L) Heynh. *Biochem. Genet.* **26,** 105–112.

Jefferson, R. A. (1987). Assaying chimeric genes in plants: The GUS gene fusion system. *Plant Mol. Biol. Rep.* **5,** 387–405.

Koncz, C., Schell, J., and Redei, G. P. (1992). T-DNA transformation and insertion mutagenesis. *In* "Methods in Arabidopsis Research" (C. Koncz, N.-H Chua, and J. Schell, eds.), pp. 224–273. River Edge, NJ: World Scientific Publishing.

Leutwiler, L., Meyerowitz, E. M., and Tobin, E. M. (1986). Structure and expression of three light-harvesting chlorophyll a/b binding protein genes in *Arabidopsis thaliana. Nucleic Acids Res.* **14,** 4051–4064.

Li, H.-M., Altschmied, L., and Chory, J. (1994). Arabidopsis mutants define downstream branches in the phototransduction pathway. *Genes Dev.* **8,** 339–349.

Meyerowitz, E. M. (1989). Arabidopsis, a useful weed. *Cell* **56,** 263–269.

Rando, R. R. (1974). Allyl alcohol induced irreversible inhibition of yeast alcohol dehydrogenase. *Biochem. Pharmacol.* **23,** 2328–2331.

Susek, R. E., Ausubel, F. M., and Chory, J. (1993). Signal transduction mutants of Arabidopsis uncouple nuclear *CAB* and *RBCS* gene expression from chloroplast development. *Cell* **74,** 787–799.

Taylor, W. C. (1989). Regulatory interactions between nuclear and plastid genomes. *Annu. Rev. Plant Physiol. Plant Mol. Biol.* **40,** 211–233.

Valvekens, D., van Montagu, M., and van Lijsebettens, M. (1988). *Agrobacterium tumefaciens*-mediated transformation of *Arabidopsis thaliana* root explants by using kanamycin selection. *Proc. Natl. Acad. Sci. U.S.A.* **85,** 5536–5540.

CHAPTER 32

Induction of Signal Transduction Pathways through Promoter Activation

R. Walden, K. Fritze, and H. Harling

Max-Planck-Institut für Züchtungsforschung
Carl-von-Linné-Weg 10
D-50829 Köln, Germany

I. Introduction

T-DNA tagging has emerged as a powerful technique for the isolation of genes from higher plants (Feldmann, 1991; Walden *et al.,* 1991; Koncz *et al.,* 1992). Based on the transfer of T-DNA from *Agrobacterium tumefacians* to the plant genome (Zambryski, 1992), T-DNA tagging capitalizes on the tendency of the T-DNA to insert preferentially into potentially transcribed regions of the plant genome (Koncz *et al.,* 1989). Insertion of the T-DNA into a transcriptional unit routinely results in a recessive mutation by virtue of gene disruption. In diploid

METHODS IN CELL BIOLOGY, VOL. 49

plants such mutations only become apparent following selfing of the mutagenized population. Moreover, the appearance of specific mutations is a matter of chance.

Possibly the most effective use of T-DNA as a tag has been demonstrated by Feldmann and co-workers using Arabidopsis seedling transformation (Feldmann *et al.,* 1989; Feldmann, 1991; Feldmann, 1992). Here populations of plants arising as progeny from selfing of inoculated individuals are screened for novel phenotypes. A wide variety of tagged genes have been isolated by this method and it is notable that many, important in controlling specific developmental pathways, could not have been isolated by other, more conventional, methods (for review, see Coomber and Feldmann, 1993).

Recently, the use of T-DNA tagging has been further refined so that dominant mutations might be generated (Hayashi *et al.,* 1992). This is accomplished by engineering the T-DNA to contain the transcriptional enhancer sequence of the 35S RNA promoter of cauliflower mosaic virus cloned as a tetramer at the right T-DNA border sequence. The idea behind the design of such a tag is that following insertion into the plant genome, expression of flanking plant genes is activated as a result of the influence of the multiple transcriptional enhancers and that overexpression produces a dominant mutation. Production of dominant mutations allows selection for a specific phenotype to be applied at the level of primary transformants. This approach has come to be known as activation tagging. Protoplast cocultivation with an Agrobacterium containing such a tag allows the production of extremely large populations of transgenic cells to which a biochemical selection can be applied. By selecting for growth of protoplasts in the absence of auxin following cocultivation, we have used this method to isolate genes functional in auxin perception/signal transduction (Hayashi *et al.,* 1992; Walden *et al.,* in preparation).

In this review, we detail the experimental protocols underlying the process of activation tagging. Although we concentrate on the use of this experimental approach to generate mutant cell (and plant) lines able to grow in culture in the absence of auxin, we also discuss the general use of this method of tagging to isolate genes whose overexpression results in a selectable phenotype.

II. Materials

A. Agrobacterium and the T-DNA Tagging Vector

The host Agrobacterium we have used is GV3101 containing the helper plasmid pMP90RK. pMP90RK encodes kanamycin and gentamycin resistance while the bacterial chromosome encodes rifampicin resistance (Koncz and Schell, 1986). The tagging vector pPCVICEn_4 HPT (Fig. 1A; Hayashi *et al.,* 1992) comprises four components:

a. the plasmid backbone containing T-DNA border sequences, origin of replication, and plasmid maintenance functions specific for Agrobacterium derived from the pPCV series of vectors (Koncz and Schell, 1986).

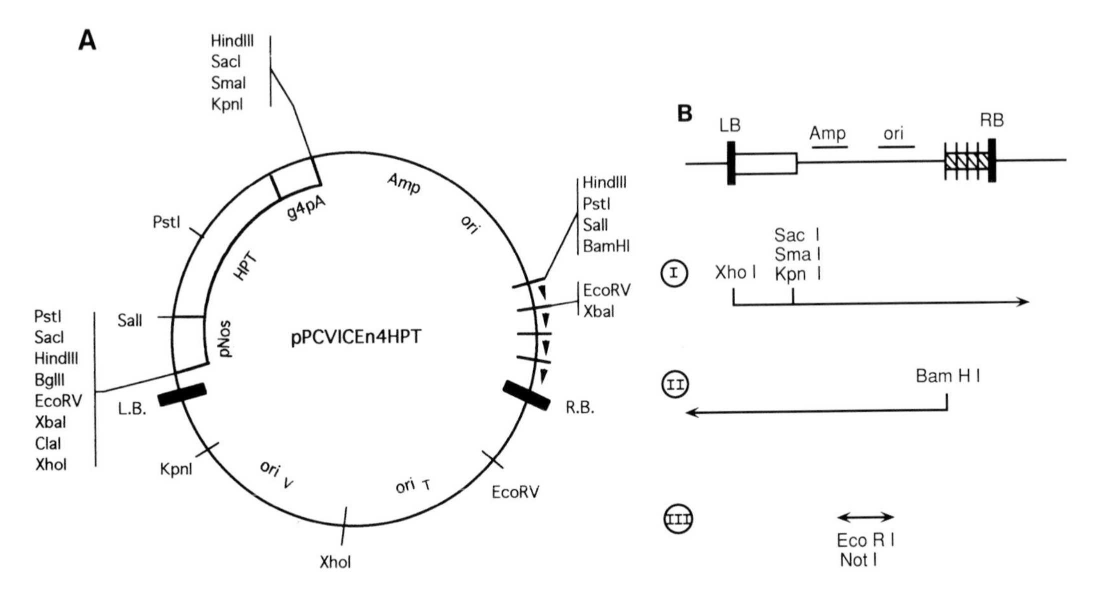

Fig. 1 Structure of the tagging vector pPCVICEn$_4$HPT. (A) Plasmid map. Functional regions and selected restriction sites are as shown. The arrowheads indicate the position of enhancer sequence derived from CaMV 35S promoter. (B) Organization of T-DNA in plant genome. Enzymes used in plasmid rescue of plant DNA to the right of the T-DNA insert (I); to the left of the insert (II), or on both sides of the insert are shown (III).

b. a hygromycin resistance gene linked to the nos promoter and the T-DNA gene 4 polyadenylation sequence derived from pGDW44 (Wing *et al.,* 1989) located at the left border sequence.

c. the sequence of the *Escherichia coli* plasmid pIC19H (Marsh *et al.,* 1984) containing an *E. coli* origin of replication and ampicillin resistance gene. In Agrobacterium the presence of the ampicillin resistance gene allows selection on carbenicillin.

d. the transcriptional enhancer sequence of the CaMV 35S promoter (−90 to −427) cloned as as a tetramer at the right border sequence.

The plasmid was introduced into GV3101 by transformation (Ebert *et al.,* 1987).

B. Plant Material

Tobacco SR1 is used throughout (Maliga *et al.,* 1975).

C. Chemicals, Enzymes, and Media

Fine chemicals are obtained from Merck AG, Darmstadt; Serva Feinbiochemika GmbH und Co., Heidelberg; Sigma Chemie GmbH, München. Enzymes for protoplasts: Serva, Heidelberg. PEG4000: Merck AG, Darmstadt. Restriction enzymes and nucleic acid-modifying enzymes are obtained from Boehringer GmbH, Mannheim; GIBCO BRL, Hamburg; New England Biolabs GmbH, Schwalbach. Culture media is obtained from Difco, Detroit; MS-salts, Sigma, München.

III. Methods

A. Bacterial Culture

The bacteria are maintained and handled using standard techniques (Draper *et al.*, 1988). We find, upon reactivation from glycerol stocks, that the tagging vector is missing from ~50% of the colonies plated on YEB media (see Table I) lacking selection. Hence following initial plating we use sequential selection on YEB containing carbenicillin (100 μg/ml), kanamycin (25 μg/ml) and/or gentamycin (40 μg/ml), and finally rifampicillin (100 μg/ml). For routine maintenance of bacteria, we culture in YEB containing carbenicillin.

B. Protoplast Cocultivation with Agrobacterium

Mesophyll protoplasts are prepared from 6- to 8-week-old (sterile) tobacco plants cultured at 22–24°C, 16 h day/8 h night on MS media (Murashige and Skoog, 1962) solidified with 1% agar. Protoplasts are isolated using a standard

Table I
Bacterial Media

YEB media	
	Beef extract, 5 g/liter
	Bacto yeast extract, 1 g/liter
	Bactopeptone, 1 g/liter
	Sucrose, 5 g/liter
pH 7.4	
Solidified with 2% agar	
Add after autoclaving and shortly before use: 2 ml/liter 1 *M* $MgSO_4$.	
LB media (Sambrook)	
	Bacto yeast extract, 5 g/liter
	Bacto tryptone, 10 g/liter
	NaCl, 5 g/liter
pH 7	
Solidified with 1.5% agar	

protocol (Negrutiu *et al.,* 1987). Briefly, leaf tissue is cut into ca. 1-cm^2 pieces and approx. 5 g of leaf material is placed in 20 ml of enzyme solution [1.5% cellulase R10; 0.5% macerozyme in 0.4 *M* K_3 media (see Table II)] and filter-sterilized. Incubation is carried out overnight at 26°C in the dark. After a 10-min mixing on an orbital shaker (~40 rpm) the solution is passed through a 100-μm sieve and divided into 12-ml plastic centrifuge tubes (Nunc). Centrifugation is carried out at ~3000 rpm in a swingout bucket centrifuge for 6 min. Cell debris and the solution underlying the floating protoplasts are carefully removed and the tube is refilled with 0.4 *M* K3 media, gently mixed, and centrifuged once more. The majority of the underlying solution is removed and the protoplasts are bulked and the yield estimated. Normally 10^6 protoplasts are obtained per 10 ml enzyme solution used.

Agrobacterium–protoplast cocultivation (Marton *et al.,* 1979) is carried out using protoplasts cultured for 4–6 days in 0.4 *M* K3 media, by which time the protoplasts should be initiating cell division. Protoplasts are incubated with a fresh culture of Agrobacterium grown in YEB media containing carbenicillin (100 μg/ml) at a density of 2×10^7 bacteria/ml to 2×10^5 protoplast/ml (i.e., 100:1) (Depicker *et al.,* 1985). The protoplast density is adjusted with 0.4 *M* K3 media and the density of bacteria judged by measuring the optical density at OD 600 nm. For 10^6 protoplasts the amount of bacteria used (in μl) is calculated as

$$\frac{100}{1.8 \times OD_{600}}.$$

Cocultivation is allowed to proceed at 26°C in the dark for 48 h. By this time, it will be clear microscopically that the bacteria have multiplied and formed large aggregates; moreover, individual bacteria will be seen adhering to the walls of individual protoplasts.

The protoplasts are washed 3× in W5 media (Table II; or seawater) at 700 rpm for 3 min in a swingout bucket rotor at room temperature. The protoplasts are resuspended in 0.4 *M* K3 media at a density of 10^6 PP/10 ml and 10^6 protoplasts are transferred to 94-mm petri dishes and cultured in 10 ml 0.4 *M* K3 media containing 500 mg/liter claforan, 15 mg/liter hygromycin, 1 mg/liter auxin, and 0.2 mg/liter kinetin. It is important that selective antibiotics be freshly made. At this point selection can be initiated. When selecting for protoplast growth in the absence of auxin the media contains kinetin alone.

Protoplasts are cultured in the light for 2 days at 26°C and then embedded in "low-melting" agarose (Shillito *et al.,* 1983). Before embedding, the concentrations of selective antibiotics and hormones are doubled so that their concentrations are maintained following addition of the agarose. For each 10^6 protoplasts embedding is carried out in a 9-mm petri dish by adding 10 ml of hand-warm 1.6% agarose solution in 0.2 *M* K3 and the resulting solidified agar is cut into quarters and transferred to a 145-mm petri dish to which 20 ml of 0.3 *M* K3 media containing selective antibiotics and hormones is added. Culture is carried out at 26°C in the light.

Table II
Plant Media

0.4 *M* K3 media	
NaH_2PO_4	150 mg/liter
$CaCl_2$	900 mg/liter
KNO_3	2500 mg/liter
NH_4NO_3	250 mg/liter
$(NH_4)_2SO_4$	134 mg/liter
$MgSO_4$	250 mg/liter
Microelements[a]	1 ml/liter
Vitamins[b]	1 ml/liter
Inositol	100 mg/liter
Xylose	250 mg/liter
Sucrose[c]	136.9 g/liter
Fe · EDTA[d]	5 ml/liter
Adjust to pH 5.8 with KOH	
MS media	
Macroelements	
NH_4NO_3	1650 mg/liter
KNO_3	1900 mg/liter
$CaCl_2 \cdot 2H_2O$	440 mg/liter
$MgSO_4 \cdot 2H_2O$	370 mg/liter
KH_2PO_4	170 mg/liter
Microelements	
Na_2EDTA	37.3 mg/liter
$FeSO_4 \cdot 7H_2O$	27.8 mg/liter
H_3BO_3	6.2 mg/liter
$MnSO_4 \cdot H_2O$	16.9 mg/liter
$ZnSO_4 \cdot 7H_2O$	8.6 mg/liter
KI	0.83 mg/liter
$Na_2MoO_4 \cdot 2H_2O$	0.25 mg/liter
$CuSO_4 \cdot 5H_2O$	25 μg/liter
$CoCl_2 \cdot 6H_2O$	25 μg/liter
Vitamins	
Myoinositol	100 mg/liter
Thiamine-HCl	0.1 mg/liter
Glycine	2.0 mg/liter
Nicotinic acid	0.5 mg/liter
Pyridoxine-HCl	0.5 mg/liter
Sucrose	10 g/liter, pH 5.8
Solidified with 10 g/liter agar	
	W5 medium
	154 m*M* NaCl
	125 m*M* $CaCl_2 \cdot 2H_2O$
	5 m*M* KCl

continues

continued

	5 m*M* glucose pH 5.6 → 6
	MaMg solution
	450 m*M* mannitol 15 m*M* $MgCl_2$ 0.1% MES pH 5.6
	PEG solution
	0.1 *M* $Ca(NO_2)_3 \cdot 4H_2O$ 0.4 *M* Mannitol 40% PEG4000 pH 7 → 9

[a] Microelement stock solution: KI, 0.83 g/liter; H_3BO_3, 6.2 g/liter; $ZnSO_4 \cdot 7H_2O$, 10.6 g/liter; $CaSO_4 \cdot 5H_2O$, 25 mg/liter; $Na_2MoO_4 \cdot 2H_2O$, 0.25 g/liter; $CoCl_2 \cdot 6H_2O$, 25 mg/liter.

[b] Vitamin stock solution: glycine, 400 mg/200 ml; thiamine-HCl, 20 mg/200 ml; nicotinic acid, 400 mg/200 ml; pyridoxine HCl, 400 mg/200 ml.

[c] 136.9 g/liter sucrose, 0.4 *M* (580–600 mOs); 34.29 g/liter sucrose, 0.1 *M*.

[d] Fe · EDTA solution: 5.57 g/liter $FeSO_4 \cdot 7H_2O$; 7.45 g/liter Na_2EDTA; boiled for 10 min.

C. Callus Formation and Plant Regeneration

Agarose segments are cultured in 145-mm petri dishes in 20 ml 0.3 *M* K3 media containing 15 mg/liter hygromycin, appropriate hormones, and the desired selective pressure. This medium is exchanged at weekly intervals, and at each change the molarity of sucrose reduced successively at 0.1 *M* intervals until 0.1 *M* is reached. Once this concentration is reached, the medium is changed every 2 weeks. In our experience, growing calli can be observed clearly 2 to 3 weeks following transformation.

Routinely we have found that shoot formation occurs spontaneously in the agarose beads in K3 media, although normally this can be obtained when callus is transferred to MS media solidified with 1% agar (and containing 0.1 mg/liter NAA; 0.5 mg/liter BAP). Shoots are allowed to develop for 2–3 weeks, excised, and placed on solid MS media + antibiotics lacking growth substances for root induction. Normally, young plants are transferred to the greenhouse 6 weeks after root formation.

D. Genetic Analysis

In the greenhouse plants are grown to maturity, during which time any obvious phenotypic changes are noted. Plants are self-pollinated and crossed with wild-type SR1. Collected seeds are sterilized (2 min 70% EtOH, 15 min 10% NaOCl + 0.1% SDS, washed 3× with sterile water), air-dried, and plated on MS containing 15 mg/liter hygromycin in 94-mm petri dishes and resistance/sensitivity to the antibiotic is scored using at least 60 individuals. Routinely we find that 50% or more of the plants segregate the hygromycin marker as a single genetic insert. Six to eight heterozygotic plant lines arising from the SR1 outcross are grown to maturity and scored in detail for phenotypic changes. These are once again self-pollinated and progeny screened for a homozygotic line. Homozygocity is confirmed by back-crossing to wild-type SR1 and testing segregation of hygromycin resistance. Homozygotic lines with a single stable T-DNA insertion displaying cosegregation of the hygromycin marker and the mutant phenotype are chosen for detailed molecular analysis. Generally, in the case of mutant lines whose protoplasts form callus in the absence of auxin, the plants themselves do not display an obvious phenotype. Hence, we have had to resort germinating seedlings of T2 and T3 populations on nonselective MS media and allowing them to grow until enough leaf material is available for protoplasting. At this point the upper stem with two or three leaves is removed and placed on MS agar containing the selective antibiotic while remaining leaf tissue is used for protoplast isolation. Independently, the ability of the stem tissue to root on hygromycin-containing media and the protoplasts to divide and grow in the absence of auxin are scored.

E. Molecular Analysis and DNA Rescue

Southern analysis is carried out using DNA isolated from young leaf tissue using standard methods (Dellaporta *et al.,* 1983). Routinely we use the hygromycin resistance gene and the sequence corresponding to the 35S RNA promoter enhancer as hybridization probes. Appropriate enzymes are used to assess copy number as well as the number of left and right border sequences (Fig. 1B). In approximately 50% of the cases studied in detail we have obtained single T-DNA inserts that were not rearranged. In the remaining cases we have observed head-to-head dimers or partial dimers. Depending on the genomic organization of the T-DNA and the position of suitable restriction sites in the plant DNA, different methods for the rescue of the flanking plant DNA potentially containing the tagged gene are available:

a. Inverse PCR (IPCR) allows the rescue of only a few hundred base pairs of plant DNA at the left or right border. Hence, chromosome walking is necessary to isolate larger plant DNA fragments, which need to be ligated to the T-DNA prior to the functional analysis.

b. DNA fragments containing a single T-DNA copy and large fragments of plant DNA at the left and right border can be isolated from a subgenomic library of the transformant. The rescued DNA is cut out of the phage's genome, self-ligated, and rescued in *E. coli* by virtue of the presence within the T-DNA of the origin of replication and ampicillin resistance contained within the T-DNA (Hayashi *et al.*, 1992).

c. Direct plasmid rescue of T-DNA and flanking plant sequences can be carried out in *E. coli* and used directly in functional analysis.

The easiest, fastest, and cheapest isolation procedure is plasmid rescue. To carry out plasmid rescue, an enzyme is selected that cuts the genomic DNA so that (*a*) a single bacterial origin of replication will be represented in the plasmid and (*b*) as much flanking plant DNA as possible is rescued. Five micrograms of plant genomic DNA is digested in a 200-μl volume with 40 units of appropriate enzyme for 4 h under conditions recommended by the manufacturer. The quality of the digest is checked on a minigel using 1 μg DNA. Digested DNA is cleaned by phenol extraction followed by ethanol precipitation. Ligation of 4 μg of DNA is carried out in a 200-μl volume using 2 Weiss units of T4 DNA ligase at 15°C overnight. The ligation reaction is ethanol-precipitated and the DNA pellet is washed three times with 70% ethanol to remove salt completely. The DNA is redissolved in 40 μl H_2O.

Electroporation is used in order to obtain maximal transformation rates using the electroporator manufacturer's instructions. We use Biorad's Gene Pulser connected to a Pulse Controller set at 25 μF, 1.6 kV, 200 Ω, and ElectroMax DH10B cells from GIBCO BRL. Twenty microliters of the electrocompetent cells are thawed on ice, mixed with 2 μl of the ligated DNA, and transferred to a precooled 0.1-cm electroporation cuvette. One pulse (approx. 4.6 ms) is given and 1 ml LB medium (Table I) is immediately pipetted into the cuvette. The medium is transferred to an Eppendorf tube and incubated at 37°C with shaking at 220 rpm for 1 h. The cells are spun down in an Eppendorf centrifuge for 20 s, the supernatant is decanted, and the cells are resuspended in the remaining droplet. The whole suspension is plated on a single LB plate containing 100 μg/ml ampicillin, which is incubated at 37°C overnight.

The number of recovered transformants varies according to the size of the plasmid to be rescued. During the whole procedure extreme care has to be taken to avoid contamination with other plasmids conferring ampicillin resistance. The recovered plasmids are analyzed by miniscreen and the organization of the rescued DNA is compared with that predicted by Southern analysis. In our laboratory, we have isolated unrearranged plasmids of up to 20 kb in this manner.

F. Functional Analysis of Rescued Plant DNA

To prove that overexpression of the isolated plant gene(s) leads to the mutant phenotype (i.e., growth in the absence of auxin), the rescued plasmid DNA is transformed again into SR1 protoplasts for functional testing. Plasmid DNA is prepared in bulk by the alkaline lysis method followed by two CsCl bandings and cleaned by *n*-butanol treatment and dialysis as described (Sambrook *et al.*, 1989). After dialysis the DNA is ethanol precipitated under sterile conditions and dissolved in sterile water at a concentration of 1 μg/ml. Rescued plant DNA is transformed by PEG-mediated DNA uptake of protoplasts (Negrutiu *et al.*, 1987). Protoplasts isolated as described above are resuspended in W5 media (Table II) and spun down by centrifugation at 700 rpm for 3 min. The final protoplast pellet is resuspended in MaMg media (Table II) to give a final concentration of 10^6 protoplasts/ml. Three hundred microliters of this suspension is used for DNA uptake. The cells are heat-shocked by incubating at 45°C for 5 min followed by cooling on ice for 2 min. After 5 min at room temperature 10 μl of the plasmid DNA solution is added to the protoplasts, followed by gentle mixing. Following a 10-min incubation at room temperature, 300 μl of PEG solution (see Table II) is added and again the contents of the tube are gently mixed. After 20 min at room temperature 4.4 ml of 0.4 *M* K3 media is added, the solution is gently mixed, and hormones, or antibiotics, are added as required (NAA 1 mg/liter; kinetin 0.2 mg/liter; kanamycin 100 mg/liter; hygromycin 15 mg/liter). The solution is gently poured into 60-mm petri dishes, which are sealed with parafilm and these are incubated at 26°C in the dark for 2 days. Subsequent culture is in continuous light at 26°C. Scoring of division can be carried out 4–5 days following isolation; at this point, if desired, the protoplasts/microcalli can be embedded. A 1.6% solution of low-melting agarose in 0.2 *M* K3 medium is melted and cooled to body (~37°C) temperature. Antibiotics and hormones are added as appropriate and 5 ml of this solution is slowly added to the petri dishes containing the protoplasts/microcalli and mixed by gentle swirling. The agarose is allowed to gel for at least an hour at room temperature. The solidified agarose is gently cut into four segments and individually transferred with a broad-blade spatula to a 94-mm petri dish and 10 ml of 0.3 *M* K3 media containing appropriate hormones and antibiotics is added. The agarose segments are cultured further in continuous light at 26°C. At weekly intervals, the media is exchanged and at each media change the molarity of sucrose is decreased, in 0.1 *M* intervals, to 0.1 *M*. Ultimately this media is changed every 2 weeks.

IV. Critical Aspects of the Procedure

The practical requirements of T-DNA tagging are:

1. The generation of large numbers of transgenic individuals to ensure that the target genome is saturated with inserts. Protoplast Agrobacterium cocultivation, with a transformation frequency of 10–20% allows this to be achieved with relative ease. Important in this procedure is that cocultivation occurs while the protoplasts are initiating cell division 4–6 days following isolation. This can be judged microscopically. To judge transformation frequency, in parallel with the tagging experiment, we carry out a cocultivation with an Agrobacterium containing a T-DNA vector encoding hygromycin resistance and culture protoplasts under standard conditions and score calli resistant to hygromycin. Agrobacterium–

protoplast cocultivation is currently only feasible with solanaceous plants where high frequencies of cell division, callus formation, and plant regeneration are routinely obtained.

2. An adequate screening procedure for a defined phenotype. The creation of a dominant mutation allows the selection of a specific phenotype at the level of primary transformant, regardless of ploidy. With cocultivation this normally implies a chemical selection at the stage of callus formation. For this selection to be effective, kill curves need to be established, using nontransformed protoplasts growing under the same conditions as those used during cocultivation. In doing this it is important to adopt a standard cell culture density, as well as standard culture conditions. Although to date we have used positive selection, screening for an enzymatic activity such as *lux* or GUS, or even the expression of endogenous genes, for example, those encoding for enzymes of the anthocyanin biosynthetic pathway, may be feasible. The central requirement to screening enzyme activity is the ease of visualization—it needs to be borne in mind that screening will entail several million calli!

3. An ability to link genetically the T-DNA insert to the observed mutation. This is central to the whole concept of T-DNA tagging. Segregation of the hygromycin resistance gene contained within the T-DNA can be used to assess the complexity of the insert. Routinely, this involves selfing and outcrossing of homozygotic individuals (discussed in Walbot, 1992). This can often be simply carried out by testing germination and normal growth of seedlings on petri dishes containing the selective antibiotic. Genetic linkage of a novel phenotype to the T-DNA in our experience has been a somewhat involved process because the majority of the mutations that we have generated are phenotypically neutral in whole plants. Hence we have had to resort to protoplast isolation and testing for growth in the absence of auxin and screening independently for hygromycin resistance. Obviously, this process is involved, labor-intensive and can only be effectively carried out with relatively limited numbers of segregating individuals. A perfect phenotype for screening would be one scorable at the stage of young plantlets, allowing testing to be carried out on petri dishes.

4. A means to isolate the tagged sequence and demonstrate complementation of the mutant phenotype. Plasmid rescue of tagged plant sequences from the genome of the mutant line is the most rapid way of obtaining the coding sequences responsible for the mutant phenotype, but it is not without complications. It is important that the genomic DNA is restricted in a way so that any plasmid obtained following ligation bears only one *E. coli* origin of replication. Hence, if multimers or parial T-DNAs are present at the site of insertion, restriction sites present within the T-DNA itself must be selected so that single replication origins are present. Another point is that following ligation of the digested plant DNA, very high rates of *E. coli* transformation are required to ensure recovering plasmids bearing plant DNA. This necessitates the use of electroporation and the use of competent cells prepared specifically for this technique. Functional

testing of rescued plant sequences is achieved simply and rapidly using the rescued plasmid DNA in PEG-mediated protoplast DNA uptake followed by subsequent culture under selective conditions. In rescuing DNAs promoting protoplast division and growth in the absence of auxin, we find that positive clones can be scored microscopically 4 to 5 days following transfection. The speed and ease of such tests have proven to be the great advantages of generating dominant mutations. Nevertheless, it should be borne in mind that rescue of the tagged genes relies on obtaining the entire (required) coding region of the gene in question. Prior to isolation there is no means of assessing directly where the gene is located with respect to left or right T-DNA border sequences, nor how far it may be from the T-DNA insert. Although initial work concerning the action of a duplication of the 35S RNA promoter enhancer indicated that a dimer greatly increased levels of expression of a promoter 2 kbp distant following transformation (Kay *et al.,* 1989), no information is available for us to judge the positional limits of such an enhancement following insertion of tetramers of the transcriptional enhancer into the genome. To complicate matters further, we are unable to judge just how much overexpression is required of a target gene in order to obtain a selectable phenotype. To date, in mutant analysis in our laboratory, we have found that the T-DNA may have inserted upstream or downstream of a target gene at distances up to 10 kb from the presumed transcriptional start site. Most of the tagged genes that we have analyzed in detail are located to the right-hand side of the right T-DNA border sequence, although we would suspect that this is no hard-and-fast rule.

V. Discussion

This review describes the practicalities of activation tagging using a T-DNA containing multiple transcriptional enhancers. The creation of dominant mutations through transcriptional activation provides two immediate advantages over other strategies of gene tagging. First, it allows the direct selection for a specific phenotype from among the population of primary transformants. Second, it eases screening for function of rescued plant sequences following transformation of wild-type cells. Coupled with Agrobacterium protoplast cocultivation, activation tagging could be applied to generate cell lines, and ultimately plant lines, selected for growth under any biochemical selection. Here we have described the use of the procedure to generate cell lines characterized by their ability to grow in culture in the absence of auxin in the media.

Similarly, we have used this approach to produce cell lines able to grow in the absence of cytokinin (Miklashevichs and Walden, unpublished) or in the presence of selective levels of an inhibitor of polyamine biosynthesis (Fritze and Walden, in preparation). This suggests that the procedure may have general application. An advantage of the approach is that the selection does not require a detailed understanding of the process under investigation. Hence the mutations obtained could be applied to study poorly understood processes, such as the molecular basis of plant hormone action for which mutants are not available at the present time.

Currently the genes that have been tagged using the outlined selection strategies are under investigation and the function of the gene products remains unknown. However, on theoretical grounds, one might envisage that a variety of tagged genes might be isolated. Where selection has been carried out for growth in the absence of a specific growth substance, by analogy with the initial work with protoplast cocultivation (Marton *et al.,* 1979), where hormone independent protoplast growth was obtained following cocultivation with wild-type Agrobacterium, one may infer that genes involved in hormone biosynthesis might be tagged. On the other hand the recent finding that protoplasts overexpressing *rolB* and *rolC* form callus in the absence of auxin and cytokinin, respectively (Walden *et al.,* 1993), would suggest that genes modifying the intracellular concentrations of active growth substances might be tagged. Finally, by analogy with cellular proto-oncogenes in animal systems, one might envisage that genes encoding proteins involved with the hormone perception/signal transducton pathway might be selected. Where positive selection is applied, genes whose products are involved in turnover of the selective agent might be obtained. Stated simply: This method of tagging is likely to result in the isolation of any gene whose product directs cell division under selective conditions. Although this may introduce an element of uncertainty into the tagging strategy, it needs to be remembered that any mutation in a little understood biological process may serve as a start to study that process.

Although, to date, we have concentrated on mutations producing growth under positive selection, screening transgenic cells for the expression of a marker gene may also be feasible and provide a means dissecting the signal transduction pathways underlying the control of gene expression. For example, a promoter directing gene expression following a specific induction (in response to stress, a pathogen or developmental cues) could be linked to a marker gene such as GUS or *lux.* This combination would be used in transformation to produce a marker plant line in which the marker gene remains unexpressed in protoplasts in the absence of the inducing factor. The marker line could then be used in activation tagging and expression of the marker gene screened for from among the secondary transformants. In such a way factors activating gene expression could be isolated. Extending this notion further, it may be feasible to use activation tagging to induce the expression of genes whose products are responsible for catalyzing biosynthetic pathways not normally active in protoplasts.

Finally, whereas in this example we have used enhancer sequences derived from a promoter generally considered to be constitutive in its mode of expression, it may be feasible to develop tagging and selection strategies based on enhancer elements responsive to specific developmental and environmental cues.

Acknowledgments

We thank Jeff Schell for support and encouragment in the development of activation tagging. The success of the approach would not have been possible without the expert technical assistance of Inge Czaja and Elke Bongartz. Our thanks go to Gisela Kobert and Frauke Furkert for preparation of the manuscript. This work has been supported by the Max-Planck-Gesellschaft and Universität Köln, Graduiertenkolleg.

References

Coomber, S. A., and Feldmann, K. A. (1993). *In* "Transgenic Plants, Vol. 1: Gene Tagging in Transgenic Plants" (S.-D. King and R. Wu, eds.), pp. 225–242. New York: Academic Press.

Dellaporta, S. L., Wood, J., and Hicks, J. B. (1983). A plant DNA minipreparation: Version II. *Plant Mol. Biol. Rep.* **1,** 19–21.

Depicker, A. G., Herman, L., Jacobs, A., Schell, J., and Van Montagu, M. (1985). Frequencies of simultaneous tranformation with different T-DNAs and their relevance to *Agrobacterium*/plant cell interaction. *Mol. Gen. Genet.* **201,** 477–484.

Draper, J., Scott, R., Armitage, P., and Walden R. (1988). "Plant Genetic Transformation and Gene Expression, A Laboratory Manual." Oxford: Blackwell.

Ebert, P. R., Ha, S. B., and An, G. (1987). Identification of an essential upstream element in the nopaline synthase promoter by stable and transient assays. *Proc. Natl. Acad. Sci.* U.S.A. **84,** 5745–5749.

Feldmann, K. A., Marks, M. D., Christianson, M. L., and Quatrano, R. S. (1989). A dwarf mutant of *Arabidopsis* generated by T-DNA insertion mutagenesis. *Science* **243,** 1351–1354.

Feldmann, K. A. (1991). T-DNA insertion mutagenesis in *Arabidopsis:* Mutational spectrum. *Plant J.* **1,** 71–82.

Feldmann, K. A. (1992). T-DNA insertion mutagenesis in *Arabidopsis:* Seed infection/transformation. *In* "Methods in Arabidopsis Research" (C. Koncz, N.-H. Chua, and J. Schell, eds.), pp. 274–289. World Scientific Singapore.

Hayashi, H., Czaja, I., Schell, J., and Walden, R. (1992). Activation of a plant gene by T-DNA tagging: Auxin independent growth *in vitro. Science* **258,** 1350–1353.

Kay, R., Chan, A., Daly, M., and McPherson, J. (1987). Duplication of CaMV 35S promoter sequences creates a strong enhancer for plant genes. *Science* **236,** 1299–1302.

Koncz, C., Martini, N., Mayerhofer, R., Koncz-Kalman, Zs., Körber, H., Rédei, G. P., and Schell, J. (1989). High-frequency T-DNA-mediated gene tagging in plants. *Proc. Natl. Acad. Sci. U.S.A.* **86,** 8467–8471.

Koncz, C., Nemeth, K., Rédei, G. P., and Schell. J. (1992). T-DNA insertional mutagenesis in Arabidopsis. *Plant Mol. Biol.* **20,** 963–976.

Koncz, C., and Schell, J. (1986). The promoter of the T_L-DNA gene 5 controls the tissue-specific expression of chimeric genes carried by a novel type of *Agrobacterium* binary vector. *Mol. Gen. Genet.* **204,** 383–396.

Maliga, P., Sz-Breznovits, A., Marton, L., and Joo, F. (1975). Non medelian Streptomycin-resistant tobacco mutant with altered chloroplasts and mitochondria. *Nature* **255,** 401–402.

Marsh, J. L., Erfle, M., and Wykes, E. J. (1984). The pIC plasmid and phage vectors with versatile cloning sites for recombinant selection by insertional inactivation. *Gene* **32,** 481–485.

Marton, L., Wullems, G. J., Molendijk, L., and Schilperoort, R. A. (1979). *In vitro* transformation of cultured cells from *Nicotiana tabacum* by *Agrobacterium tumefaciens. Nature* **277,** 129–131.

Murashige, T., and Skoog, F. (1962). A revised medium for rapid growth and bioassays with tobacco tissue cultures. *Physiol. Plant.* **15,** 473–497.

Negrutiu, I., Shillito, R., Potrykus, I., Biasini, G., and Sala, F. (1987). Hybrid genes in the analysis of transformation conditions. I. Setting up a simple method for direct gene transfer in plant protoplasts. *Plant Mol. Biol.* **8,** 363–373.

Sambrook, J., Fritsch, E. F., and Maniatis, T. (1989). "Molecular Cloning: A Laboratory Manual." Cold Spring Harbor, NY: Cold Spring Harbor Laboratory Press.

Shillito, R. D., Paszkowski, J., and Potrykus, I. (1983). Agarose plating and bead type culture technique enable and stimulate development of protoplast-derived colonies in a number of plant species. *Plant Cell Rep.* **2,** 244–247.

Walbot, V. (1992). Strategies for mutagenesis and gene cloning using transposon tagging and T-DNA insertional mutagenesis. *Annu. Rev. Plant Physiol. Plant Mol. Biol.* **43,** 49–82.

Walden, R., Czaja, I., Schmülling, T., and Schell, J. (1993). *Rol* genes alter hormonal requirements for protoplast growth and modify expression of an auxin responsive promoter. *Plant Cell Rep.* **12,** 551–554.

Walden, R., Hayashi, H., and Schell, J. (1991). T-DNA as a gene tag. *Plant J.* **1,** 281–288.

Walden, R., Koncz, C., and Schell, J. (1990). The use of gene vectors in plant molecular biology. *Methods Mol. Cell. Biol.* **1,** 175–194.

Wing, D., Koncz, C., and Schell, J. (1989). Conserved function in *Nicotiana tabacum* of a single Drosophila hsp70 promoter heat shock element when fused to a minimal T-DNA promoter. *Mol. Gen. Genet.* **219,** 9–16.

Zambryski, P. (1992). Chronicles from the Agrobacterium-plant cell DNA transfer story. *Annu. Rev. Plant Physiol. Plant Mol. Biol.* **43,** 465–490.

CHAPTER 33

In Vitro Analysis of G-Protein Functions

Hong Ma and Catherine A. Weiss
Cold Spring Harbor Laboratory
Cold Spring Harbor, New York 11724

I. Introduction

In eukaryotic cells, a variety of proteins bind guanine nucleotides; these include tubulins, ribosomal proteins, translational factors, and regulatory GTP-binding proteins (so-called G proteins). The latter group of proteins are the subject of this chapter. G proteins have been classified into two families on the basis of their subunit composition and, to some extent, of their sizes (Bourne *et al.*, 1991). The members of one family of regulatory G proteins are heterotrimeric, and they generally relay information from transmembrane receptors to intracellular effectors (Gilman, 1987; Ross, 1989; Bourne *et al.*, 1990, 1991; Simon *et al.*, 1991). Heterotrimeric G proteins consist of α, β, and γ subunits. The α subunits are generally of the sizes between 35 to 45 kDa, bind guanine nucleotides, and have a low intrinsic GTPase activity. The β and γ subunits are generally of 35–36

METHODS IN CELL BIOLOGY, VOL. 49

and 8–10 kDa, respectively, and form a tight dimeric complex. In recent years, molecular cloning has identified many genes encoding mammalian G-protein subunits (Simon *et al.,* 1991). It is now known that mammalian heterotrimeric G proteins mediate a variety of cellular responses to environmental and hormonal signals, including the hormonal regulation of cAMP levels (Gilman, 1987), sensory responses such as vision, olfaction, and taste (Stryer, 1986; Jones and Reed, 1989; McLaughlin *et al.,* 1992), and response to neurotransmitters and growth factors (Ross, 1989). Furthermore, a combination of genetic, biochemical, and molecular analyses have uncovered G-protein functions in simple eukaryotes such as the yeasts *Saccharomyces cerevisiae* and *Schizosaccharomyces pombe* (Herskowitz, 1990; Obara *et al.,* 1991; Sprague, 1991) and the slime mold *Dictyostelium discoideum* (Firtel, 1991).

The second group of regulatory G proteins comprises members that are monomeric and generally with sizes in the range 20–30 kDa; therefore, they are often referred to as monomeric or small G proteins (Hall, 1990). These can be further divided into several subfamilies. The most extensively studied ones are in the ras subfamily including the product of the *ras* proto-oncogene, which is involved in signal transmission and which may be mediated by transmembrane protein tyrosine kinases. RAS homologs in *Drosophila* and *C. elegans* are involved in signal transduction during development (Rubin, 1991; Sternberg and Horvitz, 1991). A second group consists of several mammalian rab proteins, the yeast YPT1 and SEC4 proteins, and related proteins; these are involved in vesicular transport in the secretory pathway (Bourne *et al.,* 1990; Hall, 1990; Bourne *et al.,* 1991). Another group includes the mammalian rho and rac, and the yeast CDC42 proteins, which function in cell polarity and cytoskeletal function (Hall, 1990). There are other monomeric G proteins that do not fall into these subfamilies, including the mammalian and yeast ARF and Ran proteins (Moore and Blobel, 1993).

Much has been learned about the mechanisms of action of some mammalian heterotrimeric G proteins, particularly G_s, and transductins (Gilman, 1987; Bourne, 1989; Ross, 1989; Bourne *et al.,* 1990, 1991; Simon *et al.,* 1991; Birnbaumer, 1992). These have served as models for other G proteins. The α subunit binds guanine nucleotides, and the subunit conformation and association of the heterotrimeric G proteins change depending on whether GTP or GDP is bound. The GDP-bound α subunit is associated with the $\beta\gamma$ subunits in a resting-state heterotrimer (Fig. 1A). The binding of a ligand activates a transmembrane receptor, often characterized by seven membrane spanning segments (Dohlman *et al.,*1991), which promotes the exchange of the bound GDP for a GTP. The binding of GTP to the α subunit causes a conformational change, and the α subunit–GTP complex dissociates from the $\beta\gamma$ subunits, which remain tightly bound to each other. The GTP-bound α subunit is generally referred to as being activated, and in many cases does interact with downstream effectors such as adenylate cyclase. However, in several cases the $\beta\gamma$ subunits are known to interact with effectors (Clapham and Neer, 1993). The GTPase activity of the α subunit then slowly hydrolyzes GTP to GDP and phosphate, and a conformational change

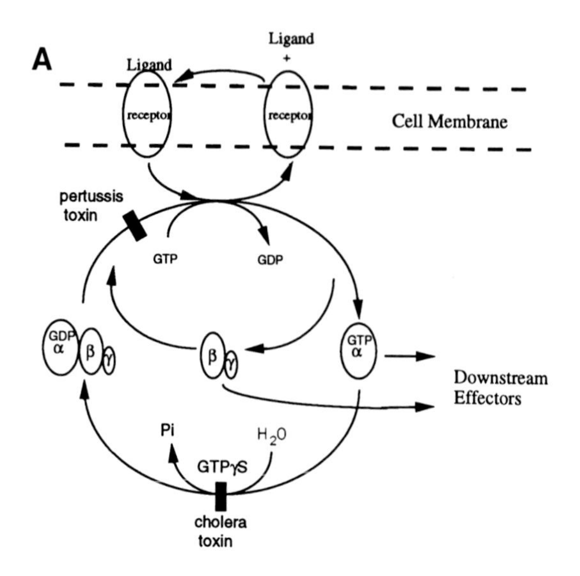

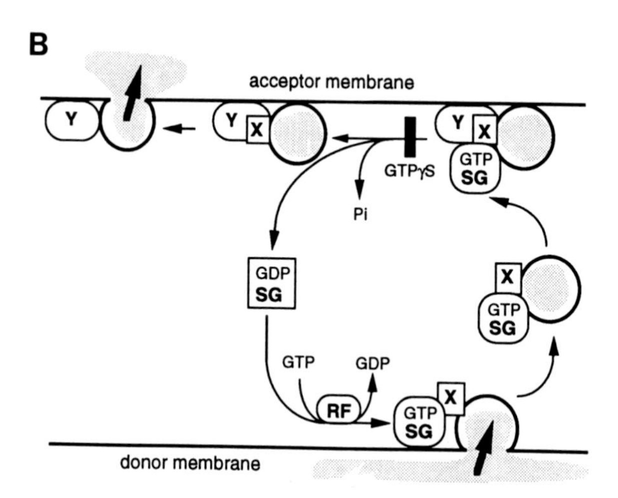

Fig. 1 Mechanisms of G protein actions. (A) Heterotrimeric G proteins composed of the α, β, γ subunits. The α and/or $\beta\gamma$ subunits may interact with a variety of effectors. (B) Small G proteins (SG) involved in secretion. Proteins X and Y are membrane-associated factors, and RF is a guanine nucleotide-releasing factor, all of which interact with the G protein. Solid bars indicate blockage by GTPγS or toxins.

allows the α subunit to reassociate with the $\beta\gamma$ subunits. It should be emphasized that the α–GTP complex, and in some cases, the resulting released $\beta\gamma$ dimer, are the molecules that activate downstream effects. Therefore, nonhydrolyzable GTP analogs, such GTPγS, and mutations reducing the GTPase activity of the α subunit, prolong the active state of heterotrimeric G proteins.

Several lines of evidence suggest that the mechanisms of the ras proteins and homologs are similar to those of the heterotrimeric G proteins (Bourne *et al.*, 1990, 1991; Hall, 1990). In other words, the GDP-bound form of ras is inactive, whereas the GTP-bound form is active. There is a significant difference between ras and heterotrimeric G proteins; ras proteins have very low intrinsic GTPase activity, which can be substantially increased by GAPs (GTPase activating pro eins). In addition, the GDP–GTP exchange of ras requires protein factors (guanine nucleotide-releasing factors) that are different from the transmembrane receptors coupled to heterotrimeric G proteins.

In contrast to heterotrimeric G proteins and ras, another mechanism is likely to operate in the action of small G proteins involved in secretion, such as the yeast SEC4 and YPT1, and mammalian rab proteins (Bourne, 1988; Walworth *et al.*, 1989; Hall, 1990). For these proteins, the GTP-bound form is required for a portion of a cyclical traffic of cellular membranes, and one GTP is required for one cycle (Fig. 1B). GTP hydrolysis is necessary for the cycle to be completed. Models have been proposed which postulate that the GTP-bound form of the small G protein associates with some factor(s) during part of the cycle, whereas the GDP-bound form associates with others. Since the normal function of these small G proteins requires the continuous cycling of GDP/GTP exchange and GTP hydrolysis, both the binding of nonhydrolyzable GTP analogs and mutations reducing GTPase activity (either in the G proteins or in the GAPs) inhibit the function of these small G proteins. The mechanism of other small G proteins, such as rho and rac, is not known.

Both the heterotrimeric and the monomeric G proteins are clearly important cellular regulators. They are present in plants and are likely to function in various processes of plant cells (see review: Ma, 1994). Indeed, a number of *in vitro* studies have provided evidence for the presence of GTP-binding proteins in various plants (Hasunuma and Funadera, 1987; Hasunuma *et al.*, 1987; Millner, 1987; Drobak *et al.*, 1988; Korolkov *et al.*, 1990; Schloss, 1990; Romero *et al.*, 1991). The combination of GTP-binding studies and immunological analysis with antibodies raised against known G protein α subunits has detected potential heterotrimeric G proteins from several plants such as zucchini (Jacobs *et al.*, 1988) and *Arabidopsis* (Blum *et al.*, 1988). In addition, biochemical evidence suggests that G proteins are involved in several plant processes, such as the swelling of wheat protoplasts (Bossen *et al.*, 1990), the formation of inositol phosphate derivatives in *Acer pseudoplatanus* (Dillenschneider *et al.*, 1986), a blue-light response in plasma membranes of etiolated pea seedlings (Warpeha *et al.*, 1991), the regulation of K^+ channel currents in cells of fava beans (Fairley-Grenot and Assmann, 1991; Li and Assmann, 1993), the cell defense response of soybean (Legendre *et al.*, 1992), and in phytochrome-mediated responses in cultured soybean cells and tomato hypocotyl cells (Neuhaus *et al.*, 1993; Romero and Lam, 1993). Furthermore, genes encoding the α and β subunits of heterotrimeric G proteins (Ma *et al.*, 1990; Ma *et al.*, 1991, Poulsen *et al.*, 1994; Weiss *et al.*, 1994) and monomeric G proteins have been isolated from several plants (Matsui *et al.*, 1989; Palme *et al.*, 1989; Anai *et al.*, 1991; Anuntalabhochai *et al.*, 1991; Sano and Youssefian, 1991; Palme *et al.*, 1992; Terryn *et al.*, 1992; Fabry *et al.*, 1993; Yang and Watson, 1993; Youssefian *et al.*, 1993).

G protein genes and their products may be analyzed in ways similar to those used for other genes, such as characterization of expression and intracellular localization using RNA *in situ* hybridization and immunodetection techniques. Because these methods are described elsewhere in this volume, they will not be repeated here. Rather, this chapter will focus on methods for biochemical studies that are unique to G proteins. We will describe several methods commonly used to detect the presence of G proteins in cell extracts or cell fractions, and discuss techniques to determine whether a G protein is involved in a particular cellular process. Examples of use of these procedures in plants will also be presented.

II. Materials

The radiolabeled nucleotides [^{35}S]GTPγS (guanosine 5′ [γ thio] triphosphate), [α-^{32}P]GTP and [γ-^{32}P]GTP (guanosine 5′ triphosphate), and [^{32}P]NAD (nicotinamide adenine dinucleotide) are purchased from NEN, Dupont. The nonradioactive nucleotides ATP, ATPγS, GTP, GDP, GTPγS, GDPβS, GMP-PNP (guanylyl-imidodiphosphate), and NAD are obtained as lithium salts from Boehringer Mannheim. Norit A is from Aldrich. Cholera toxin and pertussis toxin are from List Laboratories (Campell, CA). All other materials are of the highest grade available commercially.

III. Methods for Detecting G Proteins

A. A Renaturation Assay for GTP Binding by Small G Proteins

Because small G proteins renature easily, there is a simple method to measure GTP binding after the proteins have been separated by SDS–PAGE (Schmitt *et al.*, 1986). After separation, the gel is incubated at 4°C for 45 min in PBS (50 m*M* Na_2HPO_4/KH_2PO_4, pH 7.2, and 0.12 *M* NaCl), and the proteins are electrophoretically transferred onto a nitrocellulose filter in transfer buffer (20 m*M* Tris, 0.15 *M* glycine, and 20% methanol). The filter is washed in 10 m*M* Tris HCl, pH 7.4, 0.15 *M* NaCl, 5% BSA, and 0.05% Tween 20 for 1 h, then incubated at room temperature for 30 min in 30 ml of a buffer containing 20 m*M* Tris–HCl, pH 8, 10 m*M* $MgCl_2$, 2 m*M* DTT, 0.1% NP40, 0.3% BSA,

1 μM [α-^{32}P]GTP (3000 Ci/mmol), and 60 μg/ml of *E. coli* tRNA. Following the GTP binding, the filter is washed twice for 15 min each in 100 ml of a buffer containing 0.2% SDS, 0.5% Triton X-100, 0.5% BSA, and 0.15 *M* NaCl, and then dried; the proteins that bind GTP are visualized by autoradiography. As a ontrol, binding competition assay should be performed. The reaction mixture of preincubated with 1 m*M* cold GTP or cold ATP for 15 min before the radioactive GTP is added. A 1000-fold excess of cold GTP should completely inhibit GTP-binding, whereas the preincubation with a 1000-fold excess of ATP should have no inhibitory effect on binding. This method not only allows the detection of GTP-binding proteins, but also provides their approximate sizes. Once G proteins are detected, this assay may be used in combination with other biochemical procedures to further characterize the G protein. For example, fractionation followed by the filter assay may identify the intracellular localization of the G proteins. This procedure has been used to test for GTP binding by small G proteins from plants (Anuntalabhochai *et al.,* 1991; Wang *et al.,* 1993; Yang and Watson, 1993).

B. A GTP-Binding Assay in Solution

Although the renaturation assay is very convenient, it requires that proteins be denatured then renatured. In general, GTP-binding by native proteins in response to interactions with other proteins (e.g., receptors and effectors) cannot be analyzed using this procedure. Specifically, no heterotrimeric G protein has been shown to bind GTP using this procedure. Therefore, a general method for GTP binding is needed. It should be noted that such a method would be the least specific of G protein assays since all GTP-binding sites are not necessarily G-protein-related sites.

In principle, the GTP-binding proteins are allowed to bind a labeled GTP analog by incubation, and then the protein–nucleotide complexes are separated from the free nucleotide. Radiolabeled [^{35}S]GTPγS and a rapid filtration protocol, as described previously by Sternweis and Robishaw (1984), are generally used. Samples containing 10–100 μg of protein are assayed in 100–200 μl of reaction mixture, at a final concentration of 20 m*M* Tris–HCl, pH 8, 1 m*M* EDTA, 1 m*M* DTT, 100 m*M* NaCl, 10 m*M* $MgCl_2$ and 5 n*M* to 1 μM [^{35}S]GTPγS (1500 Ci/mmol) and incubated for 30 to 60 min at 30°C. Nonspecific binding of the radiolabeled GTP analog to proteins is measured in the same conditions but in the presence of an excess of cold GTPγS (1 m*M*). The samples are then diluted with 2 ml of buffer A (20 m*M* Tris–HCl, pH 8, 100 m*M* NaCl, and 25 m*M* $MgCl_2$), prechilled at 4°C, and filtered through a 0.45-mm nitrocellulose filter (e.g, Millipore) that has been prerinsed with buffer A. The filter-bound sample is washed rapidly (with suction) four times each with 2 ml of buffer A (additional washes do not decrease the bound radioactivity). The blank radioactivity value (without protein or with denatured protein) is generally less than 0.3% of total radioactivity used. After the filter is dried and dissolved in 2 ml of ethylene glycol monomethyl ether, the radioactivity is measured in a toluene-based scintillation fluid. Known amounts of [^{35}S]GTPγS are spotted onto the filters and counted as standards to correct for counting efficiency. Using this type of method, the presence of GTP-binding proteins has been reported in crude extracts of several plants (Hasunuma and Funadera, 1987; Blum *et al.*, 1988; Drobak *et al.*, 1988; Jacobs *et al.*, 1988). Again, as with the renaturation assay to detect small G proteins, the GTP-binding assay in solution may be used with other biochemical procedures to further analyze any GTP-binding proteins involved in a particular cellular process.

C. A GTPase Assay

The GTPase activity of G proteins affects the conformation and function of G proteins; therefore, regulation of the GTPase is an important means of controlling G protein function. For heterotrimeric G proteins, the GDP resulting from the hydrolysis of GTP remains bound to the α subunit, and the GDP–α complex associates with the $\beta\gamma$ dimer. Further hydrolysis does not occur until a new GTP replaces the bound GDP. The ligand-bound receptor interacts with the $\alpha\beta\gamma$ trimer (and not the α subunit alone), to promote the exchange of the bound GDP for a GTP; therefore, both the receptor and the $\beta\gamma$ subunits accelerate GTP hydrolysis. In the case of small G proteins, cognate GAPs stimulate the GTPase activity and downregulate G protein function. Other signaling and regulatory pathways may also modulate the GTPase activity of G proteins. Therefore, the determination of the GTPase activity is a useful way of detecting and characterizing G proteins in association with particular pathways.

The GTPase assay entails the use of radiolabeled GTP. Typically, protein samples (10 μg/ml) are incubated in a final volume of 100 μl of reaction buffer [20 m*M* Tris–HCl, pH 7.5, 5 m*M* $MgCl_2$, 1 m*M* DTT, 0.1 m*M* EDTA, 2 m*M* [γ-^{32}P]GTP (5000Ci/mmol)] at 20°C to 30°C for 10 min. The reaction is stopped by adding 0.6 ml of ice-cold 2.5% activated carbon Norit-A (Aldrich) in 20 m*M* phosphate buffer, pH 7.5, and rapid chilling. The mixture is centrifuged at 10,000 rpm for 10 min to separate the hydrolyzed radioactive phosphate from the radioactive GTP, and the amount of inorganic phosphate released is measured by counting 0.5 ml of the supernatant by liquid scintillation spectroscopy. A control to determine whether the GTPase activity is specific to GTP is performed by adding an excess (25 μM) of a nonhydrolyzable GTP analog, either GTPγS or GMP-PNP, both competitive inhibitors of the GTPase activity. The background due to nonenzymatic hydrolysis of [γ-^{32}P]GTP is measured with no protein present in the assay and is subtracted from all data. The basal GTPase activity of a sample is measured as picomoles of inorganic phosphate (P_i) released per unit of time. Comparing the basal GTPase activity of a sample to the activity measured when a stimulus of interest is applied can give an indication whether a GTP-binding protein is involved in this process. For instance, it has been shown that GTPase activity is stimulated by blue light in etiolated pea membranes, implicating a GTP-binding protein in the response to blue light (Warpeha *et al.*, 1991).

D. ADP-Ribosylation Assays

The GTP-binding and GTPase assays detect all G proteins; on the other hand, cholera and pertussis toxins offers means to detect and characterize preferentially the heterotrimeric G proteins. The α subunit of heterotrimeric G proteins, but not the small G proteins, may be labeled using these toxins and radioactively labeled NAD^+, which serves as the donor of the ADP-ribose group. G-protein α subunits sensitive to pertussis toxin have a cysteine near the carboxy terminus (usually at the fourth position from the end); thus although ADP-ribosylation by pertussis toxin is a sensitive G-protein assay, it will only identify a subset of G protein α subunits. For ADP-ribosylation experiments using pertussis toxin, the protein extracts should be prepared with protease inhibitors to minimize proteolysis and membrane-rich fractions should be used because G proteins are generally associated with membranes. The pertussis holotoxin is a hexamer of the catalytic A component (S1) and the binding B component (S2, S3, 2XS4, and S5), which facilitates the uptake of the A component by the cell (Kopf and Woolkalis, 1991). Only the A component is needed for *in vitro* studies with protein extracts. Activation of the pertussis toxin by treatment with DTT and SDS greatly increases its ADP-ribosylation activity. To activate pertussis toxin, 100 μg/ml of the toxin is incubated in 50 m*M* Hepes, pH 8, 1 mg/ml bovine serum albumin, 20 m*M* DTT, and 0.125% SDS at 30°C for 30 min (Kopf and Woolkalis, 1991). For the ADP-ribosylation reaction, the activated pertussis toxin is diluted fivefold into a reaction mix containing crude extract (5–100 μg proteins) to achieve final concentrations of 1 m*M* EDTA, 5 m*M* DTT, 10 m*M* Hepes, pH 8, 0.2 mg/ml BSA, 0.025% SDS, 20 μg/ml pertussis toxin, and 5 μ*M* [^{32}P]NAD (800Ci/mmol). The reaction mix is incubated for 10 to 60 min at 25 to 30°C, and stopped by the addition of 20% cold trichloroacetic acid and incubation on ice for 1 h. The precipitated material was collected by centrifugation, washed with ether, and dissolved in electrophoresis buffer containing 5% β-mercaptoethanol. To determine the specificity of the ADP-ribosylation, controls without the toxin or with excess nonradioactive NAD should be included; these controls should have less labeling. In addition, because pertussis toxin modifies the GDP-bound form, incubation of the protein sample with GTPγS should also reduce the ADP-ribosylation and should be included as a control.

The ADP-ribosylation by cholera toxin is considerably more complex (Gill and Woolkalis, 1991). Among the known G proteins, only G_s has been well documented as being efficiently modified by cholera toxin. G_s is ADP-ribosylated by cholera toxin on an arginine residue that is conserved among all G proteins, but other G proteins may be modified at a slower rate or not at all by the toxin (Gill and Woolkalis, 1991). These features make using cholera toxin less desirable and more prone to artifacts. Furthermore, ADP-ribosylation by cholera toxin requires a soluble factor, called the ADP-ribosylation factor (ARF), which is itself a small G protein, and is activated by the binding of GTP or GTP analogs (Gill and Woolkalis, 1991). The analog GMP–PNP is preferred over GTPγS to activate ARF, because GTPγS has a direct effect on G_s. Similar to pertussis toxin, cholera toxin is also a hexamer, and the catalytic A1 fragment can be released by treatment with DTT and SDS, as described above for the pertussis toxin (Gill and Woolkalis, 1991). This activated toxin is used at a 20-fold dilution to lower the final concentration of SDS to 0.025%. Crude extracts (containing membrane and soluble proteins) should be used for this assay, as they might contain a soluble ADP-ribosylating factor, not identified in plants yet, which should facilitate the ADP-ribosylation reaction by cholera toxin. To start the reaction, crude extracts (0.3 to 1 mg/ml of proteins) are added to the reaction mixture to produce a final concentration of 200 m*M* potassium phosphate, pH 8, 5 m*M* DTT, 2 m*M* $MgCl_2$, 50 to 100 μg/ml activated toxin, 5 μM [^{32}P]NAD (800 Ci/mmol), 0.1 m*M* GMP-PNP, and 10 m*M* thymidine and incubated at 25 to 30°C, for 30 to 60 min. The reaction is stopped as described for the pertussis toxin experiment. The gel can be stained with Coomassie blue and dried for autoradiography. It is possible to increase the amounts of toxin, NAD, and GMP-PNP threefold if the band(s) on the autoradiograph is/are weak, indicating that ADP-ribosylation has worked poorly (maybe because of a lack of ARF). According to Gill and Woolkalis (1991) under some conditions with animal G protein, all of the pertussis toxin substrates can also be labeled by cholera toxin, as they all contain arginine at the site homologous to the target site for cholera toxin. But it seems essential that the G proteins be coupled to their ligand-bound receptor and that the guanine nucleotide concentration be kept low. Proteins other than G proteins can serve as substrates for ADP-ribosylation by cholera toxin, but they are ribosylated considerably more slowly than G_s and dominate the labeling pattern only if they are very abundant. Increasing the concentration of the toxin or the NAD should readily label $G_{s\alpha}$ or an equivalent plant α subunit first. Controls to test the specificity of the ADP-ribosylation should be performed as with the pertussis toxin assay.

It must be emphasized that the toxins are only useful to identify the presence of certain classes of G proteins in an extract. To date, only one gene and its homologs encoding α subunits have been identified in plants (Ma *et al.*, 1990; Ma *et al.*, 1991; Poulsen *et al.*, 1994), and they are possible substrates for chlora toxin ADP-ribosylation but not pertussis toxin ADP-ribosylation (they lack the reactive cysteine in the carboxy terminus region), although this has not been tested directly. It is likely that other α subunit-encoding genes will be isolated in the future. Indeed a G_α subunit, which is apparently not related to the cloned G_α subunit because it can be modified by pertussis toxin and by cholera toxin, has been shown to be present in etiolated pea membranes (Warpeha *et al.*, 1991). But it is possible that, as in animals, (Simon *et al.*, 1991), plants also may have G proteins that cannot be modified by pertussis and cholera toxins and thus will not be identified using ADP-ribosylation by these toxins.

E. Ribosylation of Small G Proteins by C3 Transferase

It should be noted that some small G proteins can be ADP-ribosylated by the exoenzyme C3 transferase from *Clostridium botulinum* (Aktories *et al.*, 1990). In particular, this is the case for the rho proteins (Sekine *et al.*, 1989) and to a much lesser degree for the rac proteins (Didsbury *et al.*, 1989). In the case of the rho proteins, ADP-ribosylation by C3 transferase renders the proteins inactive (Paterson *et al.*, 1990). Although ADP-ribosylation of small G proteins has so far not been reported in plants, this assay might be helpful in the future to investigate the function of the rho-related small G proteins in plants. Unfortunately, this enzyme is not available commercially. The purification of the C3 transferase and a ribosylation assay are described in Aktories *et al.* (1988) and Ridley and Hall (1992), respectively.

IV. Analysis of G-Protein Involvement in Cellular Processes

A. Use of GTP Analogs

In addition to the detection of G proteins in particular cell extracts, the GTP analogs may be used to probe G protein functions in various cellular processes. G proteins that are involved in mediating extracellular signals, such as the heterotrimeric G proteins and the ras subfamily, are usually activated by the receptor–ligand complex. In the case of heterotrimeric G proteins, the activation involves the exchange of a bound GDP for a GTP. Therefore, the presence of a G protein in a signaling pathway may be detected as the stimulation of GTP binding by the signal. If at least a portion of the signaling pathway can be reconstituted *in vitro*, then the effect of the signal on GTP binding can be characterized using GTP binding assays described above.

In general, heterotrimeric G proteins and ras are activated by binding to GTP. For heterotrimeric G proteins, this activation is attenuated by the hydrolysis of GTP to GDP and phosphate due to the intrinsic GTPase activity of the α subunit. For monomeric G proteins, the intrinsic GTPase activity is greatly stimulated by the GTPase activating protein (GAP). Because GTP analogs such as GTPγS and GMP-PNP are not hydrolyzable, they are more potent activators of G proteins. If a signal is known or suspected for a particular cellular process, such as response to light, then guanine nucleotides may be used to mimic the signal in generating the response. Among the GTP analogs, GTPγS is the most widely used, and the discussion will be focused on it; however, it is often helpful to use GTP and more than one analog in a study to avoid potential pitfalls. If a cellular process has an *in vitro* assay, then the effects of GTP or GTP analogs can be analyzed. In general, if a micromolar concentration of GTPγS has a positive or negative effect, a G protein may be involved, because the association constant of G proteins for GTP or GTPγS is in the micromolar range. In initial studies, a wide range of concentrations (1 μM to 1 mM) of the nucleotides should be used to allow the detection of proteins that may have weaker binding to the nucleotides. Divalent metal ions are also required; usually 10–20 m*M* $MgCl_2$ is used. Controls with ATP and ATPγS should be included to exclude nonspecific nucleotide effects. Because GDP is associated with the inactive form of G proteins, GDP and GDPβS are often used as inhibitors of G protein function. The inclusion of GDP or GDP analogs in the analysis can further strengthen the case for an involvement of G proteins. If a cell-free system is not available to study a particular cellular response, but a cellular system exists where microinjection is feasible, then GTP and GTP analogs (or GDP and GDP analogs) may be used in microinjection experiments to probe the function of G proteins in the cellular pathway.

B. Use of Cholera and Pertussis Toxins

In characterization of heterotrimeric G proteins, cholera and pertussis toxins have been extremely useful but, as discussed previously, it is limited to certain classes of G proteins. Cholera toxin can ADP-ribosylate both GTP- and GDP-bound forms (Gill and Woolkalis, 1991), and the cholera toxin-catalyzed ADP-ribosylation inhibits the intrinsic GTPase activity, prolonging the activated state of the α subunit. In contrast, the pertussis toxin-catalyzed ADP-ribosylation only occurs on the GDP-bound heterotrimeric form, and the modification uncouples the G protein from the receptor (Gilman, 1987). Therefore, pertussis toxin keeps the G protein in the inactive state. These bacterial toxins can be used either *in vitro* or added to intact cells. Only the catalytic portion of the toxin is required for *in vitro* analysis; however, the holotoxin, which contains a portion capable of forming a channel to allow the passage of the catalytic portion to enter the cells, is required for use with intact cells. Similar to guanine nucleotides, the toxins may be used to associate G proteins with a particular signal and/or a cellular response. If a signal activates a G protein, then the ADP-ribosylation catalyzed by pertussis toxin should be reduced, as detected using methods described earlier. Further, a positive effect of cholera toxin on some cellular response would suggest that an activated G protein is involved in promoting the response, whereas a positive effect of pertussis toxin suggests that an activated G protein can inhibit the response. A typical experiment for studying the effects of the bacterial toxins uses about 1 μg/ml of the preactivated toxins.

Both GTP analogs and bacterial toxins have been used to probe G protein function in plant signaling pathways. In fava bean guard cells or mesophyll cells, GTPγS was found to reduce an inward or outward K^+ current, respectively, whereas GDPβS enhanced the currents (Fairley-Grenot and Assmann, 1991; Li and Assmann, 1993). Since GTPγS activates and GDPβS inhibits G proteins, these results suggest that one or more G proteins negatively regulate K^+ currents. In addition, it was found that cholera toxin inhibits both the inward K^+ current in guard cells and the outward K^+ current in mesophyll cells, further supporting the idea that a G protein negatively regulates the K^+ currents (Fairley-Grenot and

Assmann, 1991; Li and Assmann, 1993). Pertussis toxin also inhibits K^+current in guard cells, but not in mesophyll cells (Fairley-Grenot and Assmann, 1991). That pertussis toxin blocks the activation of G proteins suggests that a second G protein acts in the guard cell to regulate positively the K^+ current. In other studies, it was found using a microinjection procedure, that GTPγS (30–100 μM intracellular) and Gpp(NH)p (50–100 μM intracellular) mimic the effects of the light receptor phytochrome A on light-dependent synthesis of anthocyanin and the expression of a reporter gene (*GUS*) under the control of a light-regulated *cab* gene promoter, suggesting that a G protein may be involved in phytochrome signal transduction (Neuhaus *et al.,* 1993). In this case, cholera toxin alone had only a small effect on the light responses; however, cholera toxin in combination with a low concentration (1 μM) of GTPγS, which has no effect by itself, produced an effect similar to that of phytochrome A or 30–100 μM GTPγS (Neuhaus *et al.,* 1993). This is consistent with the knowledge that cholera toxin enhances G protein function not by activating the G protein, but by prolonging its activated state.

V. Conclusion

GTP analogs and the cholera and pertussis bacterial toxins are extremely useful tools to detect G proteins in different cellular fractions and to study the involvement of G proteins in various cellular functions. GTP analogs, particularly GTPγS, are used frequently due to the relative ease with which they can detect G proteins and probe G protein functions. However, GTP analogs are not very specific; therefore, conclusions from studies using GTP analogs are not definitive. The bacterial toxins, particularly pertussis toxin, are more specific, and they are used for analyses of heterotrimeric G proteins. Although there are limitations, these biochemical methods can provide valuable information, which complements information gained from molecular and genetic studies.

Acknowledgments

We thank Catherine Flanagan and Peter Rubinelli for comments. This work is supported by a grant to H.M. from the National Science Foundation (DCB90-04567). C.W. is supported by the Cold Spring Harbor Laboratory Robertson Fund.

References

Aktories, K., Rösener, S., Blaschke, U., and Chhatwal, G. S. (1988). Botulinum ADP ribosyltransferase C3: Purification of the enzyme and characterization of the ADP-ribosylation reaction in platelet membranes. *Eur. J. Biochem.* **172,** 445–450.

Aktories, K., Braun, U., Habermann, B., and Rösener, S. (1990). Botulinum ADP-Ribosyltransferase C3. *In* "ADP-Ribosylating Toxins and G proteins. Insights into Signal Transduction" (J. Moss and M. Vaugham, eds.), pp. 97–115. Washington, DC: American Society for Microbiology.

Anai, T., Hasegawa, K., Watanabe, Y., Uchimiya, H., Ishizaki, R., and Matsui, M. (1991). Isolation and analysis of cDNAs encoding small GTP-binding proteins of *Arabidopsis thaliana. Gene* **108,** 259–264.

Anuntalabhochai, S., Terryn, N., Van Montagu, M., and Inzé, D. (1991). Molecular characterization of an *Arabidopsis thaliana* cDNA encoding a small GTP-binding protein, Rhal. *Plant J.* **1,** 167–174.

Birnbaumer, L. (1992). Receptor-to-effector signaling through G proteins: roles for $\beta\gamma$ dimers as well as α subunits. *Cell* **71,** 1069–1072.

Blum, W., Hinsch, K.-D., Schultz, G., and Weiler, E. W. (1988). Identification of GTP-binding proteins in the plasma membrane of higher plants. *Biochem. Biophys. Res. Commun.* **156,** 954–959.

Bossen, M. E., Kendrick, R. E., and Vredenberg, W. J. (1990). The involvement of a G-protein in phytochrome-regulated, Ca^{2+}-dependent swelling of etiolated wheat protoplasts. *Physiol. Plant.* **80,** 55–62.

Bourne, H. R. (1988). Do GTPases direct membrane traffic in secretion? *Cell* **53,** 669–671.

Bourne, H. R. (1989). Who carries what message? *Nature* **337,** 504–505.

Bourne, H. R., Sanders, D. A., and McCormick, F. (1990). The GTPase superfamily: A conserved switch for diverse cell functions. *Nature* **348,** 125–132.

Bourne, H. R., Sanders, D. A., and McCormick, F. (1991). The GTPase superfamily: Conserved structure and molecular mechanism. *Nature* **349,** 117–127.

Clapham, D. E., and Neer, E. J. (1993). New roles for G-protein $\beta\gamma$-dimers in transmembrane signalling. *Nature* **365,** 403–406.

Didsbury, J., Weber, R. F., Bokoch, G. M., Evans, T., and Snyderman, R. (1989). Rac, a novel ras-related family of proteins that are botulinum toxin substrates. *J. Biol. Chem.* **264,** 16378–16382.

Dillenschneider, M., Hetherington, A., Graziana, A., Alibert, G., Berta, P., Haiech, J., and Ranjeva, R. (1986). The formation of inositol phosphate derivatives by isolated membranes from *Acer psudoplatanus* is stimulated by guanine nucleotides. *FEBS Lett.* **208,** 413–417.

Dohlman, H. G., Thorner, J., Caron, M. G., and Lefkowitz, R. J. (1991). Model system for the study of seven-transmembrane-segment receptors. *Ann. Rev. Biochem.* **60,** 653–688.

Drobak, B. K., Allan, E. F., Comerford, J. G., Roberts, R., and Dawson, A. P. (1988). Presence of guanine nucleotide-binding proteins in a plant hypoctyl fraction. *Biochem. Biophys. Res. Commun.* **150,** 899–903.

Fabry, S., Jacobsen, A., Huber, H., Palme, K., and Schmitt, R. (1993). Structure, expression, and phylogeneic relationships of a family of *ypt* genes ecoding small G-proteins in the green alga *Volvox carteri. Curr. Genet.* **24,** 229–240.

Fairley-Grenot, K., and Assmann, S. M. (1991). Evidence for G-protein regulation of inward K^+ channel current in guard cells of fava bean. *Plant Cell* **3,** 1037–1044.

Firtel, R. A. (1991). Signal transduction pathways controlling multicellular development in *Dictyostelium. Trends Genet.* **7,** 381–388.

Gill, D. M., and Woolkalis, M. J. (1991). Cholera toxin-catalyzed [^{32}P]ADP-ribosylation of proteins. *Methods Enzymol.* **195,** 267–280.

Gilman, A. G. (1987). G proteins: Transducers of receptor-generated signals. *Annu. Rev. Biochem.* **56,** 615–649.

Hall, A. (1990). The cellular functions of small GTP-binding proteins. *Science* **249,** 634–640.

Hasunuma, K., and Funadera, K. (1987). GTP-binding protein(s) in green plant, *Lemna paucicostata. Biochem. Biophys. Res. Commun.* **143,** 908–912.

Hasunuma, K., Furukawa, K., Tomita, K., Mukai, C., and Nakamura, T. (1987). GTP-binding proteins in etiolated epicotyls of *Pisum sativum* (Alaska) seedlings. *Biochem. Biophys. Res. Commun.* **148,** 133–139.

Herskowitz, I. (1990). A regulatory hierarchy for cell specialization in yeast. *Nature* **342,** 749–757.

Jacobs, M., Thelen, M. P., Farndale, R. W., Astle, M. C., and Rubery, P. H. (1988). Specific guanine nucleotide binding by membranes from *Cucurbita pepo* seedlings. *Biochem. Biophys. Res. Commun.* **155,** 1478–1484.

Jones, D. T., and Reed, R. R. (1989). G_{olf}: An olfactory neuron specific-G protein involved in odorant signal transduction. *Science* **244,** 790–795.

Kopf, G. S., and Woolkalis, M. J. (1991). ADP-ribosylation of G proteins with Pertussis toxin. *Methods Enzymol.* **195,** 257–266.

Korolkov, S. N., Garnovskaya, M. N., Basov, A. S., Chunaev, A. S., and Dumler, I. L. (1990). The detection and characterization of G-proteins in the eyespot of *Chlamydomonas reinhardtii. FEBS Lett.* **270,** 132–134.

Legendre, L., Heinstein, P. F., and Low, P. S. (1992). Evidence for participation of GTP-binding proteins in elicitation of the rapid oxidative burst in cultured soybean cells. *J. Biol. Chem.* **267,** 20140–20147.

Li, W., and Assmann, S. (1993). Characterization of a G-protein-regulated outward K^+ current in mesophyll cells of *Vicia faba* L. *Proc. Natl. Acad. Sci. U.S.A.* **90,** 262–266.

Ma, H. (1994). GTP-binding proteins in plants: New members of an old family. *Plant Mol. Biol.* **26,** 1611–1636.

Ma, H., Yanofsky, M. F., and Meyerowitz, E. M. (1990). Molecular cloning and characterization of *GPA1,* a G protein α subunit gene from *Arabidopsis thaliana. Proc. Natl. Acad. Sci. U.S.A.* **87,** 3821–3825.

Ma, H., Yanofsky, M. F., and Huang, H. (1991). Isolation and sequence analysis of *TGA1* cDNAs encoding a tomato G protein α subunit. *Gene* **107,** 189–195.

Matsui, M., Sasamoto, S., Kunieda, T., Nomura, N., and Ryotaro, I. (1989). Cloning of *ara,* a putative *Arabidopsis thaliana* gene homologous to the ras-related gene family. *Gene* **76,** 313–319.

McLaughlin, S. K., McKinnon, P. J., and Margolskee, R. F. (1992). Gustducin is a taste-cell-specific G protein closely related to the transducins. *Nature* **357,** 563–569.

Millner, P. A. (1987). Are guanine-binding proteins involved in regulation of thylakoid protein kinase activity? *FEBS Lett.* **226,** 155–160.

Moore, M. S., and Blobel, G. (1993). The GTP-binding protein Ran/TC4 is required for protein import into the nucleus. *Nature* **365,** 661–663.

Neuhaus, G., Bowler, C., Kern, R., and Chua, N.-H. (1993). Calcium/calmodulin-dependent and -independent phytochrome signal transduction pathways. *Cell* **73,** 937–952.

Obara, T., Nakafuku, M., Yamamoto, M., and Kaziro, Y. (1991). Isolation and characterization of a gene encoding a G-protein α subunit from *Schizosaccharomyces pombi:* Involvement in mating and sporulation pathways. *Proc. Natl. Acad. Sci. U.S.A.* **88,** 5877–5881.

Palme, K., Diefenthal, T., Sander, C., Vingron, M., and Schell, J. (1989). Identification of guanine nucleotide-binding proteins in plants: Structural analysis and evolutionary comparison of the *ras*-related *ypt* gene family from *Zea mays. In* "The Guanine Nucleotide Binding Protein: Common Structural and Functional Properties" (L. Bosch, B. Kraal, and A. Parmeggiani, eds.), pp. 273–284. New York: Plenum.

Palme, K., Diefenthal, T., Vingron, M., Sander, C., and Schell, J. (1992). Molecular cloning and structural analysis of genes from *Zea mays* (L), coding for members of the *ras*-related *ypt* gene family. *Proc. Natl. Acad. Sci. U.S.A.* **89,** 787–791.

Paterson, H. F., Self, A. J., Garrett, M. D., Aktories, K., and Hall, A. (1990). Microinjection of recombinant $p21^{rho}$ induces rapid changes in cell morphology. *J. Cell Biol.* **111,** 1001–1007.

Poulsen, C., Mai, X. M., and Borg, S. (1994). A *Lotus japonicus* cDNA encoding an α subunit of a heterotrimeric G-protein. *Plant Physiol.* **105,** 1453–1454.

Ridley, A. J., and Hall, A. (1992). The small GTP-binding protein rho regulates the assembly of focal adhesions and actin stress fibers in response to growth factors. *Cell* **70,** 389–399.

Romero, L. C., and Lam, E. (1993). Guanine nucleotide binding protein involvement in early steps of phytochrome-regulated gene expression. *Proc. Natl. Acad. Sci. U.S.A.* **90,** 1465–1469.

Romero, L. C., Sommer, D., Gotor, C., and Song, P.-S. (1991). G-protein in etiolated *Avena* seedlings: Possible phytochrome regulation. *FEBS Lett.* **282,** 341–346.

Ross, E. M. (1989). Signal sorting and amplification through G protein-coupled receptors. *Neuron* **3,** 141–152.

Rubin, G. M. (1991). Signal transduction and the fate of the R7 photoreceptor in *Drosophila. Trends Genet.* **7,** 372–377.

Sano, H., and Youssefian, S. (1991). A novel *ras*-related *rgpl* gene encoding a GTP-binding protein has reduced expression in 5-azacytidine induced dwarf rice. *Mol. Gen. Genet.* **228,** 227–232.

Schloss, J. A. (1990). A chlamydomonas gene encodes a G protein β subunit-like polypeptide *Mol. Gen. Genet.* **221,** 443–452.

Schmitt, H. D., Wagner, P., Pfaff, E., and Gallwitz, D. (1986). The *ras*-related *YPT1* gene product in yeast: A GTP-binding protein that might be involved in microtubule organization. *Cell* **47,** 401–412.

Sekine, A., Fujiwara, M., and Narumiya, S. (1989). Asparagine residue in the *rho* gene product is the modification site for botulinum ADP-ribosyltransferase. *J. Biol. Chem.* **264,** 8602–8605.

Simon, M. I., Strathmann, M. P., and Gautam, N. (1991). Diversity of G proteins in signal transduction. *Science* **252,** 802–808.

Sprague, G. F., Jr. (1991). Signal transduction in yeast mating. *Trends Genet.* **7,** 393–397.

Sternberg, P. W., and Horvitz, H. R. (1991). Signal transduction during *C. elegans* vulval induction. *Trends Genet.* **7,** 366–371.

Sternweis, P. C., and Robishaw, J. D. (1984). Isolation of two proteins with high affinity for guanine nucleotides from membranes of bovine brain. *J. Biol. Chem.* **259,** 13806–13813.

Stryer, L. (1986). Cyclic GMP cascade of vision. *Annu. Rev. Neurosci.* **9,** 87–119.

Terryn, N., Anuntalabhochai, S., Van Montagu, M., and Inzé, D. (1992). Analysis of a *Nicotiana plumbaginifolia* cDNA encoding a novel small GTP-binding protein *FEBS Lett.* **299,** 287–290.

Walworth, N. C., Goud, B., Kabcenell, A K., and Novick, P. J. (1989). Mutational analysis of SEC4 suggests a cyclical mechanism for the regulation of vesicular traffic. *EMBO J.* **8,** 1685–1693.

Wang, M., Sedee, N. J. A., Heidekamp, F., and Snaar-Jagalska, B. E. (1993). Detection of GTP-binding proteins in barley aleurone protoplasts. *FEBS Lett.* **329,** 245–248.

Warpeha, K. M. F., Hamm, H. E., Rasenick, M. M., and Kaufman, L. S. (1991). A blue-light-activated GTP-binding protein in the plasma membranes of etiolated peas. *Proc. Natl. Acad. Sci. U.S.A.* **88,** 8925–8929.

Weiss, C. A., Garnaat, C. W., Mukai, K., Hu, Y., and Ma, H. (1994). Isolation of cDNAs encoding guanine nucleotide-binding protein β-subunit homologues from maize (ZGB1) and *Arabidopsis* (AGB1). *Proc. Natl. Acad. Sci. U.S.A.* **91,** 9554–9558.

Yang, Z., and Watson, J. C. (1993). Molecular cloning and characterization of rho, a ras-related small GTP-binding protein from the garden pea. *Proc. Natl. Acad. Sci. U.S.A.* **90,** 8732–8736.

Youssefian, S., Nakamura, M., and Sano, H. (1993). Molecular characterization of *rgp2,* a gene encoding a small GTP-binding protein from rice. *Mol. Gen. Genet.* **237,** 187–192.

CHAPTER 34

Production of Recombinant Plant Calmodulin and Its Use to Detect Calmodulin-Binding Proteins

Birong Liao and Raymond E. Zielinski

Department of Plant Biology
University of Illinois
1201 W. Gregory Drive
Urbana, Illinois 61801

I. Introduction

Calmodulin (CaM) is a major intracellular receptor for second messenger Ca^{2+} signals and is expressed in every cell of all eukaryotes, including plants (reviewed recently by Poovaiah and Reddy, 1993; Roberts and Harmon, 1992). CaM transduces these signals by binding four Ca^{2+}, and binding to and altering the activities

METHODS IN CELL BIOLOGY, VOL. 49

of a variety of enzymatic, cytoskeletal, and structural proteins. A major portion of our current understanding of Ca^{2+}- and CaM-dependent regulation of cellular function has emerged from the identification and subsequent characterization of these CaM-binding proteins (CaM-BP), which serve as response elements distal to CaM in Ca^{2+}-mediated signal transduction pathways. However, the preponderance of well-characterized examples of CaM-regulated proteins is of animal origin. Clearly, determining the identities of the target proteins with which CaM interacts is an issue of fundamental importance if we are to understand the mechanisms by which second messenger Ca^{2+} signals are transduced in plant cells.

Molecular recognition and biochemical regulation in a variety of cellular systems are dictated by the interaction of relatively short peptide sequences. The Ca^{2+}-dependent regulatory effects exerted by CaM over its protein response element targets are initiated typically via the ability of CaM to bind with high affinity to positively charged peptides that adopt an amphiphilic α-helical structure (O'Neil and DeGrado, 1989). The basic amphiphilic α-helical peptides with which CaM interacts have been shown experimentally to be as short as 17 amino acids and the minimum length for binding has been postulated to be 14 residues (Ikura *et al.,* 1992). The high-affinity (K_d values typically in the range 1 to 200 nM) and specificity of CaM for binding its polypeptide targets and the ability of the CaM-binding domains of these proteins to renature following denaturation during SDS–polyacrylamide gel electrophoresis (SDS–PAGE) have been exploited numerous times to identify and characterize CaM-regulated proteins in animal cells (e.g., Billingsley *et al.,* 1985; Walker *et al.,* 1993). These methods have only recently been employed to characterize CaM-BP of plant origin (Ling and Assmann, 1992) and to isolate cDNA clones from expression libraries of plant origin (Baum *et al.,* 1993; Watillon *et al.,* 1992; Reddy *et al.,* 1993). In this report, we present methods to detect plant CaM-binding proteins that exploit the simplicity with which recombinant plant CaM can be purified in milligram amounts from modest-sized cultures of induced *Escherichia coli* and labeled with a variety of reporters, which offer the advantages of sensitive detection of CaM-binding proteins and relatively low toxicity.

II. Materials

A. Bacterial Strains

E. coli host strains BL21(DE3) (Studier *et al.,* 1990) and XL-1blue and Y1090 were obtained from Novagen and Stratagene, respectively. Recombinant λgt 11 phage containing a cloned calcineurin α-subunit insert (Kincaid *et al.,* 1988) were generously provided by Randall Kincaid.

B. Chemicals

Casein (I-block) and disodium 3-(4-methoxyspiro[1,2-dioxetane-3,2′-(5′-chloro) tricyclo[3.3.1.1^{3,7}]-decan]-4-yl)phenyl phosphate (CSPD) were purchased from Tropix (Bedford, MA). Biotinyl-ε-aminocaproic acid *N*-hydroxysuccinimide ester (biotin-X-NHS) was from Calbiochem (La Jolla, CA). Alkaline phosphatase–avidin D and avidin D–agarose were purchased from Vector Laboratories (Burlingame, CA). Calf intestinal alkaline phosphatase (CaM-free) was obtained from Boehringer-Mannheim (Indianapolis, IN). Succinimidyl 4-(*N*-maleimidomethyl) cyclohexane-1-carboxylate(SMCC), dimethyl formamide (DMF), and 2-mercaptoethylamine were from Pierce (Rockford, IL). DNase I, calcineurin, nitro blue tetrazolium (NBT), and 5-bromo-4-chloro-3-indolyl phosphate (BCIP) were from Sigma (St. Louis, MO); IPTG was from Promega (Madison, WI). Electrophoretic supplies, gelatin, SDS–PAGE molecular weight standards and biotinylated SDS–PAGE standards, and Tween-20 were purchased from Bio-Rad (Richmond, CA).

C. Other Materials and Equipment

Centricon-30 ultrafiltration units were obtained from Amicon. Nytran membranes were purchased from Schleicher and Schuell. PhotoGene chemiluminescence development folders and Reflection autoradiographic film were obtained from GIBCO BRL (Bethesda, MD) and DuPont (Wilmington, DE), respectively. The electrophorectic protein blotter (GENIE blotter) and power supply were from Idea Scientific (Minneapolis, MN).

III. Methods

A. A Plant CaM Expression Vector

A full-length *Arabidopsis thaliana* CaM cDNA (CaM-2, Ling *et al.*, 1991) was cloned into an *Nde*I–*Eco*RI-cleaved pET5a vector (Studier *et al.*, 1990), as shown in Fig. 1a. Before cloning, an *Nde*I recognition sequence was introduced into the CaM translational start site by PCR using a degenerate start site primer (M. C. Gawienowski and R. E. Zielinski, unpublished). Bacterial strains harboring pETCaM-2 and a variety of other CaM sequences have been highly stable in our hands (at least 99% of the bacteria retain the expression plasmids) according to the assay recommended by Studier *et al.* (1990); similarly, all CaM proteins and site-directed mutants we have tested can be handled and labeled using the methods described here. Thus, the assumption implicit in the procedures we describe in this article is that virtually all recombinant plant CaM proteins can be purified and derivatized similarly to those derived from pETCaM-2.

B. Purifying Recombinant CaM

For CaM purification, the procedure of Roberts *et al.* (1985) was used with the following modifications. (1) A single, fresh colony of recombinant bacteria

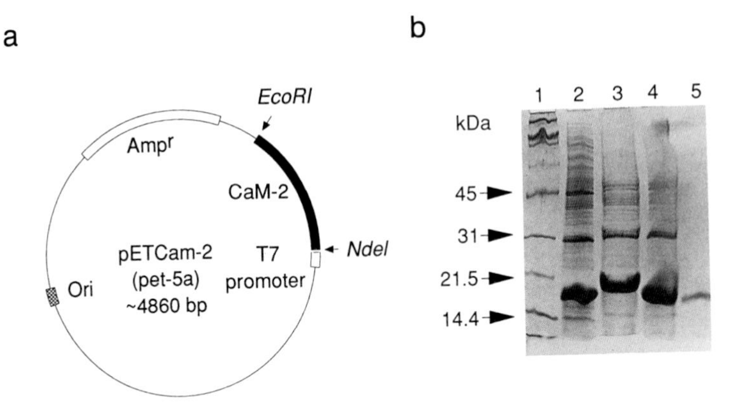

Fig. 1 (a) The design of an expression vector engineered for production of recombinant plant CaM in *E. coli.* An *Nde*I restriction site was engineered by PCR to span the initiator methionine codon of an *Arabidopsis* CaM-2 cDNA. An *Nde*I–*Eco*RI restriction fragment of the CaM-2 cDNA was subcloned into pET-5a to form pETCaM-2, which directs the expression of unfused CaM protein in *E. coli* BL21(DE3). (b) SDS–polyacrylamide gel electrophoresis of protein fractions derived from different stages of a typical recombinant CaM purification from an induced, overproducing strain of bacteria. Lane 1: molecular mass standards; lane 2: crude extract of soluble proteins (20 μg); lane 3: 55% $(NH_4)_2SO_4$-soluble proteins (20 μg); lane 4: pH 4 precipitate (20 μg); lane 5: EDTA eluate from phenyl–Sepharose (2 μg).

was inoculated into 25 ml NZCYM medium containing 25 μg/ml ampicillin and cultured at 37°C with 300 rpm shaking until the A_{550} of the culture reached 0.6. This culture was used to inoculate 1100 ml of NZCYM medium previously warmed to 37°C and the incubation was continued at 37°C with shaking. When the A_{550} of the large culture reached 0.6–0.8, IPTG was added to a final concentration of 1 m*M* and the culture was allowed to continue growing for 3 h. (2) During protein extraction from the induced cells, DNase I concentration was reduced to 45 units/ml during cell lysis. (3) Increased yields of recombinant CaM produced by the pETCaM vector necessitated increasing the size of the phenyl–Sepharose affinity column in the final purification step from 1 to 10 ml, which increased the yield of purified protein proportionally. Typically, we were able to isolate 20 to 40 mg of CaM per liter of induced bacterial culture. The purity of CaM was greater than 95% as judged by SDS–PAGE as shown in Fig. 1b (lane 5) and by direct amino acid sequencing (data not shown). Under the conditions of growth and induction described above, we find that recombinant CaM produced from pETCaM expression plasmids routinely accounts for about 20 to 50% of the total extractable soluble protein (Fig. 1b, lane 2).

C. Purifying ^{35}S-Labeled Recombinant CaM (^{35}S-CaM)

The procedure of Fromm and Chua (1992) was used with some modifications: (1) Chloramphenicol was omitted from the culture because we used the more permissive BL21(DE3) bacterial host; (2) M9 medium of Studier *et al.* (1990) was used instead of the M9 medium of Maniatis *et al.* (1989), because BL21(DE3) does not grow measurably in sulfur-free medium; (3) labeling was performed using ^{35}S-Translabel (ICN, Costa Mesa, CA) instead of [^{35}S]-methionine; (4) CaM bound to phenyl–Sepharose affinity columns was eluted with at least 5 column-volumes of elution buffer (25 m*M* Tris–HCl, pH 7.5, 2 m*M* EGTA). Typical yields were 250–350 μg CaM per 50 ml bacterial culture with a specific activity of 3×10^6 cpm/μg; this represents half the yield of protein, but double the specific activity compared with cells labeled using [^{35}S]-methionine.

D. Conjugating CaM with Alkaline Phosphatase (AP-CaM)

Our method is based on the results of Walker *et al.* (1993), except that we have taken advantage of the fact that plant CaM possesses a single cysteine residue that can be modified with heterobifunctional crosslinking reagents to conjugate CaM with a reporter molecule at a single, well-defined site. Alkaline phosphatase (approximately 3 mg) was dialyzed exhaustively versus conjugation buffer (25 m*M* Hepes/NaOH pH 7.4, 1 m*M* $MgCl_2$, 0.1 m*M* $ZnCl_2$) at 4°C, and then concentrated to a final volume of 100 μl using a Centricon-30 filter. The protein was mixed with 1 μl of 200 m*M* SMCC in DMF and incubated for 30 min at 25°C (this represents a 10-fold molar excess of SMCC to 69-kDa alkaline phosphatase monomers). The reaction was stopped by diluting the mixture with 2 ml of ice-cold cross-linking buffer (25 m*M* Hepes/NaOH, pH 7.4, 150 m*M* NaCl, 1 m*M* $MgCl_2$, 0.1 m*M* $ZnCl_2$), and the activated alkaline phosphatase was then concentrated using a Centricon-30 filter to a final volume of 100 μl. An equal volume of purified CaM (700 μg, 42 nmol) suspended in cross-linking buffer was then mixed with the SMCC-AP and the mixture incubated for 2 h at room temperature. Following the cross-linking reaction, unreacted SMCC-AP molecules were inactivated by adding 2-mercaptoethylamine to the reaction mixture at a final concentration of 1 m*M* and continuing the room temperature incubation for 20 min. Final clean-up of the reaction was performed by diluting the reaction mixture with 2 ml of ice-cold cross-linking buffer and concentrating the proteins using a Centricon-30 filter.

Figure 2a shows a model of AP-CaM, illustrating the nature of the heterobifunctional crosslinking arm joining the polypeptides, whereas Fig 2b qualitatively traces a cross-linking experiment by SDS–PAGE analysis of protein at different stages of the procedure. Lane 4 of Fig. 2b illustrates our typical result that alkaline phosphatase monomers are present that are cross-linked to one (20%), two (40%), or zero (40%) molecules of CaM in the final preparation. AP-CaM can be stored at 4°C for at least 3 months without significant loss of activity.

E. Biotinylating Recombinant CaM (Bio-CaM)

These methods are based on the procedures originally used by Billingsley *et al.* (1985). Biotin-X-NHS ester was dissolved in *N,N*-dimethylformamide (DMF)

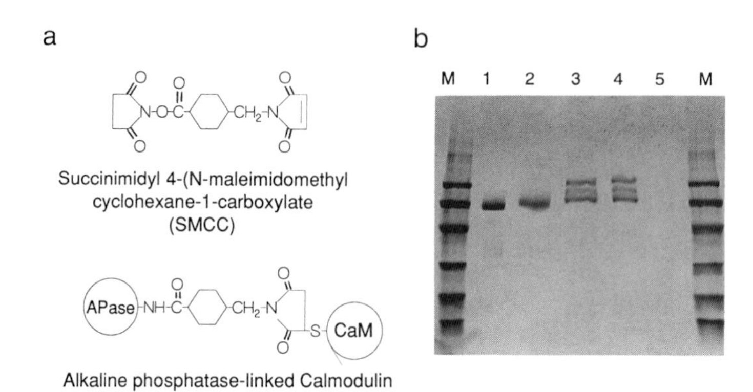

Fig. 2 (a) Generalized structure of CaM covalently coupled to calf intestinal alkaline phosphatase via the heterobifunctional NHS cross-linker, SMCC. (b) SDS–polyacrylamide gel assay of CaM–alkaline phosphatase cross-linking reactions. Lanes M: molecular mass standards; lane 1: dialyzed alkaline phosphatase (2 μg); lane 2: SMCC-modified alkaline phosphatase (2 μg); lanes 3 and 4: alkaline phosphatase-conjugated CaM (equivalent to 2 μg of alkaline phosphatase) before and after final filtration through Centricon-30, respectively; lane 5: retentate from Centricon-30 filtration, which should contain all the unconjugated CaM from the reaction mixture.

at a concentration of 25 mg/ml. CaM was dissolved in 100 m*M* Hepes/NaOH, pH 8.5, at a concentration of 2 mg/ml. To 1 ml of CaM-2 solution, 8 μl of biotin-X-NHS was added. The reaction was incubated at room temperature for 2 h with slow shaking on a rocker platform. The reaction was stopped by adding in 5 μl of ethanolamine. The biotin–CaM conjugate (Bio-CaM) was dialyzed three times against phosphate buffered saline (PBS) to remove unreacted biotin-X-NHS ester. Percentage biotinylation of CaM was assayed by diluting 20 μl of the conjugate into 380 μl of PBS and equally dividing the sample into two tubes. Two hundred microliters of the dilution were passed through a 1.0-ml avidin D agarose column that was previously washed with 10 ml of PBS. Eight hundred microliter of PBS was used to elute the unmodified CaM. The wash and flow-through were collected and amount of protein was assayed using the Bio-Rad protein assay solution. The fraction of CaM that was biotinylated was estimated by the difference in the amount of proteins before and after passing through the avidin D–agarose column divided by the amount of protein before the column chromatography. Normally, 80 to 100% of the input CaM was biotinylated and retained on the avidin D–agarose column. CaM derivatized in this manner can be stored for 6 months at 4°C.

F. Detecting CaM-Binding Proteins

1. Electrophoretic Fractionation and Blotting

Protein fractions to be tested for CaM-binding activity were separated by electrophoresis in 10–20% gradient SDS–polyacrylamide gels. Electrophoresis was carried out in a Mini-PROTEAN II cell (Bio-Rad). Proteins were transferred to Nytran membranes for 1 h at 24 V in a GENIE blotter using Tris–glycine (no methanol) as transfer buffer.

2. Detecting CaM–Protein Interaction Following SDS–PAGE

After blotting, membranes were blocked with 2% casein (I-block) in either buffer A (CaM-binding buffer: 50 m*M* Tris–HCl, 150 m*M* NaCl, 1 m*M* $CaCl_2$, pH 7.5) or buffer B (EDTA buffer: 50 m*M* Tris–HCl, 150 m*M* NaCl, 5 m*M* EDTA, pH 7.5). For protein detection with ^{35}S-CaM, membranes were incubated with 3.2 μg/ml ^{35}S-CaM overnight in buffer A containing 0.5% gelatin, 0.05% Tween-20, and 0.02% NaN_3 and subsequently washed three times (5 min each) with buffer A. The membranes were dried at 37°C and exposed to X-ray films for 2 to 10 days. The labeled CaM could be reused as long as it was stored at 4°C with addition of cycloheximide (10 μg/ml) and chloramphenicol (25 μg/ml).

For protein detection with AP-CaM, membranes were incubated with the conjugate at a concentration of 3.2 μg/ml (the estimated concentration of CaM in the AP-CaM conjugate) in buffer A or B containing 0.5% gelatin, 0.05% Tween-20, and 0.02% NaN_3 for 1 h and washed five times (5 min each) in the same buffer but without CaM, and finally washed five times in assay buffer (0.1 *M* diethanolamine pH 10, 1 m*M* $MgCl_2$, 0.02% NaN_3). Chemiluminescence detection was carried out by incubating the membranes with 0.25 m*M* CSPD in assay buffer for 5 min, then the membranes were briefly blotted on a piece of filter paper and wrapped in development folders. The membranes were exposed to X-ray film for 3 to 10 min. Both the AP-CaM conjugate and the CSPD reagent can be reused for several weeks when stored at 4°C.

For protein detection with Bio-CaM, membranes were incubated with 10 μg/ml of derivatized CaM in buffer A or B containing 0.5% gelatin, 0.05% Tween-20, and 0.02% NaN_3 for 1 h and washed two times (10 min each) in the same buffer without CaM. The membranes were subsequently incubated with alkaline phosphatase–avidin D (1:3000 dilution) in the same buffer for 1 h. For chemiluminescence detection of protein–Bio-CaM complexes, the same procedures as those for AP-CaM were used except that films were exposed for 20–30 min. For conventional colorimetric reaction with Bio-CaM, membranes were washed in buffer A or B containing 0.5% gelatin, 0.05% Tween-20, and 0.02% NaN_3 after reacting the proteins with Bio-CaM, and then washed three times (5 min each) in 100 m*M* Tris–HCl, 100 m*M* NaCl, 5 m*M* $MgCl_2$, pH 9.5; CaM-binding proteins were detected by adding fresh buffer containing 0.17 mg/ml nitro blue tetrazolium (NBT) and 0.08 mg/ml 5-bromo-4-chloro-3-indolyl phosphate (BCIP) and incubating the mixture for 30 min.

3. Screening cDNA Expression Libraries

The method of Fromm and Chua (1992) was used, except that (1) Nytran filters were used to immobilize the recombinant proteins; (2) recombinant protein production was induced by incubating filters on phage lawns overnight (about 12 h) at 37°C; and (3) filters were blocked with 2% gelatin in buffer A. To detect CaM-BP with AP-CaM, the conditions described above for electrophoretically transferred proteins were used.

IV. Critical Aspects of the Procedures

One of the most critical aspects of the procedure to detect CaM-binding proteins separated by SDS–PAGE is the efficiency with which the binding proteins are transferred to solid supports. Ling and Assmann (1992) reported that the use of alkaline pH CAPS-based buffers in a wire-electrode-type electrophoretic transfer apparatus greatly enhanced the sensitivity of their CaM-binding protein assays. Although this system has been successful in our hands, we find the best system for protein transfer to membranes has been an apparatus that utilizes plate-type electrodes, minimal buffer volume, and a high electrical field and Tris–glycine (no methanol) buffer. Clearly, the issue of vital importance at this step is to maximize the transfer of protein from the gel to the solid support medium. These conditions should be established empirically using the available transfer apparatus and power supplies before initiating experiments to detect CaM-binding proteins.

To detect CaM-binding proteins using ^{35}S-CaM in either expression library screening experiments or following separation by SDS–PAGE, it is crucial to label and purify sufficient amounts of CaM with the highest possible specific activity. We have compared the growth of BL21(DE3) bacterial cells harboring the pET-CaM expression plasmid in the M9 media of Studier *et al.* (1990) and of Maniatis *et al.* (1989), and found that BL21(DE3) cells would not grow in the sulfur-free M9 recipe of Maniatis *et al.* (1989). We attempted several experiments in which sulfur-free medium was supplemented with various mixtures of ^{35}S-labeled and cold Na_2SO_4, but we were not able to supply BL21(DE3) cells with sufficient amounts of $Na_2{}^{35}SO_4$ to meet both criteria of high specific activity and protein yield because of the amount of radioisotope required. As a more cost-efficient compromise, we first grew the bacteria in the M9 medium of Studier *et al.* (1990) to an A_{600} of 0.8–1, and then induced the bacteria with IPTG and added [^{35}S]methionine or -Translabel. At this point, endogenous sulfur in the medium is growth-limiting, and thus, uptake and incorporation of ^{35}S-labeled amino acids into recombinant CaM is very efficient. This approach enabled us to obtain 250–350 μg of CaM per 20-ml culture with a specific activity of 1–1.5 $\times$ 10^6 cpm/μg using [^{35}S]methionine, and approximately the same mass of CaM, but with a specific activity of 3 $\times$ 10^6 cpm/μg, using ^{35}S-Translabel in a 50-ml culture.

For screening cDNA expression libraries for clones encoding CaM-binding proteins, it is crucial to minimize the background. The conditions described here for both ^{35}S-CaM and AP-CaM are sufficiently stringent and reproducible to facilitate their use in screening recombinant phage. However, when we used Bio-CaM as probe to screen cDNA expression libraries or positive controls harboring cDNAs encoding known CaM-regulated proteins, we found that the background signals made it impossible to distinguish between the positive and the negative controls. This is probably due to high level of endogenous biotin in the plating bacteria, because the background was somewhat bacterial strain-dependent. We have tried to block filters with avidin to mask endogenous biotin before probing, but the level of residual avidin on the filters was high enough to mask the positive controls. Thus, we do not consider Bio-CaM to be a sufficiently reliable ligand to screen expression libraries in the bacterial strains XL-1blue and Y1090, even though it is a sensitive and reliable reagent for detecting CaM-binding proteins fractionated by SDS–PAGE.

V. Results

The utility of the different methods we have described for labeling CaM to use as a probe for detecting CaM-binding proteins can be illustrated using two applications, which involve detecting CaM-binding activity in protein fractions after separation by SDS–PAGE and in induced lysates of recombinant bacteriophage harboring cDNA expression libraries.

Figure 3 shows the results of an experiment in which crude protein fractions prepared from etiolated or green pea plants and known amounts of the CaM-regulated phosphoprotein phosphatase, calcineurin, were separated by SDS–PAGE and probed with derivatized CaM proteins. Although CaM-binding activity can be detected with each of the CaM probes described, the qualitative spectrum of proteins recognized and the level of detection sensitivity varies widely. In terms of both sensitivity and speed detection, AP-CaM is clearly the probe of choice. Using known amounts of calcineurin as a standard, we estimate that the limits of detection of CaM-binding activity are 100 pg for AP-CaM, 1 ng for Bio-CaM using chemiluminescent detection, 10 ng for Bio-CaM using colorimetric reagents, and 30 ng using ^{35}S-CaM (labeled with [^{35}S]methionine). It should be noted that the sensitivity of ^{35}S-CaM labeled with ^{35}S-Translabel is expected to be close to that of Bio-CaM detected with the colorimetric reagents NBT and BCIP, but the speed with which the results are obtained is still greatly in favor of Bio-CaM. In most, but not all, cases, binding of labeled CaM to the immobilized proteins is dependent on the presence of Ca^{2+}.

Although the Bio-CaM and ^{35}S-CaM probes qualitatively recognize a similar spectrum of CaM-binding proteins, different polypeptides appear to be detected with different levels of efficiency. Even more dramatic is the difference between the spectrum of CaM-binding proteins detected between AP-CaM and those revealed by all other CaM probes tested (e.g., compare the patterns observed in Figs. 3a and 3c, lanes 3 and 4). These results are probably a consequence of steric hindrance caused by the AP reporter moiety, which prevents or greatly

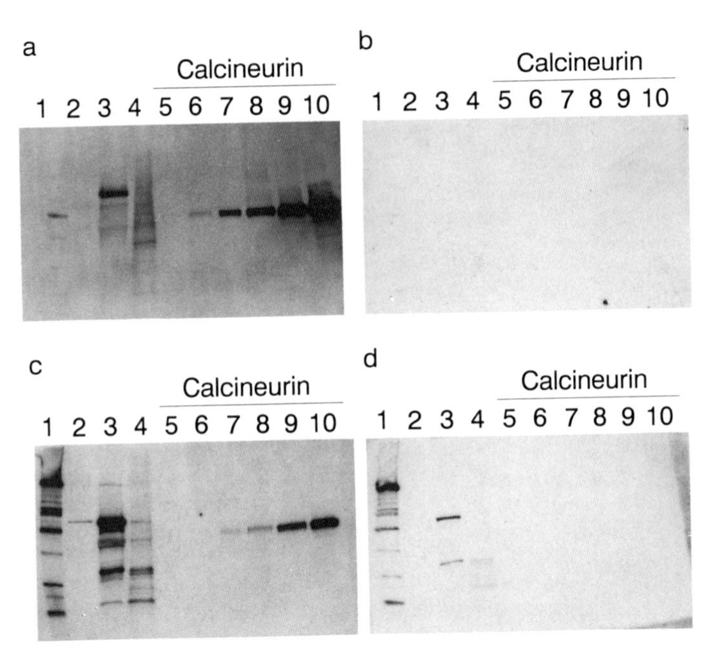

Fig. 3 Detection of CaM-binding proteins following SDS–PAGE fractionation and the limits of sensitivity of the method using CaM probes derivatized as described in the text. Detection with AP-CaM in presence of Ca^{2+} (a) or EDTA (b). Detection with Bio-CaM and chemiluminescent reagent in the presence of Ca^{2+} (c) or EDTA (d). Detection with Bio-CaM and colorimetric reagents in the presence of Ca^{2+} (e). Detection with ^{35}S-CaM labeled with [^{35}S]methionine (f). Protein profiles of samples after (g) or before (h) electrotransfer. Lane 1 (a, b): prestained molecular weight standard (low-range, Bio-Rad); lane 1 (f, g, h, also lane 7 of h): molecular weight standard (low range, Bio-Rad); lane 1 (c, d, e): biotinylated molecular weight standard (low range, Bio-Rad); lane 2: 1 μg purified rubisco; lane 3: crude, soluble protein extract from etiolated pea seedlings; lane 4: pea leaf soluble proteins at an intermediate stage in the purification of NAD kinase; lanes 5–10 (a–g): 0.1, 1, 10, 30, 100, 300 ng calcineurin, respectively; lanes 5–6 (h): 300, 100 ng calcineurin, respectively.

reduces the ability of AP-CaM to interact with certain proteins. These results are consistent with a variety of site-directed mutagenesis (e.g., Craig *et al.*, 1987), genetic (e.g., Ohya and Botstein, 1994), and chemical modification studies (e.g., Mann and Vanaman, 1989), which have indicated that different regions of CaM are critical for its interaction with different CaM-regulated proteins. Thus, one practical advantage of the differential interaction of ^{35}S-CaM, Bio-CaM, and AP-CaM with CaM-binding proteins is that they can be used to identify biochemically different classes of CaM-binding proteins.

Because of the differences in the CaM-binding proteins recognized by recombinant CaM labeled with different reporter molecules, we have generally favored performing primary screens of cDNA expression libraries with ^{35}S-CaM, despite the limitation that it is the least sensitive method for detecting CaM–protein interaction. This is based on three primary considerations: first, ^{35}S-CaM should

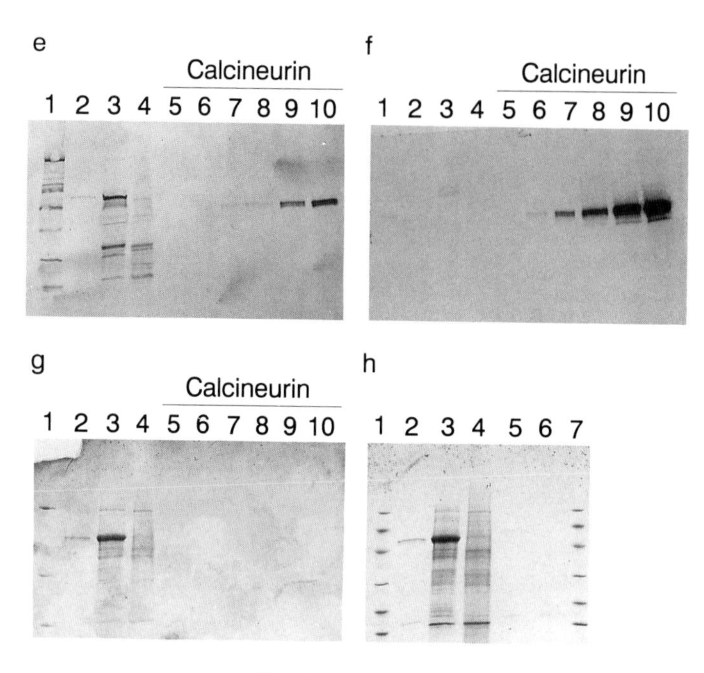

Fig. 3 (*continued*).

interact with the broadest spectrum of CaM-binding proteins because there is no steric hindrance from bulky reporter groups; second, ^{35}S-CaM produces low backgrounds, which minimizes the selection of false positives; and third, the backgrounds we have generally observed using Bio-CaM, whose spectrum of protein recognition is similar to that of ^{35}S-CaM, is unacceptably high for reproducibly screening recombinant phage libraries. In these experiments, labeling CaM using ^{35}S-Translabel yields probes that provide the best signal-to-background ratios, and clear autoradiographic exposures of plaque screens are normally obtained within 2 days.

Once primary screening experiments have identified phage harboring cDNAs encoding putative CaM-binding proteins, however, secondary screenings can be performed using both ^{35}S-CaM and AP-CaM. Figure 4 shows the result of a control experiment in which recombinant phage harboring a calcineurin α-subunit cDNA insert (Kincaid *et al.*, 1988) were screening using ^{35}S-CaM and AP-CaM. In these lower density screenings, AP-CaM provides an alternative means for rapid screening with only moderate to low levels of background. An additional bonus of this method is that, because of the different qualitative spectrum of AP-CaM interaction with CaM-binding proteins compared with ^{35}S-CaM, different classes of CaM-binding proteins can be recognized during the process of library screening. This will assist in sorting the recombinant sequences and minimizing the numbers of clones that must be analyzed by cross-hybridiza-

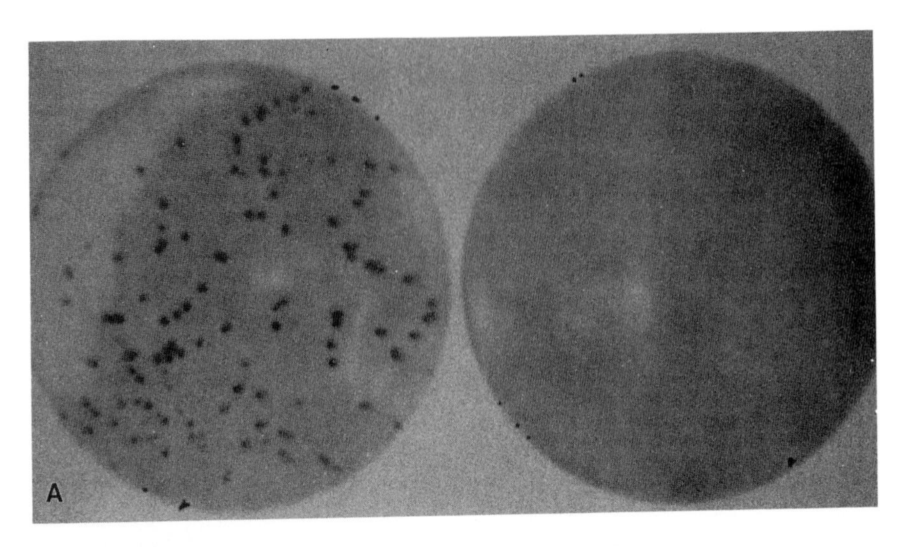

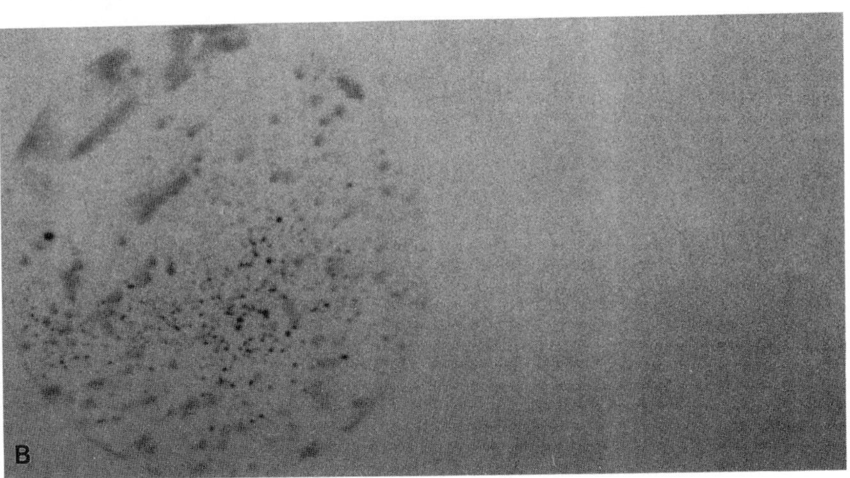

Fig. 4 Screening of recombinant phage from a λgt11 cDNA expression library using (A) AP-CaM or (B) ^{35}S-CaM labeled with [^{35}S]methionine. Left panel: a positive control recombinant phage harboring a calcineurin α-subunit cDNA insert; right panel: negative control phage. Autoradiographic exposures were for (A) 5 min and (B) 2 days.

tion and DNA sequencing. A different strategy to grouping CaM-binding protein cDNA clones is to analyze the interaction of the proteins they encode with CaM after inducing protein production in lysogens or after subcloning the cDNA inserts in expression vectors. Although more time-consuming than plaque-based assays, this method is compatible with all the recombinant CaM probes because binding is performed on extracted proteins after fractionating them by SDS–

PAGE. Using these methods, we have isolated over 100 potential cDNA clones encoding CaM-binding proteins from various *Arabidopsis* cDNA expression libraries (B. Liao, A. Singh and R. E. Zielinski, unpublished data). Preliminary sequence analyses of a limited number of these cDNAs indicate that they represent a wide variety of CaM-binding proteins, including homologs of known CaM-regulated proteins from animals and some that may be unique to higher plant systems. Thus, the tools described in this report should prove to be invaluable in the identification and biochemical characterization of the protein response elements involved in the early steps in Ca^{2+}-based signal transduction pathways in plants.

Acknowledgment

This work was supported by a grant from the National Science Foundation (MCB 92-05702) to R.E.Z.

References

Baum, G., Chen, Y., Arazi, T., Takatsuji, H., and Fromm, H. (1993). A plant glutamate decarboxylase containing a calmodulin binding domain. *J. Biol. Chem.* **268,** 19610–19617.

Billingsley, M. L., Pennypacker, K. R., Hoover, C. G., Brigati, D. L., and Kincaid, R. L. (1985). A rapid and sensitive method for detection and quantification of calcineurin and calmodulin-binding proteins using biotinylated calmodulin. *Proc. Natl. Acad. Sci. U.S.A.* **82,** 7585–7589.

Craig, T. A., Watterson, D. M., Prendergast, F. G., Haiech, J., and Roberts, D. M. (1987). Site-specific mutagenesis of the α-helices of calmodulin. Effects of altering a charge cluster in the helix that links the two halves of calmodulin. *J. Biol. Chem.* **262,** 3278–3284.

Fromm, H., and Chua, N.-H. (1992). Cloning of plant cDNAs encoding calmodulin-binding proteins using ^{35}S-labeled recombinant calmodulin as a probe. *Plant Mol. Biol. Rep.* **10,** 199–206.

Ikura, M., Clore, G. M., Gronenborn, A. M., Zhu, G., Klee, C. B., and Bax, A. (1992). Solution structure of a calmodulin-target peptide complex by multidimensional NMR. *Science* **256,** 632–638.

Kincaid, R. L., Nightingale, M. S., and Martin, B. M. (1988). Characterization of a cDNA clone encoding the calmodulin-binding domain of mouse brain calcineurin. *Proc. Natl. Acad. Sci. U.S.A.* **85,** 8983–8987.

Ling, V., and Assmann, S. M. (1992). Cellular distribution of calmodulin and calmodulin-binding proteins in *Vicia faba* L. *Plant Physiol.* **100,** 970–978.

Ling, V., Perera, I., and Zielinski, R. E. (1991). Primary structures of *Arabidopsis* calmodulin isoforms deduced from the sequences of cDNA clones. *Plant Physiol.* **96,** 1196–1202.

Maniatis, T., Fritsch, E. F., and Sambrook, J. (1989). "Molecular Cloning: A Laboratory Manual." p. A.3. Cold Spring Harbor, NY: Cold Spring Harbor Laboratory Press,

Mann, D. M., and Vanaman, T. C. (1989). Topographical mapping of calmodulin-target enzyme interaction domains. *J. Biol. Chem.* **264,** 2373–2378.

Ohya, Y., and Botstein, D. (1994). Diverse essential functions revealed by complementing yeast calmodulin mutants. *Science* **263,** 963–966.

O'Neil, K. T., and DeGrado, W. F. (1989). How calmodulin binds its targets: Sequence independent recognition of amphiphilic α-helices. *Trends Biochem. Sci.* **15,** 59–64.

Poovaiah, B. W., and Reddy, A. S. N. (1993). Calcium and signal transduction in plants. *CRC Crit. Rev. Plant Sci.* **12,** 185–211.

Reddy, A. S. N., Takezawa, D., Fromm, H., and Poovaiah, B. W. (1993). Isolation and characterization of two cDNAs that encode for calmodulin-binding proteins from corn root tips. *Plant Sci.* **94,** 109–117.

Roberts, D. M., Crea, R., Malecha, M., Alvarado-Urbina, G., Chiarello, R. H., Watterson, D. M. (1985). Chemical synthesis and expression of a calmodulin gene designed for site-specific mutagenesis. *Biochemistry* **24,** 5090–5098.

Roberts, D. M., and Harmon, A. C. (1992). Calcium-modulated proteins: targets of intracellular calcium signals in higher plants. *Annu. Rev. Plant Physiol. Mol. Biol.* **43,** 375–414.

Studier, F. W., Rosenberg, A. H., Dunn, J. J., and Dubendorf, J. W. (1990). Use of T7 RNA polymerase to direct expression of cloned genes. *Methods Enzymol.* **185,** 60–89.

Walker, R. G., Hudspeth, A. J., and Gillespie, P. G. (1993). Calmodulin and calmodulin-binding proteins in hair bundles. *Proc. Natl. Acad. Sci. U.S.A.* **90,** 2807–2811.

Watillon, B., Kettmann, R., Boxus, P., and Burny, A. (1992). Cloning and characterization of an apple (*Malus domestica* (L.)) cDNA encoding a calmodulin-binding protein domain similar to the calmodulin-binding region of type-II mammalian Ca^{2+}/calmodulin-dependent protein kinase. *Plant Sci.* **81,** 227–235.

CHAPTER 35

Analysis of the Light Signaling Pathway in Stomatal Guard Cells

Ken-Ichiro Shimazaki* **and Toshinori Kinoshita†**

* Biological Laboratory
College of General Education
Kyushu University
Ropponmatsu, Fukuoka 810, Japan

† Department of Biology
Faculty of Science
Kyushu University
Hakozaki, Fukuoka 812, Japan

I. Introduction

Stomatal aperture, which regulates gas exchange between leaves and the atmosphere, is modulated by volume changes in guard cell pairs. Guard cells surrounding the stomatal pore respond to external stimuli, such as light, growth regulators (abscisic acid, auxin), Ca^{2+}, CO_2, and air pollutants, and these responses act to

METHODS IN CELL BIOLOGY, VOL. 49

optimize growth conditions for plants (Willmer, 1983; Zeiger, 1983). The cells depend heavily on signal transduction mechanisms by which the external stimuli are transduced into intracellular signals (Assmann, 1993).

Light is the most important environmental signal for guard cells as well as for the whole plant. Blue light induces stomatal opening. It creates a proton electrochemical gradient across the guard cell plasma membrane, by signaling the activation of the proton pump (Assmann *et al.*, 1985; Shimazaki *et al.*, 1986), and this drives uptake of K^+ through a voltage-gated K^+ channel (Schroeder *et al.*, 1987). Although blue light responses such as phototropism, heliotropism, movement of chloroplasts and pulvini, suppression of hypocotyl elongation, and stomatal opening are ubiquitous in the plant kingdom, the molecular mechanisms of these responses have not been clarified. Investigation of the signal transduction process involved in the blue light response of stomata may provide clues to elucidate the mechanisms underlying light-dependent, transmembrane signaling in plant cells.

In this chapter, we describe methods for the isolation of epidermal layers and guard cell protoplasts, to provide the basic materials for the study of the physiology and biochemistry of stomata. We provide a description of the use of pharmacological tools as probes of the blue light signaling pathway in stomata. Protein phosphorylation and dephosphorylation are known to play a key role when the external stimuli are transduced into intracellular signals in all organisms. Methods for the measurement of phosphorylation and dephosphorylation of guard cell proteins in response to light will also be described.

There have been extensive studies on the molecular mechanisms of signal transduction involved in the process of stomatal closing, using techniques of electrophysiology and cell biology (Assmann, 1993). For more-general methods for the study of stomata, readers are referred to Weyers and Meidner (1990).

II. Materials and Methods

A. Preparation of Epidermal Peels

Commelina benghalensis plants grown for 4 to 8 weeks in a greenhouse 22°–30°C) are kept in the dark for 14 h before peeling. Leaf strips (5-mm width, 4-cm length) are excised with a razor blade parallel to the veins, and the epidermis is peeled from the abaxial side under dim orange light. As reported by Weyers and Travis (1981) for *C. communis,* the epidermal cells of *C. benghalensis* are damaged and show reduced responsiveness to light, if the angle of peeling is acute rather than obtuse. The strips of epidermis obtained are floated on distilled water (cuticular side up), and are cut with small ceramic scissors in the water by holding the end of the epidermis with forceps. The resultant isolated epidermal strips (5 × 5 mm) are stored in distilled water in the dark until use; most of the stomata are closed. Preparation of epidermal layers of *C. communis* and *Vicia faba* suitable for investigation of stomatal movement can be found in Schwartz and Zeiger (1984) and Weyers and Meidner (1990).

B. Isolation of Guard Cell Protoplasts from *Vicia faba*

Methods for the isolation of guard cell protoplasts from onion and tobacco were first reported by Zeiger and Hepler (1976), and from *V. faba* and *C. communis* on a large scale by Schnabl *et al.* (1978), Shimazaki *et al.* (1982), and Fitzsimons and Weyers (1983).

1. Slow Method

The abaxial epidermis is peeled from 4- to 8-week-old *Vicia* leaves (about 100 leaves) using a wide-edged forceps in distilled water. Green portions attached to isolated epidermis are removed with a sharp-edged forceps and the epidermal strips are accumulated in ice-cold distilled water. The accumulated epidermal peels are cut with ceramic scissors and treated by ultrasonication (Ultrasonic disrupter, Tomy Model UD-201, Tokyo) for 20 s to remove contaminating mesophyll cells and to destroy epidermal cells. Cell fragments are washed out with distilled water on 200-μm nylon mesh. The retained epidermal material is transferred to an osmoticum comprising 0.25 *M* mannitol, 1 m*M* $CaCl_2$, and 4% Onozuka R-10, pH 5.4. Incubation is continued for 1 h at 20°C with shaking (50 strokes/min). The digested epidermal strips are rinsed with 0.35 *M* mannitol and 1 m*M* $CaCl_2$ on a nylon mesh (58 μm), and then transferred into a medium containing 4% Cellulase Onozuka R-10, 0.35 *M* mannitol, 2.5 m*M* $CaCl_2$, 0.5% BSA, and 20 μg/ml chloramphenicol. Incubation is continued with gentle shaking (30 strokes/min) for 14 h at 20°C. The digestion medium is passed through a membrane filter (pore size = 0.22 μm, Fuji Film Co., Tokyo) to remove bacteria. Released protoplasts are passed through a nylon mesh (25 μm) and collected by low-speed centrifugation for 5 min ($110 \times g$). The protoplast pellet is washed twice with 0.4 *M* mannitol and 1 m*M* $CaCl_2$, and the protoplasts are stored in the dark on ice before use.

2. Fast Method

The first-step digestion of the epidermis is done for 40 min at 27°C (110 strokes/min) in a medium containing 0.02% Pectolyase Y-23 (Seishin Pharmaceutical Industry Co., Japan), 2% Cellulase Onozuka RS (Yakult Pharmaceutical Industry Co., Japan), 0.2% BSA, 1 μg/ml pepstatin A, 0.25 *M* mannitol, and 1 m*M* $CaCl_2$ (pH 5.5) (Gotow *et al.,* 1984). For the second-step digestion, the mannitol concentration is raised to 0.4 *M*, while the other ingredients remain the same as described in Sction II,B,1. The digestion is performed for 90 min (40 strokes/min).

3. Blender Method

The blender method has the advantage of being applicable to many kinds of plant species because it avoids time-consuming peeling (Kruse *et al.*, 1989). The essence of this method is to isolate the epidermis by mechanical separation from other tissue in a Waring blender. Midveins and veins of *Vicia* leaves are removed with scissors or a razor blade, and the leaves are cut into small pieces (10 × 10 mm). Leaf pieces are homogenized at room temperature in a solution of 10%Ficoll, 5 m*M* $CaCl_2$ and 0.1% polyvinylpyrrolidone (K-30). Homogenization conditions vary from 7000 rpm for 3 min to 20,000 rpm for 50 s, depending on plant age and species. Epidermal peels are washed thoroughly with tap-water on nylon mesh (200 μm), and are then subjected to the enzymatic digestion procedures described previously. Mesophyll and xylem fragments are sometimes difficult to eliminate from the final protoplast preparation. Such contaminants can be removed by discontinuous, Percoll density-gradient centrifugation (400 × *g*, 5 min); *Vicia* protoplasts are usually recovered in a band between 50 and 90% Percoll. Guard cell protoplasts can be isolated from *Commelina communis, Chlorophytum, Nicotiana glauca,* and *Zea mays* by this method. (Kruse *et al.*, 1989).

C. Measurements of Stomatal Opening and Swelling of Guard Cell Protoplasts

Stomatal opening is determined by measuring apertures in the epidermis of *C. benghalensis* using an inverted microscope (Nikon Diaphot TMD) equipped with a precalibrated ocular micrometer. Four to six epidermal strips (5 × 5 mm) are floated on incubation medium (cuticular side up) in a small petri dish (16-mm diameter, 2.5 ml). The medium comprises 10 m*M* Mes–NaOH (pH 6.1), 30 m*M* KCl, and 0.1 m*M* $CaCl_2$. The petri dish is placed directly on a flat glass bottle (thickness 5 cm), which contains distilled water, and is illuminated with blue light from the top through a light guide, and with red light from the bottom. A heat-absorbing filter (thickness 4 mm) was inserted between the red light source and the glass bottle. Blue light is obtained by passing the light from a halogen lamp (Sylvania EFR 150W) through a blue glass filter (Corning 5-60). Red light is obtained by passing the light from a halogen lamp (Sylvania EXR 300 W) through a red glass filter (Corning 2-61). The suggested light intensity is 600 μmol m^{-2} s^{-1} for red light and 15 μmol m^{-2} s^{-1} for blue light. During illumination of the epidermis for extended periods (more than 1 h), a drop of distilled water is added to the incubation medium. It is possible to determine the apertures of 60 to 80 stomata within 6 min.

Swelling of guard cell protoplasts corresponds to the opening of stomata (Zeiger and Hepler, 1977). The diameters of guard cell protoplasts can be determined by taking a photograph of the protoplasts using light microscopy at magnification of 400×, and cell volume can be calculated on the assumption that the protoplasts are perfect spheres (Gotow *et al.*, 1984). Guard cell protoplasts (0.5 ml, 0.5 × 10^6 cells/ml) from *Vicia* are incubated in 0.4 *M* mannitol, 10 m*M*

KCl, 1 m*M* $CaCl_2$ and 10 m*M* Mes–NaOH (pH 6.2) under light or with fusicoccin (FC) for the indicated periods, with gentle stirring at 24°C.

Recently, a sophisticated method to determine the diameter of guard cell protoplasts has been developed using a microscope attached to a digitizing CCD camera, connected to an image processor (Amodeo *et al.*, 1992). This method has made it possible to determine the diameter of 10 to 15 protoplasts within 30 s.

D. Measurement of Blue Light-Dependent Proton Pumping in Guard Cell Protoplasts

Blue light-dependent proton pumping by guard cell protoplasts is measured by the pH decrease in the suspension of guard cell protoplasts using a dual-beam protocol (Shimazaki *et al.*, 1986). The reaction mixture (1.0 ml) consists of 0.125 m*M* Mes–NaOH (pH 6.0), 1 m*M* $CaCl_2$, 0.4 *M* mannitol, 10 m*M* KCl in which are suspended the guard cell protoplasts (40–80 μg as soluble protein). Red light at 600 μmol $m^{-2}s^{-1}$ is obtained from a tungsten lamp by passing light through a glass cut-off filter (Corning 2-61). Blue light is provided by a tungsten lamp through a glass filter (Corning 5-60) at 100 μmol $m^{-2}s^{-1}$ for 30 s. The pH of the suspension is monitored with a glass pH electrode connected to a pH meter (Beckman ϕ71) and recorded on a chart recorder. Frequently, the pH electrode records an artificial pH change in response to blue light illumination. To prevent this, an orange filter (cinemoid 5A) must be attached to the electrode facing the blue light.

E. Measurement of Protein Phosphorylation and Dephosphorylation in Guard Cells

1. One-Dimensional SDS–Polyacrylamide Gel Electrophoresis Followed by Autoradiography

Guard cell protoplasts are incubated in 0.39 *M* mannitol, 1 m*M* $CaCl_2$, 10 m*M* Mes–NaOH (pH 6.1), 10 m*M* KCl, and 1850 kBq of $^{32}P_i$. The mixture is assembled and kept in the dark, and then illuminated for the indicated periods. The reaction is terminated by the addition of solubilization medium to an aliquot of the protoplast suspension. The final solubilized sample (70 μl) comprises 10 m*M* Tris–HCl (pH 8), 1 m*M* EDTA, 2% SDS, 10% sucrose, 5% 2-mercaptoethanol, 0.004% Coomassie brilliant blue, 1 m*M* PMSF, 2 μg/ml leupeptin, and the protoplasts (30 μg protein). To facilitate solubilization, the samples are heated in hot water at 95°C for 5 min and then stored on ice until use.

Solubilized samples are subjected to SDS–PAGE according to the method of Laemmli (1970). The separation gel contains 12.5 and 7.5% polyacrylamide for low- and high-molecular-weight proteins, respectively. The stacking gel contained 4% polyacrylamide. After electrophoresis, the gel is stained in a solution of 0.25% Coomassie brilliant blue, 50% methanol, and 10% acetic acid for 20 min, destained in 25% ethanol and 7% acetic acid for 3 h, and then dried on a gel-drier. Autoradiography is carried out by exposing Fuji RX film to the dried gels for 12 to 48 h at room temperature.

2. Two-Dimensional Gel Electrophoresis

The two-dimensional gel electrophoresis method reported by O'Farrell (1975) can separate more than 1000 polypeptides. The method combines isoelectric focusing in the first dimension and SDS–PAGE in the second. Since separated polypeptides migrate according to their isoelectric point pH (pI), and the pI of individual polypeptides changes upon protein phosphorylation, the occurrence of protein phosphorylation can be detected as a mobility shift of the polypeptide. Although the method gives high resolution with a pI in the range of pH 4–7, it is difficult to resolve proteins that are either more basic or more acidic. We adopted nonequilibrium pH gradient electrophoresis (NEPHGE) (O'Farrell *et al.*, 1977) by which proteins with wider pI values (pH 3.5 to 10) can be separated. Furthermore, the method was modified to solubilize membranes of guard cells according to the method by Hurkman and Tanaka (1986).

An Aliquot of the protoplast suspension (200 μg protein), having been illuminated with blue or red light for the indicated time periods, is mixed with 50% TCA (final concentration of 10% TCA) to terminate the reaction. After 10 min, the mixture is centrifuged at 11,000 rpm for 15 min, and the resulting pellet is suspended in 4% SDS, 2% 2-mercaptoethanol, 20% glycerol, and 2 m*M* PMSF in 100 m*M* Tris–HCl (pH 8.5). The sample is heated for 3 min at 80°C and solubilized using vigorous mixing. Four volumes of cold acetone (−20°C) are added, and the centrifugation is repeated. The pellet is dried and solubilized in 50 μl of a solution containing 9.5 *M* urea (Schwarz/Mann, Biotech, Inc.), 2% Nonidet P-40 (Nacalai, Tesque, Inc., Kyoto, Japan), 5% 2-mercaptoethanol, and 5% Ampholine (pH 3.5/10, Pharmacia LKB, Sweden). The solubilized sample is subjected to isoelectric focusing, and the reaction is terminated before reaching equilibrium. The gel mixture contains 9.2 *M* urea, 2% Nonidet P-40, 4% acrylamide (Bio-Rad), 0.2% bisacrylamide (Bio-Rad), and 2% Ampholine (pH 3.5/10). The mixture is poured into a glass tube (2.5 × 130 mm) and the gel is polymerized by addition of 10 μl of 10% ammonium persulfate and 7 μl N,N,N^1,N^1,-tetramethylenediamine (TEMED) to 10 ml of the mixture. Solubilized guard cell proteins (200 μg) are loaded on top of the gel, the solution (10 μl) of 6 *M* urea and 2% Ampholine (pH 3.5/10) is overlaid further. Electrophoresis is carried out at constant voltage using 100 V for 30 min, 300 V for 30min, 500 V for 30 min, and finally 700 V for 2 h. The anode at the top is covered with 0.01 *M* H_3PO_4 and the cathode on the bottom is 0.02 *M* NaOH. After electrophoresis, the gels containing separated proteins are equilibrated with a solution of 2.3% SDS, 5% 2-mercaptoethanol, 10% glycerol, and 63 m*M* Tris–HCl (pH 6.8) for 30 min at 40°C. The equilibrated gel is attached to the top of a slab gel with 1% agarose (Schwarz/Mann, Biotech) prepared in the equilibration solution and is subjected to SDS–PAGE on the slab gel

($1 \times 130 \times 140$ mm) according to the method of Laemmli (1970). Polypeptides on the slab gel are stained with silver (Sil-best stain, Nacalai Tesque, Kyoto, Japan). The protein content is determined by the method of Bradford (1976).

III. Results and Discussion

Guard cell protoplasts appear as a pair of spheres surrounding the stomatal pore, similar to their appearance within the intact epidermis (Fig. 1A). Epidermal strips in the digestion medium are passed through a wide-mouth 10-ml glass pipet by repeated (20 to 30 times) resuspension, to release the protoplasts. Isolated protoplasts are shown in Fig. 1B.

When a suspension of guard cell protoplasts is illuminated by red light (600 μmol $m^{-2}s^{-1}$), high alkalinization due to CO_2 uptake is observed (Fig. 2a). The pH shows an almost constant value after about 50 min of illumination. A short pulse of blue light (100 μmol $m^{-2}s^{-1}$, 3 0 s) superimposed on the background red light is given. The pH decrease starts about 25 s after blue light illumination and is sustained for more than 10 min after the pulse (Shimazaki *et al.*, 1986). Since the pH decrease shows a time course similar to that of the blue light-dependent ion pumping measured by whole-cell patch clamping (Assmann *et al.*, 1985), the pH decrease seems to be due to electrogenic proton pumping.

Blue light seems to induce stomatal opening by activating the plasma membrane proton pump; however, the mechanism by which the perception of blue light is transduced into the pump activation is not known. Recent investigations have suggested that protein phosphorylation carried out by protein kinases is one of the key events in the signal transduction process in both plant and animal cells. Various kinds of protein kinase inhibitors have been developed to investi-

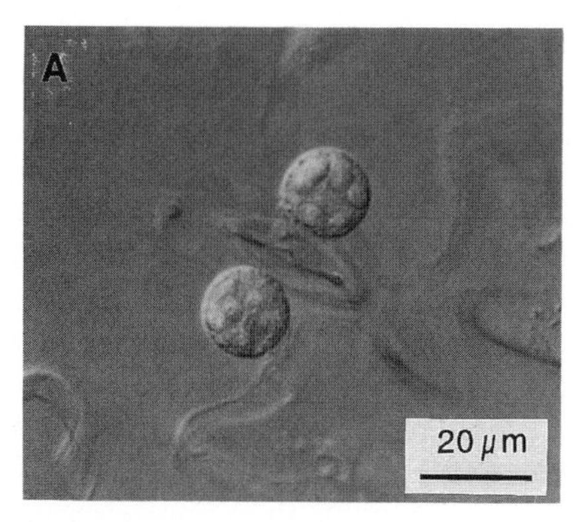

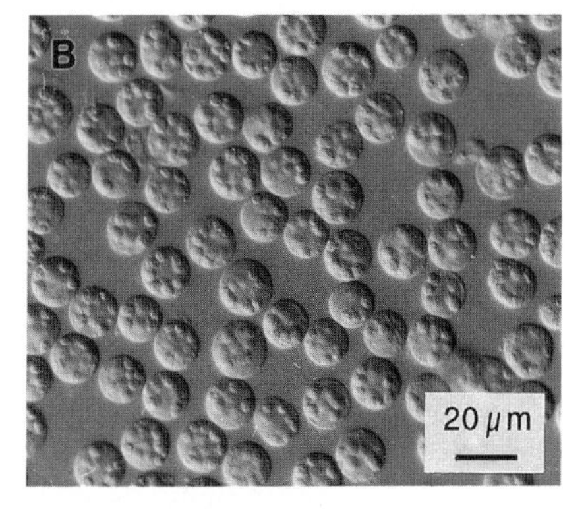

Fig. 1 Guard cell protoplasts formed at the stomatal pore of *Vicia faba* (A), and isolated guard cell protoplasts (B). Chloroplasts can be seen clearly in the protoplasts.

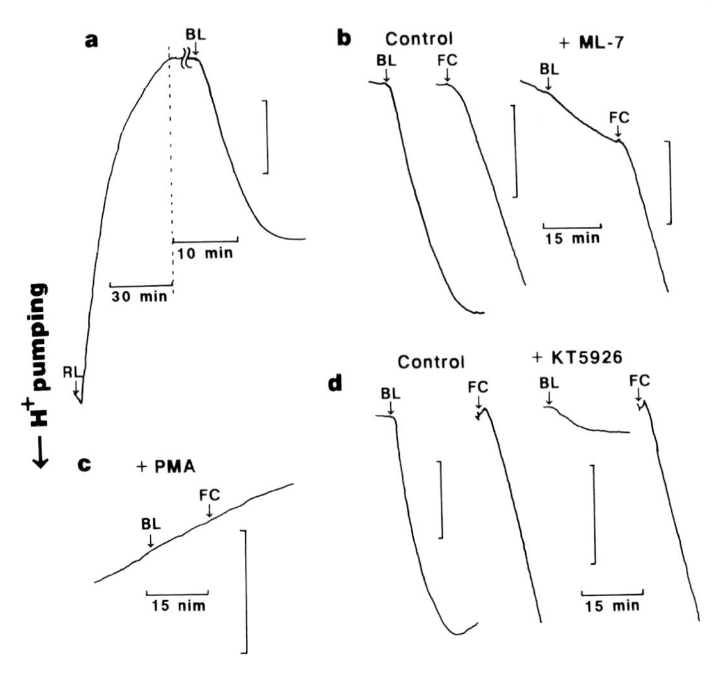

Fig. 2 Blue light-dependent proton pumping in *Vicia* guard cell protoplasts. (a) A large alkalinization elicited by red light (RL), and acidification (pH decrease) elicited by a pulse of blue light (100 μmol $m^{-2}s^{-1}$, 30 s), in a suspension of guard cell protoplasts. (b) Effect of ML-7. (c) Effect of PMA. (d) Effect of KT5926. Concentrations of ML-7, KT5926, PMA, and FC were 100, 10, 5 and 10 μM, respectively (for details, see text).

gate the role of kinases in animal cells (Table I), although these inhibitors have not been tested extensively in plant cells.

Table II shows the effects of these inhibitors on the magnitude of blue light-dependent proton pumping in *Vicia* guard cell protoplasts. Table III documents effects of inhibitors on stomatal opening in the epidermis of *C. benghalensis.* Both blue light-dependent proton pumping and light-dependent stomatal opening are suppressed markedly by inhibitors of myosin light chain kinase (MLCK), such as ML-9, ML-7, and KT5926. Other inhibitors of protein kinases have little or no effect. These results indicate that MLCK may be involved in the blue light response of stomata (Shimazaki *et al.,* 1992). All inhibitors tested (Table II) have been shown to permeate efficiently across the plasma membrane in animal cells.

A nonspecific effect of the inhibitors on the guard cells has not been excluded. Specificity of the inhibitor action can be tested using fusicoccin. Since FC is an activator of the proton pump, we can expect that FC would induce both the proton pumping and the stomatal opening in the presence of inhibitor.

Blue light-dependent proton pumping was inhibited by ML-7 and KT5926, but further addition of fusicoccin induced proton pumping to a level similar to

Table I
Properties of Various Kinds of Protein Kinase Inhibitors

	Inhibitor						
	H7	H-8	KN-62	ML-9	ML-7	K-252a	KT5926
Enzyme affected	[inhibition constant, K_i (μM)]						
Protein kinase C	6.0[a]	15[a]	>100[b]	54[c]	42[c]	0.025[d]	0.723[e]
cAMP-dependent protein kinase	3.0	1.2	>100	32	21	0.016	1.200
cGMP-dependent protein kinase	5.8	0.48	—	—	—	0.020	0.158
Myosin light-chain kinase	97	68	>100	3.8	0.3	0.020	0.018
Calmodulin kinase II	—	—	0.9	—	—	—	—

Data from [a]Hidaka *et al.* (1984), [b]Tokumitsu *et al.* (1990), [c]Saitoh *et al.* (1987), [d]Nakanishi *et al.* (1988), and [e]Nakanishi *et al.* (1990).

that observed in the absence of inhibitors (Fig. 2b, 2d). This suggests that ML-7 and KT5926 do not affect either the proton pump or the metabolic activity of the guard cells, although they do affect the blue light signaling pathway in stomata (Shimazaki *et al.,* 1993). In contrast, phenylmercuric acetate (PMA) at 5 μM inhibits proton pumping, but the addition of FC does not induce further proton pumping (Fig. 2c).

Stomata open upon illumination with both red and blue light, with apertures ranging from 8 to 10 μm. The opening is suppressed by ML-7, but the stomata open widely after the addition of FC. In contrast, PMA suppresses stomatal opening in *Commelina* epidermis, and further addition of FC does not induce stomatal opening (Table III).

Figure 3a shows polypeptide profiles of guard cell protoplasts after SDS–PAGE stained with Coomassie brilliant blue. There is no difference between protoplast polypeptides kept in the dark and those kept under red light. Autoradiograms of the lanes shown in Fig. 3a are shown in Fig. 3b. Several proteins with apparent molecular masses of 42, 40, 34, 32, 26, and 19 kDa are phosphorylated in the dark. Dephosphorylation of a 26-kDa protein is induced by red light. A very low intensity of monochromatic far-red light (730 nm, 0.5 μmol $m^{-2}s^{-1}$) is effective for dephosphorylation (not shown). Several lines of evidence suggest that the 26-kDa protein is the light-harvesting chl *a/b* protein complex of photosystem II (Kinoshita *et al.,* 1993). Figure 4a shows the polypeptide profile of guard cells that had been illuminated by red light, separated by two-dimensional electrophoresis. A large number of acidic proteins of guard cell protoplasts are found in

Table II
Inhibition of Blue Light-Dependent Proton Pumping

Inhibitor	Concentration (μM)	Magnitude of H^+-pumping (nmol H^+/μg protein/pulse)
H-7	0	0.301
	200	0.266
H-8	0	0.331
	200	0.321
KN-62	0	0.368
	50	0.360
ML-9	0	0.619
	50	0.279
ML-7	0	0.300
	50	0.073
K-252a	0	0.486
	1	0.116
	10	0.047
KT5926	0	0.386
	1	0.078
	10	0.036
PMA	0	0.465
	2.5	0.106

slab gels, although separation of individual polypeptides is often unsatisfactory in the acidic region. Figure 4b documents effects of a pulse of blue light on the polypeptide profile in guard cell protoplasts. A 80-kDa protein (arrows) is shifted to a more acidic region by blue light (Fig. 4b). This mobility shift is inhibited completely by ML-7, which suppresses blue light-dependent proton pumping (Fig. 4c), suggesting that the 80-kDa protein is phosphorylated. It might be involved in signal transduction processes of the blue light response of stomata.

Table III
Induction of Stomatal Opening in *Commelina benghalensis* Epidermis by FC in the Presence of ML-7 or PMA

Inhibitor	Concentration (μM)	Stomatal aperture (μM)	FC-induced stomatal aperture (μM)
ML-7	0	7.86 ± 3.21	11.98 ± 1.68
	100	1.71 ± 1.94	11.16 ± 2.99
PMA	0	9.98 ± 2.83	12.12 ± 1.65
	5	3.60 ± 1.20	3.06 ± 1.46

Note. ML-7 and PMA were added to the bathing solution 5 min before illumination or addition of FC. Incubation was performed for 2 h under white light.

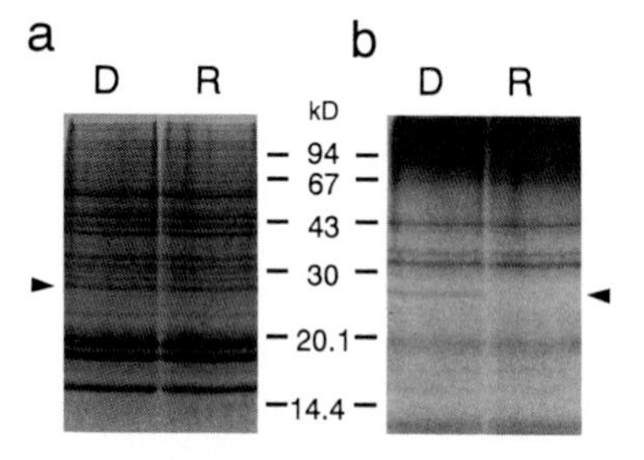

Fig. 3 Protein phosphorylation and dephosphorylation of guard cell protoplasts of *Vicia faba*. (a) Polypeptide profiles of guard cell protoplasts separated by SDS–PAGE. (b) Autoradiograms of guard cell protoplasts polypeptides separated by SDS–PAGE. Guard cell protoplasts were incubated with $^{32}P_i$ in the dark (D), and then illuminated with red light for 20 min (R). Arrowheads indicate the 26-kDa protein.

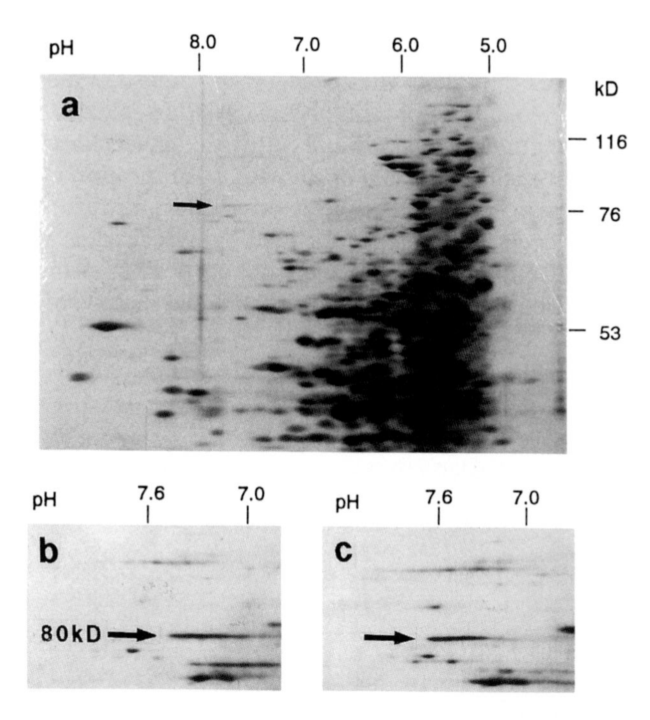

Fig. 4 Protein patterns of *Vicia* guard cell protoplasts separated by two-dimensional gel electrophoresis. (a) Guard cell protoplasts were illuminated with red light. (b) Mobility shift of 80-kDa protein induced by a pulse of blue light. The reaction was terminated 2 min after the initiation of a pulse of blue light under the background red light, when the rate of proton pumping was at its maximum. (c) As for (b) except in the presence of 100 μM ML-7. Reactions were terminated by 50% TCA. The polypeptides were located using silver staining.

Although the mobility shift is found, direct evidence for protein phosphorylation should be obtained with ^{32}P.

IV. Conclusions and Perspectives

In this chapter, we have described the use of stomatal guard cell protoplasts as a model system for studying the signal transduction mechanism underlying the light response of plant cells. The application of pharmacological tools that had been extensively developed for studies of animal cells was adopted to help elucidate the mechanisms of the signal transduction system in guard cells. Problems may be encountered because of nonspecific actions of the commonly used inhibitors on the behavior of the cells. However, since the terminal target of the blue light signal seems to be the plasma membrane H^+-ATPase of guard cells, FC, an activator of H^+-ATPase, may be used to investigate whether the cell metabolism has been disturbed by the inhibitors. Biochemical analysis reveals precise and definite properties of individual components, but such studies do not always indicate the function of the component *in vivo*. Pharmacological agents that affect the specific component are most useful in such cases.

The study of protein phosphorylation induced by blue light should become a powerful tool to study and clarify the molecular mechanisms through which blue light elicits responses of stomata. Identification of such phosphorylated proteins in guard cells will make it possible to analyze the process biochemically and molecularly. Evidence for blue light-dependent protein phosphorylation found by two-dimensional gel electrophoresis that is suppressed by the MLCK inhibitor may be an initial step in elucidating the cascade of blue light signaling in stomata.

References

Amodeo, G., Srivastava, A., and Zeiger, E. (1992). *Plant Physiol.* **100,** 1567–1570.

Assmann, S. M. (1993). *Annu. Rev. Cell Biol.* **9,** 345–373.

Assmann, S. M., Simoncini, L., and Schroeder, J. I. (1985). *Nature* **318,** 285–287.

Bradford, M. M. (1976). *Anal. Biochem.* **72,** 248–254.

Fitzsimons, P. J., and Weyers, J. D. B. (1983). *J. Exp. Bot.* **138,** 55–66.

Gotow, K., Shimazaki, K., Kondo, N., and Syono, K. (1984). *Plant Cell Physiol.* **25,** 671–675.

Hidaka, H., Inagaki, M., Kawamoto, S., and Sasaki. Y. (1984). *Biochemistry* **23,** 5036–5041.

Hurkman, W. J., and Tanaka, C. K. (1986). *Plant Physiol.* **81,** 802–806.

Kinoshita, T., Shimazaki, K., and Nishimura, M. (1983). *Plant Physiol.* **102,** 917–923.

Kruse, T., Tallman, G., and Zeiger, E. (1989). *Plant Physiol.* **90,** 1382–1386.

Laemmli, U. K. (1970). *Nature* **227,** 680–685.

Nakanishi, S., Yamada, K., Kase, H., Nakamura, S., and Nonomura, Y. (1988). *J. Biol. Chem.* **263,** 6215–6219.

Nakanishi, S., Yamada, K., Iwanishi, K., Kuroda, K., and Kase, H. (1990). *Mol. Pharmacol.* **37,** 482–488.

O'Farrell, P. H. (1975). *J. Biol. Chem.* **250,** 4007–4021.

O'Farrell, P. Z., Goodman, H. M., and O'Farrell, P. H. (1977). *Cell* **12,** 1133–1142.

Saitoh, M., Ishikawa, T., Matsushima, S., Naka, M., and Hidaka, H. (1987). *J. Biol. Chem.* **262,** 7796–7801.

Schnabl, H., Bornman, C. H., and Ziegler, H. (1978). *Planta* **143,** 33–39.

Schroeder, J. I., Raschke, K., and Neher, E. (1987). *Proc. Natl. Acad. Sci. U.S.A.* **84,** 4108–4112.

Schwartz, A., and Zeiger, E. (1984). *Planta* **161,** 129–136.

Shimazaki, K., Gotow, K., and Kondo, N. (1982). *Plant Cell Physiol.* **23,** 871–879.

Shimazaki, K., Iino, M., and Zeiger, E. (1986). *Nature* **319,** 324–326.

Shimazaki, K., Kinoshita, T., and Nishimura, M. (1992). *Plant Physiol.* **99,** 1416–1421.

Shimazaki, K., Kinoshita, T., and Nishimura, M. (1993). *Plant Cell Physiol.* **34,** 1321–1327.

Tokumitsu, H., Chijiwa, T., Hagiware, M., Mizutani, A., Terasawa, M., and Hidaka, H. (1990). *J. Biol. Chem.* **265,** 4315–4320.

Weyers, J., and Meidner, H. (1990). "Methods in Stomatal Research." Longman, Scientific & Technical, UK.

Weyers, J. D. B., and Travis, A. J. (1981). *J. Exp. Bot.* **32,** 837–850.

Willmer, C. M. (1983). "Stomata." London: Longman.

Zeiger, E. (1983). *Annu. Rev. Plant Physiol.* **34,** 441–475.

Zeiger, E., and Hepler, P. K. (1976). *Plant Physiol.* **58,** 492–498.

Zeiger, E., and Hepler, P. K. (1977). *Science* **196,** 887–889.

CHAPTER 36

Immunocytochemical Localization of Receptor Protein Kinases in Plants

Veronica P. Counihan, Thomas E. Phillips, and John C. Walker
Division of Biological Sciences
University of Missouri
Columbia, Missouri 65211

I. Introduction

Immunocytochemistry is a powerful technique that has been used extensively in cellular studies of animals and plants. Our experiences with the immunocytochemical localization of the tissue-specific and subcellular distribution of the receptor-like protein kinase ZmPK1 illustrates the value of the technique in characterization of the polypeptide products of cloned genes of unknown function. The gene encoding ZmPK1 is representative of a number of genes from plants that appear to encode transmembrane proteins with intrinsic protein kinase activity (Walker and Zhang, 1990; Stein *et al.*, 1991; Chang *et al.*, 1992; Goring and Rothstein, 1992; Kohorn *et al.*, 1992; Tobias *et al.*, 1992; Walker, 1993). These receptor protein kinases have sequence motifs diagnostic of serine/threonine protein kinases and an overall architecture reminiscent of transmembrane receptor protein kinases. Additionally, serine/threonine-specific kinase activity has been demonstrated *in vitro* for kinase-domain fusion proteins of several potential receptor kinases (Chang *et al.*, 1992; Goring and Rothstein, 1992; Stein and Nasrallah, 1993). Given the protein kinase activity and overall similarity to animal receptor protein kinases, it is likely that ZmPK1 and other plant transmembrane protein kinases act as cell surface receptors in plants. However, recent evidence suggests that transmembrane serine–threonine protein kinases from yeast are present in the endoplasmic reticulum, and function in signaling between the endoplasmic reticulum and the nucleus. (Nikawa and Yamashita, 1992; Cox *et al.*, 1993; Mori *et al.*, 1993). These potential receptor protein kinases are similar in overall structure to the receptor-like protein kinase of plants. The possibility that not all transmembrane protein kinases of plants function at the plasma membrane requires the confirmation of ultrastructural localization.

Receptor activity has yet to be demonstrated for any of the receptor-like protein kinases of plants. Ligands have not yet been isolated, and the specific roles played by individual receptors in signal transduction pathways have not been established. Immunocytochemical techniques have been useful in demonstrating interactions between receptor protein kinases and their extracellular ligands in mammalian systems (Schlessinger *et al.*, 1978; Haigler *et al.*, 1979), and have allowed analysis of their cellular processing after internalization (Felder *et al.*, 1990). Examination of the cell- and tissue-specific localization of similar potential receptors in plants may provide insights into their specific function, as well as provide basic information about possible ligands.

This chapter will present a guide to immunocytochemical techniques useful in localization of receptor-like protein kinases. A protocol relevant to the examination of the tissue distribution of a receptor-like protein kinase, utilizing paraffin-embedded tissue, will be described. Protocols allowing higher resolution examination of subcellular distribution at the light and electron microscopy levels using resin-embedded tissues will also be described.

A. Fixation

The techniques of fixation and immunocytochemistry are not as well defined in plants as in animals. Published protocols for plant material often vary widely in terms of fixation reagents, buffering systems, and duration of fixation. In creating a fixation protocol for immunocytochemistry it is essential not only to review the literature pertaining to the tissue and antigen of interest but also to have an understanding of the underlying theory of fixation. Van den Bosch (1991) and Hermann (1988) offer helpful reviews of immunocytochemistry of plant tissue at the electron microscopic level. Additionally, Berlyn and Miksche (1976) offer theory and practical techniques relating to fixation and paraffin embedding of plant material, which may be applied to immunocytochemical studies. It is important to note that protocols that work successfully for the immunolocalization of one antigen may not allow the localization of a second antigen. Published protocols should not be expected to provide immediate localization of an antigen, but instead provide a starting point for adequate fixation, which may then be altered to allow retention of the antigen. The protocols to be described here are for the immunolocalization of a transmembrane protein kinase of maize. Application of these protocols to other species of plants, particularly dicots, or dissimilar antigens may require changes in the composition of fixative and length of fixation and infiltration.

B. Antibody Detection

The choice of primary antibody can directly affect the success of immunolocalization studies. Whether a particular antibody will be useful for immunocytochemistry must be determined empirically. Crosslinking produced by fixation may obsure both three-dimensional and linear epitopes. Additionally, protein denaturation may occur when organic solvents or acids (e.g., ethanol, acetone, acetic acid) are used as fixatives or dehydrants.

Before use in immunocytochemistry, antibodies must be tested for crossreactivity with cellular components other than the antigen of interest. Immunoblots of total cellular extracts are a useful preliminary step in analyzing crossreactivity. Appropriate immunocytochemical controls include the use of preimmune antisera, competition with excess antigen, and the omission of primary or secondary antigen.

Affinity-purified antibodies are useful for immunocytochemistry in that the opportunity for nonspecific interactions is greatly reduced compared to crude polyclonal antiserum. The primary antibodies used in the protocols described here are affinity-purified polyclonals raised against a 13-mer peptide conjugated to keyhole limpet hemocyanin. The peptide corresponds to a hydrophilic region of the extracellular domain of ZmPK1.

There are several choices available for the detection of the primary antibody, including secondary antibodies tagged with fluorescent labels, enzymes such as alkaline phosphatase, or colloidal gold. We have utilized gold-linked antibodies for several reasons. First, light level and EM level results may be correlated easily when similar processing and detection schemes are used. Second, light level detection and silver enhancement of bound secondary antibodies are very straightforward, inexpensive, and quick. This technique is reproducible and reagents are available in kit form (Amersham). No specialized equipment is needed to process sections, and, unlike fluorescence methods, the technique may be done in the light. This makes silver-enhanced gold detection a technique that is useful for the lab that, like ours, is not dedicated solely to immunocytochemistry. Although reflected or epipolarized light allows more sensitive detection (Cornelese-ten Velde *et al.*, 1990), silver-enhanced gold may be viewed by standard brightfield optics.

II. Immunolocalization in Paraffin-Embedded Tissue by Light Microscopy

A. Rationale

Tissue processed in an aldehyde-based fixative and embedded in paraffin is particularly useful for the examination of organ- and tissue-specific expression of the receptor protein kinase, ZmPK1. There are several other choices available for localization at this level, including cryosectioning, with minimal fixation of sectioned tissue, and microwave stabilization of tissue with no chemical fixation (Kok and Boon, 1990); both of these are advantageous when maximal retention of antigenicity is necessary. Paraffin embedding of aldehyde-fixed tissue was chosen over other techniques because of the increased structural preservation of the tissue. Reactivity with antibodies of interest was retained.

B. Preparation of Tissue

1. Fixation

We have used three fixation procedures with success in the localization of ZmPK1 in paraffin-embedded tissue. The first uses the common botanical fixative FAA, a mixture of formalin, acetic acid, and ethanol. The fixative is commonly used in anatomical studies to preserve the overall architecture of plant tissues. Tissues fixed in this manner tend to section easily. This fixative acts through a combination of crosslinking and precipitation of proteins, and results in disruption of the cytoplasm (Berlyn and Miksche, 1976). FAA does not allow more than a general pattern of tissue distribution to be observed. The inability of this fixative to preserve subcellular structures prevents its use in any subsequent electron microscopic studies. FAA is adequate for determining the organ and tissue distribution of a particular antigen. The second fixative we have used is Bouin's fixative, a picric-acid based fixative that provides good preservation of root tips. The third fixative used successfully is freshly depolymerized paraformaldehyde in Hepes buffer (HBF). This fixative results in excellent preservation of tissue, but does not section quite as easily as FAA- or Bouin's-fixed tissue. Typically, we fix 5-day-old maize root tips in FAA, Bouin's, or HBF for 2 h to overnight at 4°C under vacuum. Older tissue, such as stems and mature leaves, and desiccated tissue is fixed in FAA and often require extended fixation and dehydration periods, of up to 3 days. After this fixation period, tissue that remains floating in the fixative is discarded. Tissue fixed in HBF is then washed in Hepes buffer and slowly dehydrated stepwise; tissue fixed in Bouin's is washed in water. Tissue fixed in FAA is not washed, but immediately dehydrated, starting at 50% ethanol.

Tissue is dehydrated through ethanol, cleared with *tert*-butyl alcohol (TBA), and embedded in Paraplast. We have utilized TBA as paraffin solvent because in our hands it results in much better sectioning qualities for maize tissue than does xylene, the most commonly used paraffin clearing agent. However, like xylene, TBA is a health hazard and should be handled in a fume hood. Additionally, TBA has a low flash point, and care must be taken when melting it. The tissue is then infiltrated with Paraplast. For root tips, overnight infiltration is adequate; but an extended infiltration period may be required (2 to 3 days) for older tissues and embryos. Following infiltration, the tissue is embedded in flat molds and placed at −20°C to solidify. The standard fixation and embedding protocols are listed in Table I.

Table I
Processing Schedule for Light-Level Immunocytochemistry Using HBF or Bouin's Fixation[a]

Process	Time
Fixation at 4°C	1 h to overnight or longer, depending on tissue
Wash tissue[b]	3 washes of 20 min each
10% ethanol at 4°C	1/2 h
20% ethanol at 4°C	1/2 h
30% ethanol at 4°C	1/2 h
40% ethanol at 4°C	1/2 h
50% ethanol at 4°C	1/2 h
60% ethanol at 4°C	1/2 h
70% ethanol at 4°C	1/2 h (may be held in 70% overnight)
80% ethanol at 4°C	1 h
95% ethanol at 4°C	1 h
100% ethanol at 4°C	1 h
100% ethanol at 4°C	1 h
1:1 ethanol:TBA at 27°C	1 h
1:2 ethanol:TBA at 27°C	1 h
100% TBA at 27°C	1 h
100% TBA at 27°C	1 h
1:1 TBA:Paraplast at 50°C	1 h
1:2 TBA:Paraplast at 50°C	1 h
100% Paraplast at 50°C	1 h
100% Paraplast at 50°C	Overnight to 3 days
Transfer to embedding molds	

[a] FAA Schedule: same as HBF/Bouin's except dehydration starts at 50% ethanol, directly from fixative.

[b] Use Hepes buffer for HBF fixation and water for Bouin's fixation.

2. Sectioning

Paraffin blocks are allowed to warm to room temperature and sectioned into 8-μm ribbons on a standard microtome. The sections are placed onto droplets of degassed water on clean, uncoated or aminopropyltriethoxysilane (APTS)-treated slides and heated overnight at 42°C to allow decompression of the sections and adherence to the slides. Uncoated slides are advantageous in that they result in minimal nonspecific binding of immunocytochemical reagents and subsequent background. After extended incubation periods, however, sections may be lost from these slides. Tissue adheres exceedingly well to slides treated with APTS, but an increase in background staining of the slide can result.

C. Immunocytochemistry

Slides are dewaxed in two 5- to 10-min changes of Hemo-De (Fisher) followed by 100% ethanol, 95, 70, and 50% ethanol, and two changes of dH_2O. Slides are drained individually, and individual sections are encircled using a PAP pen (Electron Microscopy Sciences). The PAP pen creates a hydrophobic barrier that minimizes the amounts of reagents needed. On APTS-coated slides the hydrophobicity of the slide surface can eliminate the need to use a PAP pen. The sections are then immediately covered with phosphate-buffered saline (PBS; Harlow and Lane, 1988) plus 0.2% sodium azide, until all slides have been treated. At no time during subsequent processing should the sections be allowed to dry out. The slides are then treated with blocking solution (see formulations section). The sections are blocked for 20 min at room temperature in a humid chamber. We use an airtight Tupperware box, lined with water-dampened paper toweling. The slides are then drained and immediately treated with the primary antibody diluted in blocking solution. The correct dilution must be determined using a dilution series; a starting point is to use a dilution that is 10× more concentrated than that used for immunoblot analysis. Each slide is gently covered with a piece of Parafilm and incubated at room temperature overnight. The slides are then gently washed three times (5 min per wash) with PBS/azide. The secondary incubation with gold-linked anti-rabbit IgG (Auroprobe LM, Amersham; diluted 1/40) is done for 1 h at room temperature. Slides are again washed in PBS/azide, as above; following this the slides are washed gently in water. The protocol is summarized as follows:

1. Dewax: take slides through two 5- to 10-min changes of Hemo-De (or xylene) and through an ethanol series (100, 95, 70% ethanol) into distilled water. Encircle sections with PAP pen; hold slides in PBS/azide.
2. Cover sections with droplets of blocking buffer; gently cover slides with Parafilm. Incubate sections at room temperature 20 min.
3. Drain slides; cover sections immediately with primary antibody diluted in blocking buffer. Cover slides with Parafilm; incubate overnight in humidity chamber.

4. Drain slides; wash three times (5 min per wash) in PBS/azide.

5. Drain slides; cover sections immediately with secondary antibody (gold-linked) diluted 1/40. Cover slides with Parafilm; incubate for 1 h in humid chamber.

6. Drain slides; wash three times (5 min per wash) in PBS/azide.

7. Wash slides three times (5 min per wash) in H_2O. Sections are now ready for silver enhancement.

D. Silver Enhancement

Silver enhancement is a technique to increase the size of individual bound gold particles so that they are visible at low magnification. Silver enhancement acts through the formation of silver deposits onto gold particles, which serve as nucleation sites. For some abundant antigens, enhancement may not be necessary for visualization, particularly at high magnification (Cornelese-ten Velde and Prins, 1990). However, for our antigen, silver enhancement is necessary and produces clear results with a high signal-to-noise ratio.

We utilize the IntenSE M kit (Amersham) for silver enhancement following the manufacturer's directions. The reagents are quite temperature sensitive; development time will vary with the temperature of the working environment. At 22°C, we have found a development time of 6–7 min to give good results for our antibody. In some cases, particularly with low-abundance antigens, it may be necessary to perform two rounds of development. In this case we have found that the first round of enhancement should not exceed 5 min, and the second round, following a wash of the slide in water to remove reagents, should be observed closely, so that random precipitation of silver does not occur. Optimal enhancement in our hands occurs at 4 to 5 min. After development is complete, slides should again be washed thoroughly in water. We have noticed that residual silver may appear on the slides if they have not been adequately washed; this precipitant is not immediately visible. After thorough washing, slides are mounted in a commercially available mounting medium (Gelmount, Fisher) or in Airvol mounting medium (Klymkowsky and Hanken, 1991) and dried overnight at room temperature.

The silver enhancement protocol is as follows:

1. Mix silver enhancement reagent (according to manufacturer's directions) and apply to sections; incubate at room temperature. Sections may be monitored occasionally under a dissecting scope; enhancement should be complete by 6–7 min. Wash slides immediately after enhancement in copious amounts of H_2O).

2. If necessary, repeat step 1, using freshly mixed enhancement reagents; limit second enhancement to approximately 5 min.

3. Mount sections with aqueous mounting medium; let dry at least 4 h before viewing.

E. Microscopy

Silver-enhanced sections are viewed under brightfield or reflected light illumination. Under brightfield, silver staining is visible as a dark black precipitant; under reflected or polarized light, bright punctate staining stands out more clearly against a dark background. Figure 1 shows a 5-day-old root tip, fixed with FAA, embedded in paraffin, and subjected to immunocytochemistry using a ZmPK1-specific antibody.

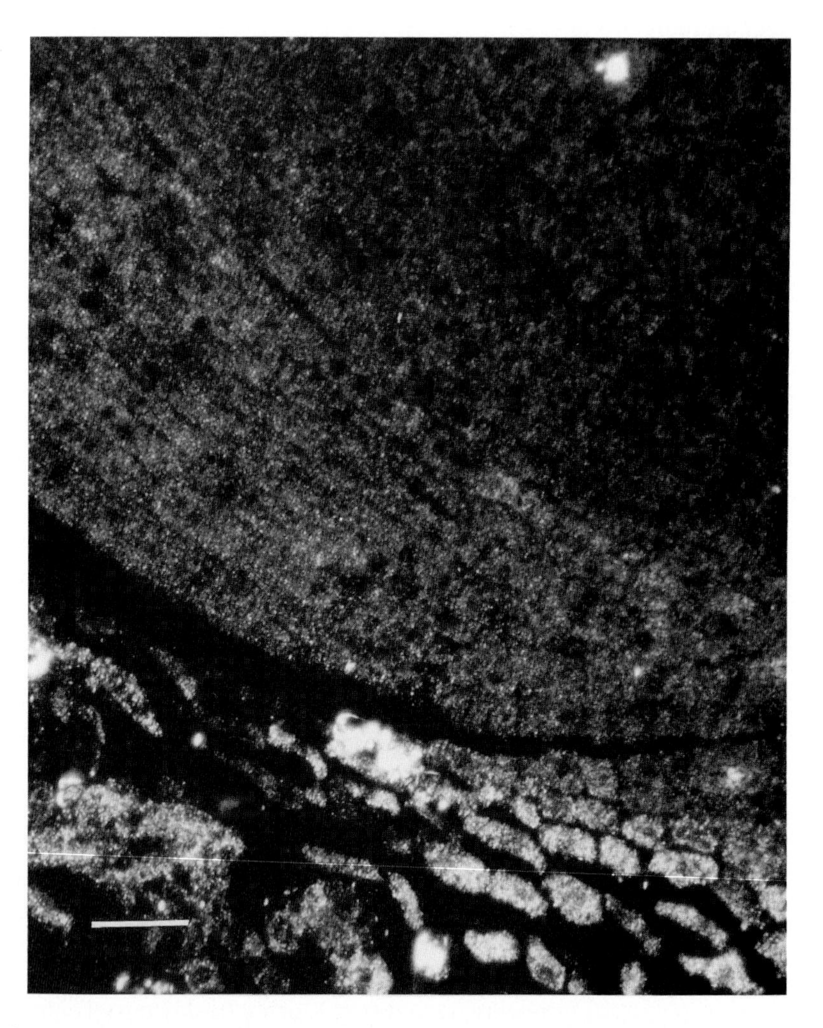

Fig. 1 Eight-micrometer section of root tip fixed in FAA and embedded in paraffin. This section was reacted with ZmPK1-specific primary antibody, colloidal gold-linked secondary antibody, and two rounds of silver enhancement, and viewed by epipolarized optics. Staining is most evident at the periphery of the outer root cap cells, but is also apparent in cells of the root cortex and elsewhere. Magnification: 200; bar, 5 μm.

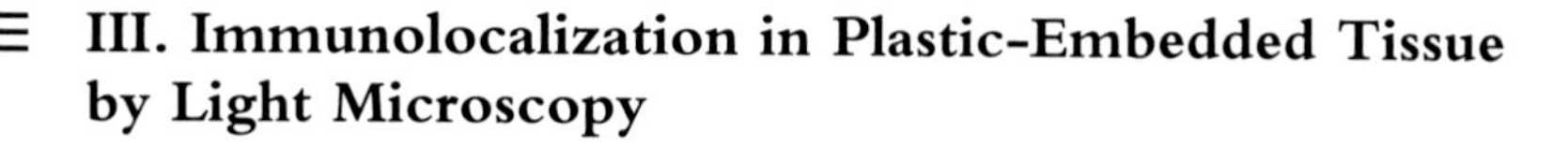

III. Immunolocalization in Plastic-Embedded Tissue by Light Microscopy

A. Rationale

Advantages of embedding in plastic resins include substantial improvements in tissue morphology and preservation. At this level, the subcellular localization of an antigen may be defined. However, a major disadvantage of tissue embedded in this manner is that the plastic matrix may obstruct the interaction of antibody and epitope in immunocytochemical studies. This is very much the case with traditional embedding agents such as Spurr's. Spurr's resin has been used successfully, however, for immunolocalization studies in plants, particularly when periodate acid treatment of sections is utilized (Craig and Goodchild, 1984). A variety of hydrophilic resins, designed especially for immunocytochemistry, such as LR White (medium or hard grade; Electron Microscopy Sciences) and Lowicryl K4M and HM20 (Polysciences), are available and should be used in addition to or in place of Spurr's resin. These resins differ among themselves in physical characteristics, such as hydrophobicity and hardness, which affect their sectioning ability. We have LR White in both the medium and the hard grades, and Lowicryls HM20 and K4M successfully for immunocytochemical studies of ZmPK1. For maize root tips we have found LR White (hard grade) to provide the best sectioning characteristics.

B. Preparation of Tissue

Small (1 mm^3) pieces of tissue are fixed in HBF for 2 h to overnight at 4°C. The tissue is then washed three times (20 min per wash) in Hepes buffer, dehydrated, and infiltrated. We have found that prolonged infiltrations with LR White, under vacuum for 3 days, with daily changes of fresh resin, provides the best sectioning qualities for maize root tips. This extended infiltration period is probably not necessary for most nonlignified dicotyledonous tissues.

After infiltration, the tissue is oriented and embedded in fresh LR White placed in BEEM capsules or gelatin capsules, and polymerized at 60°C overnight. Tissue is processed according to the schedule below:

1. Aliquot freshly prepared fixative into glass scintillation vials etched with a diamond marker to provide permanent identification. Chill fixative on ice.
2. Cut 1-mm^3 sections of tissue into freshly prepared fixative (chilled on ice), using a double-edged razor blade. Fix 2 h to overnight at 4°C.
3. Discard any pieces of tissue that remain floating. Decant fixative and replace immediately with wash buffer. Repeat wash at 20-min intervals, for a total of three washes.
4. Dehydration—Tissue is placed into 10% ethanol (on ice) for 20 min. Dehydration is continued stepwise (20, 30, 40, 50, 60, 70, 80, 90% ethanol) at 20-min intervals. Tissue is then taken through three changes of 100% ethanol; a freshly opened bottle of ethanol should be used for this step.

5. Infiltration

1:1 Ethanol : LR White	1 h, on ice
1:2 Ethanol : LR White	1 h, on ice
100% LR White	1 h, on ice
100% LR White	1 h, on ice
100% LR White	overnight to 3 days under vacuum at room temperature

6. Embedding—Samples are oriented and embedded in fresh LR White, using gelatin capsules or BEEM capsules. Samples are polymerized overnight at 56°C. The embedded tissue may be sectioned at thicknesses ranging from 0.5 to 2 μm with a glass knife, using an ultramicrotome. These sections are transferred onto a droplet of water on aminopropyl silane-treated slides and heated at 60°C until the water evaporates. The slides then may be used in immunocytochemical studies.

C. Immunocytochemistry

Plastic sections (0.5–2 μm) are incubated for 20 min in PBS; tissue is then blocked and incubated with primary and secondary antibody as described previously for paraffin-embedded tissue. The slides should be treated with a PAP pen to conserve reagents. Silver enhancement of the gold-linked secondary antibody is limited to a single round of enhancement. In our experience, best results are obtained when the enhancement period is limited to 4 min. Increased enhancement results in background staining that is visible at higher magnification, particularly using reflected or polarized light optics. Figure 2 shows a 2-μm-thick section of root tip embedded in LR White and subjected to immunocytochemistry. The pattern of staining seen is much more defined than the FAA-fixed, paraffin-embedded tissue shown in Fig. 1.

IV. Immunolocalization by Electron Microscopy

For localization at the electron microscopic level we employ LR White (hard grade)-embedded tissue that has been previously analyzed at the light level (as described in Section III). Electron microscopic immunolocalization should not normally be attempted if an antigen fails to be detected at the light microscopic level in resin-embedded tissue. Thin sections with a silver-gray interference color are collected with a loop (Electron Microscopy Sciences) and placed onto 400-mesh nickel grids (Electron Microscopy Sciences) that have been freshly cleaned with acetone, and treated with grid adhesive (Grid Coat, Electron Microscopy Sciences). For immunocytochemical studies, grids are blocked by floating each grid initially in a droplet of PBS, then in blocking buffer for 20 min. Grids are then placed into droplets of primary antibody. As our affinity-purified polyclonal antibodies to ZmPK1 are of low titer, we use a dilution of 1/10 for this step. To

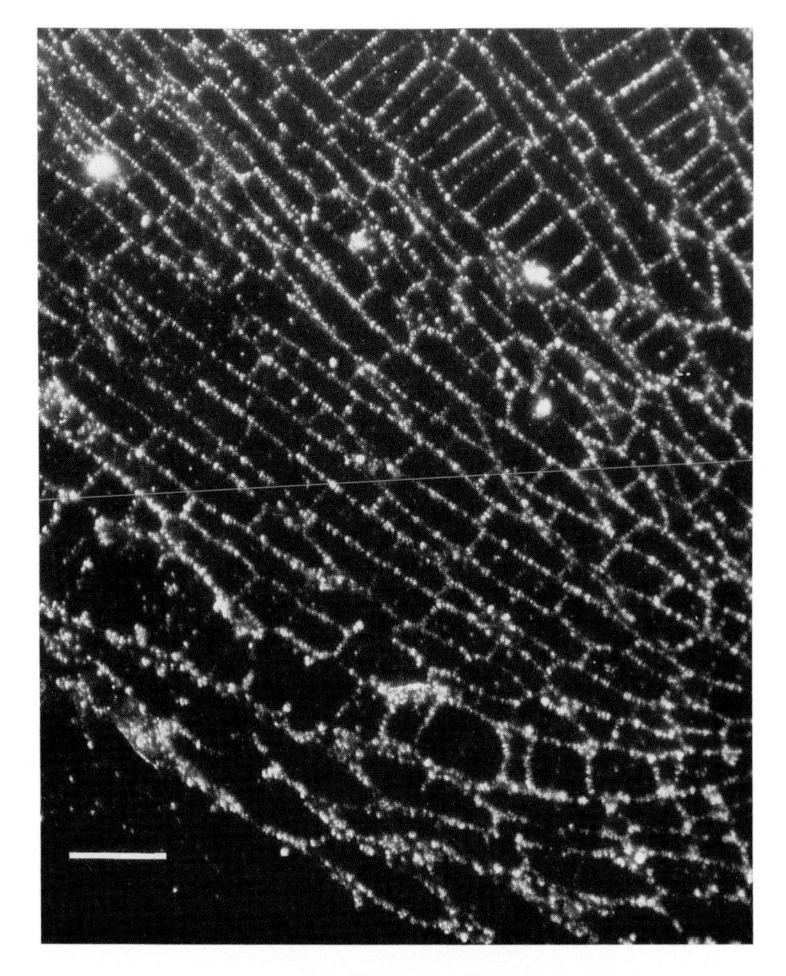

Fig. 2 Section (2-μm) of HBF-fixed, LR White-embedded tissue, subjected to ZmPK1-specific immunocytochemistry, with a single round of silver enhancement. Staining is evident in all cell types of the root tip. Magnification: 400; bar, 5 μm.

provide a humid environment during antibody incubations, the grids are placed on Parafilm in a disposable Petri dish, lined along its periphery with water saturated Kimwipes. The primary incubation is done at room temperature, overnight. The grids are then rinsed in sequential droplets of distilled water. After each rinse, droplets clinging to the grid or forceps are removed by gently touching the forceps only with a small piece of filter paper. The sections are then placed into secondary antibody (Auroprobe EM colloidal gold-linked anti-primary antibody, Amersham), diluted in blocking buffer. We use 10-nm gold, diluted 1/25, as recommended by the manufacturer. After a 1-h room temperature incubation, the grids are thoroughly rinsed as described above and stained to increase contrast. We stain sequentially with uranyl magnesium acetate (10 min) and Reynold's lead citrate (1 min) (Frisch and Phillips, 1990), using the droplet technique described earlier, rinsing thoroughly after staining in each reagent. Because of the absence of en bloc staining with uranyl acetate and osmium tetroxide, this tissue lacks the contrast that is typical of conventionally processed tissue. We have found an increase in contrast may be obtained by staining for 5 min in a droplet of 1% potassium permanganate solution after the uranyl acetate/ Reynold's lead citrate steps. Figure 3 shows a silver section of LR White-embedded tissue subjected to immunocytochemistry using a ZmPK1-specific antibody.

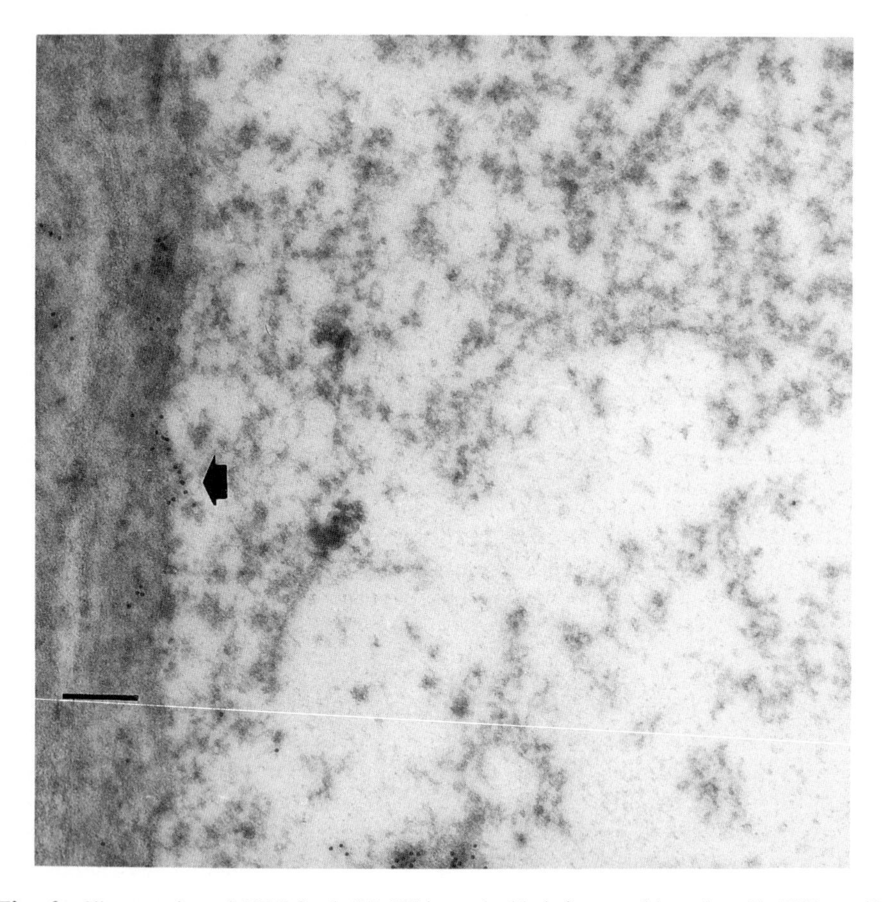

Fig. 3 Silver section of HBF-fixed, LR White-embedded tissue, subjected to ZmPK1-specific immunocytochemistry, using 10-nm colloidal gold-linked IgG as secondary antibody. Staining is evident at the plasma membrane (arrow), as expected for ZmPK1. Magnification: 20,000; bar, 150 nm.

V. Formulations

FAA (formalin–acetic alcohol; Berlyn and Miksche, 1976): 50 ml of ethanol (95%); 5 ml glacial acetic acid; 10 ml formaldehyde (37% solution); 35 ml H_2O.

Hepes fix base (5× stock solution): 0.15 M Hepes, pH 6.8, 0.35 *M* NaCl, 10 m*M* $CaCl_2$

Hepes wash buffer: 30 m*M* Hepes, pH 6.8, 70 m*M* NaCl, 2 m*M* $CaCl_2$

Preparation: Dilute hepes fix base fivefold.

HBF fixative (Hepes-buffered formaldehyde): 70 m*M* NaCl, 30 m*M* Hepes, pH 6.8, 2 m*M* $CaCl_2$, 2% freshly depolymerized formaldehyde.

Preparation of 25 ml fixative: Heat 10 ml H_2O to 60°C in a fume hood. While stirring slowly, add 0.5 g of paraformaldehyde. After heating mixture for approximately 5 min, slowly add 0.2 *N* NaOH, dropwise, until the paraformaldehyde depolymerizes and goes into solution. Use as little NaOH as possible to depolymerize paraformaldehyde. Cool solution; add 5 ml Hepes fix base (5× stock solution). Adjust pH to 6.8 with HCl if necessary. Bring to 25-ml final volume with H_2O.

Bouin's fixative (Berlyn and Miksche, 1976): 5 ml of glacial acetic acid; 25 ml of 37% formaldehyde; 75 ml of a saturated aqueous picric acid stock.

(Note: picric acid is explosive when dry, and must be stored as a saturated aqueous solution.)

Blocking solution: 10% normal goat serum (Sigma), plus 10% bovine serum albumin (Sigma), in phosphate-buffered saline, pH 7. Aliquot and store at −20°C.

Airvol mounting medium (modification of Klymkowsky and Hanken, 1991): Dissolve 10 g of Airvol (polyvinyl alcohol; Air Products, Inc., Allentown, PA) in 40 ml 50 m*M* Tris, pH 8. Stir overnight at room temperature to dissolve. Add 20 ml glycerol. Aliquot into 10-ml syringes and store at −20°C. Thawed aliquots have a shelf-life of 2 weeks at room temperature.

APTS slide coating (modification of O'Keefe et al., 1991): Clean slides are dipped twice into a solution of 2% aminopropyltriethoxysilane in acetone, then in two changes of acetone. Slides are then dipped in distilled water and allowed to air-dry. Slides must be absolutely spotless before dipping; clean in soapy water followed by a chromic acid bath and rinse in distilled water.

Potassium permanganate: 1% $KMnO_4$, made fresh in H_2O. Centrifuge at 10,000× *g* for 20 min before use.

VI. Conclusions

Immunocytochemistry, using paraffin- or LR White-embedded tissue and silver-enhanced gold staining is a straightforward technique requiring little specialized apparatus. This technique has been useful in allowing researchers involved in molecular biological aspects of receptor protein kinase structure and function to confirm the predicted localization of an expected cell surface receptor and to begin to explore aspects of this receptor's ultrastructural and tissue-specific localization.

Acknowledgments

We thank the Molecular Cytology Core Facility of the University of Missouri for assistance with the immunocytochemistry. Studies described here have been supported by the National Science Foundation (MCB-9105388), the University of Missouri Food for the 21st Century Program, and a USDA National Needs Fellowship and Sigma Xi Grant-in-Aid-of-Research to V.C.

References

Berlyn, G. P., and Miksche, J. P. (1976). "Botanical Microtechnique and Cytochemistry." Ames: Iowa State Univ. Press.

Chang, C., Schaller, G. E., Patterson, S. E., Kwok, S. F., Meyerowitz, E. M., and Bleeker, A. B. (1992). The TMK1 gene from Arabidopsis codes for a protein with structural and biochemical characteristics of a receptor protein kinase. *Plant Cell* **4,** 1263–1271.

Cornelese-ten Velde, I., and Prins, F. A. (1990). New sensitive light microscopical detection of colloidal gold on ultrathin sections by reflection contrast microscopy. *Histochem.* **94,** 61–71.

Cornelese-ten Velde, I., Bonnet, J., Tanke, H. J., and Ploem, J. S. (1990). Reflection contrast microscopy performed on epi-illumination microscope stands: comparison of reflection contrast- and epi-polarization microscopy. *J. Microsc.* **159,** 1–13.

Cox, J. S., Shamu, C. E., and Walter, P. (1993). Transcriptional induction of genes encoding endoplasmic reticulum resident proteins requires a transmembrane protein kinase. *Cell* **73,** 1197–1206.

Craig, S., and Goodchild, D. J. (1984). Periodate-acid treatment of sections permits on-grid immunogold localization of pea seed vicilin in ER and Golgi. *Protoplasma* **122,** 35–44.

Felder, S., Miller, K., Moehren, G., Ullrich, A., Schlessinger, J., and Hopkins, C. R. (1990). Kinase activity controls the sorting of the epidermal growth factor receptor within the multivesicular body. *Cell* **61,** 623–634.

Frisch, E. B., and Phillips, T. E. (1990). Lectin binding patterns to plasmalemmal glycoconjugates of goblet cells undergoing differentiation *in vitro*. *J. Electron Microsc. Tech.* **16**(1), 25–36.

Goring, D. R., and Rothstein, S. J. (1992). The S-locus receptor kinase gene in a self-incompatible Brassica napus line encodes a functional serine/threonine kinase. *Plant Cell* **4,** 1273–1281.

Haigler, H. T., McKanna, J. A., and Cohen, S. (1979). Direct visualization of the binding and internalization of epidermal growth factor in human carcinoma cells A-431. *Proc. Natl. Acad. Sci. U.S.A.* **75,** 3317–3321.

Harlow, E., and Lane, D. (1988). "Antibodies: A Laboratory Manual." Cold Spring Harbor, NY: Cold Spring Harbor Laboratory Press.

Hermann, E. M. (1988). Immunocytochemical localization of macromolecules with the electron microscope. *Annu. Rev. Plant Physiol. Plant Mol. Biol.* **39,** 139–155.

Kohorn, B. D., Lane, S., and Smith, T. A. (1992). An Arabidopsis serine/threonine kinase homologue with an epidermal growth factor repeat selected in yeast for its specificity for a thylakoid membrane protein. *Proc. Natl. Acad. Sci. U.S.A.* **89,** 10989–10992.

Kok, L. P., and Boon, M. E. (1990). Microwaves for microscopy. *J. Microsc.* **158,** 291–322.

Klymkowsky, M. W., and Hanken, J. (1991). Whole mount staining of Xenopus and other vertebrates. *Methods Cell Biol.* **36,** 419–441.

Mori, K., Ma, W., Gething, M.-J., and Sambrook, J. (1993). A transmembrane protein with a $cdc2^+$/CDC28-related kinase activity is required for signaling from the ER to the nucleus. *Cell* **74,** 743–756.

Nikawa, J., and Yamashita, S. (1992). *IRE1* encodes a putative protein kinase containing a membrane-spanning domain and is required for inositol phototropy in Saccharomyces cerevisiae. *Mol. Microbiol.* **6,** 1441–1446.

O'Keefe, H. P., Melton, D. A., Ferreiro, B., and Kintner, C. (1991). In situ hybridization. *Methods Cell Biol.* **36,** 443–463.

Schlessinger, J., Shecter, Y., Willingham, M. C., and Pastan, I. (1978). Direct visualization of binding aggregation, and internalization of insulin and epidermal growth factor on living fibroblastic cells. *Proc. Natl. Acad. Sci. U.S.A.* **75,** 2659–2663.

Stein, J. C., and Nasrallah, J. B. (1993). A plant receptor-like gene, the S-locus receptor kinase of *Brassica oleracea* L., encodes a functional serine/threonine kinase. *Plant Physiol.* **101,** 1103–1106.

Stein, J. C., Howlett, B., Boyes, D. C., Nasrallah, M. E., and Nasrallah, J. B. (1991). Molecular cloning of a putative receptor protein kinase gene encoded at the self-incompatibility locus of *Brassica oleracea. Proc. Natl. Acad. Sci. U.S.A.* **88,** 8816–8820.

Tobias, C. M., Howlett, B., and Nasrallah, J. M. (1992). An Arabidopsis thaliana gene with sequence similarity to the S-locus receptor kinase of *Brassica oleracea. Plant Physiol.* **99,** 284–290.

Van den Bosch, K. A. (1991). Immunogold labelling. *In* "Electron Microscopy of Plant Cells" (J. L. Hall and C. Hawes, eds.), pp. 181–218. London: Academic Press.

Walker, J. C. (1993). Receptor-like kinase genes of Arabidopsis thaliana. *Plant J.* **3,** 451–456.

Walker, J. C., and Zhang, R. (1990). Relationship of a putative receptor protein kinase from maize to the S-locus glycoproteins of Brassica. *Nature* **345,** 743–746.

CHAPTER 37

Expression and Assay of Autophosphorylation of Recombinant Protein Kinases

Mark A. Horn and John C. Walker

Division of Biological Sciences
University of Missouri
Columbia, Missouri 65211

I. Introducton

Protein kinases have been found to play an important role in many signaling processes in a variety of organisms. A large number of cDNA's coding for many different types of protein kinases have been identified in plants (for a recent comprehensive review see Hunter, 1991). Although protein kinases are present in a large number of diverse organisms, their amounts are often low within the cells in which they function. The low levels of these enzymes, along with intracellular compartmentalization, can impede the isolation of protein kinases from plant tissues via classical biochemical techniques. One way to circumvent these problems is to express the protein kinase, or a portion of the protein kinase of interest, in a heterologous expression systems (such as *Escherichia coli*), and to characterize their enzyme activity *in vitro*. This chapter outlines the various factors that must be considered when designing such an experimental system.

II. Materials

The following materials or their equivalent are required to study recombinant protein kinases.

Expression vectors:
- T7 expression vector(s) (Novagen, Madison, WI)
- pMal expression vector(s) (New England Biolabs, Beverly, MA)
- pGEX expression vector(s) (Pharmacia, Milwaukee, WI)

Protease-deficient *E. coli* strains:
- *E. coli* BL21(DE3) (Novagen, Madison, WI)
- *E. coli* DH5a (Clontech, Palo Alto, CA)
- *E. coli* PR745 (New England Biolabs, Beverly, MA)

Affinity matrices for fusion protein purification:
- Glutathione agarose (Sigma, St. Louis, MO)
- Amylose agarose (New England Biolabs, Beverly, MA)

Specialized equipment:
- Sonicator, Cell disruptor, Model 375 (Heat Systems Ultrasonics, Plain view, NY)
- Hunter thin-layer electrophoresis unit (C.B .S. Scientific Co., Del Mar, CA)
- 100-μm 20 $\times$-cm microcrystalline cellulose glass-backed thin-layer electro phoresis plates without fluorescent indicators (E. M. Science, Gibbs town, NJ)

III. Selecting the Region of a Protein Kinase Molecule to Express

A. The Full-Length Protein Kinase Molecule

In every case, it would be ideal to express the complete, full-length molecule of interest in a heterologous expression system. Unfortunately, one of the inherent limitations of heterologous protein expression in *E. coli* is that transmembrane proteins are not expressed at high levels and sometimes are even toxic to the growth of the bacteria. This toxicity appears to arise from the presence of the transmembrane domain of the molecule being expressed. We have observed that the expression in *E. coli* of either the extracellular or the intracellular domain of one plant receptor-like protein kinases, RLK5 (Walker, 1993), results in the production of a large amount of active protein. On the other hand, no attempt to express the full-length, transmembrane domain-containing molecule has resulted in detectable protein production. In addition to toxicity questions, proteins expressed in prokaryotic systems lack post-translational modifications such as complicated disulfide bond formation, glycosylation, and acylation.

B. The Catalytic Domain of the Protein Kinase Molecule

When deciding which region of the molecule to express you must consider the characteristics of the molecule that you wish to study. In our case, we have been primarily interested in studying the autophosphorylation of a group of receptor-like protein kinases from plants. Therefore it is sufficient to study the kinetic characteristics of the putative catalytic domain of the molecule(s) of interest. Similar approaches have been used in the characterization of several different protein kinases in animal systems, such as the insulin receptor (Kohanski, 1993; Wente *et al.,* 1990). These studies indicate that the catalytic properties of the truncated insulin receptor are similar, if not identical, to that of the intact insulin receptor (Kohanski, 1993; Wente *et al.,* 1990). In addition, the catalytic domain of such protein kinases do not require any of the post-translational modifications required for the production of functional full-length receptor molecules. The genetic boundaries of a protein kinase catalytic domain are defined as being bounded at the amino terminal by the amino acid that falls 7 residues upstream from the Gly–X–Gly–X–X–Gly consensus sequence, and at the carboxyl terminal by a set of hydrophobic residues that lie 10–18 amino acids downstream from the invariant Arg residue (Hanks and Quinn, 1991). Although expression of the catalytic domain in *E. coli* can be helpful in demonstrating protein kinase activity, this method may not be satisfactory for examining the interaction of a regulatory domain with the catalytic domain.

IV. Choosing the Best Expression Vector

A. Employing Expression Vectors Containing the T7 Promoter

In choosing the optimal expression vector for a given application, one must consider the amount of protein produced by the expression system, and the ability to easily purify the protein of interest. An efficient promoter available for *E. coli* expression systems is the viral T7 promoter (Studier *et al.,* 1990). This promoter has three main advantages; it is easily inducible, results in the addition of very few extra N-terminal amino acids to the protein of choice, and yields a high amount of the heterologous protein. Unfortunately, the protein produced in such systems must be purified by classical biochemical methods.

B. The pGEX family of Expression Vectors

One way to circumvent the problems in purification of expressed proteins, which are inherent to the T7 promoter systems, is to express the protein of interest as a fusion protein. The fusion protein should possess a domain with properties that simplify purification of the desired protein. One of the first fusion proteins to be employed is the glutathione-S-transferase (GST) protein (Smith and Johnson, 1988). In the pGEX vectors (Pharmacia), expression of the fusion protein containing both the GST protein and the protein of interest is under the control of the *lac* promoter and is therefore inducible by adding IPTG. The purification of the fusion protein exploits the ability of the GST protein and any GST fusion protein to bind to a glutathione–agarose column. This interaction is of sufficient avidity to allow for the retention of the fusion protein while washing away unwanted proteins. The fusion protein is subsequently released by addition of reduced glutathione. Several commercially available GST fusion protein expression vectors have been developed. These contain a variety of multiple cloning sites as well as sequences coding for oligopeptide proteolysis sites, allowing efficient separation of the protein of interest from the fusion protein. In our hands, the pGEX2T vector, expressed in PR745 cells, normally results in a yield of between 1 and 10 mg of the fusion protein per liter of cells.

C. The pMal Family of Expression Vectors

The pMal family of expression vectors (New England Biolabs) employs the maltose binding protein (MBP) as a fusion protein (Guan *et al.*, 1988). This expression system is also under the control of the *lac* promoter. The expressed fusion proteins are purified via affinity chromatography on an amylose–agarose column. In addition, a wide variety of expression vectors have been developed that possess different multiple cloning sites and encode different oligopeptide proteolytic cleavage sites. In our hands, this vector usually yields substantially more fusion protein (between 5 and 30 mg of protein per liter) than other expression systems.

V. Choice of *E. coli* Strains for Heterologous Protein Expression

A. *E. coli* BL21(DE3)

In contrast to the situation with the other expression vectors described in this chapter (pGEX and pMAL) that use the *lac* promoter and the *E. coli* host

RNA polymerase, the T7 promoter-driven expression vectors have an obligate requirement for the T7 RNA polymerase gene. *E. coli* BL21(DE3) cells contain a λ prophage gene that carries the T7 RNA polymerase gene (Studier *et al.*, 1990).

B. *E. coli* DH5α

Before considering any other strain of *E. coli* for heterologous protein expression the DH5α strain should be tried. Some fusion proteins that are produced at high levels, and that do not contain oligopeptide sites recognized by *E. coli* proteases, can be successfully expressed in DH5α. If an expression experiment results in the production of small amounts of fusion protein or in proteolytically degraded fusion protein, one should then turn to an *E. coli* strain that is protease deficient.

C. *E. coli* PR745

This strain of *E. coli* lacks a functional lon protease. This protease not only degrades fusion proteins but also seems to be responsible for the activation of other bacterial proteases. We routinely use this strain for the expression of fusion proteins.

VI. Isolation of Fusion Proteins

A. Induction of Fusion Protein Production

Many recent publications have described a variety of procedures for induction of fusion protein expression using IPTG (Winograd *et al.*, 1993). Instead of individually analyzing each procedure, we describe the method that seems to work most efficiently for the production of RLK5 containing fusion proteins. Cells are grown to a OD_{600} of 0.8. IPTG is added to a final concentration of 0.1 m*M* and the cells are allowed to produce fusion protein at room temperature overnight (approximately 8 h). We have found with all fusion proteins we have worked with that inducing the cells at room temperature results in a substantial increase in the proportion of fusion protein present in the soluble state.

B. Disruption of Cells and Release of Soluble Fusion Proteins

The cells were collected by centrifugation (7000 × *g*, 10 min), suspended in 50 ml of the appropriate lysis buffer (50 m*M* Hepes, pH 7.4, 150 m*M* NaCl, 10 m*M* EDTA, 1 m*M* DTT, 200 μ*M* PMSF for GST fusion proteins and 10 m*M* Na_2PO_4, pH 7.2, 0.5 *M* NaCl, 0.25% Tween-20, 10 m*M* 2-ME, 10 m*M* EDTA, 10 m*M* EGTA, 200 μ*M* PMSF for MBP fusion proteins) and frozen overnight at −20°C. The samples were thawed at room temperature, additional PMSF was added (200 μM), and the cells were lysed in 25-ml aliquots via sonication for 5 min. Triton X-100 was added to a final concentration of 1% and insoluble material was removed by centrifugation (10,000 $\times$ *g*, 20 min).

C. Affinity Purification of Fusion Proteins

The entire cleared cell extract, containing the fusion protein, was added to 10 ml of a 10% w/v solution of the proper affinity matrix (glutathione–agarose for GST fusion proteins and amylose–agarose for MBP fusion proteins) and incubated for 30 min at 4°C. The agarose beads were then collected via centrifugation 1000 $\times$ *g* for 5 min and were washed three times with 10 ml of lysis buffer. The gel was then resuspended in 30 ml of lysis buffer and poured into a column. The recombinant protein was eluted by adding a solution containing 15 m*M* glutathione in 50 m*M* Hepes, pH 8, for GST fusion proteins or 50 m*M* Hepes, pH 7.4, 0.5 *M* NaCl, 10 m*M* 2-ME, and 10 m*M* maltose for MBP fusion proteins, individual fractions were collected, and protein concentrations were determined by measuring absorbance at 280 nm.

VII. Demonstration of Protein Kinase Activity

A. Protein Kinase Activity in Purified Fusion Proteins

In order to be useful for biochemical characterization the fusion protein containing the catalytic domain of the protein kinase of interest must be purifiable in an enzymatically active state. To determine whether a protein can autophos phorylate, a small amount of the protein kinase of interest is incubated in protein kinase buffer (50 m*M* Hepes, pH 7.4, 10 m*M* $MgCl_2$, 10 m*M* $MnCl_2$, 1 m*M* DTT, 10 μM [γ-^{32}P]ATP (10,000 cpm/pmol ATP)) for the desired time period. Although this buffer works well for the protein kinases we study, other protein kinases may require different levels of specific components (i.e., Ca^{+2}, higher ATP concentrations, specific substrates). After incubation is complete, an equal volume of electrophoresis sample buffer is added (Laemmli, 1970). The sample is denatured and reduced at 70°C for 30 min to avoid nonenzymatic phosphorylation (Schieven and Martin, 1988). The proteins are separated via SDS–PAGE and the phosphorylated species detected via autoradiography. Figure 1A shows an example of the results of such an experiment. The two different fusion protein constructs of the catalytic domain of RLK5 possess autophosphorylation activity. In addition, neither the fusion protein formed by expressing the reverse orientation of the DNA coding for the catalytic domain or a mutant, catalytically inactive, catalytic domain shows kinase activity. Although most protein kinases are active in the purified isolated form, some protein kinases may be active only *in vivo* or in freshly isolated bacterial extracts. Therefore if the purified protein kinase of interest does not appear to have any protein kinase activity, it may be useful

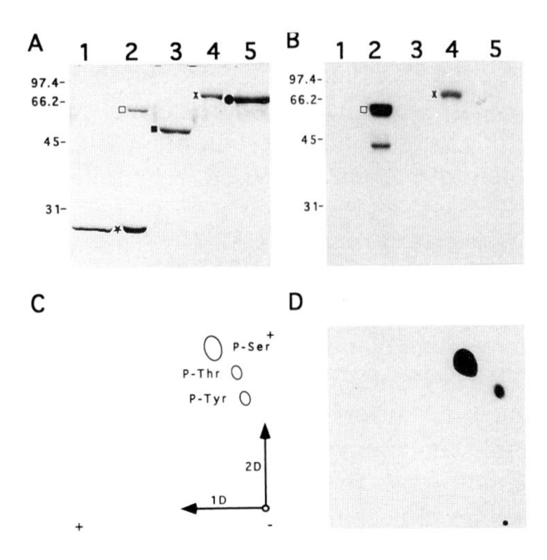

Fig. 1 Expression and *in vitro* autophosphorylation of RLK5 fusion proteins. Fusion proteins were purified from IPTG-induced *E. coli* cells containing a recombinant RLK5 catalytic domain expression plasmid. The fusion proteins, 2 μg, were then incubated in kinase buffer containing 10 μM [γ-^{32}P]ATP (10^5 cpm/pmol ATP) for 30 min at room temperature. After electrophoresis, the resulting gel was stained with Coomassie blue, destained, and dried and the radioactive species detected via autoradiography. Phosphoamino acid analysis was accomplished as indicated in Section V,II,B. (A) Coomassie blue-stained 12.5% SDS–PAGE gel. Lane 1, A glutathione S-transferase; reverse orientation of the catalytic domain of RLK5 fusion protein (★); Lane 2, A glutathione S-transferase; sense orientation of the catalytic domain of RLK5 fusion protein (□); Lane 3, A maltose-binding protein; reverse orientation of the catalytic domain of RLK5 fusion protein (■); Lane 4, A maltose-binding protein; sense orientation of the catalytic domain of RLK5 fusion protein (X); Lane 5, A maltose-binding protein; mutant, kinetically inactive, catalytic domain of RLK5 fusion protein (●). (B) An autoradiogram of the gel in (A), illustrating ^{32}P-labeled glutathione S-transferase; sense orientation of the catalytic domain of RLK5 fusion protein (□) and maltose-binding protein; sense orientation of the catalytic domain of RLK5 fusion protein (X). (C) Illustration of the positions of the phosphoamino acid standards after two-demensional electrophoresis and ninhydrin staining. (D) Autoradiogram of the maltose-binding protein; sense orientation of the catalytic domain of RLK5 fusion protein phosphoamino acids.

to investigate its activity *in vivo*. This can most readily be accomplished using *E. coli* cells carrying the expression plasmid of interest, which are first incubated for a period of time with radioactive P_i and then induced with IPTG for fusion protein expression. After induction, the fusion protein is purified, and should be radioactive, if it can undergo autophosphorylation.

B. Determining the Precise Amino Acid(s) Phosphorylated

After determining that a protein kinase has activity, it is informative to determine which amino acid (serine, threonine, or tyrosine) it phosphorylates. This is most easily accomplished by two-dimensional thin-layer electrophoresis (2D-TLE) of a HCl digest of the protein that has autophosphorylated in the presence of [γ-^{32}P]ATP. The procedure normally employed (Boyle *et al.*, 1991) is basically as follows: a Coomassie blue-stained band containing the autophosphorylated protein of interest is excised, rehydrated in 50 m*M* NH_4HCO_3, 0.1% SDS, and 0.5% 2-ME, ground with a small pestle, boiled for 5 min, and extracted by agitation at 37°C for at least 1 h. The protein is precipitated by adding 20 μg of BSA and solid TCA to 20% (w/v), followed by incubation at −20°C for 1 h and at −70°C for 1 h. The precipitate is collected by centrifugation and the TCA removed via lyophilization. The sample is hydrolyzed in 50 μl 6 *N* HCl for 1 h at 110°C. The HCl is removed via lyophilization, and the amino acids are resuspended in buffer, pH 1.9 (2.2% formic acid, 7.8% acetic acid). An amount of sample containing approximately 200 cpm of ^{32}P-labeled hydrolyzed protein and nonradioactive phosphoamino acid standards (1 part of a 1 mg/ml solution of phosphoserine, phosphothreonine, and phosphotyrosine to 15 parts of hydrolyzed protein) is applied in the lower right-hand side of a 100-μm 20 × 20-cm microcrystalline cellulose glass-backed thin-layer electrophoresis plate without fluorescent indicators (for example, No. 5716; E. M. Science, Gibbstown, NJ).

The actual electrophoresis takes place in a Hunter thin-layer electrophoresis unit (HTLE 7000; CBS Scientific, Inc., Del Mar, CA). The first dimension of the electrophoresis takes place in the horizontal direction in buffer, pH 1.9 (2.2% formic acid, 7.8% acetic acid) for 20 min at 1.5 kV. The second dimension of the electrophoresis takes place in the vertical dimension in buffer, pH 3.5 (5% acetic acid, 0.5% pyridin) for 16 min at 1.3 kV. After electrophoresis is complete, the plate is dried in an oven at 65°C for 30 min. The phosphoamino acid standards are detected by spraying the TLC plate with 0.25% (w/v) ninhydrin in acetone followed by incubation at 65°C for 15 min to develop the ninhydrin phosphoamino acid staining. After detecting the standards, the plate is placed on film to detect the radioactive phosphoamino acids. Figure 1B is an illustration of a typical analysis of an autophosphorylated catalytic domain of RLK5-containing fusion proteins. This figure illustrates that the catalytic domain of RLK5-containing fusion proteins are autophosphorylated on serine/threonine residues at a ratio of 10 : 1.

VIII. Determining the Number of Autophosphorylation Sites

Many protein kinases possess regulatory autophosphorylation sites. Phosphorylation of these different sites may serve to upregulate, downregulate, or change the substrate specificity of the catalytic domain of the protein kinase. The number of phosphorylation sites can be approximated by determining the number of radioactive phosphopeptides generated in a tryptic digest of an autophosphorylated protein kinase. This approximation is often valid because proteins are digested by trypsin into fragments that contain one or a small number of autophosphorylatable amino acids. The electrophoretic analysis is performed as described in (Boyle *et al.*, 1991) and is basically as follows. A band containing the ^{32}P-labeled protein to be analyzed is excised from a dried Coomassie-stained SDS–PAGE gel and extracted repeatedly into a buffer containing 50 m*M* ammonium bicarbonate (pH 7.3–7.6), 0.5% (w/v) SDS, and 0.1% (v/v) 2-mercaptoethanol. The peptides in this sample are precipitated by adding solid TCA to 20%. The dried TCA pellet is oxidized in 50 μl of cold performic acid for 30 min. The performic acid is removed by lyophilization and the resulting pellet is dissolved in 50 m*M* ammonium bicarbonate and cleaved with trypsin (10% w/w) for 4 h at 37°C. The sample is lyophilized to dryness, followed by repeated resuspension in buffer, pH 1.9, and lyophilization. Approximately 2000 cpm of the sample is applied in a small volume onto a 100 μm 20 $\times$ 20-cm microcrystalline cellulose glass-backed plates without fluorescent idicators (for example, No. 5716; E. M. Science, Gibbstown, NJ). The tryptic phosphopeptides are separated by electrophoresis in the first direction (pH 1.9, 1.5 kV, 30 min) followed by ascending thin-layer chromatography in phosphopeptide buffer (*n*-butanol : pyridine : acetic acid : water (75 : 50 : 15 : 60)). After electrophoresis, the radioactive species are detected by autoradiography. Figure 2 illustrates a typical 2D-TLE analysis of a tryptic phosphopeptide map obtained from autophosphorylated glutathione *S*-transferase; RLK5 catalytic domain fusion protein.

IX. Discussion and Conclusions

The expression of recombinant protein kinases in *E. coli* is a simple and inexpensive way to produce milligram amounts of an active protein kinase from a cloned gene. These recombinant enzymes are useful tools to examine the biochemical properties of any cloned protein kinase. To facilitate purification, we have chosen to construct fusion proteins using commercially available expression vectors. These fusion proteins contain a protein tag that allows that recombinant enzyme to be purified by affinity chromatography. Fusion proteins are not only easy to purify but the addition of a well-characterized protein tag often helps the solubility and stability of the recombinant protein. To further enhance the recovery of these recombinant enzymes we have used host strains that are protease deficient and growth conditions that favor the recovery of soluble fusion protein. To ensure that the catalytic properties of the expressed proteins are not unduly influenced by the affinity tag, or its purification, we have compared the activities of two different recombinant fusion proteins that have the same protein kinase catalytic domains. Our analyses demonstrate that the protein kinase fusions that we have studied have essentially identical enzymatic properties. The availability of large amounts of protein kinase has allowed us to determine the intrinsic biochemical properties and sites of autophosphorylation of a plant protein kinase that had not been previously characterized. Although these studies were limited to *in vitro* analyses with a nonnative form of the protein kinase,

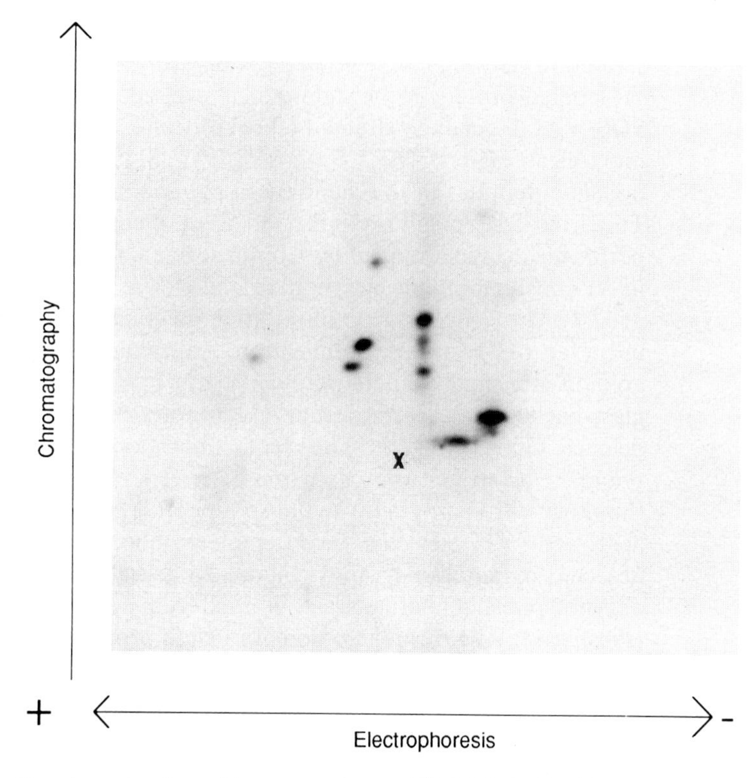

Fig. 2 Two-dimensional peptide map analysis of ^{32}P-labeled glutathione S-transferase; sense-orientation of the catalytic domain of RLK5 fusion protein. The fusion protein was isolated and autophosphorylated to a specific activity of 1000 cpm/μg. The labeled protein was cleaved with trypsin (10% w/w) O/N at 37°C. The phosphotryptic peptides (2000 cpm) were loaded onto the cellulose plate at the position marked (x). Samples were resolved horizontally by electrophoresis at pH 1.9 for 45 min at 1.5 kV and vertically by ascending chromatography in phosphochromatography buffer (37.5% *n*-butanol, 25% pyridine, 7.5% acetic acid). Radioactive species were detected via autoradiography.

the recombinant enzymes provide a useful tool to characterize the intrinsic catalytic characteristics of the enzyme of interest and should assist in our understanding of the function and biochemical properties of the native enzyme isolated from plants.

References

Boyle, W. J., Van Der Geer, P., and Hunter, T. (1991). Phosphopeptide mapping and phosphoamino acid analysis by two-dimensional separation on thin-layer cellulose plates. *In* "Methods of Enzymology" (T. Hunter and B. M. Sefton, eds.), Vol. 201, pp. 110–149. New York: Academic Press.

Guan, C. D., Ping, L., Riggs, P. D., and Inouye, H. (1988). Vectors that facilitate the expression and purification of foreign peptides in *Escherichia coli* by fusion to maltose-binding protein. *Gene* **67,** 21–30.

Hanks, S. K., and Quinn, A. E. (1991). Protein kinase catalytic domain sequence database: Identification of conserved features of primary structure and classification of family members. *In* "Methods of Enzymology" (T. Hunter and B. M. Sefton, eds.), Vol. 200, pp. 38–62. New York: Academic Press.

Hunter, T. (1991). Protein kinase classification. *In* "Methods of Enzymology" (T. Hunter and B. M. Sefton, eds.), Vol. 200, pp. 3–37. New York: Academic Press.

Kohanski, R. (1993). Insulin receptor autophosphorylation. I. Autophosphorylation kinetics of the native receptor and its cytoplasmic kinase domain. *Biochemistry* **32,** 5766–5772.

Laemmli, U. K. (1970). Cleavage of structural proteins during the assembly of the head of bacteriophage T4. *Nature* (*London*) **227,** 660–685.

Schieven, G., and Martin, G. S. (1988). Nonenzymatic phosphorylation of tyrosine and serine by ATP is catalyzed by manganese but not magnesium *J. Biol. Chem.* **263,** 15590–15593.

Smith, D. B., and Johnson, K. S. (1988). Single-step purification of polypeptides expressed in *Escherichia coli* as fusions with glutathione-S-transferase. *Gene* **67,** 31–40.

Studier, W. F., Rosenberg, A. H., Dunn, J. J., and Dubendorff, J. W. (1990). Use of T7 RNA polymerase to direct expression of cloned genes. *In* "Methods of Enzymology" (D. V. Goeddel, ed.), Vol. 185, pp. 60–89. New York: Academic Press.

Walker, J. C. (1993). Receptor-like protein kinase genes of *Arabidopsis thaliana. The Plant J.* **3,** 451–456.

Wente, S. R., Villalba, M., Schramm, V. L., and Rosen, O. M. (1990). Mn^{2+}-binding properties of a recombinant protein-tyrosine kinase derived from the human insulin receptor. *Proc. Natl. Acad. Sci. U. S. A.* **87,** 2805–2809.

Winograd, E., Pulido, M. A., and Wasserman, M. (1993). Production of DNA-recombinant polypeptides by tac-inducible vectors using micromolar concentrations of IPTG. *Biotechniques* **14,** 886–890.

CHAPTER 38

Transmembrane Signaling and Phosphoinositides

Myeon H. Cho and Wendy F. Boss

Botany Department
North Carolina State University
Raleigh, North Carolina 27695-7612

I. Introduction

Inositol phospholipids are important mediators of cell metabolism. These negatively charged polyphosphorylated phospholipids can function as direct effectors of alterations to the activities of membrane enzymes as well as the source of the second messengers, inositol trisphosphate (IP_3), and diacylglycerol (DAG). Although there is a plethora of researchers working on phosphatidylinositol bisphosphate (PIP_2) metabolism in animal cells, very few researchers work on PIP_2 metabolism in plant cells. There are two major reasons for this. One is that it is more difficult to analyze inositol phospholipids and inositol phosphates in higher plants than in animals; two, there is a dearth of evidence thus far to indicate that IP_3 is a second messenger in higher plants. Both problems derive,

METHODS IN CELL BIOLOGY, VOL. 49

in part, from the fact that PIP_2 levels are relatively low in all the higher plants studied (Hetherington and Drøbak, 1992; Drøbak, 1992; Gross and Boss, 1993; Drøbak, 1993). This does not mean, however, that inositol phospholipids are not important in plants. They are present and their metabolism has been shown to respond rapidly to external stimuli (Morse *et al.,* 1987; Einspahr *et al.,* 1988; Memon and Boss, 1990; Chen and Boss, 1990; Tan and Boss, 1992; Cho and Boss, 1993). Furthermore, evidence is accumulating to suggest that the inositol phospholipids in higher plants act as direct effectors of membrane and cytoskeletal proteins (Chen and Boss, 1991; Tan and Boss, 1992; Gross and Boss, 1993; Yang *et al.,* 1993; Drøbak, 1993; Yang and Boss, 1994).

Our goal in writing this chapter is to convince the reader that one can monitor inositol phospholipid metabolism in plants, but that it must be done carefully in order to be able to interpret the results. We have described briefly the protocols used in our laboratory and have given some background and perspective. Many of these procedures were developed by other researchers in the field, and the reader is encourage to read the seminal references cited.

II. Materials

Higher plant cells and algae grown in suspension culture and cut segments of higher plant tissue are the most common sources of material for labeling studies (Boss and Massel, 1985; Morse *et al.,* 1987; Einspahr *et al.,* 1988; Chen and Boss, 1990; Cho and Boss, 1993). Using cells grown in suspension culture has several advantages: (1) the cells can be labeled *in vivo* without injury; (2) relatively uniform cells can be grown in large quantities; (3) the cells can be grown through several cell division cycles in a defined culture medium; (4) they can be harvested rapidly. The disadvantage is that one cannot easily see a change in morphology in response to most stimuli. The carrot cell line we have used most frequently was originally derived from *Daucus carota* embryogenic callus and was subsequently cultured and selected on the basis of the fusion potential of the protoplasts (Boss *et al.,* 1984; Wheeler and Boss, 1989; Chen and Boss, 1990). By comparison to the usually large vacuolated and rapidly growing suspension culture cells, these cells grow more slowly and in tight clusters. They readily incorporate $[^3H]$inositol into phosphatidylinositol (PI), lysoPI, and phosphatidylinositol monophosphate (PIP), and $[^3H]$lysoPIP and $[^3H]PIP_2$ can be detected with time (Wheeler and Boss, 1987; van Breemen *et al.,* 1990 and Figs. 1A and 1B).

Algae provide a good system to study inositol phospholipid metabolism (Irvine *et al.,* 1989; Einspahr and Thompson, 1990; Quarmby *et al.,* (1992). This is not only because of the ease of growing and labeling algae but also because they appear to synthesize relatively high levels of PIP_2 compared to higher plants (Irvine *et al.,* 1989; Gross and Boss, 1993).

Studies of cut plant segments are often limited by the uptake of the $[^3H]$inositol or $^{32}P_i$ into the tissues of interest. Light and rapid air circulation encourage

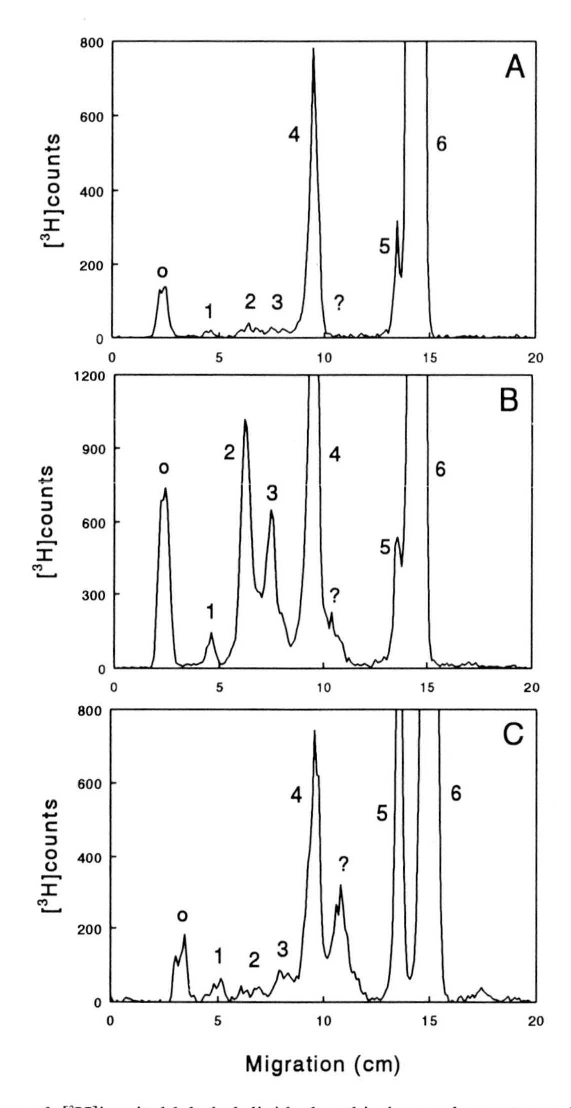

Fig. 1 Separation of [^{3}H]inositol-labeled lipids by thin-layer chromatography using $CHCl_3$: $MeOH:NH_4OH:H_2O$ (86:76:6:16, v/v/v/v) as a solvent and analyzing with a Bioscan System 500 imaging scanner. (A) [^{3}H]Inositol-labeled lipids from carrot cells incubated with [^{3}H]inositol (1 μCi/0.04 g fresh wt/ml conditioned medium) for 4 h. (B) [^{3}H]Inositol-labeled lipids from carrot cells incubated with [^{3}H]inositol (0.4 μ Ci/0.02 g fresh wt/ml conditioned medium) for 18 h. (C) [^{3}H]Inositol-labeled lipids from a petunia leaf incubated in a solution of [^{3}H]inositol (2 μCi/ml H_2O) overnight in a growth chamber under constant fluorescent light (o, origin; 1, PIP_2; 2, lysoPIP_1; 3, lysoPIP_u; 4, PIP; ?, unknown inositol lipid; 5, lysoPI; 6, PI).

transpiration and enhance [^{3}H]inositol incorporation into the lipids of leaves. With many plant tissues, multiple inositol-labeled lipids are present (Fig. 1C), some of which have not been identified and many of which will comigrate if the proper solvent system is not chosen (Boss, 1989; Rincón and Boss, 1990; Cho *et al.,* 1992). More importantly, according to Coté and Crain (1992) a major disadvantage in using cut segments for comparative studies of inositol phospholipid metabolism is that the incorporation of label can vary several-fold in the control tissue alone, especially with short-term labeling. This can make it impossible to quantitate differences resulting from treatments.

III. Methods and Critical Aspects of the Procedures

A. Labeling Inositol Phospholipids with ^{32}P

$^{32}P_i$ and myo[2-^{3}H]inositol are the most common radioisotopes used to label the inositol phospholipids. $^{32}P_i$ labels phospholipids, sugar phosphates, nucleotides, and other cellular metabolites that can interfere with the analysis of the inositol phospholipids and inositol phosphates. With short-term labeling (min), however, the primary ^{32}P-labeled lipids formed are PIP_2, PIP, and PA, and thus the inositol lipids and their metabolites are easier to resolve (Coté and Crain, 1992; Einspahr *et al.,* 1988). We have found that ^{32}P incorporation into PIP_2 saturates after approximately 10 min with the carrot cells. The major drawback to using short-term labeling is that the stimulus applied may effect [^{32}P]P_i uptake or the levels of [^{32}P]ATP within the cell and thereby affect the recovery of [^{32}P]PIP or PIP_2 without affecting phospholipid turnover. In addition, differences in the uptake of the label among tissue samples prior to applying the stimulus are more pronounced with short-term labeling (Coté and Crain, 1992).

B. Labeling Inositol Phospholipids with *myo*[2-^{3}H]Inositol

myo[2-^{3}H]Inositol is a more selective means of labeling the inositol phospholipids and inositol phosphates *in vivo* than $^{32}P_i$. Cells must be labeled to equilibrium for the data to be interpreted as changes in mass, and this is usually not achieved unless the cells are labeled for several cell division cycles. However, one can use [^{3}H]inositol to monitor effectively the degradation of inositol phospholipids and the accumulation of [^{3}H]inositol phosphates.

For most of our studies we have labeled carrot suspension culture cells with *myo*[2-^{3}H]inositol (0.2 μCi ml^{-1} for lipid analysis and 0.4 μCi ml^{-1} for inositol phosphate analysis) for 18 h. The cells are grown in inositol-free medium and the [^{3}H]inositol is added to the cells (approximately 0.25 g fresh wt in 25 ml^{-1} of medium) 3 days after transfer (early log phase of growth). For short-term labeling (2 to 4 h) 1 to 2 μCi ml^{-1} is added. As with the ^{32}P, short-term labeling studies have the advantage of yielding a higher percentage of the ^{3}H in PIP (compare Figs. 1A and 1B). However, with short-term [^{3}H]inositol labeling one must determine whether the stimulus or treatment used affects the biosynthesis of PI and the biogenesis of PIP and PIP_2 as well as uptake and incorporation of [^{3}H]inositol.

C. Extraction and Separation of Inositol Phospholipids

It should be pointed out that no single extraction procedure will be satisfactory in all respects, and that the procedure of choice will depend on the measurements required. The efficacy of extraction should be determined by following recoveries of radioactive standards added to tissue extracts following termination.

The process of harvesting the cells or tissue can alter the metabolism of the inositol phospholipids and affect the interpretation of the data; therefore, careful controls must be done. We normally harvest the carrot cells by brief centrifugation ($200 \times g$ for 30 s) and immediately add ice-cold extraction medium.

The acid extraction method is most commonly used for inositol phospholipids. A detailed description is given by Cho *et al.* (1992). A critical factor is the ratio of organic solvent to aqueous sample. We usually use 0.05 to 0.1 g fresh wt of cells or tissue or 0.1 ml of membranes per 1.5 ml of ice-cold $CHCl_3$: MeOH (1:2, v/v). Cells or tissue samples are vortexed well and placed on ice for 20 to 30 min to enhance the extraction. The samples are warmed to 25°C and the following solutions are added sequentially with vortexing: 0.5 ml of 0.1 *M* EDTA (pH 4.4), 0.5 ml of 2.4 *N* HCl, and 0.5 ml of $CHCl_3$. The samples are centrifuged for 6 min at $2000 \times g$ and the lower phase is removed. The upper phase is reextracted two more times with $CHCl_3$ and the combined lower phases are back-extracted with 2 ml of MeOH:1 *N* HCl (1:1, v/v) two times. For the final wash, the lower phase is removed carefully so not to include any aqueous, upper phase. The lipid samples are dried *in vacuo* (water aspirator) and stored under nitrogen until analyzed. Samples are reconstituted in $CHCl_3$:MeoH (2:1, v/v), spotted on Whatman LK5-D thin-layer plates that are presoaked in 1% potassium oxalate, and dried in a microwave oven 10 min. The plates are developed in $CHCl_3$:MeOH:NH_4OH:H_2O (86:76:6:16, v/v/v/v). A visible marker NBD-PA (Avanti Polar Lipids) is used to monitor the migration of the lipids. When NBD-PA reaches 15 cm, PI is just below it and the other inositol phospholipids will be well separated. The lysolipids and other inositol labeled lipids will migrate very close to PI, PIP, and PIP_2; therefore, it is essential to run standards. Internal standards should be run from time to time especially if one has different amounts of lipids or treatments that affect the normal migration of the lipids.

HPLC also can be used to separate effectively the inositol phospholipids (Coté *et al.,* 1990). Our experience has been that thin-layer chromatography allows us to compare several treatments (up to 10 samples per plate) under identical conditions, and once the lipids have been separated, they can be analyzed and quantitated reliably with an imaging scanner. In addition, there is much less repair and upkeep (essentially none) for an imaging scanner relative to an HPLC.

If thin-layer chromatolography is used, an imaging scanner is essential to resolve and quantitate reproducibly the [^{3}H]inositol lipids. The plant [^{3}H]inositol phospholipids cannot be detected well enough by autoradiography even with enhancers. In addition, because there are so many [^{3}H]inositol-labeled lipids it is difficult to identify and scrape reproducibly PIP and PIP_2 from the plates.

D. Extraction Procedures for Inositol Phosphates

For extraction of the water-soluble inositol phosphates from tissues, methods routinely used include chloroform/methanol, chloroform/methanol/HCl (as for the lipids), perchloric acid followed by neutralization by KOH or by FREON/octylamine, and trichloroacetic acid with neutralization by diethy ether. For extraction of acid-labile, cyclic inositol phosphates, a mixture of phenol, chloroform, and methanol is used (Hawkins *et al.,* 1987). To ensure good recovery of inositol phosphates, a small amount of phytic acid hydrolysate should be added (Wreggett and Irvine, 1987).

We have used the method described by Kirk *et al.* (1990), which is briefly described below. Perchloric acid containing 1 mg/ml phytic acid carrier is added to the cells to give a final concentration of 4% (v/v) perchloric acid. The cells are placed on ice for 10 min prior to inositol phosphate analysis (Kirk *et al.,* 1990). The precipitated protein is centrifuged ($>1000 \times g$) for 5 min. The supernatant is saved and the perchloric acid therein is removed by a modification (Shears *et al.,* 1987) of a method first described by Sharps and McCarl (1982). One volume of the perchlorate-quenched supernatant is added to 0.08 vol of 50 m*M* EDTA (pH 7, with NaOH) followed by 1.5 vol of freshly mixed 1:1 (v/v) 1,1,2-trichlorotrifluoroethane : tri-*n*-octylamine, all of which must be cool but not frozen (i.e., kept just above ice, but not in ice). The samples are mixed vigorously in a tightly sealed tube and centrifuged at $1000 \times g$ for 5 min at 4°C. The largest possible proportion of the neutralized upper phase is saved but the precise amount, as with all phase separates, will depend upon the volumes used and the internal diameter of the tubes. Ice-cold water may be added to the lower phase in a volume equal to that of the removed upper phase to enhance recovery. After further mixing and centrifugation, the upper phase is again withdrawn and combined with the earlier extract. After perchloric acid extraction and neutralization, the recovered supernatants can be stored at −20°C for up to 2 months.

E. Inositol Phosphate Analysis

There are several separation methods used to analyze inositol phosphates. Descending paper chromatography, paper ionophoresis, and gravity-fed anion-exchange column chromatography will not adequately resolve all the inositol phosphate isomers and other inositol metabolites in whole plant extracts (Rincón *et al.*, 1989; Coté *et al.*, 1990). Anion-exchange HPLC (Irvine *et al.*, 1985) is capable of resolving positional isomers of the inositol phosphates as well as the plant metabolites (Coté *et al.*, 1987) and also can be used for the separation of cyclic inositol phosphates.

For the anion-exchange HPLC analysis, we use an Adsorbosphere 5 μ-SAX HPLC column (Alltech Associates, Deerfield, IL) eluted with a slight modification of the salt gradient previously described (Menniti *et al.*, 1990) and generated from water and buffer (1 *M* ammonium dihydrogen phosphate, pH 3.35, with phosphoric acid): 0 to 10 min, 0% buffer; 10 to 85 min the buffer increased linearly from 0 to 35%; 85 to 130 min, the buffer increased linearly from 35 to 80%. Half-minute fractions are collected for 80 min, and 1-min fractions are collected thereafter. Scintillant is added to each of the fractions, and the radioactivity is assessed. Each sample also should contain an internal standard (e.g., $[^{14}C]$-I(1,3,4)P_3) to account for run-to-run variability.

HPLC is the only method that can resolve all the different inositol phosphates. Some disadvantages are that it is very time-consuming (each run can take up to 2 h), it is expensive (in terms of equipment, columns, and scintillation fluid), and only a small number of samples can be analyzed on one column.

A specific binding assay for the measurement of I(1,4,5)P_3 mass has been developed, based on displacement of $[^3H]$-I(1,4,5)P_3 from specific binding proteins in bovine adrenal cortex (Challis *et al.*, 1988; Palmer *et al.*, 1989). The assay is easy, and large numbers of samples can be processed simultaneously. However, the ability of ATP and many other normal intracellular components to displace I(1,4,5)P_3 from its binding site can pose considerable problems for measurement of I(1,4,5)P_3 in cell extracts (Nunn and Taylor, 1990). Rigorous controls are essential and have been described (Challis *et al.*, 1990). The advantages of the binding assay are that it is very sensitive (pmol of IP_3 can be detected), and it measures IP_3 mass without relying on uptake or incorporation of a radiolabel. The disadvantages are the potential for nonspecific binding and the expense of the commercially available kits.

F. *In Vitro* Measurements of Inositol Phospholipid Metabolism

One best kept secret is that *in vitro* lipid phosphorylation is easier to analyze and interpret than protein phosphorylation. This is because of the limited number of lipid substrates and, therefore, of products formed. The ease of analysis and consistency of the results have been major factors in contributing to several laboratories focusing on *in vitro* studies.

Inositol phospholipid kinases and lipases have been characterized extensively by Marianne Sommarin and Anna Stina Sandelius. The assay conditions, with minor modifications, are briefly described below. The reader is encouraged to read their many papers for specifics on the effects of cation, detergents, pH, and other assay conditions (Sandelius and Sommarin, 1986; Sommarin and Sandelius, 1988; Melin *et al.,* 1992; for review see Sandelius and Sommarin, 1990).

1. PI 4 and PIP 5 Kinase Assays

PI and PIP kinase activities should be measured in the absence and presence of exogenous substrates, and careful time course studies of reaction rates as well as treatment times should be done for each new system and stimulus. To measure enzyme activity, isolated membranes (15 to 40 μg protein) are resuspended in 40 μl of 30 m*M* TrisMes buffer (pH 6.5) containing 15 m*M* $MgCl_2$. Phosphorylation is started by adding 10 μl of ATP stock solution, which contained 10 μCi of [γ-^{32}P]ATP (7000 Ci $mmol^{-1}$), 5 m*M* ATP, 0.05% (v/v) Triton X-100, and 5 m*M* Na_2MoO_4 in 30 m*M* TrisMes containing 15 m*M* $MgCl_2$ (pH 6.5), to give a final concentration of 1 m*M* ATP, 1 m*M* Na_2MoO_4, and 0.01% Triton X-100. Na_2MoO_4 is added as a nonspecific phosphatase inhibitor. When exogenous substrates are added, the PI and PIP are presolubilized at a concentration of 5 mg/ml in 2% Triton X-100. The substrate stock solution is dded to give 25 μg of PI or PIP and a final concentration of 0.2% Triton X-100. With the high Triton, the pH is increased to 8 for optimal activity (Sommarin and Sandelius, 1988). The reaction tubes are shaken vigorously at 25°C, and after 10 min, the reaction is stopped by adding 1.5 ml of ice-cold $CHCl_3$: MeOH (1:2, v/v). The lipids are extracted and analyzed as described in Section III,C and by Cho *et al.* (1992).

The major product formed by higher plant membranes using endogenous substrate is phosphatidic acid (PA). PA can be anywhere from 70 to 90% of the ^{32}P product formed. DAG kinase is inhibited by detergent (Lundberg and Sommarin, 1992), and thus, less PA is formed when exogenous PI or PIP is added in Triton micelles. We have not detected any PI 3-kinase activity *in vitro;* however, the 3-kinase also is inhibited by Triton and, therefore, may have been inactivated. Because several products can be formed and because under some conditions (e.g., high concentrations of Ca^{2+} and/or Mn^{2+}) pyrophosphates of PIP and PIP_2 can form nonenzymatically (Gumber and Lowenstein, 1986), it is important to analyze the products.

2. PIP and PIP_2 Phospholipase C Assay

PIP and PIP_2 phospholipase C (PLC) activity is assayed according to the method of Melin *et al.* (1992). The standard reaction mixture contains 50 m*M* TrisHCl (pH 6), 20 μ*M* Ca^{2+} [a $CaCl_2$/EGTA mixture is used as described by Marks and Maxfield (1991)], 0.2 m*M* PIP or PIP_2, and 4 to 6 μg of membrane protein in a final volume of 50 μl. It is important not to use excess membrane. The reaction rate is proportional to the amount of enzyme up to 6 μg of plasma membrane protein (Melin *et al.,* 1987). The reaction is started by the addition of 10 μl of PIP or PIP_2 stock solution containing [^{3}H]inositol PIP (1100 dpm

$nmol^{-1}$) in 0.1% deoxycholate. The stock solution is prepared by drying an aliquot of the lipid substrate in $CHCl_3$ under a stream of nitrogen followed by sonication in 0.1% sodium deoxycholate for 10 min. The reaction is stopped after 5 min at 25°C by addition of 1 ml of $CHCl_3$: MeOH (2 : 1, v/v). After addition of 250 μl of 1 *N* HCl, vortexing, and brief centrifugation in a table-top centrifuge, the radioactive reaction products are recovered in the upper phase, analyzed by ion exchange chromatography on a Dowex AG 1-X8 column (Berridge *et al.,* 1983), and quantitated by liquid scintillation counting.

The aqueous products must be analyzed to substantiate that hydrolysis is caused by a C-type lipase. We use a slight modification of the procedure of Berridge *et al.* (1983) as described by Rincon *et al.* (1989). Aqueous samples are diluted with 10 ml deionized H_2O and applied onto 1-ml Dowex 1-X8 columns (formate form; Bio-Rad). The loaded columns are washed with 10 ml of deionized H_2O. Fractions of approximately 1 ml are collected by sequential elution with 10 ml of 5 m*M* sodium tetraborate + 60 m*M* sodium formate to elute glycerolphosphoinositol; 0.2 *M* ammonium formate + 0.1 *M* formic acid for IP; 0.4 *M* ammonium formate + 0.1 *M* formic acid for IP_2, and 1 *M* ammonium formate + 0.1 *M* formic acid for IP_3. The ion-exchange resin exhibits batch variation, so it is essential to check the elution profiles with inositol phosphate standards. The columns can be regenerated for a limited number of times (<5) by washing the column with 20 ml 2 *M* ammonium formate + 0.1 *M* formic acid, followed by 20 ml water.

IV. Conclusions and Perspectives

PIP and PIP_2 are present in plants; however, their precise roles in regulating cell metabolism are unknown. One limitation in studying plant inositol phospholipid metabolism has been the plethora of inositol lipids and metabolites relative to PIP and PIP_2. Furthermore, only a few cells within a tissue may be responding to a given stimulus and only a small pool of the PIP or PIP_2 within those cells may be turning over. Thus, in studying PIP and PIP_2 metabolism, one should identify the stimulus-sensitive pool and find a means of selectively labeling it in the most responsive cells or tissue. Inhibitor studies can be useful in studying metabolic pathways; however, no inhibitor is specific and it is unacceptable to interpret the results of inhibitor studies as indicative of PIP_2 turnover without showing changes in both the inositol phospholipids and the inositol phosphates. Careful analyses of the metabolites are essential.

In vitro studies of enzyme activity should not be overlooked. Differences in the specific activities of enzymes involved in inositol phospholipid biosynthesis have been shown to persist in isolated membranes (Chen and Boss, 1990; Memon and Boss, 1990; Tan and Boss, 1992; Cho *et al.,* 1993). These differences can result from modification of the enzyme or a regulatory component or a change in the distribution of the enzyme or regulatory component and may reflect a change in the physiological state of the cell.

Time course measurements are crucial to delineating the sequence of events in a stimulus–response pathway. Thus far, no one has demonstrated an increase in cytosolic calcium following a stimulus-induced increase in PIP_2 turnover in higher plants, and the *in vitro* data indicate that changes in cytosolic calcium could initiate the hydrolysis of PIP_2 or PIP (Melin *et al.,* 1992). In addition, activation of PI 4-kinase by the protein activator PIK-A49 is dependent on the phosphorylation of PIK-A49 by a calcium-dependent protein kinase (Yang and Boss, 1994). This means that an increase in cytosolic calcium could initiate an increase in PIP and PIP_2 turnover.

Virtually nothing is known about the regulation of the interactions among the extracellular matrix, plasma membrane, and cytoskeleton in plants. PIP and PIP_2 can bind actin-binding proteins (Aderem, 1992) and can activate membrane ATPases (Memon *et al.,* 1989; Chen and Boss, 1991). In addition, PIK-A49 is an actin-bundling protein and has translational elongation factor-1α activity (Yang *et al.,* 1993). Thus, the inositol phospholipids may provide a mechanism for membrane and cytoskeletal interaction. This opens up a new area for plant research. As the enzymes in the pathway are purified and the genes encoding them are identified, it is hoped that we will gain further insights into the regulation of inositol phospholipid metabolism and signal transduction in plants.

Acknowledgments

This work has been supported by grants from the National Science Foundation and by the North Carolina Agricultural Research Service.

References

Aderem, A. (1992). Signal transduction and the actin cytoskeleton: the roles of MARCKS and profilin. *Trends Biochem. Sci.* **17,** 438–443.

Berridge, M. J., Dawson, R. M. C., Downes, C. P., Heslop, J. P., and Irvine, R. F. (1983). Changes in the levels of inositol phosphates after agonist-dependent hydrolysis of membrane phosphoinositides. *Biochem J.* **212,** 473–482.

Boss, W. F. (1989). Plant phosphoinositide metabolism: A potential mechanism for signal transduction. *In* "Second Messengers in Plant Growth and Development." (W. F. Boss and D. J. Morré, eds.), pp. 29–56. New York: Alan R. Liss.

Boss. W. F., Grimes, H. D., and Brightman, A. O. (1984). Calcium-induced fusion of fusogenic wild carrot protoplasts. *Protoplasma.* **120,** 209–215.

Boss, W. F., and Massel, M. O. (1985). Polyphosphoinositides are present in plant tissue culture cells. *Biochem. Biophys. Res. Commun.* **132,** 1018–1023.

Challis, R. A. J., Batty, I., and Nahorski, S. R. (1988). Mass measurements of inositol 1.4,5-trisphosphate in rat cerebral cortex slices using a radioreceptor assay: Effects of neurotransmitters and depolarization. *Biochem. Biophys. Res. Commun.* **157,** 421–427.

Challis, R. A. J., Chilvers, E. R., Willcocks, A. L., and Narhorski, S. R. (1990). Heterogeneity of [^{3}H]inositol 1,4,5-trisphosphate binding sites in adrenal-cortical membranes. Characterization and validation of a radioreceptor assay. *Biochem J.* **265,** 421–427.

Chen, Q., and Boss, W. F. (1990). Short-term treatment with cell wall degrading enzymes increases the inositol phospholipid kinase and vanadate-sensitive ATPase activity. *Plant Physiol.* **94,** 1820–1829.

Chen, Q., and Boss, W. F. (1991). Neomycin inhibits the PIP and PIP_2 stimulation of plasma membrane ATPase of carrot cells. *Plant Physiol.* **96,** 340–343.

Cho, M. H., Chen, Q., Okpodu, C. M., and Boss, W. F. (1992). Separating and detecting inositol phospholipids. *LC·GC* **10,** 464–468.

Cho, M. H., Shears, S. B., and Boss, W. F. (1993). Changes in phosphatidylinositol metabolism in response to hyperosmotic stress in *Daucus carota* L. cells grown in suspension culture. *Plant Physiol.* **103,** 637–647.

Coté, G. G., Morse, M. J., Crain, R. C., and Satter, R. L. (1987). Isolation of soluble metabolites of the phosphatidylinositol cycle from *Samanea saman. Plant Cell Rep.* **6,** 352–355.

Coté, G. G., Satter, R. L., Morse, M. J., and Crain, R. L. (1990). Extraction, separation, and characterization of the metabolites of the inositol phospholipid cycle. *In* "Inositol Metabolism in Plants" (D. J. Morré, W. F. Boss, and F. A. Loewus, ed.), pp. 113–137. New York: Wiley-Liss.

Coté, G. G., and Crain, R. C. (1992). Artifactual elevation of the apparent levels of phosphatidic acid and phosphatidylinositol 4,5-bisphosphate during short-term labeling of plant tissue with radioactive precursor. *Plant Physiol.* **100,** 1042–1043.

Drøbak, B. K. (1992). The plant phosphoinositide system. *Biochem J.* **288,** 697–712.

Drøbak, B. K. (1993). Plant phosphoinositides and intracellular signaling. *Plant Physiol.* **102,** 705–709.

Einspahr, K. J., Peeler, T. C., and Thompson, Jr., G. A. (1988). Rapid changes in polyphosphoinositide metabolism associated with the response of *Dunaliella salina* to hypoosmotic shock. *J. Biol. Chem.* **263,** 5775–5779.

Einspahr, K. J., and Thompson, Jr., G. A. (1990). Transmembrane signalling via phosphatidylinositol 4,5-bisphosphate hydrolysis in plants. *Plant Physiol.* **93,** 361–366.

Gross, W., and Boss, W. F. (1993). Inositol phospholipids and signal transduction. *In* "Control of Plant Gene Expression" (D. P. S. Verma, ed.), pp. 17–32. Caldwell, NJ: The Telford Press.

Gumber, S. B., and Lowenstein, J. M. (1986). Non-enzymic phosphorylation of polyphosphoinositides and phosphatidic acid is catalysed by bivalent metal ions. *Biochem. J.* **235,** 617–619.

Hawkins, P. T., Berrie, C. P., Morris, A. J., and Downes, C. P. (1987). Inositol 1,2-cyclic 4,5-trisphosphate is not a product of muscarinic receptor-stimulated phosphatidylinositol 4,5-bisphosphate hydrolysis in rat parotid glands. *Biochem. J.* **243,** 211–218.

Hetherington, A. M., and Drøbak, B. K. (1992). Inositol-containing lipids in higher plants. *Prog. Lipid Res.* **31,** 53–63.

Irvine, R. F., Angga rd, E. E., Letcher, A. J., and Downes, C. P. (1985). Metabolism of inositol 1,4,5-trisphosphate and inositol 1,3,4-trisphosphate in rat parotid glands. *Biochem. J.* **229,** 505–511.

Irvine, R. F., Letcher, A. J., Lander, D. J., Drøbak, B. K., Dawson, A. P., and Musgrave, A. (1989). Phosphatidylinositol(4,5)bisphosphate and phosphatidylinositol(4)phosphate in plant tissues. *Plant Physiol.* **89,** 888–892.

Kirk, C. J., Morris, A. J., and Shears, S. B. (1990). Inositol phosphate second messenger. *In* "Peptide Hormone Action. A Practical Approach" (K. Siddle and J. C. Hutton, ed.), pp. 151–184. Oxford: IRL Press.

Lundberg, G. A., and Sommarin, M. (1992). Diacylglycerol kinase in plasma membranes from wheat. *Biochim. Biophys. Acta* **1123,** 177–183.

Marks, P. W., and Maxfield, F. R. (1991). Preparation of solutions with free calcium concentration in the nanomolar range using 1,2-bis(o-aminophenoxy)ethane-N,N,N′,N′-tetraacetic acid. *Anal. Biochem.* **193,** 61–71.

Melin, P. M., Sommarin, M., Sandelius, A. S., and Jergil, B. (1987). Identification of Ca^{2+}-stimulated polyphosphoinositide phospholipase C in isolated plant plasma membranes. *FEBS Lett.* **223,** 87–91.

Melin, P. M., Pical, C., Jergil, B., and Sommarin, M. (1992). Polyphosphoinositide phospholipase C in wheat root plasma membranes. Partial purification and characterization. *Biochim. Biophys. Acta* **1123,** 163–169.

Memon, A. R., Chen, Q., and Boss, W. F. (1989). Inositol phospholipids activate plasma membrane ATPase in plants. *Biochem. Biophys. Res. Commun.* **162,** 1295–1301.

Memon, A. R., and Boss, W. F. (1990). Rapid light-induced changes in phosphoinositide kinase and H^+-ATPase in plasma membrane of sunflower hypocotyls. *J. Biol. Chem.* 14817–14821.

Menniti, F. S., Oliver, K. G., Nogimori, K., Obie, J. F., Shears, S. B., and Putney, Jr., J. W. (1990). Origins of *myo*-inositol tetrakisphosphates in agonist-stimulated rat pancreatoma cells. Stimulation by bombesin of *myo*-inositol 1,3,4,5,6-pentakisphosphate breakdown to *myo*-inositol 3,4,5,6-tetrakisphosphate. *J. Biol. Chem.* **265,** 11167–11176.

Morse, M. J., Crain, R. C., and Satter, R. L. (1987). Light-stimulated inositol phospholipid turnover in *Samanea saman* leaf pulvini. *Proc. Natl. Acad. Sci. U.S.A.* **84,** 7075–7078.

Nunn, D. L., and Taylor, C. W. (1990). Liver inositol 1,4,5-trisphosphate-binding sites are the Ca^{2+}-mobilizing receptors. *Biochem. J.* **270,** 227–232.

Palmer, S., Hughes, K. T., Lee, D. Y., and Wakelam, M. J. O. (1989). Development of a novel Ins(1,4,5)P_3 specific binding assay. *Cell Signal* **1,** 147–153.

Quarmby, L. M., Yueh, Y. G., Cheshire, J. L., Keller, L. R., Snell, W. J., and Crain, R. C. (1992). Inositol phospholipid metabolism may trigger flagellar excision in *Chlamydomonas reinhardtii. J. Cell Biol.* **116,** 737–744.

Rincón, M., Chen, Q., and Boss, W. F. (1989). Characterization of inositol phosphates in carrot (*Daucus carota* L.) cells. *Plant Physiol.* **89,** 126–132.

Rincón, M., and Boss, W. F. (1990). Second-messenger role of phosphoinositides. *In* "Inositol Metabolism in Plants" (D. J. Morré, W. F. Boss, and F. A. Loewus, eds.), pp. 173–200. New York: Wiley-Liss.

Sandelius, A. S., and Sommarin, M. (1986). Phosphorylation of phosphatidylinositol in isolated plant membranes. *FEBS Lett.* **201,** 282–286.

Sandelius, A. S., and Sommarin, M. (1990). Membrane-localized reactions involved in polyphosphoinositide turnover in plants. *In* "Inositol Metabolism in Plants" (D. J. Morré, W. F. Boss, and F. A. Loewus, eds.), pp. 139–161. New York: Wiley-Liss.

Sharps, E. D., and McCarl, R. L. (1982). A high-performance liquid chromatographic method to measure ^{32}P incorporation into phosphorylated metabolites in cultured cells. *Anal. Biochem.* **124,** 421–424.

Shears, S. B., Storey, D. J., Morris, A. J., Cubitt, A. B., Parry, J. B., Michell, R. H., and Kirk, C. J. (1987). Dephosphorylation of *myo*-inositol 1,4,5-trisphosphate and *myo*-inositol 1,3,4-trisphosphate. *Biochem. J.* **242,** 393–402.

Sommarin, M., and Sandelius, A. S. (1988). Phosphatidylinositol and phosphatidylinositol phosphate kinases in plant plasma membranes. *Biochim. Biophys. Acta* **958,** 268–278.

Tan, Z., and Boss, W. F. (1992). Association of phosphatidylinositol kinase, phosphatidylinositol monophosphate kinase, and diacylglycerol kinase with the cytoskeleton and F-actin fractions of carrot (*Daucus carota* L.) cells grown in suspension culture. *Plant Physiol.* **100,** 2116–2120.

van Breemen, R. B., Wheeler, J. J., and Boss, W. F. (1990). Identification of carrot inositol phospholipids by fast atom bombardment mass spectrometry. *Lipids* **25,** 328–334.

Wheeler, J. J., and Boss, W. F. (1987). Polyphosphoinositides are present in plasma membranes isolated from fusogenic carrot cells. *Plant Physiol.* **85,** 389–392.

Wheeler, J. J., and Boss, W. F. (1989). The presence of *sn*-1-palmitoyl lysophosphatidylinositol monophosphate correlates positively with the fusion-permissive state of the plasma membrane of fusogenic carrot cells grown in suspension culture. *Biochim. Biophys. Acta* **984,** 33–40.

Wreggett, K. A., and Irvine, R. F. (1987). A rapid separation method for inositol phosphates and their isomers. *Biochem. J.* **245,** 655–660.

Yang, W., Burkhart, W., Cavallius, J., Merrick, W. C., and Boss, W. F. (1993). Purification and characterization of a phosphatidylinositol 4-kinase activator in carrot cells. *J. Biol. Chem.* **268,** 392–398.

Yang, W., and Boss, W. F. (1994). Regulation of phosphatidylinositol 4-kinase biosynthesis by the protein activator, PIK-A49. Activation requires phosphorylation of PIK-A49. *J. Biol. Chem.,* **269,** 3852–3857.

INDEX

B

C

D

H

I

X

Y

Z

VOLUMES IN SERIES

Founding Series Editor
DAVID M. PRESCOTT

Volume 1 (1964)
Methods in Cell Physiology
Edited by David M. Prescott

Volume 2 (1966)
Methods in Cell Physiology
Edited by David M. Prescott

Volume 3 (1968)
Methods in Cell Physiology
Edited by David M. Prescott

Volume 4 (1970)
Methods in Cell Physiology
Edited by David M. Prescott

Volume 5 (1972)
Methods in Cell Physiology
Edited by David M. Prescott

Volume 6 (1973)
Methods in Cell Physiology
Edited by David M. Prescott

Volume 7 (1973)
Methods in Cell Biology
Edited by David M. Prescott

Volume 8 (1974)
Methods in Cell Biology
Edited by David M. Prescott

Volume 9 (1975)
Methods in Cell Biology
Edited by David M. Prescott

Volume 10 (1975)
Methods in Cell Biology
Edited by David M. Prescott

Volume 11 (1975)
Yeast Cells
Edited by David M. Prescott

Volume 12 (1975)
Yeast Cells
Edited by David M. Prescott

Volume 13 (1976)
Methods in Cell Biology
Edited by David M. Prescott

Volume 14 (1976)
Methods in Cell Biology
Edited by David M. Prescott

Volume 15 (1977)
Methods in Cell Biology
Edited by David M. Prescott

Volume 16 (1977)
Chromatin and Chromosomal Protein Research I
Edited by Gary Stein, Janet Stein, and Lewis J. Kleinsmith

Volume 17 (1978)
Chromatin and Chromosomal Protein Research II
Edited by Gary Stein, Janet Stein, and Lewis J. Kleinsmith

Volume 18 (1978)
Chromatin and Chromosomal Protein Research III
Edited by Gary Stein, Janet Stein, and Lewis J. Kleinsmith

Volume 19 (1978)
Chromatin and Chromosomal Protein Research IV
Edited by Gary Stein, Janet Stein, and Lewis J. Kleinsmith

Volume 20 (1978)
Methods in Cell Biology
Edited by David M. Prescott

Advisory Board Chairman
KEITH R. PORTER

Volume 21A (1980)
Normal Human Tissue and Cell Culture, Part A: Respiratory, Cardiovascular, and Integumentary Systems
Edited by Curtis C. Harris, Benjamin F. Trump, and Gary D. Stoner

Volume 21B (1980)
Normal Human Tissue and Cell Culture, Part B: Endocrine, Urogenital, and Gastrointestinal Systems
Edited by Curtis C. Harris, Benjamin F. Trump, and Gary D. Stoner

Volume 22 (1981)
Three-Dimensional Ultrastructure in Biology
Edited by James N. Turner

Volume 23 (1981)
Basic Mechanisms of Cellular Secretion
Edited by Arthur R. Hand and Constance Oliver

Volume 24 (1982)
The Cytoskeleton, Part A: Cytoskeletal Proteins, Isolation and Characterization
Edited by Leslie Wilson

Volume 25 (1982)
The Cytoskeleton, Part B: Biological Systems and *in Vitro* Models
Edited by Leslie Wilson

Volume 26 (1982)
Prenatal Diagnosis: Cell Biological Approaches
Edited by Samuel A. Latt and Gretchen J. Darlington

Series Editor
LESLIE WILSON

Volume 27 (1986)
Echinoderm Gametes and Embryos
Edited by Thomas E. Schroeder

Volume 28 (1987)
***Dictyostelium discoideum:* Molecular Approaches to Cell Biology**
Edited by James A. Spudich

Volume 29 (1989)
Fluorescence Microscopy of Living Cells in Culture, Part A: Fluorescent Analogs, Labeling Cells, and Basic Microscopy
Edited by Yu-Li Wang and D. Lansing Taylor

Volume 30 (1989)
Fluorescence Microscopy of Living Cells in Culture, Part B: Quantitative Fluorescence Microscopy—Imaging and Spectroscopy
Edited by D. Lansing Taylor and Yu-Li Wang

Series Editors

LESLIE WILSON AND PAUL MATSUDAIRA